Psychopharmacology

Drugs, the Brain, and Behavior

Psychopharmacology

DRUGS, THE BRAIN, AND BEHAVIOR

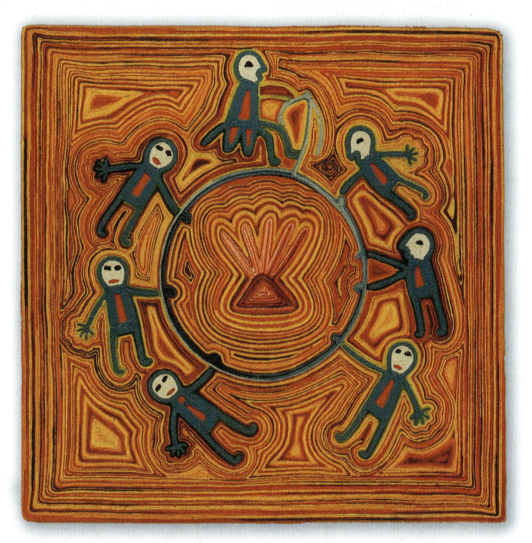

Jerrold S. Meyer

University of Massachusetts

Linda F. Quenzer

University of Hartford

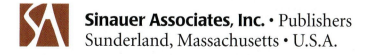

Sinauer Associates, Inc. • Publishers
Sunderland, Massachusetts • U.S.A.

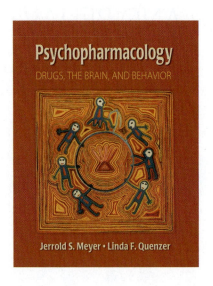

About the Cover

On the cover: The Huichol Indians of Mexico have been using the peyote cactus in religious ceremonies since pre-Columbian times. This yarn painting portrays a peyote ceremony with six communicants and a shaman (at top) surrounding a fire that represents Tatewari, the first shaman. Yarn painting is a traditional art form that involves pressing colored yarn onto a board covered with beeswax.
Image courtesy of Roshi Joan Halifax, Upaya.

Psychopharmacology: Drugs, the Brain, and Behavior

Copyright ©2005 by Sinauer Associates, Inc.
All rights reserved. This book may not be reproduced in whole or in part without permission from the publisher.

For information, address:
 Sinauer Associates, 23 Plumtree Road, Sunderland, MA 01375 U.S.A.
 FAX: 413-549-1118
 E-mail: publish@sinauer.com
 Internet: www.sinauer.com

Library of Congress Cataloging-in-Publication Data

Meyer, Jerrold S., 1947-
  Psychopharmacology : drugs, the brain, and behavior / Jerrold S. Meyer,
Linda F. Quenzer.
     p. cm.
  ISBN 0-87893-534-7
  1. Psychopharmacology. 2. Brain chemistry. I. Quenzer, Linda F.
   II. Title.

RM315.M478 2005
615'.78—dc22   2004020935

 5 4 3 2

To Robert S. Feldman - teacher, mentor, and friend

Brief Contents

Contents

Chemical Signaling by Neurotransmitters and Hormones 63

Methods of Research in Neurobehavioral Pharmacology 89

Catecholamines 119

6 Acetylcholine and Serotonin 139

7 Glutamate and GABA 163

Drug Abuse, Dependence, and Addiction 185

Alcohol 215

10   *The Opiates*   245

11   *Psychomotor Stimulants: Cocaine and the Amphetamines*   275

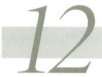

Nicotine and Caffeine 303

13 *Marijuana and the Cannabinoids* 327

14 *Hallucinogens, PCP, and Ketamine* 347

15 Inhalants, GHB, and Anabolic–Androgenic Steroids 365

16 Affective Disorders 385

17 *Anxiety Disorders* 411

18 *Schizophrenia* 441

Preface

For thousands of years, humans have used psychoactive substances to modify their perceptions and mood. Throughout most of this period, plants were the sole source of these powerful mind-altering agents, and the agents themselves remained shrouded in mystery. However, things began to change dramatically with the birth of modern chemistry in the nineteenth century. First, chemists could now extract, purify, and identify the active ingredients that conferred psychoactive properties on a particular plant species. Second, the growing sophistication of chemical synthesis techniques allowed medicinal chemists to develop new drugs that could be used to treat various diseases, including mental disorders. Most recently, powerful techniques of biochemistry and of cellular and molecular biology have provided insights into the mechanisms of drug action that would have been unimaginable just a few decades ago.

Indeed, the rate of new discovery in psychopharmacology has reached breathtaking proportions. A bibliographic search of the National Library of Medicine found that during 2003 alone, over 1,700 scientific articles were published that contained the word "alcohol" in the title. You, the student, are fortunate to be studying psychopharmacology at such an exciting time. One aim of our book is to convey that excitement as you begin your exploration of the many psychoactive drugs and their uses. Another key aim is to help you learn not merely what various substances do in terms of their subjective and behavioral effects, but also how these effects occur. Our underlying philosophy is that a full appreciation of psychopharmacology requires some understanding of the mechanisms of drug action. This philosophy is reflected in the organization of this book as well as the depth of coverage given to mechanistic studies in both humans and relevant animal models.

The present book grew out of a more advanced text, *Principles of Neuropsychopharmacology*, authored by us together with our former colleague and mentor, Robert S. Feldman (now retired). However, *Psychopharmacology: Drugs, the Brain, and Behavior* is much more than just a condensed and updated version of our earlier book. We

have striven to engage your interest with a variety of new features, including chapter-opening vignettes, breakout boxes presenting novel or cutting-edge topics for special discussion, and many full-color photographs and illustrations depicting important concepts and experimental data. We have also used a balanced approach to convey the full breadth of our field, ranging from historical accounts of drug use, to clinical and preclinical behavioral studies, to the latest research on drug receptors and on drug effects in genetically engineered mice.

Psychopharmacology: Drugs, the Brain, and Behavior is divided into four sections. Chapters 1 through 4 provide extensive foundation materials, including the basic principles of pharmacology, neurophysiology and neuroanatomy, synaptic transmission, and research methods in psychopharmacology. Chapters 5 through 7 describe key features of major neurotransmitter systems, including the catecholamines, serotonin, acetylcholine, glutamate and GABA. These are the neurotransmitters most commonly associated with psychoactive drug effects. Chapters 8 through 15 discuss theories and mechanisms of drug addiction, with comprehensive coverage of all major substances of abuse. Chapters 16 through 18 consider the biochemical bases of psychopathology and the drugs used to treat disorders of mood, anxiety disorders, and schizophrenia. There is an outline at the beginning of each chapter that shows the organization of the chapter. These outlines should be useful to instructors for determining class reading assignments and to students for identifying the major topics covered in each chapter.

Although the use of psychoactive drugs is not a recent phenomenon, never before has a society become so dependent on these substances, whether for their mood-altering properties in recreational settings or for the remarkable benefits they provide to so many psychiatric patients. *Psychopharmacology: Drugs, the Brain, and Behavior* will help you understand the characteristics of psychoactive drugs, their psychological and behavioral effects, and the mechanisms by which such effects occur. We trust that you will enjoy reading the book as much as we have enjoyed writing it.

ACKNOWLEDGMENTS

This book is the culmination of the efforts of many dedicated people who contributed their ideas and their hard work to the project. First and foremost, we acknowledge the excellent editorial supervision of Graig Donini with the able assistance of production editors Kathaleen Emerson, Sydney Carroll, and Mara Silver. Together, you were a great team that kept us on task (though not always on deadline) and raised our spirits when the going got tough. David McIntyre did a superb job of seeking out just the right photographs for the book, as well as creating a few of his own when needed. We are indebted to other key staff members of Sinauer Associates who worked on this project, including Chris Small, Joan Gemme, and Jefferson Johnson. We would like to acknowledge Peter Farley, the first editor on this project, who encouraged us to develop an undergraduate version of the "big book," and we also thank Mark Williams for his beautiful artwork, Mark Via for copyediting, and Margaret Trombley for her contributions to the glossary.

The following reviewers contributed many excellent suggestions for improving the book:

James Appel, University of South Carolina
Gregory Berns, Emory University
M. Imad Damaj, Virginia Commonwealth
  University
Shelly Dickinson, St. Olaf College
Russell Frohardt, St. Edward's University
Judith E. Grisel, Furman University
Shannon Harding, Fairfield University
Ronald M. Harris Warwick, Cornell University
Carl L. Hart, Columbia University
Michael Kerchner, Washington College
Karen Parfitt, Pomona College
William Pizzi, Northeastern Illinois University
Franca Placenza, University of Toronto
Keith Trujillo, California State University,
  San Marcos

Ellen Incillo, Tony Guilliano, Scott Meek, and Lorraine Wolpert provided valuable feedback early in the preparation of the manuscript. Finally, we are indebted to our spouses, Melinda and Ray, who supported and encouraged us and who willingly sacrificed so much of our time together during this lengthy project. Linda also thanks her son, Alex Rosati, who provided invaluable insights into the style of presentation and assisted with the early art production.

Supplements to Accompany Psychopharmacology

Instructor's Resource CD

Available to qualified adopters of the textbook, the *Psychopharmacology* Instructor's Resource CD (ISBN 0-87893-535-5) contains all of the figures (art and photos) and tables from the textbook. All are provided both as high-resolution and low-resolution JPEG images, and have been formatted, sized, and color-corrected for optimal image quality when projected in the classroom. In addition, a ready-to-use Microsoft® PowerPoint® presentation of all figures and tables is provided for each chapter of the textbook.

Test Bank

Included on the Instructor's Resource CD is the *Psychopharmacology* Test Bank. The test bank includes 50 test questions per chapter, consisting of approximately 40 multiple choice and 10 short answer. The questions have been designed to provide instructors with a good selection of factual and conceptual questions, at a range of difficulty levels. The test bank is provided as Microsoft® Word® files.

Psychopharmacology

Drugs, the Brain, and Behavior

1 *Principles of Pharmacology*

Although we intuitively feel that we know what a drug is, its definition changes from culture to culture and even within a culture over time. Drugs may be herbal antidotes and vitamins, expensive prescription medications, or illicit substances used for recreation. Although we like to think that we understand drug effects, there are cases when responses to drugs seem quite bizarre and unpredictable. Here are a few examples:

Poison arrow toxins Curare is a natural product taken from trees and bushes by South American hunters to tip their poison arrows. The drug paralyzes the animal and quickly depresses respiration and causes death. Isn't it odd that although the curare remains in the animal tissue and is not destroyed by cooking, the hunters do not experience any of the drug's effects when consuming the meat?

Urine testing Drug testing for marijuana use is becoming increasingly common in schools and on the job. But how can a urine test detect the drug in an individual after only one administration and long after intoxication is ended?

Failed birth control pills Women taking certain medications such as carbamazepine to control their epileptic seizures show a significantly higher occurrence of "failures" in their oral contraceptives, leading to unwanted pregnancies. Under what circumstances could using certain prescription drugs increase a woman's probability of pregnancy?

Ordinary foods as poisons Have you heard of strange cases in which food becomes quite toxic? Foods rich in tyramine—cheddar, Roquefort, and Camembert cheeses, pickled herring, red wine, beer, and chicken livers—may suddenly cause a dangerous increase in blood pressure, cardiac arrhythmias, and fatal cerebral hemorrhage if consumed in combination with certain antidepressant medications. How can a normal diet interact with prescription drugs in such a dangerous manner?

Unexpected overdose Approximately 1% of all heroin addicts in the United States die from heroin overdose each year. In many instances the fatal dose was no different from the one the addict used just the day before. How could the same dose that the individual used safely for weeks and weeks suddenly become so lethal?

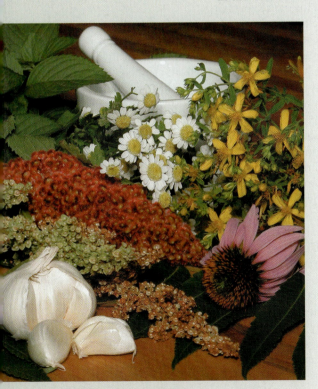

Commonly available plants and roots have a long history of medicinal use.

Are the preceding examples real medical mysteries, or can basic understanding of the principles of pharmacology explain the unusual effects observed? As you read this chapter, you will be able to unravel these surprising puzzles. The chapter begins with a consideration of physiological factors that determine how much of the drug we ingest gets into the blood, how quickly that happens, and how long the drug remains active. The second part of the chapter deals with drug–receptor dynamics; that is, how the drug interacts with proteins in nerve cell membranes to initiate biobehavioral effects.

Pharmacology: The Science of Drug Action

Pharmacology is the scientific study of the actions of drugs and their effects on a living organism. Until the beginning of the last century, pharmacology studied drugs that were almost all naturally occurring substances. The importance of plants to the lives of ancient man is well documented. Writings from as early as 1500 B.C. describe plant-based medicines used in Egypt and in India. The Ebers Papyrus describes the preparation and use of more than 700 remedies for ailments as varied as crocodile bites, baldness, constipation, headache, and heart disease. Of course, many of these treatments included elements of magic and incantation, but there are also references to some modern drugs such as castor oil and opium. The Chinese also have a very long and extensive tradition in the use of herbal remedies that continues today. World Health Organization estimates suggest that in modern times, as many as 80% of the people in developing countries are totally dependent on herbs or plant-derived medicinals. And in the United States, modern herbal medicines or drugs based on natural products represent half of the top 25 drugs on the market (Hollinger, 1997). Box 1.1 discusses the benefits and dangers of herbal remedies.

Placed in historical context, drug development in the United States is in its infancy. Nevertheless, the rapid introduction of many new drugs by the pharmaceutical industry has forced the formation of several specialized areas of pharmacology. Two of these areas are of particular interest to us. **Neuropharmacology** is concerned with drug-induced changes in the functioning of cells in the nervous system, while **psychopharmacology** emphasizes drug-induced changes in mood, thinking, and behavior. In combination, the goal of **neuropsychopharmacology** is to identify chemical substances that act upon the nervous system to alter behavior that is disturbed due to injury, disease, or environmental factors. Additionally, neuropsychopharmacologists are interested in understanding the neurobiology of behavior, utilizing chemical agents as probes.

When we speak of **drug action,** we are referring to the specific molecular changes produced by a drug when it binds to a particular target site or receptor. These molecular changes lead to more widespread alterations in physiological or psychological functions, which we consider **drug effects.** The site of drug action may be very different from the site of drug effect. For example, atropine is a drug used in ophthalmology to dilate the pupil of the eye before eye exams. Atropine has a site of action (the eye muscles of the iris) that is close to the site of its ultimate effect (widening the pupil), so it is administered directly to the eye. In comparison, morphine applied to the eye itself has no effect. Yet when it is taken internally, the drug's action on the brain leads to "pinpoint" pupils. Clearly, for morphine, the site of effect is far distant from its initial action.

Keep in mind that because drugs act at a variety of target sites, they always have multiple effects. Some may be **therapeutic effects,** meaning that the drug–receptor interaction produces desired physical or behavioral changes. All other effects produced are referred to as **side effects,** and they vary in severity from mildly annoying to distressing and dangerous. For example, amphetamine-like drugs produce alertness and insomnia, increased heart rate, and decreased appetite. Drugs in this class reduce the occurrence of spontaneous sleep episodes, characteristic of the disorder called narcolepsy, but produce anorexia (loss of appetite) as the primary side effect. In contrast, the same drug may be used as a prescription diet control in weight reduction programs. In such cases, insomnia and hyperactivity are frequently disturbing side effects. Thus the therapeutic and side effects change depending on the desired outcome.

The drug effects we have described so far have been **specific drug effects,** defined as those based on the physical and biochemical interactions of a drug with a target site in living tissue. In contrast, **nonspecific drug effects** are those that are based not on the chemical activity of a drug–receptor interaction but on certain unique characteristics of the individual. It is quite clear that an individual's background (e.g., drug-taking experience), present mood, expectations of drug effect, perceptions of the drug-taking situation, attitude toward the administering physician, and other factors influence the outcome of drug use. Nonspecific drug effects help to explain why the same individual self-administering the same amount of ethyl alcohol may experience a sense of being lighthearted and gregarious on one occasion and depressed and melancholy on another. The basis for such a phenomenon may well be the varied neurochemical state existing in the individual at different times, over which specific drug effects are superimposed.

One common example of nonspecific effects is that of the **placebo.** Many of you will automatically think of a placebo as a "fake" pill. A placebo *is* in fact a pharmacologically inert compound administered to an individual; however, in many instances it has not only therapeutic effects but side effects as well. Just as many of the symptoms of illness may have psychogenic or emotional origins, belief in a drug may pro-

BOX 1.1   Pharmacology in Action

Herbal Medicine— Panacea or Hazard?

Would you be likely to drink a tea of dried stem barks of *Strychnosmyrotoides* to combat malaria or subject yourself to bee stings to get a mega-dose of natural steroids to relieve the signs of arthritis or chew kaolin (white clay) to relieve morning sickness? Probably not, but plants and other natural products have a long history of medicinal use and still play a significant role in modern healing systems. There are many examples of the historical role of plants in medicine.

The modern herbalist administering mistletoe for epilepsy, hypertension, and hormone imbalance reflects the early Roman use of mistletoe for seizures, to heal ulcers, and to enhance fertility in women. Much of early medical treatment was undertaken by priest doctors or shamans who included elements of magic and the supernatural into the therapeutic regimen. But even in modern times, in much of the world healers with a special understanding of plants and of sacred artifacts supply the therapeutic treatments for the community. Their skill comes from experience (trial and error) and knowledge passed down from previous generations.

Many of the ancient healing plants continue to play a role in modern society as a source of conventional therapeutic agents, as with the extraction of morphine from the opium poppy. Until the 1960s childhood leukemia was almost certainly fatal. But a chemotherapeutic drug made from the Madagascar rosy periwinkle has raised the long-term survival rate to over 90% (Swerdlow, 2000). Digitalis (used to treat heart failure) comes from the leaves of the foxglove plant, and ephedrine (used for a variety of respiratory conditions) comes from the ephedra plant.

Besides using the plant extracts themselves, drug developers frequently use natural products as templates for synthetic or semisynthetic pharmaceuticals. Many Westerners are turning toward herbal remedies because they are perceived as being gentler and more natural and having fewer side effects. Today, scientists join with shamans in a search for healing plants that treat cancer, prevent heart disease, stop pain, and cure other ailments.

Shaman Pharmaceuticals was formed in the early 1990s as a consortium of larger drug companies with the goal of supporting increased acquisition and evaluation of plant materials, particularly from the tropical rain forests endangered by exploitation (Hollinger, 1997). Although these changes reflect a new interest in preserving biodiversity and the cultural history that goes with it, the amount of money spent on producing plant-based prescription medications is limited by the fact that plant evaluation requires a huge investment of time and money with

often limited outcome. Also, modern Western emphasis on genetic research focuses on understanding the pathological process in a particular disease and attempting to design a molecule (synthetic) that repairs it. These factors limit the enthusiasm for research into ethnobotony.

As wonderful as the discoveries have been, there is a dark side to herbal remedies. Despite consumers' enthusiasm for medicinal herbs, many scientists and medical practitioners feel that herbs need far more regulation. Many think that Americans are engaged in a vast, uncontrolled experiment. Some estimates suggest that 12.1% of Americans spent over $5 billion in 1997 alone (Swerdlow, 2000) on herbal remedies that have not been evaluated by the Food and Drug Administration (FDA). Because herbal medicines are classified as dietary supplements, the FDA does not monitor the quality control of the many products on the market.

Lacking such control, the concentration and purity, as well as the effectiveness, of a particular herbal medi-

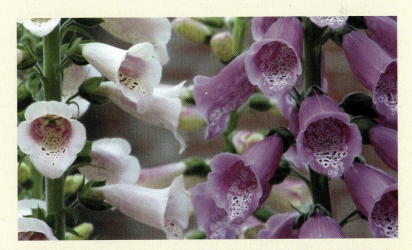

Foxglove (*Digitalis purpurea*) is the source of the cardiotonic drug digitalis. Potency can vary greatly according to growing conditions, and an overdose can be fatal, so safe preparations from foxglove leaves require standardization with modern pharmacological techniques.

(continued on next page)

BOX 1.1 (continued)

cine vary from brand to brand and even between batches produced by the same manufacturer. Those who use herbal medications or dietary supplements must do so at their own risk, and those risks may be all too real. Dietary supplements have been known to cause serious asthma attacks, blood clots, liver scarring, impotence, kidney failure, and seizures. Some herbal supplements interact in dangerous ways with physician-prescribed medications and may pose a special hazard if used before surgical procedures.

Although it is clear that plants contain biologically active chemicals, it is still unclear if any particular herbal product is in fact more effective than a placebo. The single greatest difficulty in the evaluation process is the fact that in most cases scientists have been unable to identify which chemical or combination of chemicals is responsible for the reduction of blood pressure, relief of pain, or improvement in mood. The active ingredient in the herb has not been extracted for identification.

In order to run trials of effectiveness, one needs to administer the same dose of the active ingredient to each subject before making objective measurements and also demonstrate dose-dependent pharmacological effects. Unfortunately, the concentration remains unspecified in herbal preparations. If a particular individual finds that an herb is effective in reducing his depression, for example, he will not know what dose was taken nor whether the preparation will contain the same dose the next time he purchases it.

When screened, some herbal preparations have been found to contain none of what is listed on the label. Unfortunately, even products from highly reputable manufacturers are variable, because the final effective concentration will depend on factors such as plant growing conditions, portions of the plants utilized, and even how long the herbal preparation has been sitting on the store shelf. In an examination of ginseng products, a 10-fold difference in the active ingredient was found despite the labeled content being identical. In other cases, analysis of herbal medicines sold in California showed that 32% contained at least one drug or contaminant—including lead, arsenic, and mercury—not listed on the label. The dietary supplement L-tryptophan was removed from the market when 36 people died and 1500 became seriously ill, apparently due to the 63 contaminants found in the preparation (Brody, 1998).

Other critics of herbal remedies also contend that the confidence in limited side effects is naive. Since the herbs contain dilute, biologically active chemicals, they will certainly produce some effects that are undesirable or dangerous and there is the risk of potential interactions with other drugs. Self-medication with St. John's wort, for example, has been shown to alter the blood levels of prescription antidepressants and other drugs, and is known to interact with medications used to treat HIV infection. More recently, concern has been raised over self-medication with estrogen-containing products, which may be particularly hazardous to women with estrogen-sensitive tumors. Herbal remedies thus represent both a boon to good health and a potential hazard.

---

duce real physiological effects despite the lack of chemical activity. The effects are not limited to the individual's subjective evaluation of relief, but include measurable physiological changes such as altered gastric acid secretion, blood vessel dilation, hormonal changes, and so forth.

In a classic study, two groups of patients with ulcers were each given a placebo. In the first group, the medication was provided by a physician who assured the patients that the drug would provide relief. The second group also received the placebo, but it was administered by a nurse who described it as experimental in nature. In group 1, 70% of the patients found significant relief, while in group 2, only 25% were helped by the "drug" (Levine, 1973).

In pharmacology, the placebo is essential to the design of experiments evaluating the effectiveness of new medications because it eliminates the influence of expectation on the part of the patient. This control group is identical to the experimental group in all ways, and the subjects are unaware of the substitution of an inactive substance (e.g., a sugar pill or saline injection) for the test medication. Comparison of the two groups provides information on the effectiveness of the drug beyond subject expectation.

The large contribution of nonspecific factors and the high and variable incidence of placebo responders make the **double-blind experiment** highly desirable. In these experiments, neither the patient nor the observer knows what treatment the patient has received. Such precautions ensure that the results of any given treatment will not be colored by overt or covert prejudices on the part of either the patient or the observer. If you would like to read more about the use of placebos in both clinical research and therapeutics and the associated ethical dilemmas, refer to the articles by Brown (1998) and Rothman and Michels (1994).

Throughout this chapter we will be using examples that include both therapeutic and recreational drugs that affect mood and behavior. Since there are usually several names for the same substance, it may be helpful to understand how drugs are named (Box 1.2).

Pharmacokinetic Factors Determining Drug Action

Although it is safe to assume that the chemical structure of a drug determines its action, it quickly becomes clear that additional factors are also powerful contributors. The dose of the drug administered is clearly important, but more important is the amount of drug in the blood that is free to bind at specific target sites (**bioavailability**) to elicit drug action. The following sections of this chapter describe in detail the dynamic factors that contribute to bioavailability. Collectively, these factors constitute the **pharmacokinetic** component of drug action; they are listed below and illustrated in Figure 1.1.

1. *Routes of administration.* How and where a drug is administered determines how quickly and how completely the drug is absorbed into the blood.
2. *Absorption and distribution.* Because a drug rarely acts where it initially contacts the body, it must pass through a variety of cell membranes and enter the blood plasma, which transports the drug to virtually all of the cells in the body.
3. *Binding.* Once in the blood plasma, some drug molecules move to tissues to bind to active target sites (receptors). While in the blood, a drug may also bind (**depot binding**) to plasma proteins or may be stored temporarily in bone or fat, where it is inactive.
4. *Inactivation.* Drug inactivation, or **biotransformation,** occurs primarily as a result of metabolic processes in the liver. The amount of drug in the body at any one time is dependent on the dynamic balance between absorption and inactivation. Therefore, inactivation influences both the intensity and duration of drug effects.
5. *Excretion.* The liver metabolites are eliminated from the body with the urine or feces. Some drugs are excreted in an unaltered form by the kidneys.

Although these topics will be discussed sequentially in the following pages, keep in mind that in the living organism, these factors are at work simultaneously. In addition to bioavailability, the drug effect experienced will also depend on how rapidly the drug reaches its target, the frequency and history of prior drug use (see the discussion on tolerance later in the chapter) and, finally, nonspecific factors that are characteristics of the individual and his environment.

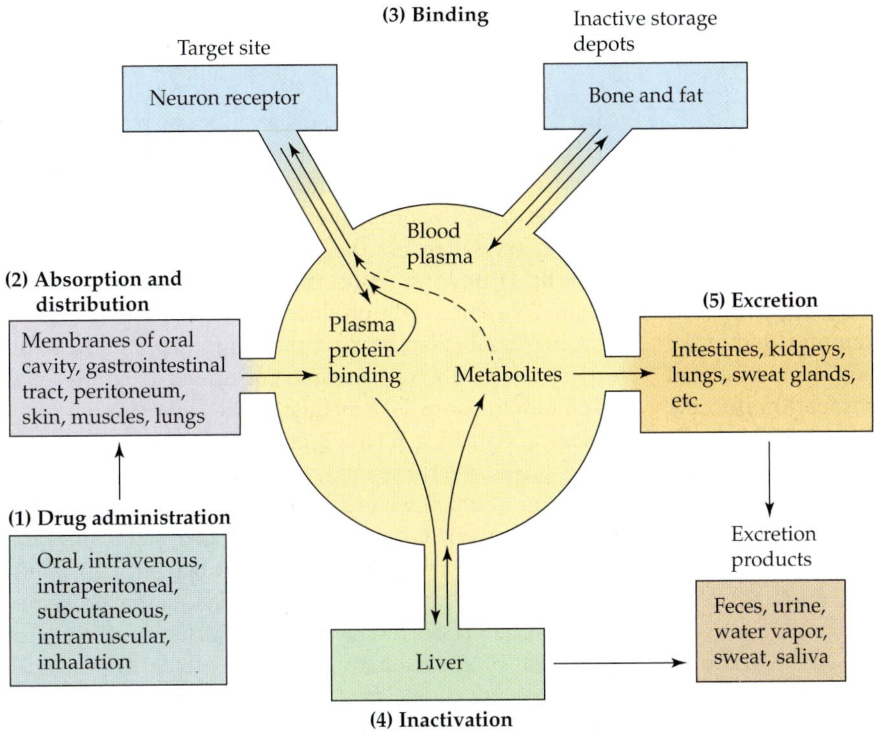

Methods of drug administration influence the onset of drug action

The route of administration of a drug determines how much drug reaches its site of action and how quickly the drug effect occurs. **Oral administration (PO)** is the most popular route for taking drugs because it is safe, self-administered, economical, and avoids the complications and discomfort of injection methods. Drugs that are taken orally come in the form of capsules, pills, tablets, or liquid, but to be effective, the drug must dissolve in stomach fluids and pass through the stomach wall to reach blood capillaries. In addition, the drug must be resistant to destruction by stomach acid and stomach

Figure 1.1 Pharmacokinetic factors that determine bioavailability of drugs From the site of administration (1), the drug moves through cell membranes to be absorbed into the blood (2), where it circulates to all cells in the body. Some of the drug molecules may bind to inactive sites such as plasma proteins or storage depots (3) and some to receptors in target tissue. Blood-borne drug molecules also enter the liver (4), where they may be transformed into metabolites and travel to the kidneys and other discharge sites for ultimate excretion (5) from the body.

BOX 1.2 Pharmacology in Action

Naming Drugs

Drug names can be a confusing issue for many people because drugs that are sold commercially, either by prescription or over the counter, usually have four or more different kinds of names. All drugs have a chemical name that is a complete chemical description suitable for synthesizing by an organic chemist. Chemical names are rather clumsy and rarely used except in a laboratory setting. In contrast, generic names (also called nonproprietary names) are official names of drugs and are listed in the United States Pharmacopeia (USP).

These names are a much shorter form of the chemical name but are still unique for that drug. For example, one popular antianxiety drug has the chemical name 7-chloro-1,3-dihydro-1-methyl-3-phenyl-2H-1,4-benzodiazepin-2-one and the generic name diazepam. The brand name, or trade name, of that drug (Valium) specifies a particular manufacturer and a formulation. A brand name is trademarked and copyrighted by an individual company, which means that it has an exclusive right to advertise and sell that drug.

Slang or street names of commonly abused drugs are an additional way to identify a particular chemical.

Unfortunately, the names change over time and vary with geographic locations and particular groups of people. In addition, there is no way to know the chemical characteristics of the substance in question. Some terms are used in popular films or television and become more generally familiar, such as "crack" or "ice," but most disappear as quickly as they appeared. The National Institute on Drug Abuse has compiled a list of over 150 street names for marijuana and over 75 for cocaine, including coke, big C, nose candy, snow, white girl, happydust, pearl, freeze, doing the line, and many others.

---

enzymes that are important for normal digestion. Insulin is one drug that can be destroyed by digestive processes and for that reason cannot be administered orally.

The movement of the drug from the site of administration to the blood circulation is called **absorption.** Although some drugs are absorbed from the stomach, the majority of drugs are not fully absorbed until they reach the small intestine. Many factors influence how quickly the stomach empties its contents into the small intestine and hence determine the ultimate rate of absorption. For example, food in the stomach, particularly if it is fatty, will slow the movement of the drug into the intestine, delaying absorption into the blood. The amount of food, the physical activity of the individual, and many other factors make it difficult to predict how quickly the drug will reach the intestine. In addition, all the drug absorbed from the stomach and intestine into the blood goes directly to the liver on its way to the general circulation. Liver metabolism of some of the drug molecules will reduce the amount of available drug before it reaches the general circulation. This phenomenon, called the **first-pass effect,** is shown in Figure 1.2. Because of these factors, oral administration produces drug plasma levels that are more irregular and unpredictable and rise more slowly than the other methods of administration.

Intravenous (IV) injection is the most rapid and accurate method of drug administration since a precise quantity of the agent is placed directly into the blood and the passage through cell membranes such as the stomach wall is eliminated (see Figure 1.2). However, the quick onset of drug effect

with IV injection is also a potential hazard. An overdose or a dangerous allergic reaction to the drug leaves little time for corrective measures, and the drug cannot be removed from the body as it can be from the stomach by stomach pumping.

For drug abusers, IV administration provides a more dramatic subjective drug experience than self-administration in other ways, because the drug reaches the brain almost instantly. Drug users report that intravenous injection of a cocaine solution usually produces an intense "rush" or "flash" of pure pleasure that lasts for approximately 10 minutes. This experience rarely occurs when cocaine is taken orally or taken into the nostrils (snorting; see the discusssion on topical administration). However, intravenous use of street drugs poses several special hazards. First, drugs that are impure or of unknown quality provide uncertain doses, and toxic reactions are common. Second, lack of sterile injection equipment and aseptic techniques can lead to infections such as hepatitis, HIV, and endocarditis (inflammation of the lining of the heart). Fortunately, many cities have implemented free needle programs that significantly reduce the probability of cross infection. Third, many drug abusers attempt to dissolve drugs that have insoluble filler materials that, when injected, may be trapped in small blood vessels in the lungs, leading to reduced respiratory capacity or death.

An alternative to the IV procedure is **intramuscular (IM)** injection, which has the advantage of slower and more even absorption over a period of time. Drugs administered by this method are usually absorbed within 10 to 30 minutes. Absorption can be slowed down by combining the drug with

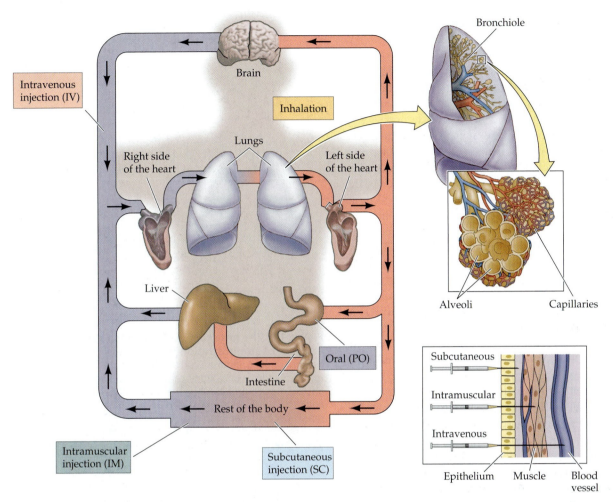

Figure 1.2 Routes of drug administration First-pass effect. Drugs administered orally are absorbed into the blood that must pass through the liver before reaching the general circulation. Some drug molecules may be destroyed in the liver before they can reach target tissues. (Inset) Pulmonary absorption through capillaries in the alveoli. Rapid absorption following inhalation occurs because the large surface area of the lungs and the rich capillary networks provide efficient exchange of gases to and from the blood. (Inset) Methods of administration by injection. The speed of absorption of drug molecules from administration sites depends upon the amount of blood circulating to that area.

a second drug that constricts blood vessels, because the rate of drug absorption is dependent upon the rate of blood flow to the muscle (see Figure 1.2). To provide slower sustained action, the drug may be injected as a suspension in vegetable oil. For example, IM injection of medroxyprogesterone acetate (Depo-Provera) provides effective contraception for 3 to 6 months without the need to take daily pills. One disadvantage of IM administration is that in some cases the injection solution can be quite irritating and cause significant muscle discomfort.

Intraperitoneal (IP) injection is rarely used with humans, but is the most common route of administration for small laboratory animals. The drug is injected through the abdominal wall into the peritoneal cavity, the space that surrounds the abdominal organs. IP injection produces rapid effects, but not as rapid as IV. Variability in absorption occurs depending on where (within the peritoneum) the drug is placed.

In **subcutaneous (SC)** administration, the drug is injected just below the skin (see Figure 1.2) and is absorbed at a rate dependent on blood flow to the site. Absorption is usually fairly slow and steady, but there can be considerable variability. Rubbing the skin to dilate blood vessels in the immediate area increases the rate of absorption. Injection of a drug in a nonaqueous solution (such as peanut oil) or implantation of a drug pellet or delivery device further slows the rate of absorption. Subcutaneous implantation of drug-containing pellets is most often used to administer hormones. One contraceptive drug (Implanon) used in Europe may soon become available in the United States. Its hormones are contained in a single small capsule that is implanted through a small incision just under the skin of the upper arm. A woman is protected from pregnancy for a 3-year period unless the device is removed.

Inhalation of drugs, such as those used to treat asthma attacks, allows the drug to be absorbed into the blood by passing through the lungs. Absorption is very rapid because the area of the pulmonary absorbing surfaces is large and rich with capillaries (see Figure 1.2). The effect on the brain is very rapid because the blood from the capillaries of the lungs goes straight to the brain without returning to the heart first.

Inhalation is a method preferred for self-administration in cases when oral absorption is too slow and much of the active drug is destroyed before reaching the brain. Nicotine released from the tobacco of a cigarette by heat into the smoke produces a very rapid rise in blood level and rapid central nervous system (CNS) effects, which peak in a matter of minutes. Tetrahydrocannabinol (THC), an active ingredient of marijuana, and crack cocaine are also rapidly absorbed after smoking. In addition to the inherent dangers of the drugs themselves, disadvantages of inhalation include irritation of the nasal passages and damage to the lungs by small particles that may be included in the inhaled material.

Topical application of drugs to the mucous membranes such as the conjunctiva of the eye, nasopharynx, vagina, colon, and urethra generally provides local drug effects. However, some topically administered drugs can be readily absorbed into the general circulation, leading to widespread effects. Direct application of finely powdered cocaine to the nasal mucosa by sniffing leads to rapid absorption, producing profound effects on the CNS that peak in about 15 to 30 minutes. Cocaine addicts whose nasal mucosa has been damaged by chronic cocaine "snorting" may resort to the application of the drug to the rectum, vagina, or penis.

Although the skin provides an effective barrier to the diffusion of water-soluble drugs, certain lipid-soluble substances (i.e., those that dissolve in fat) are capable of penetrating slowly. **Transdermal** (i.e., through the skin) drug administration with skin patches provides a controlled and sustained delivery of drug at a preprogrammed rate. The patches consist of a polymer matrix embedded with the drug in high concentration. Transdermal delivery is now a common way to prevent motion sickness with scopolamine and to reduce cigarette craving with nicotine patches.

Special injection methods must be used for some drugs that act on nerve cells because a cellular barrier, the blood–brain barrier (discussed later in the chapter), prevents or slows the passage of the drugs from the blood into neural tissue. For example, **epidural** injection is used when spinal anesthetics are administered directly into the cerebrospinal fluid surrounding the spinal cord of a mother during childbirth, bypassing the blood–brain barrier. In animal experiments, a microsyringe or cannula is employed, which enables precise drug injection into discrete areas of

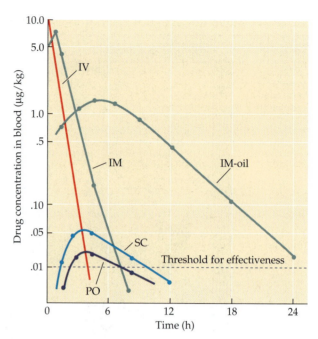

Figure 1.3   The time course of drug blood level depends on route of administration The blood level of the same amount of drug administered by different procedures to the same individual varies significantly. Intravenous (IV) produces an instantaneous peak when the drug is placed into the blood and rapid decline. Intramuscular (IM) administration produces rapid absorption and rapid decline, although IM administration in oil (IM-oil) shows slower absorption and gradual decline. Slow absorption following subcutaneous (SC) administration means some of the drug is metabolized before absorption is complete. For that reason, no sharp peak occurs and overall blood levels are lower. Oral (PO) administration produces the lowest blood levels and a relatively short time over threshold for effectiveness in this instance. (After Levine, 1973.)

brain tissue (**intracranial**) or into the cerebrospinal fluid–filled chambers, the ventricles (**intracerebroventricular**). In this way experimenters can study the electrophysiological, biochemical, or behavioral effects of drugs on particular nerve cell groups. This method is described in Chapter 4.

Because the route of administration significantly alters the rate of absorption, blood levels of the same dose of a drug administered by different routes vary significantly. Figure 1.3 compares the drug concentrations in blood over time for various routes of administration. Keep in mind that the peak level for each method reflects not only the differences in absorption rate but also the fact that slow absorption provides opportunity for liver metabolism to act on some of the drug molecules before absorption is complete. The advantages and disadvantages of selected methods of administration are summarized in Table 1.1.

TABLE 1.1 **Advantages and Disadvantages of Selected Routes of Drug Administration**

Route of administration	Advantages	Disadvantages
Oral (PO)	Safe; self-administered; economical; no needle-related complications	Slow and highly variable absorption; subject to first-pass metabolism; less predictable blood levels
Intravenous (IV)	Most rapid; most accurate blood concentration	Overdose danger; cannot be readily reversed; requires sterile needles and medical technique
Intramuscular (IM)	Slow and even absorption	Localized irritation at site of injection; needs sterile equipment
Subcutaneous (SC)	Slow and prolonged absorption	Variable absorption depending on blood flow
Inhalation	Large absorption surface; very rapid onset; no injection equipment needed	Irritation of nasal passages; small particles inhaled may damage lungs
Topical	Localized action and effects; easy to self-administer	May be absorbed into general circulation
Transdermal	Controlled and prolonged absorption	Local irritation; useful only for lipid soluble drugs
Epidural	Bypasses blood–brain barrier; very rapid effect on CNS	Not reversible; needs trained anesthesiologist; possible nerve damage

Multiple factors modify drug absorption

Once the drug has been administered, it is absorbed from the site of administration into the blood to be circulated throughout the body and ultimately to the brain, which is the primary target site for **psychoactive drugs** (i.e., those drugs that have an effect on thinking, mood, and behavior). We have already shown that the rate of absorption is dependent on several factors. Clearly, the route of administration alters absorption because it determines the area of the absorbing surface, the number of cell layers between the site of administration and blood, the amount of drug destroyed by metabolism or digestive processes, and the extent of binding to food or inert complexes. Absorption is also dependent on drug concentration, which is in part determined by individual differences in age, sex, and body size. Finally, absorption is dependent on the solubility and ionization of the drug.

Transport across membranes   Perhaps the single most important factor in determining plasma drug levels is the rate of passage of the drug through the various cell layers (and their respective membranes) between the site of administration and the blood. To understand this process, we need to look more carefully at cell membranes.

Cell membranes are made up primarily of complex lipid (fat) molecules called **phospholipids,** which have a negatively charged region at one end and two uncharged lipid tails (Figure 1.4A). These molecules are arranged in a bilayer with their phosphate ends forming two almost continuous sheets filled with fatty material (Figure 1.4B). In this configuration, the charged heads are in contact with both the aqueous intracellular fluid and the aqueous extracellular fluid. The proteins that are found inserted in the phospholipid bilayer have func-

tions that will be described later (see Chapter 3). The molecular characteristics of the cell membrane prevent most molecules from passing through unless they are soluble in fat.

Lipid-soluble drugs   Drugs with high lipid solubility move through cell membranes by **passive diffusion,** leaving the water in the blood or stomach juices and entering the lipid layers of membranes. Movement across the membranes is always in a direction from higher to lower concentration. The larger the concentration difference on each side of the membrane (called the **concentration gradient**), the more rapid is the diffusion. Lipid solubility increases the absorption of drug into the blood and also determines how readily a drug will pass the lipid barriers to enter the brain. For example, the narcotic drug heroin is a simple modification of the parent compound morphine. Heroin, or diacetylmorphine, is more soluble in lipid than is morphine and penetrates into brain tissue more readily, thus having a quicker onset of action and more potent reinforcing properties.

Ionized drugs   Most drugs are not readily lipid soluble because they are weak acids or weak bases that can become ionized when dissolved in water. Just as common table salt (NaCl) produces positively charged ions (Na^+) and negatively charged ions (Cl^-) when dissolved in water, many drugs form two charged (ionized) particles when placed in water. While NaCl is a strong electrolyte, which causes it to almost entirely dissociate in water, most drugs are only partially ionized when dissolved in water. The extent of the **ionization** depends on two factors: the relative acidity/alkalinity (pH) of the solution and an intrinsic property of the molecule (pK_a).

Acidity or alkalinity is expressed as pH, which is described on a scale of 1 to 14, with 7 being neutral. Acidic solutions

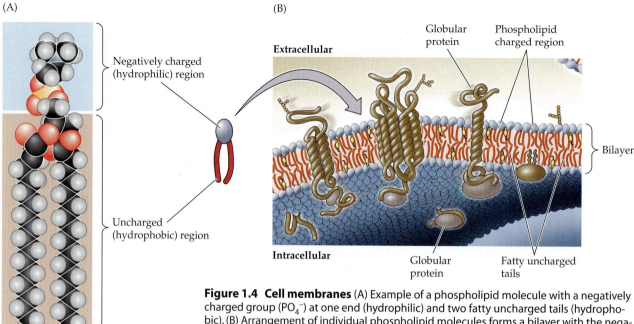

(A)

Negatively charged (hydrophilic) region

Uncharged (hydrophobic) region

(B)

Extracellular

Globular protein

Phospholipid charged region

Bilayer

Intracellular

Globular protein

Fatty uncharged tails

Figure 1.4 Cell membranes (A) Example of a phospholipid molecule with a negatively charged group (PO_4^-) at one end (hydrophilic) and two fatty uncharged tails (hydrophobic). (B) Arrangement of individual phospholipid molecules forms a bilayer with the negatively charged heads attracted to the water molecules of both the intracellular and extracellular fluids. The fatty tails of the molecules are tucked within the two charged layers and have no contact with aqueous fluid. Embedded in the bilayer are protein molecules that serve as receptors or channels.

have a lower pH, and alkaline (basic) solutions have a pH greater than 7.0. Drugs are dissolved in body fluids that differ in pH (Table 1.2), and these differences play a role in drug ionization and movement from one body fluid compartment to another, for example, from the stomach to the bloodstream or from the bloodstream into the kidney urine.

The second factor determining ionization is a characteristic of the drug molecule. The pK_a of a drug represents the pH of the aqueous solution in which that drug would be 50% ionized and 50% non-ionized. In general, drugs that are weak acids ionize more readily in an alkaline environment and become less ionized in an acidic environment. The reverse is true of drugs that are weak bases. If we put the weak acid aspirin (acetylsalicylic acid) into stomach acid, it will remain primarily in a non-ionized form (Figure 1.5).

TABLE 1.2 pH of Body Fluids

Fluid	pH
Stomach fluid	1.0–3.0
Small intestine	5.0–6.6
Blood	7.35–7.45
Kidney urine	4.5–7.5
Saliva	6.2–7.2
CSF	7.3–7.4

The lack of electrical charge makes the drug more lipid soluble and hence readily absorbed from the stomach to the blood. In the intestine, where the pH is around 5.0 to 6.0, ionization increases and absorption through that membrane is reduced compared to that of the stomach.

This raises the question of why aspirin molecules do not move from the stomach to the blood and back to the stomach again. In our example, aspirin in the acidic gastric fluid is primarily in the non-ionized form and thus passes through the stomach wall into the blood. In blood (pH 7.4), however, aspirin becomes more ionized; it is said to be "trapped" within the blood and does not return to the stomach. Meanwhile, the circulation moves the aspirin molecules away from their concentrated site at the stomach to maintain a concentration gradient that favors drug absorption.

Drugs that are highly charged in both acidic and basic environments are very poorly absorbed from the gastrointestinal tract and cannot be administered orally. The first of the medical mysteries proposed at the start of this chapter is now solved. South American hunters readily eat the flesh of game killed with curare-poisoned arrows because the drug does not leave the digestive system to enter their blood.

Other factors Factors other than ionization also have a significant influence on absorption. For instance, the much greater surface area of the small intestine and the slower movement of material through the intestine, as compared to

get sites in a given unit of time. The average dose of a drug is typically based on the response of individuals between the ages of 18 and 65 who weigh 150 pounds. However, for people who are very lean or obese, the average dose may be inappropriate because of variations in the ratio of fat to water in the body. For these individuals, body surface area, which reflects both size and weight, may be a better basis for determining drug dose. The sex of the individual also plays a part in determining plasma drug level because in the female, adipose tissue, relative to water, represents a larger proportion of the total body weight. Overall, the total fluid volume, which contains the drug, is relatively smaller in women than in men, producing a higher drug concentration at the target site in women. It should be obvious also that the smaller fluid volume of a child means that a standard dose of a drug will be more concentrated and, therefore, will produce a greater drug effect.

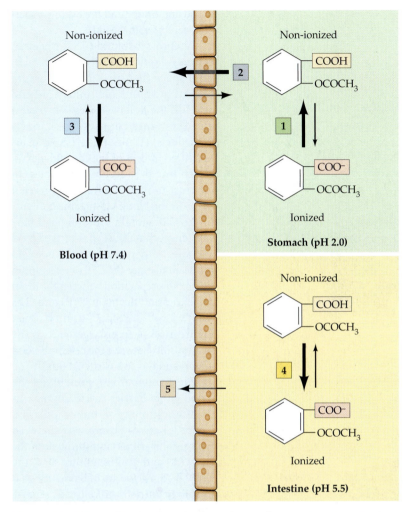

Figure 1.5 Effect of ionization on drug absorption On the right side of the cell barrier in stomach acid (pH 2.0), the aspirin molecules tend to remain in the non-ionized form (1), which promotes the passage of the drug through the cell walls (2) to the blood. Once the intact aspirin molecules reach the blood (pH 7.4), they ionize (3) and are "trapped" in the blood to be circulated throughout the body. In the lower portion of the figure, when the aspirin has reached the intestine, it tends to dissociate to a greater extent (4) in the more basic pH. Its more ionized form reduces passage (5) through the cells to the blood, so absorption from intestine is slower than from the stomach.

Drug distribution is limited by selective barriers

Regardless of the route of administration, once the drug has entered the blood, it is carried throughout the body within 1 or 2 minutes and can have an action at any number of receptor sites. In general, those parts of the body that have the most blood flow will have the highest concentration of drug. Since blood capillaries have numerous pores, most drugs can move from blood and enter body tissues regardless of lipid solubility, unless they are bound to protein (see the discussion on depot binding later in this chapter). High concentrations of drugs will be found in the heart, brain, kidneys, and liver. Because the brain receives about 20% of the blood that leaves the heart, lipid-soluble drugs are readily distributed to brain tissue. However, the blood–brain barrier limits the movement of ionized molecules from the blood to the brain.

Blood–brain barrier   Blood plasma is supplied by a dense network of blood vessels that permeates the entire brain. This system supplies brain cells with oxygen, glucose, and amino acids, and also carries away carbon dioxide and other waste products. Despite the vital role the blood circulation plays in cerebral function, many substances found in blood fluctuate significantly and would have disruptive effects on brain cell activity if materials were transferred freely between

the stomach, provide a much greater opportunity for absorption of all drugs. Therefore, the rate at which the stomach empties into the intestine very often is the significant rate-limiting factor. For this reason, medication is often prescribed to be taken before meals and with sufficient fluid to move the drug through the stomach and into the intestine.

Since drug absorption is closely related to the concentration of the drug in body fluids (e.g., stomach), it should certainly be no surprise to you that the drug dosage required to achieve a desired effect is directly related to the size of the individual. In general, the larger the individual, the more diluted the drug will be in his larger fluid volume, and less drug will reach the tar-

(A)

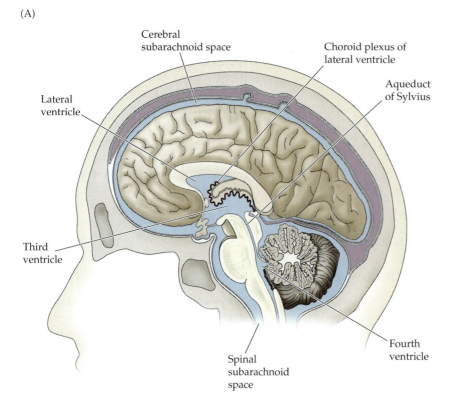

Cerebral subarachnoid space

Choroid plexus of lateral ventricle

Aqueduct of Sylvius

Lateral ventricle

Third ventricle

Spinal subarachnoid space

Fourth ventricle

(B)

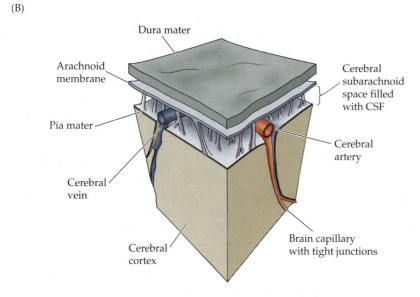

Dura mater

Arachnoid membrane

Cerebral subarachnoid space filled with CSF

Pia mater

Cerebral artery

Cerebral vein

Cerebral cortex

Brain capillary with tight junctions

Figure 1.6 Distribution of cerebrospinal fluid
(A) The CSF (blue) is manufactured by the choroid plexus within the cerebral ventricles. In addition to filling the ventricles and their connecting aqueducts, CSF fills the space between the arachnoid membrane and the pia mater (subarachnoid space) to cushion the brain against trauma. (B) Enlarged diagram to show detail of CSF-filled subarachnoid space and the relationship to cerebral blood vessels. Notice how blood vessels penetrate the brain tissue.

blood and brain (and the brain's associated cerebrospinal fluid).

Cerebrospinal fluid (CSF) is a clear, colorless liquid that fills the subarachnoid space that surrounds the entire bulk of the brain and spinal cord and also fills the hollow spaces (ventricles) and their interconnecting channels (aqueducts) (Figure 1.6A). CSF is manufactured by cells of the choroid plexus, which line the cerebral ventricles. In contrast to the wide fluctuations that occur in the blood plasma, the contents of the CSF remain quite stable. Many substances that diffuse out of the blood and affect other organs in the body do not seem to enter the CSF or affect brain tissue. This separation between the brain capillaries and the brain/CSF comprises what we call the blood–brain barrier. Figure 1.6B is an enlargement of the relationship between the cerebral blood vessels and the cerebrospinal fluid.

The principal component of the blood–brain barrier is actually the distinct morphology of brain capillaries. Figure 1.7 shows a comparison between typical capillaries found throughout the body (A) and capillaries that serve the CNS (B). Since the job of blood vessels is to deliver nutrients to cells and remove waste, the walls of typical capillaries are made up of endothelial cells that have both small gaps (**intercellular clefts**) as well as larger openings (**fenestrations**) through which molecules can pass. In addition, general capillaries have **pinocytotic vesicles** that envelop and transport larger molecules through the capillary wall. In contrast, in brain capillaries, the intercellular clefts are closed because the adjoining edges of the endothelial cells are fused, forming **tight junctions.** Also, fenestrations are absent and pinocytotic vesicles are rare. Although lipid-soluble materials can pass through the walls of the blood vessels, most materials are moved from the blood of brain capillaries by special transporters. Surrounding brain capillaries are numerous glial feet, extensions of the glial cells called **astrocytes.** It is likely that the close interface of astrocytes with both nerve cells and

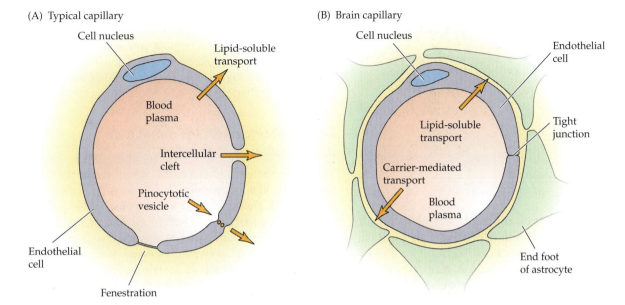

(A) Typical capillary

Cell nucleus

Lipid-soluble transport

Blood plasma

Intercellular cleft

Pinocytotic vesicle

Endothelial cell

Fenestration

(B) Brain capillary

Cell nucleus

Endothelial cell

Tight junction

Lipid-soluble transport

Carrier-mediated transport

Blood plasma

End foot of astrocyte

Figure 1.7 Cross section of typical capillaries and brain capillaries (A) The capillaries found throughout the body have characteristics that encourage the movement of materials between the blood and surrounding cells. (B) Brain capillaries minimize movement of water-soluble molecules through the blood vessel wall because there are essentially no large or small clefts or pinocytotic sites. (After Oldendorf, 1975.)

brain capillaries provides the astrocytes with a unique opportunity to modify neuron function.

Before we go on, we should emphasize that the blood–brain barrier is selectively permeable, not impermeable. Although the barrier does reduce diffusion of water-soluble (i.e., ionized) molecules, it does not impede lipid-soluble molecules.

Finally, the blood–brain barrier is not complete. Several brain areas are not isolated from materials in the blood. One of these is the **area postrema**, or CTZ (chemical trigger zone), which is located in the medulla of the brain stem. This area, the "vomiting center," causes vomiting when toxic substances are detected in the blood. The interaction between blood and brain is necessary to efficiently couple a toxic stimulus and the potentially lifesaving response. A second area is the **median eminence** of the hypothalamus. Capillary fenestrations in this brain region allow neurohormones manufactured by the hypothalamus to move into the blood traveling to the pituitary gland. These neurohormones, or releasing factors (for example, growth hormone–releasing factor), regulate anterior pituitary hormone secretion. Chapter 3 discusses the hypothalamic factors more fully. A limited blood–brain barrier exists in other regions of the brain wherever a functional interaction (e.g., blood monitoring) is required between the blood and neural tissue.

The limited permeability of the blood–brain barrier is important to psychopharmacology because we need to know which drugs remain non-ionized at plasma pH and readily enter the CNS and which drugs circulate only throughout the rest of the body. Minor differences in drug molecules are responsible for a relative selectivity of drug action. For example, physostigmine readily crosses the blood–brain barrier and is useful for treating the intoxication caused by some agricultural pesticides. It does so by increasing the availability of the neurotransmitter acetylcholine. In contrast, the structurally related but highly ionized drug neostigmine is excluded from the brain and increases acetylcholine only peripherally. Its restriction by the blood–brain barrier means that neostigmine can be used to treat the muscle disease myasthenia gravis, without significant CNS side effects, but it would not be effective in treating pesticide-induced intoxication.

Placental barrier A second barrier, unique to women, occurs between the blood circulation of a pregnant mother and that of her fetus. The placenta, which connects the fetus with the mother's uterine wall, is the means by which nutrients from the digestion of food, O_2, CO_2, fetal waste products, and drugs are exchanged. As is true for other cell membranes, lipid-soluble substances diffuse easily and water-soluble substances pass less easily. The potential for transfer of drugs from mother to fetus has very important implications for the health and well-being of the developing child. Potentially damaging effects on the fetus can be divided into two categories: acute toxicity and teratogenic effects.

The fetus may experience acute toxicity in utero following exposure to the disproportionately high drug blood level of its mother. In addition, after birth, any drug remaining in the newborn's circulation is likely to have a dramatic and pro-

TABLE 1.3 Periods of Maximum Teratogenic Sensitivity for Several Organ Systems in the Human Fetus

Organ system	Days after fertilization
Brain	15–60
Eye	15–40
Genitalia	35–60
Heart	15–40
Limbs	25–35

longed action because of slow and incomplete metabolism. It is well known that opiates such as heroin readily reach the fetal circulation, and that newborn infants of heroin- or methadone-addicted mothers experience many of the signs of opiate withdrawal. Certain tranquilizers, gaseous anesthetics, alcohol, many barbiturates, and cocaine all readily pass into fetal circulation to cause acute toxicity. In addition, alcohol, cocaine, and the carbon monoxide in cigarette smoke all deprive the fetus of oxygen. Such drugs pose special problems because they are readily accessible and widely used.

Teratogens are agents that induce developmental abnormalities in the fetus. The effects of teratogens such as drugs (both therapeutic and illicit), exposure to X-rays, and some maternal infections (e.g., German measles) are dependent on the timing of exposure. The fetus is most susceptible to damaging effects during the first trimester of pregnancy, because it is during this period that many of the fetal organ systems are formed. Each organ system is maximally sensitive to damaging effects during its time of cell differentiation (Table 1.3). Many drugs can have damaging effects on the fetus despite minimal adverse effects in the mother. For example, the vitamin A–related substance isotretinoin, which is a popular prescription acne medication (Accutane), produces serious birth defects and must be avoided by sexually active young women. Past experience has taught us that the evaluation of drug safety must include evaluation of potential fetal effects as well as effects on adults. Furthermore, since teratogenic effects are most severe during the time before pregnancy is typically recognized, use of any drug known to be teratogenic in animals should be avoided by women of childbearing age.

Depot binding alters the magnitude and duration of drug action

We already know that after a drug is absorbed into the blood from its site of administration, it circulates throughout the body. Thus, high concentrations of drug may be found in all organs that are well supplied with blood. In addition to these reservoirs, drug binding occurs at inactive sites where no measurable biological effect is initiated. Such sites, called **drug depots,** include plasma protein (e.g., albumin), muscle, and fat. Any drug molecules tied up in these depots cannot reach active sites nor be metabolized by the liver. However, the drug binding is reversible, so the drug remains bound only until the blood level drops, causing it to unbind gradually and circulate in the plasma.

The binding of a drug to inactive sites (**depot binding**) has significant effects on the magnitude and duration of drug action. Some of these effects are summarized in Table 1.4. First, depot binding reduces the concentration of drug at its sites of action because only freely circulating (unbound) drug can pass across membranes. For a drug that binds readily to depot sites, its onset of action may be delayed and its effects reduced because the number of drug molecules reaching the target tissue is dependent upon its release from inactive sites. Also, individual differences in the amount of depot binding explains in part why some people are more sensitive to a particular drug than others.

Second, since binding to albumin, fat, and muscle is rather nonselective, many drugs with similar physiochemical characteristics compete with each other for these sites. Such competition may lead to much-higher-than-expected

TABLE 1.4 Effects of Drug Depot Binding on Therapeutic Outcome

Depot-binding characteristics	Therapeutic outcome
Rapid binding to depots before reaching target tissue	Slower onset and reduced effects

Individual differences in amount of binding	Varying effects:
	  High binding means less free drug, so some people seem to need higher doses
	  Low binding means more free drug, so these individuals seem more sensitive

Competition among drugs for depot-binding sites	Higher-than-expected blood levels of the displaced drug, possibly causing greater side effects, even toxicity
Bound drug is not metabolized	Drug remains in the body for prolonged action
Binding to depots follows the rapid action at targets (redistribution)	Rapid termination of drug action

free drug blood level of the displaced drug, producing a drug overdose. For example, the antiseizure drug phenytoin is highly protein bound, but aspirin can displace some of the phenytoin molecules from the binding sites because aspirin binds more readily. When phenytoin is displaced from plasma protein by aspirin, the elevated drug level may be responsible for unexpected side effects or toxicity. Many psychoactive drugs, including the antidepressant fluoxetine (Prozac) and the tranquilizer diazepam (Valium), show extensive (over 90% of the drug molecules) plasma protein binding and may contribute to drug interactions.

Third, bound drug molecules cannot be altered by liver enzymes because the drug is not free to leave the blood to enter liver cells for metabolism. For this reason, depot binding frequently prolongs the time that the drug remains in the body. This phenomenon explains why some drugs, such as THC, which is stored in fat and only slowly released, can be detected in urine for many days after a single dose. Such slow release means that an individual could test positive for urinary THC (one active ingredient in marijuana) without experiencing the cognitive effects at that time. As we suggested in the beginning of the chapter, the prolonged presence of drugs in body fat and inert depots makes preemployment and student drug testing possible.

Finally, depots may be responsible for terminating a drug's action, as in the case of the rapid-acting CNS depressant thiopental. Thiopental, a barbiturate used for intravenous anesthesia, is highly lipid soluble, so the rapid onset of sedation is due to the drug's entry to the brain. However, the deep sedation does not last very long because the blood level falls rapidly as a result of redistribution of the drug to other tissues, causing thiopental to move from the brain to the blood to maintain equilibrium. High levels of thiopental can be found in the brain 30 seconds after IV infusion. However, within 5 minutes brain levels of the drug have dropped to threshold anesthetic concentrations. In this way, thiopental induces sleep almost instantaneously but is effective for only about 5 minutes, followed by rapid recovery.

Biotransformation and elimination of drugs contributes to bioavailability

Drugs are eliminated from the body by the combined action of several mechanisms, including biotransformation (metabolism) of the drug and excretion of the metabolites that have been formed.

Drug clearance   Drug clearance from the blood usually occurs exponentially and is referred to as **first-order kinetics.** Exponential elimination means that a constant fraction (50%) of the free drug in the blood is removed in each time interval. This model assumes that when blood levels are high, clearance occurs more rapidly, and as blood levels drop, the rate of clearance also is reduced. The amount of time required for removal

of 50% of the drug in blood is called the **half-life,** or $t_{1/2}$. Figure 1.8 provides an example of the half-life determination for the stimulant dextroamphetamine (Dexedrine), a drug used to treat attention deficit disorder. Although this drug is essentially eliminated after 6 half-lives (6×10 hours), many psychoactive drugs have half-lives of several days, so clearance may take weeks after even a single dose. A list of the half-lives of some common drugs is provided in Table 1.5.

Although most drugs are cleared from the blood by first-order kinetics, under certain conditions some drugs are eliminated according to the zero-order model. **Zero-order kinetics** means that drug molecules are cleared at a constant rate regardless of drug concentration. Ethyl alcohol is one drug that is eliminated by zero-order kinetics when administered in high doses. Alcohol is removed from the body at approximately 10 to 15 ml/hour, or 1.0 ounce of 100-proof alcohol per hour.

Biotransformation by liver microsomal enzymes   Most drugs are chemically altered by the body before they are

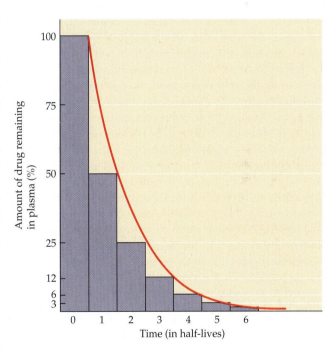

Figure 1.8 First-order kinetics of drug clearance Exponential elimination of drug from the blood occurs when clearance during a fixed time interval is always 50% of the drug remaining in blood. For example, the half-life of orally administered dextroamphetamine (Dexedrine) is approximately 10 hours. Therefore, 10 hours (1 half-life) after the peak plasma concentration has been reached, the drug concentration is reduced to about 50% of its initial value. After 20 and 30 hours (i.e., 2 and 3 half-lives) have elapsed, the concentration is reduced to 25% and 12.5%, respectively. After 6 half-lives, the drug is essentially eliminated, with 1.6% remaining. The curve representing the rate of clearance is steeper early on when the rate is more rapid and becomes more shallow as the rate of clearance decreases.

TABLE 1.5 Half-Life of Some Common Drugs

Drug	Trade/Street name	Half-life
Cocaine	Coke, Big C, snow	0.5–1.5 hours
Nicotine	Tobacco	2 hours
THC	Marijuana	20–30 hours
Acetylsalicylic acid	Aspirin	3–4 hours
Ibuprofen	Advil	3–4 hours
Naproxen	Aleve	12 hours
Sertraline	Zoloft	2–3 days
Fluoxetine	Prozac	7–9 days
Morphine	Morphine	1.5–2 hours

excreted. The chemical changes are catalyzed by enzymes and can occur in many tissues and organs, including the stomach, intestine, blood plasma, kidney, and brain. However, the greatest number of chemical changes, which we call drug metabolism or **biotransformation,** occur in the liver.

There are two major types of biotransformation. Type I biotransformations are sometimes called phase I, because these reactions often occur before a second metabolic step. Phase I changes involve *nonsynthetic* modification of the drug molecule by oxidation, reduction, or hydrolysis. Oxidation is by far the most common reaction; it usually produces a metabolite that is less lipid soluble and is often less active, but it may produce a metabolite with equal or even greater activity than the parent drug. Type II, or phase II, modifications are *synthetic* reactions that require the combination (called conjugations) of the drug with some small molecule such as glucuronide, sulfate, or methyl groups. Glucuronide conjugation is particularly important for inactivating psychoactive drugs. These metabolic products are less lipid soluble because they are highly ionized and are almost always biologically inactive. In summary, the two phases of drug biotransformation ultimately produce one or more inactive metabolites, which are water soluble so that they can be excreted more readily than the parent drug. The metabolites formed in the liver are returned to the circulation, and are subsequently filtered out by the kidneys, or they may be

excreted into bile and eliminated with the feces. Those metabolites that are active also return to the circulation and may have additional action on target tissues before being further metabolized into inactive products. Obviously, drugs that are converted into active metabolites have a prolonged duration of action. Table 1.6 shows several examples of the varied effects of phase I and phase II metabolism. The sedative drug phenobarbital is rapidly inactivated by phase I metabolism. In contrast, aspirin is converted first to an active metabolite by phase I metabolism, but phase II action produces an inactive compound. Morphine does not undergo phase I metabolism but is inactivated by phase II reactions. Finally, diazepam (Valium), a long-lasting antianxiety drug, has several active metabolites before a phase II inactivation.

The liver enzymes primarily responsible for metabolizing psychoactive drugs are located on the smooth endoplasmic reticulum, which is a network of tubules within the liver cell cytoplasm. They are often called **microsomal enzymes** because they exhibit particular characteristics on biochemical analysis. The microsomal enzymes lack specificity and can metabolize a wide variety of compounds including toxins ingested with food or environmental pollutants. Among the most important liver microsomal enzymes is the **cytochrome P450** enzyme family. The more than 30 members of this class of enzyme are responsible for oxidizing a majority of psychoactive drugs, including antidepressants, morphine, and amphetamine.

Factors influencing drug metabolism   The enzymes of the liver are of particular interest to psychopharmacologists because several factors significantly influence the rate of biotransformation. These factors alter the magnitude and duration of drug effects and are responsible for significant drug interactions and individual differences in response to drugs. These factors include (1) enzyme induction; (2) enzyme inhibition; (3) drug competition; and (4) individual differences in age, gender, and genetics.

Many psychoactive drugs, when used repeatedly, cause an increase in liver enzymes (called **enzyme induction**). The increased enzymes not only cause the drugs to speed up their own rate of biotransformation, but they can also increase the rate of metabolism of all other drugs modified by them. For

TABLE 1.6 Varied Effects of Phase I and Phase II Metabolism

Active drug	Active metabolites and inactive metabolites[a]			
Phenobarbital	——————————— Phase I ———————————→	Hydroxyphenobarbital		
Aspirin	—— Phase I ——→ **Salicylic acid**	—— Phase II ——→ Salicyclic-glucuronide		
Morphine	——————————— Phase II ———————————→	Morphine-6-glucuronide		
Diazepam	—— Phase I ——→ **Desmethyldiazepam**	—— Phase I ——→ **Oxazepam**	—— Phase II ——→ Oxazepam-glucuronide	

[a]Bold terms indicate active metabolites.

example, repeated use of the antiseizure drug carbamazepine (Tegretol) increases the number of cytochrome P450 enzyme molecules, leading to more rapid metabolism of carbamazepine and other drugs, producing a lower blood level and reduced biological effect. Among the drugs metabolized by the same enzyme are oral contraceptives. For this reason, if carbamazepine is prescribed to a woman taking oral contraceptives, either the hormone dose must be increased or an alternative means of birth control used (Zajecka, 1993). As you saw at the beginning of this chapter, failure to increase the dose leads to higher rates of unwanted pregnancy.

Another common example is cigarette smoke, which also increases certain cytochrome P450 enzymes. People who are heavy smokers may need higher doses of those drugs, such as antidepressants and caffeine that are metabolized by the same enzyme. Such changes in drug metabolism and elimination explain in part why some drugs lose their effectiveness with repeated use—a phenomenon known as tolerance (see the discussion on tolerance later in the chapter)—and also cause a reduced action of other drugs (cross tolerance). Clearly, an individual's drug-taking history can have a major impact on the effectiveness of the drugs he or she currently takes.

In contrast to drug-induced induction of liver enzymes, some drugs directly inhibit the action of enzymes (**enzyme inhibition**), which reduces the metabolism of other drugs taken at the same time. In such cases one would experience a much more intense or prolonged drug effect. Monoamine oxidase inhibitors, used to treat depression, act in the brain by preventing the destruction of neurotransmitters by the enzyme monoamine oxidase. The same enzyme is found in the liver, where it is responsible for metabolizing a variety of drugs. Inhibiting enzyme function means impaired metabolism (and elevated blood levels) of many drugs, including opiates, alcohol, aspirin, and others. In addition, the enzyme normally metabolizes amines such as tyramine, which is found in red wine, beer, some cheeses, and other foods. When individuals who are taking these antidepressants eat foods rich in tyramine, toxic high blood pressure and cardiac arrhythmias can occur, making normal foods potentially life-threatening. The opening paragraph of this chapter mentions this "food toxicity," and more detail is provided in Chapter 15.

A second type of inhibition, based on **drug competition** for the enzyme, occurs for drugs that share a metabolic system. Since there are a limited number of enzyme molecules, an elevated concentration of either drug reduces the metabolic rate of the second, causing potentially toxic levels. Cytochrome P450 metabolism of alcohol leads to higher-than-normal brain levels of other sedative–hypnotics, for example, barbiturates or Valium, when administered at the same time, producing a potentially dangerous drug interaction.

Finally, differences in drug metabolism due to genetic and environmental factors can explain why some individuals seem to be extremely sensitive to certain drugs while others may need much higher doses than normal to achieve an effect.

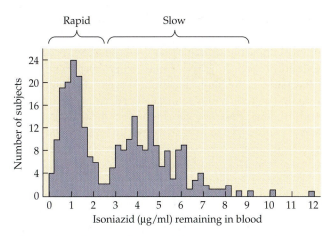

Figure 1.9 Two genetic populations for isoniazid metabolism Six hours after oral administration of isoniazid to 267 subjects, blood levels of the drug were measured. The bimodal frequency distribution shows that one subpopulation of subjects were rapid metabolizers and had an average of 1 μg/ml remaining in the blood. A second portion of the population were much slower metabolizers and had an average of 4 to 5 μg/ml of drug remaining. Note that several subjects had extremely slow metabolism, making them very likely to show toxic side effects, particularly if the drug were taken chronically. (After Evans, 1960.)

Over 40 years ago, the first **genetic polymorphisms** (genetic variations among individuals that produce multiple forms of a given protein) for drug-metabolizing enzymes were identified. Large variations, for instance, were found in the rate of acetylation of isoniazid, a drug used to treat tuberculosis and subsequently found to relieve depression. Acetylation is a conjugation reaction in which an acetyl group is attached to the drug. In the early experiment, blood levels of isoniazid were measured 6 hours after its oral administration to 267 subjects. The bimodal distribution in Figure 1.9 clearly shows that some individuals metabolized much of the drug during the 6 hours ("rapid inactivators"), while a second group ("slow inactivators") eliminated far less drug and are thus more likely to develop toxic side effects at normal doses. In addition to isoniazid, the metabolism of more than a dozen related drugs and chemicals are also affected by these genetic variations. It is significant that 44 to 54% of American Caucasians and African Americans, 60% of Europeans, 10% of Asians, and only 5% of Eskimos are slow inactivators (Levine, 1973). Other enzymes also show wide genetic differences. For example, approximately 50% of certain Asian groups (Chinese, Japanese, and Koreans) have reduced capacity to metabolize acetaldehyde, which is an intermediary metabolic step in the breakdown of alcohol. The resulting elevation in acetaldehyde causes facial flushing, tachycardia, drop in blood pressure, and sometimes nausea and vomiting. The reduced metabolic capacity is caused by a specific mutation in the gene for aldehyde dehydrogenase (Wall and Ehelers, 1995).

In addition to variations in genes, other individual differences influence metabolism. Significant changes in nutrition or in liver function, as accompany various diseases, lead to significantly higher drug blood levels and prolonged and exaggerated effects. Additionally, advanced age is often accompanied by a reduced ability to metabolize drugs, while children under the age of two also have insufficient metabolic capacity and are vulnerable to drug overdoses. In addition, both the young and elderly have reduced kidney function, so clearance of drugs is much slower. Gender differences also exist in drug metabolism. For example, the stomach enzymes that metabolize alcohol before it reaches the bloodstream are far less effective in women than in men. This means that for an identical dose, a woman will have a much higher concentration of alcohol reaching her blood to produce biological effects. If you would like to read more about some of the clinical concerns of differences in drug metabolism, see Applegate (1999).

Renal excretion   Although drugs can be excreted from the body in the breath, sweat, saliva, feces, or breast milk, the most important route of elimination is in the urine. Therefore, the primary organ of elimination is the kidney. The kidneys are a pair of organs each about the size of a fist. They are responsible for filtering materials out of the blood and excreting the waste products, while returning necessary substances, such as water, glucose, sodium, potassium, and chloride, to the blood. Liver biotransformation of drugs into ionized (water-soluble) molecules traps the metabolites in the kidney tubules so that they can be excreted with waste products in the urine.

Section Summary

A drug's effects are determined by (1) how much of the drug reaches its target sites, where it has biological action; and (2) how quickly it reaches those sites. The pharmacokinetic factors that determine bioavailability include the method of administration, rate of absorption and distribution, binding at inactive sites, biotransformation, and excretion. These factors interact, so that as a drug is being absorbed and distributed throughout the body to act at target sites, some of its molecules are simultaneously being bound to inactive sites, while others are metabolized and excreted. The route of administration is significant because it determines both onset and duration of drug action. The method of administration influences absorption of the drug because it determines the area of the absorbing surface, the number of cell layers the drug must pass through, and the extent of first-pass metabolism. Each of the methods described has distinct advantages and disadvantages.

Absorption is not dependent only on administration method but also on the solubility and ionization of the drug and individual differences in age, sex, and body size, which contribute to the concentration of the drug. Lipid-soluble drugs are not ionized and readily pass through fatty membranes at a rate dependent on the concentration gradient. Drugs that are weak acids tend to remain un-ionized (lipid soluble) in acidic body fluids like stomach juices; they are more readily absorbed there than in the more alkaline intestinal fluid, where ionization of weak acids increases and absorption is reduced. Drugs that are weak bases are more ionized in the acidic stomach fluid, so they are absorbed less readily there than from the more basic intestine, where ionization is reduced and the drugs become more lipid soluble.

Once a drug is in the blood, it is distributed to all the organs of the body, as determined by the extent of blood flow to the tissue. The CNS has a lower drug concentration than would be expected because the blood–brain barrier reduces the exposure of brain and spinal cord to water-soluble molecules. The brain capillaries that constitute the blood–brain barrier have very few pores to allow drug molecules to leave the circulation and affect the neural tissue. Although the placental barrier separates maternal and fetal circulation, it does not impede passage of most drug molecules, so the developing fetus is exposed to most drugs consumed by the mother. Numerous drugs, particularly those ingested during the first trimester of pregnancy, are capable of interfering with fetal organ development. Once in general circulation, some drug molecules bind to inactive depots, where they cannot act at target sites nor be metabolized. Depot binding is responsible for modifying the onset and duration of drug effect.

In addition to the absorption and distribution of a drug in the body, the rate of degradation and elimination is equally important in determining bioavailability. Drugs are most often biotransformed by liver enzymes (e.g., cytochrome P450) that produce products for excretion that are inactive and more water soluble. Phase I metabolism involves oxidation, reduction, or hydrolysis and produces an ionized metabolite that may be inactive, equally active, or more active than the parent drug. Phase II metabolism involves the conjugation of the drug with a simple molecule provided by the body, such as glucuronide or sulfate. Products of phase II metabolism are always inactive and more water soluble. The kidney is most often responsible for filtration of metabolites from the blood before excretion with the urine. Alternatively, the metabolites may be excreted into bile and eliminated with the feces.

Several factors that influence drug metabolism and elimination are significant to psychopharmacologists because they are responsible for many drug interactions and also explain why some individuals respond differently to drugs.

1. Liver enzymes can be induced (increased) by some classes of drugs given repeatedly. More enzyme means more-efficient metabolism, which reduces blood levels of drug and reduces the intensity and/or duration of its effects.

2. Some drugs directly impair liver enzyme action, so any drug normally metabolized by that enzyme will remain in the body for longer periods of time, producing prolonged drug effects.

3. The limited number of enzymes also means that if two drugs share a metabolic system, then the two will compete for biotransformation, causing elevated blood levels of one or the other or both drugs.

4. Individuals who are very sensitive or very resistant to drug effects may differ genetically in the efficiency of the metabolic enzymes. Rapid metabolizers will appear to be less responsive to the drug, while slow metabolizers may show greater response, increased side effects, or toxicity.

In addition to genetic differences, differences in age, sex, nutrition, and organ (e.g., kidney and liver) function also are responsible for varying rates of biotransformation.

Pharmacodynamics: Drug–Receptor Interactions

Pharmacodynamics is the study of the physiological and biochemical interaction of drug molecules with the target tissue that is responsible for the ultimate drug effects. Drugs can be classified into a wide variety of categories (Box 1.3), but all the drugs we are concerned with affect cell function in target tissue by acting on receptors. Knowing which receptors a drug acts on and where the receptors are located is crucial to understanding what actions and side effects will be produced.

Receptors, large protein molecules located either on the surface of or within cells, are the initial sites of action of a biologically active agent such as a neurotransmitter, hormone, or drug (all referred to as ligands). A **ligand** is defined as any molecule that binds to a receptor with some selectivity. Because most drugs do not readily pass into neurons, neuropharmacology is most often interested in receptors found on the outside of cells that relay information through the membrane to affect intracellular processes (Figure 1.10A). Which of the many possible intracellular changes occurs depends upon whether the receptor is coupled to an ion channel or to a G protein (see Chapter 3). The essence of neuropharmacology is to identify drugs that can act at neurotransmitter receptors to enhance or reduce the normal functioning of the cell and bring about a clinically useful effect.

A second type of receptor is found within the target cell, either in the cytoplasm (as for the glucocorticoids) or in the nucleus (e.g., sex steroid receptors). Most of the hormones that act on the brain to influence neural events utilize this type of receptor. Hormonal binding to intracellular receptors alters cell function by triggering changes in the expression of

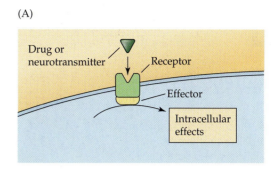

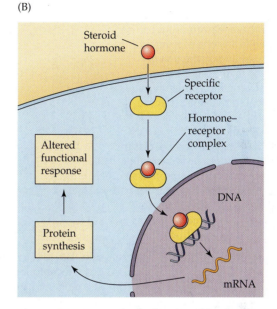

Figure 1.10 Two principal types of receptors (A) Most drugs and neurotransmitters remain outside the cell and bind to receptors on the exterior cell surface. When these receptors are activated, they initiate changes in an effector, which causes intracellular changes, such as movement of ions or changes in enzyme activity. (B) Many hormones are capable of entering the cell before acting on an intracellular receptor that changes the expression of specific genes within the nucleus. The altered protein synthesis in turn leads to changes in cell function.

the genetic material within the nucleus, producing differences in protein synthesis (Figure 1.10B). Sex hormones act in this way to facilitate mating behavior and other activities related to reproduction. This mechanism is described more fully in Chapter 3.

Extracellular and intracellular receptors have several common features

Several characteristics are common to receptors in general. The ability to recognize specific molecular shapes is one very important characteristic. The usual analogy of a lock and key suggests that only a limited group of neurochemicals or drugs

BOX 1.3 Pharmacology in Action

Drug Categories

As we have already learned earlier in this chapter, all drugs have multiple effects, which vary with dose and bioavailability, the nature of the receptors occupied, and the drug-taking history (e.g., tolerance) of the individual. For these reasons drugs can be categorized in any one of several classes depending on the trait of interest. One might classify drugs according to chemical structure, medical use, legal status, neurochemical effects, abuse potential, behavioral effects, and many other categories. Amphetamine may be described as a CNS stimulant (based on increased brain activity and behavioral arousal), an anorectic used for diet control (medical use), a sympathomimetic (because it neurochemically mimics the effects of the sympathetic nervous system), or a Schedule III drug (a controlled substance based on the federal government's assessment of abuse potential). Since we are particularly interested in brain function and behavior, the classification used in this text emphasizes CNS action and behavioral effects.

CNS stimulants produce increased electrical activity in the brain and behavioral arousal, alertness, and a sense of well-being in the individual. Among the drugs in this class are amphetamine, cocaine, and methylphenidate (Ritalin), as well as the methylxanthines, which include caffeine, theophylline, and theobromine. Nicotine may also be included here because of its activating effect on CNS neurons, although behaviorally for some individuals the drug clearly has a calming effect. Classification is also complicated by the fact that drug effects are dose-dependent and drugs occasionally produce dramatically different effects at different doses. Low and moderate doses of amphetamine, for example,

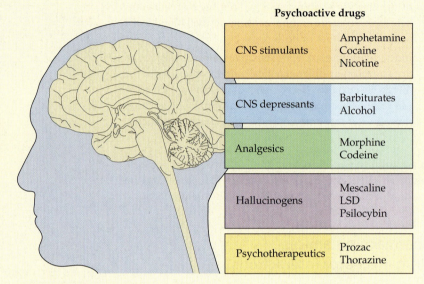

Psychoactive drugs

CNS stimulants	Amphetamine Cocaine Nicotine
CNS depressants	Barbiturates Alcohol
Analgesics	Morphine Codeine
Hallucinogens	Mescaline LSD Psilocybin
Psychotherapeutics	Prozac Thorazine

stimulate physical activity, but at high doses locomotion may be reduced and replaced by meaningless stereotyped, repetitive acts that have clear psychotic characteristics.

CNS depressants include a variety of drugs that depress CNS function and behavior to cause a sense of relaxation and drowsiness. Some of the sedative–hypnotics are useful for these sedating qualities and in their ability to relieve anxiety or induce sleep. At high doses more profound mental clouding occurs, along with loss of coordination, intoxication, and coma. The significant drugs in this group include the barbiturates (such as Seconal), the benzodiazepines (including Valium), and ethyl alcohol, all of which will be considered in later chapters. Some might include marijuana in this class because of its relaxing and depressant qualities at low doses, although at higher doses hallucinogenic characteristics may occur prominently.

The analgesics are drugs that frequently have CNS-depressant quali-

ties, although their principal effect is to reduce the perception of pain. The most important drugs in this class are the narcotics. Narcotics, or opiates, such as morphine, heroin, or codeine, are derived from the opium poppy; the synthetic narcotics (called opioids) include meperidine (Demerol), methadone, and fentanyl. All of the opiate-like drugs produce relaxation and sleep as well as analgesia. Under some circumstances these drugs also produce a powerful sense of euphoria and a desire to continue drug administration. Nonnarcotic analgesics, of course, also belong in this class but have little effect on behavior and do not produce relaxation or sleep. These include aspirin, acetaminophen (Tylenol), and ibuprofen (Motrin).

The hallucinogens, or mind-altering drugs, are often called "psychedelics" because their primary effect is to alter one's perceptions, leading to vivid visual illusions or distortions of objects and body image. As a group, these drugs produce a wide variety of effects on

BOX 1.3 (continued)

brain chemistry and neural activity. They include many naturally occurring substances such as mescaline and psilocybin. Certainly LSD belongs in this class, as does MDMA (street name: ecstasy). The drug PCP (street name: angel dust) and its analog ketamine (street name: special K), which is used as an animal sedative, might belong in the class of CNS depressants, but their ability to cause profound hallucinogenic experiences and their use as a model for psychotic behavior prompts their placement in this category.

Psychotherapeutic drugs as a classification is intended to suggest that some psychoactive drugs are used almost entirely to treat clinical disorders of mood or behavior: the antipsy-

chotics, antidepressants, and mood stabilizers. These drugs have distinctly different mechanisms of action and are rarely found in use outside the therapeutic realm. The antipsychotics reduce symptoms of schizophrenia, including hallucinations and bizarre behavior. Some examples include haloperidol (Haldol) and chlorpromazine (Thorazine). The antidepressants also belong in this classification; they are used to treat disorders of mood. Among the most familiar are amitriptyline (Elavil), sertraline (Zoloft), and fluoxetine (Prozac). While drugs in this class reverse the symptoms of clinical depression, they do not produce the effects of CNS stimulants nor do they produce euphoria. Finally, the mood

stabilizers reduce the dramatic mood swings between mania and depression that characterize bipolar disorder. Lithium carbonate (Lithonate) is still most often prescribed, but valproate (Depakote) and carbamazepine (Tegretol) are increasingly popular. Each of these types of drugs will be described in subsequent chapters of this text.

Clearly, many of the drugs you may be interested in have not been mentioned: hormones such as the anabolic steroids and contraceptives, the inhalants including household products and glues, and others. Many of these would require special categories for classification, but this text will address some of those topics in Chapter 14.

---

can bind to a particular receptor protein to initiate a cellular response. These neurochemicals are called **agonists.** Molecules that have the best chemical "fit" (i.e., have the highest **affinity**) attach most readily to the receptor. However, just as one may put a key in a lock but not be able to turn it, so too a ligand may be recognized by a receptor, but may not initiate a biological action. Such ligands are considered to have low **efficacy.** These molecules are called **antagonists** because not only do they produce no cellular effect after binding, but by binding to the receptor they prevent an "active" ligand from binding; hence they "block" the receptor (Figure 1.11).

A second significant feature of receptors is that the binding or attachment of the specific ligand is temporary. When the ligand dissociates (i.e., separates) from the receptor, it has further opportunity to attach once again. Third, ligands binding to the receptor produce a physical change in the three-dimensional shape of the protein, initiating a series of intracellular events that ultimately generates a biobehavioral effect. How much intracellular activity occurs depends on the number of interactions with the receptor as well as the ability of the ligand to alter the shape of the receptor, which reflects its efficacy.

Fourth, although we tend to think about receptors as a permanent characteristic of cells, these proteins in fact have a life cycle just as other cell proteins do. Not only is there a normal life span for receptors, but receptors are modified both in number (long-term regulation) and in sensitivity (more rapid regulation via second messengers). Long-term regulation, called **up-regulation** when receptor numbers increase or **down-regulation** when receptors are reduced in number, reflects compensatory changes following prolonged absence of receptor agonists or chronic activation of the receptor, respectively.

This phenomenon was initially observed in muscle, where it was found that if the nerve serving a particular muscle was cut (thereby eliminating the release of the neurotransmitter from the nerve endings), a compensatory increase in neurotransmitter receptors occurred over the muscle surface. More recently, the same phenomenon has been found in the CNS not only when nerves are severed but also when nerve activity is chroni-

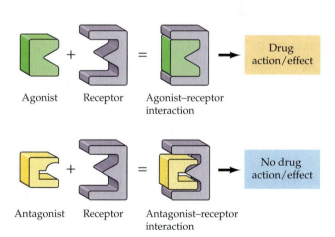

Figure 1.11 Agonist and antagonist interactions with receptors The agonist molecule has an excellent fit for the receptor (high affinity) and produces a significant biological response (high efficacy). The antagonist in this case fits less well and also has very low efficacy. Note that if both the agonist and antagonist are present simultaneously, they will compete to fit into the same receptor, producing a partial drug effect. (After Carroll, 1996.)

cally reduced by drugs. For instance, chronic use of receptor antagonists leads to subsequent up-regulation of receptors. Likewise, drugs that activate a nerve pathway or act as agonists at the receptor cause a reduction in receptor proteins if they are administered repeatedly. In each case, change in receptor number requires 1 to 2 weeks of altered activity. Changes in sensitivity due to second messenger-induced function is far more rapid. These changes will be discussed more fully in Chapter 3.

Finally, we have already learned that once drugs are absorbed, they are distributed throughout the body, where there are multiple sites of action (receptors) that mediate different biobehavioral effects. However, a given drug's receptor proteins may have different characteristics in different target tissues. These varied receptors, called **receptor subtypes,** will be covered more extensively later in the book. The goal of neuropharmacology is to design drugs that bind with greater affinity to one receptor subtype so as to initiate a very selective therapeutic effect, without acting on related receptor subtypes and producing side effects. For instance, in Table 1.7 you can see that caffeine works on the xanthine receptor subtype in the CNS to produce alertness more effectively than the xanthines found in tea (theophylline) or cocoa (theobromine). In contrast, theophylline is the most active of the three in stimulating the heart and causing increased urine output (diuresis).

TABLE 1.7 Relative Biological Activity of Xanthines[a]

Biological effects	Caffeine	Theophylline	Theobromine
CNS stimulation	1	2	3
Cardiac stimulation	3	1	2
Respiratory stimulation	1	2	3
Skeletal muscle stimulation	1	2	3
Diuresis	3	1	2

Source: From Richie, 1975.

[a]Each drug acts more effectively on some xanthine receptor subtypes than others. 1 = most active; 3 = least active.

If we were to graph the effects of several pain-relieving drugs, we might find a relationship similar to the one shown in Figure 1.13. The first three curves show the dose–response characteristics for hydromorphine, morphine, and codeine—all drugs from the opiate analgesic class. For each drug, increasing the concentration produces greater analgesia (elevation in pain threshold) until the maximum response is achieved. The absolute amount of drug necessary to produce a specific effect indicates the drug's **potency.** The differences in potency among the three drugs can be seen by comparing the ED_{50} for each drug. Hydromorphine requires approximately 2 mg, while morphine needs 10 mg to achieve the same effect and codeine needs more than 100 mg. Therefore, morphine is more potent than codeine and hydromorphine is more potent

Dose–response curves describe receptor activity

One important method used to evaluate receptor activity is the **dose–response curve,** which describes the amount of biological or behavioral effect (response) for a given drug concentration (dose). A typical curve is shown in Figure 1.12. When plotted on semilog scale, the curve takes on a classic S-shape. At low doses, the drug-induced effect is slight, because very few receptors are occupied. In fact, the threshold dose is the smallest dose that produces a measurable effect. As the dose of the drug is increased, more receptors are activated and a greater biological response occurs. The ED_{50} (50% effective dose) is the dose that produces half the maximal effect, and the maximum response occurs at a dose at which we assume the receptors are fully occupied* (we might call it the ED_{100}).

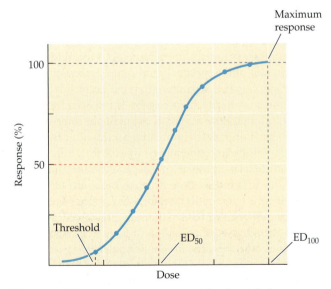

Figure 1.12 Dose–response curve The classic S-shape describes the gradual increase in biological response that occurs with increasing doses of a drug (drug–receptor activation). Threshold is the dose producing the smallest measurable response. The dose at which the maximum response is achieved is the ED_{100} (100% effective dose), while the ED_{50} is the dose that effectively produces 50% of the maximum response.

---

*This assumption is not warranted in all cases, however, such as in those models of receptor pharmacology describing "spare receptors." Those interested in the complexities of receptor occupancy theory should refer to a standard textbook in pharmacology.

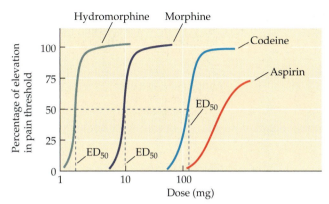

Figure 1.13 Dose–response curves for four analgesic agents Each curve represents the increase in pain threshold (the magnitude of painful stimulus required to elicit a withdrawal response) as a function of dose. The ED_{50} for hydromorphine, morphine, and codeine help compare potency. The linear portions of the curves for the opiate analgesics are parallel, suggesting they work through the same mechanism. Aspirin is not an opiate and relieves pain by a very different mechanism of action, so the shape of the curve is distinct. In addition, aspirin's maximum effectiveness never reaches the level of the opiates. (After Levine, 1983.)

than either. The relative position of the curves on the *x*-axis indicates potency and reflects the affinity of each drug for the receptor that mediates the measured response. Although the three differ in affinity for the receptor, each reaches the same maximum on the *y*-axis, indicating that they have identical efficacy. The fact that the linear portions of the curves are parallel to one another indicates that they are working by the same mechanism. Although the concept of potency provides some means of comparison, its practical use is limited. As you can see, a lower-potency drug is frequently just as effective and requires only a somewhat higher dose. If the low-potency drug also produces fewer side effects or is less expensive, then it may in fact be the preferred drug. You might consider these issues the next time a drug advertisement makes claims for being the most potent of its kind available.

Figure 1.13 also shows the dose–response for aspirin. In contrast to the first three drugs, aspirin is not an opioid, and the distinctive shape of its dose–response curve shows that although aspirin also relieves pain, it does not act on the same receptors or work by the same mechanism. In addition, regardless of how much aspirin is administered, it never achieves the same efficacy as the opiates.

The therapeutic index calculates drug safety

Among the multiple responses to any drug, some are undesirable or even dangerous side effects and need to be evaluated carefully in a therapeutic situation. For example, Figure 1.14 depicts three distinct pharmacological effects produced

by drug A, which is prescribed to reduce anxiety. The blue curve shows the number of individuals who experience reduced anxiety at various doses of the drug. The purple curve shows the number of persons suffering respiratory depression (a toxic effect) from various doses of the same drug. Comparing the ED_{50} for relieving anxiety (i.e., the dose at which 50% of the population show reduced anxiety) and the TD_{50} (50% toxic dose; the dose at which 50% of the population experiences a particular toxic effect) for respiratory depression, you can see that for most individuals the toxic dose is much higher than the dose producing the desired effect. An alternative interpretation is that at the dose needed to provide significant clinical relief to many patients (50%), almost none of the patients would be likely to experience respiratory depression. Therefore, pharmacologists would say the drug has a relatively favorable **therapeutic index** ($TI = TD_{50}/ED_{50}$). In contrast, the dose of drug A that produces sedation and mental clouding (red curve) is not very different from the ED_{50}. That small difference means that there is a high probability that a dose effective in reducing anxiety is likely to also produce significant mental clouding and sedation, which may represent serious side effects for many people who might use the drug.

Receptor antagonists compete with agonists for binding sites

We have already introduced the concept of receptor antagonists: those drugs that compete with agonists to bind to

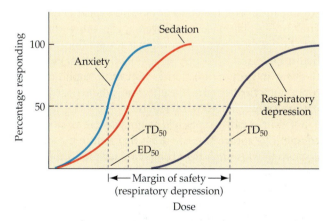

Figure 1.14 Comparison of ED_{50} and TD_{50} The therapeutic index is calculated by comparing the dose of drug required to produce a toxic effect in 50% of the individuals (TD_{50}) with the dose that is effective for 50% (ED_{50}). Each drug may have several therapeutic indices based on the toxic effects or side effects that are of concern. Since the optimum condition is to have an effective dose that is very low and not have toxicity except at very high doses, the TI will be large for a safer drug. The figure shows a large margin of safety for an antianxiety drug that can produce respiratory depression.

receptors but fail to initiate an intracellular effect, thereby reducing the effect of the agonists. These are called **competitive antagonists.** As the name implies, they can be displaced from those sites by an excess of the agonist, because an increased concentration of active drug can compete more effectively for the fixed number of receptors. A simple example will clarify. If we assume that the agonist and antagonist have similar affinities for the receptor, then if 100 molecules of drug and 100 molecules of antagonist were both present at the receptor, the probability of an agonist acting on the receptor would be 1 to 1. If drug molecules were increased to 1000, the odds of agonist binding rise to 10 to 1; at 1,000,000 agonist molecules, the odds favor agonist binding by 10,000 to 1. Certainly at that point the presence of the antagonist is of no consequence to the biobehavioral effect measured.

Figure 1.15A illustrates the effect of a competitive antagonist, naloxone, on the analgesic effect of morphine. The blue line shows a typical dose–response curve for the analgesic effect of morphine. When the subjects were pretreated with naloxone, the dose–response curve shifted to the right (red line), demonstrating that for any given dose of morphine, the naloxone-pretreated subjects showed less analgesia. The addition of naloxone diminished the potency of morphine. The figure also shows that the inhibitory action of naloxone was overcome by increasing the amount of morphine administered; that is, the same maximum effect (analgesia) was achieved, but more morphine was required. If you look at the chemical structures of the two drugs in Figure 10.3, you will see the striking similarity and understand how the two drugs compete to be recognized by the same receptor protein.

We have emphasized receptor antagonism because, in combination with the concept of dose-dependency, it is a vital tool in pharmacology. If we want to know whether a specific ligand–receptor interaction is responsible for a particular biological effect, the biological effect must be shown to occur in proportion to the amount of ligand present (dose) and, furthermore, the effect must be reduced in the presence of a competitive antagonist.

Of course, other types of antagonism can occur. **Noncompetitive antagonists** are drugs that reduce the effect of agonists in ways other than competing for the receptor. For example, a noncompetitive antagonist may impair agonist action by binding to a portion of the receptor other than the agonist binding site, by disturbing the cell membrane supporting the receptor, or by interfering with the intracellular processes that were initiated by the agonist–receptor association. Figure 1.15B illustrates the effect of a noncompetitive antagonist on the analgesic effect of morphine. In general, the shape of the dose–response curve will be distorted and the same maximum effect is not likely to be reached.

Furthermore, although pharmacologists are concerned with molecular actions at the receptor, biobehavioral inter-

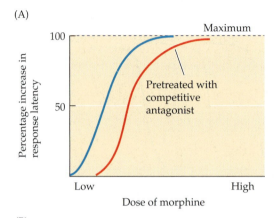

(A)

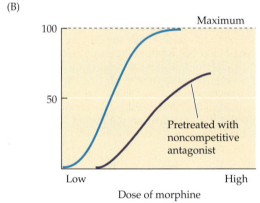

(B)

Figure 1.15 Drug antagonism (A) The effect of a competitive antagonist (naloxone) on the analgesic effect of morphine. The addition of a competitive antagonist essentially reduces the agonist's potency, as shown by the parallel shift of the dose–response curve to the right. (B) In contrast, adding a noncompetitive antagonist usually produces a distinct change in the shape of the dose–response curve, showing that it does not act at the same receptor site. Also, regardless of the increase in morphine, the maximum efficacy is never reached.

actions can also result in several different possible outcomes. **Physiological antagonism** (Figure 1.16A) involves two drugs that act in two distinct manners but interact in such a way that they reduce each other's effectiveness in the body. For example, one drug may act on receptors in the heart to increase heart rate, while the second may act on distinct receptors in the brain stem to slow heart rate. Clearly, two agents may have **additive effects** if the outcome equals the sum of the two individual effects (Figure 1.16B). Finally, **potentiation** refers to the situation in which the combination of two drugs produces effects that are greater than the sum of their individual effects (Figure 1.16C). Potentiation often involves issues of pharmacokinetics such as altered metabolic rate or competition for depot binding, which may elevate free drug blood levels in unexpected ways.

(A) Physiological antagonism

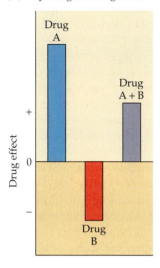

Figure 1.16 Possible results of the interaction of two drugs (A) Physiological antagonism results when two drugs produce opposite effects and reduce each other's effectiveness. (B) Additive effects occur when the combined drug effect equals the sum of each alone. (C) Potentiation is said to occur when the combined drug effects are greater than the sum of the individual drug effects.

(B) Additive effects

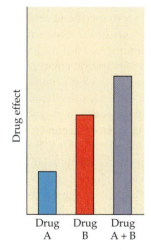

(C) Potentiation

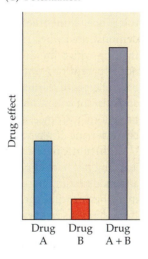

Biobehavioral Effects of Chronic Drug Use

Many prescription and over-the-counter drugs are taken on a regular basis for chronic medical or psychiatric conditions. These drugs are taken for periods of weeks, months, or even years. Recreational drugs also are most often used repeatedly rather than on only a single occasion. When a drug is used on several occasions (i.e., chronically administered), changes in the magnitude of response to the drug frequently occur. Most often the response diminishes with chronic use (tolerance), but occasionally the effects are increased (sensitization). In some cases, selected effects of a particular drug decrease while others increase in magnitude, as is true for the stimulant drug amphetamine. It should be clear that an individual's drug-taking history has a significant influence on drug action.

Repeated drug exposure can cause tolerance

Drug **tolerance** is defined as a diminished response to drug administration after repeated exposure to that drug. In other words, tolerance has developed when increasingly larger doses of a given drug must be administered to obtain the same magnitude of biological effect that occurred with the original dose. The development of tolerance to one drug can also diminish the effectiveness of a second drug. This phenomenon, called **cross-tolerance,** is the basis for a number of drug interactions. For example, the effective anticonvulsant dose of phenobarbital is significantly larger in a patient who has a history of chronic alcohol use than in a patient who has not developed tolerance to alcohol.

Characteristics of tolerance   Although the appearance of tolerance varies, several general features are worth mentioning. These characteristics are summarized in Table 1.8. First, as is true for biological processes in general, tolerance is reversible; that is, it gradually diminishes if you stop using the drug. Additionally, the extent of tolerance that develops is dependent on the pattern of drug administration: the dose and frequency of drug use as well as the environment in which it occurs. Chronic heroin users may take as much as 1800 mg without ill effects, despite the fact that the lethal range for a novice heroin user is 200 to 400 mg.

However, regardless of dose and frequency, some drugs induce tolerance relatively rapidly (LSD), while others take weeks of chronic use (barbiturates) or never cause significant tolerance (antipsychotics). In some cases tolerance even develops during a single administration, as when an individual experiences significantly greater effects of alcohol as his blood level rises than he experiences several hours later when his blood level has fallen to the same point. This form of tolerance is called **acute tolerance.**

Also, it is important to be aware that not all biobehavioral effects of a particular drug demonstrate tolerance equally.

TABLE 1.8 Significant Characteristics of Tolerance

Reversible when drug use stops
Dependent on dose and frequency of drug use and drug-taking environment
May occur rapidly, or after long periods of chronic use, or never
Not all effects of a drug show the same amount of tolerance
Several different mechanisms explain multiple forms of tolerance

For example, morphine-induced nausea and vomiting show rapid development of tolerance, but the constipating effects of the drug rarely diminish even after long-term use. Sometimes the uneven development of tolerance is beneficial, as when tolerance develops for the side effects of a drug but not for its therapeutic effects. At other times, the uneven development of tolerance poses a hazard, as when a drug's desired effects diminish, requiring increased doses, but the lethal or toxic effects do not show tolerance. Chronic barbiturate use is one such example. As more drug is taken to achieve the desired effect, the dose gets increasingly close to the lethal dose that causes respiratory depression.

Finally, several types of tolerance exist and have distinct mechanisms. Although some drugs never induce tolerance at all, others may cause several types (refer to Table 1.9 for examples). The three principal forms are drug disposition tolerance, pharmacodynamic tolerance, and behavioral tolerance.

Drug disposition tolerance (metabolic tolerance)
Drug disposition tolerance, or **metabolic tolerance,** occurs when repeated use of a drug reduces the amount of that drug available at the target tissue. The most common form of drug disposition tolerance occurs when drugs increase their own rate of metabolism. It is clear that many drugs are capable of liver microsomal enzyme induction (see the discussion on biotransformation earlier in this chapter), which results in increased metabolic capacity. A more-efficient metabolism reduces the amount of drug available to target tissue and diminishes drug effects. All drugs metabolized by the induced enzyme family will likewise show a reduced effect (cross-tolerance). Drug disposition tolerance requires repeated administration over time in order for protein synthesis to build new enzyme proteins. Well-documented examples of inducers of liver enzymes such as cytochrome P450 include drugs from many classes: the sedative phenobarbital, the antibiotic rifampicin, the antiseizure medication phenytoin, cigarette smoke, and anabolic steroids.

Pharmacodynamic tolerance
The most dramatic form of tolerance that develops to the central actions of certain drugs cannot be explained on the basis of altered metabolism or altered concentration of drug reaching the brain. **Pharmacodynamic tolerance** occurs when changes in nerve cell function compensate for the continued presence of the drug. In an earlier section we described the normal response to chronic receptor activation as receptor down-regulation. Once receptors have down-regulated, a given amount of drug will have fewer receptors to act on and therefore produce less of a biological effect. Compensatory up-regulation (increased receptor number) occurs in cases where receptor activation is chronically reduced. Other cellular adjustments to chronic drug use will be described in later chapters dealing with individual agents such as ethanol, amphetamine, caffeine, and others.

Behavioral tolerance
Although many instances of tolerance can be attributed to cell physiology and chemistry, a behavioral component involving learning and adaptation has been demonstrated by numerous investigators. **Behavioral tolerance** (sometimes called context-specific tolerance) is demonstrated when tolerance occurs in the same environment in which the drug was administered but tolerance is not apparent or is much reduced in a novel environment. Several types of learning (habituation, classical conditioning, and operant conditioning) play a part in the development of behavioral tolerance, as well as in the withdrawal syndrome characteristic of physical dependence (see Chapter 8).

Habituation, the simplest form of learning, involves learning *not* to respond to a repetitious stimulus. Initially, any sudden stimulus (e.g., a loud noise) interferes with ongoing behavior while the individual orients to the novel event. If the stimulus is repeated a number of times with no significant consequence, the normal behavior continues undisrupted. In an analogous way, the first administration of a drug may alter ongoing behavior, but repeated exposure to the drug effects will alter the behavior less and less. Since

TABLE 1.9 Types of Tolerance Exhibited by Selected Drugs

Drug or drug class	Drug disposition tolerance	Pharmacodynamic tolerance	Behavioral tolerance
Barbiturates	+	+	+
Alcohol	+	+	+
Morphine	+	+	+
Amphetamine	–	+	+
Cocaine	–	+	+
Caffeine	–	+	?
Nicotine	–	+	?
LSD	–	+	–

habituation-induced tolerance disappears in a novel environment, it is unlikely that enzyme or receptor changes are responsible.

Pavlovian, or **classical conditioning,** plays an important role in drug use and in tolerance. In the original experiments with Pavlov's dogs, the meaningless bell (neutral stimulus) was presented immediately before the presentation of the meat (unconditioned stimulus), which elicited reflexive salivation (unconditioned response). Following repeated pairings, the bell took on the characteristic of a conditioned stimulus, because presented alone it could elicit salivation, now a conditioned response. Since many psychoactive drugs elicit reflexive effects such as cortical arousal, elevated blood pressure, or euphoria, they can act like unconditioned stimuli, and the drug-taking procedure or stimuli in the environment may become conditioned stimuli that elicit a conditioned response even before the drug is administered (Figure 1.17). These results may explain why the various rituals and procedures of drug procurement and use may elicit reinforcing effects similar to those of the drug itself. An example of this phenomenon is the "needle freak," who by act of injection alone derives significant morphine-like effects. Why the conditioned response is similar to the unconditioned response in some cases and different from (even opposite)

the unconditioned response in other cases is not entirely clear. Nevertheless, both occurrences are well documented.

Siegel (1985) suggests that tolerance is at least in part due to the learning of an association between the effects of a given drug and the environmental cues that reliably precede the drug effects. To explain tolerance development, the "anticipatory" response (conditioned response) must be compensatory in nature. That is, the environment associated with the administration of the drug elicits physiological responses opposite to the effect of the drug. For instance, in animals repeatedly experiencing the hyperthermic effects of injected morphine, the injection procedure alone *in the same environment* leads to a compensatory drop in body temperature. Figure 1.18 shows the results of a study of two groups of rats that had an identical course of morphine injections (5 mg/kg SC for 10 days) that would normally produce evidence of tolerance to the hyperthermic effect. On test day, the rats given morphine in the identical environment (the "Same" animals) showed the expected decrease in hyperthermia, an indication of tolerance. Animals given morphine in a novel environment (the "Different" animals) did not show the same extent of tolerance. The conclusion drawn is that classically conditioned environmental responses contribute to the development of tolerance to morphine. Some researchers believe that environmentally induced tolerance may explain why addicts who use their drug in a new envi-

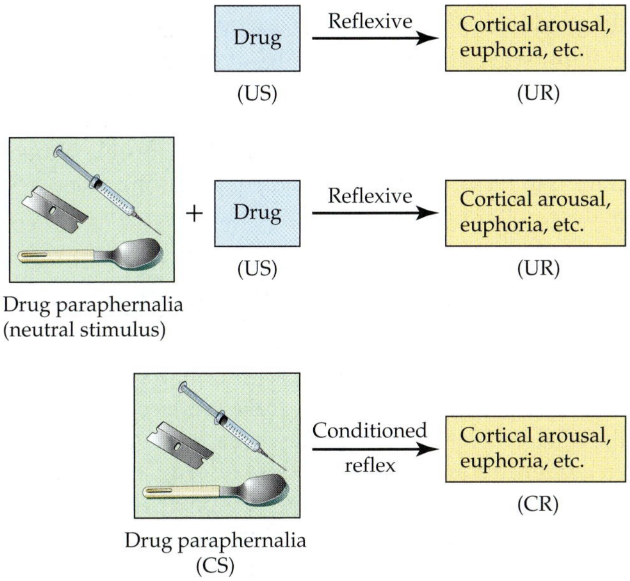

Figure 1.17 Classical conditioning of drug-related cues Although drug-taking equipment and the immediate environment is initially a meaningless stimulus to the individual, its repeated pairing with the drug (unconditioned stimulus; US), which naturally elicits euphoria, arousal, or other desirable effects (unconditioned response; UR), gives the drug-taking equipment new meaning. Ultimately the equipment and environment alone (now a conditioned stimulus; CS) could elicit drug effects (conditioned response; CR) in the absence of the drug.

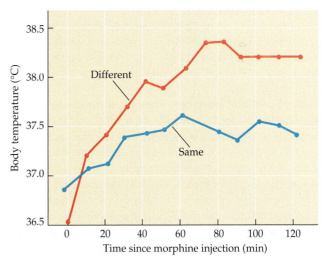

Figure 1.18 Tolerance to morphine-induced hyperthermia Following an identical series of prior morphine injections (5 mg/kg SC for 10 days), rats were tested with a morphine injection and changes in body temperature were measured for the next two hours. One group of rats was given the morphine in the same environment in which they were previously treated ("Same"), and the second group were tested in a novel environment ("Different"). The animals treated in the same environment show much less hyperthermia, which indicates tolerance. (After Siegel, 1978b.)

ronment or alter their drug-taking routine may suddenly show much greater response to the same dose of the drug they had used the day before. This phenomenon may explain at least some of the fatal drug overdoses that were described at the beginning of the chapter. Although environment is clearly significant in drug tolerance, keep in mind that the neural changes that underlie learning or behavioral tolerance are subtle alterations in physiology that may be similar to pharmacodynamic tolerance.

The appearance of tolerance to a psychoactive drug is often manifested in a task in which **operant conditioning** plays some part. For example, Leblanc et al. (1976) showed that alcohol administration (2.5 g/kg IP) to rats initially disrupted the performance of traversing a moving belt, but repeated administrations had less and less effect. The improved performance could be identified as a type of tolerance, but the apparent tolerance could be due to the learning of a new skill (the ability to run a treadmill while under the influence of the drug), which we would expect to improve with practice. How do we know that the improvement is not due to changes in metabolic rate or pharmacodynamic tolerance? The answer can be found by adding a second group of animals, who had the same number of alcohol treatments and the same number of practice sessions on the treadmill, but the drug was administered *after* each practice session. If the tolerance in the first group was due to metabolic changes, the extent of tolerance in the two groups should have been identical, but in fact the second group showed significantly less tolerance. The same type of tolerance is demonstrated by the alcoholic who learns to maneuver fairly efficiently while highly intoxicated to avoid detection, whereas a less experienced alcohol abuser with the same blood alcohol level may appear behaviorally to be quite intoxicated.

State-dependent learning   **State-dependent learning** is a concept that is closely related to behavioral tolerance. Tasks learned in the presence of a psychoactive drug may subsequently be performed better in the drugged state than in the nondrugged state. Conversely, learning acquired in the nondrugged state may be more available in the nondrugged state. This phenomenon, which has been called state-dependent learning, illustrates the difficulty in transferring learned performance from a drugged to a nondrugged condition (Figure 1.19). An example of this is the alcoholic who during a binge hides his supply of liquor for later consumption, but is unable to find it while he is sober (in the nondrugged state). Once he has returned to the alcoholic state, he can readily locate his cache.

One explanation for state dependency is that the drug effect may become part of the environmental "set"; that is, it may assume the properties of a stimulus itself. A drugged subject learns to perform a particular task in relationship to all the internal and external cues in the environment, includ-

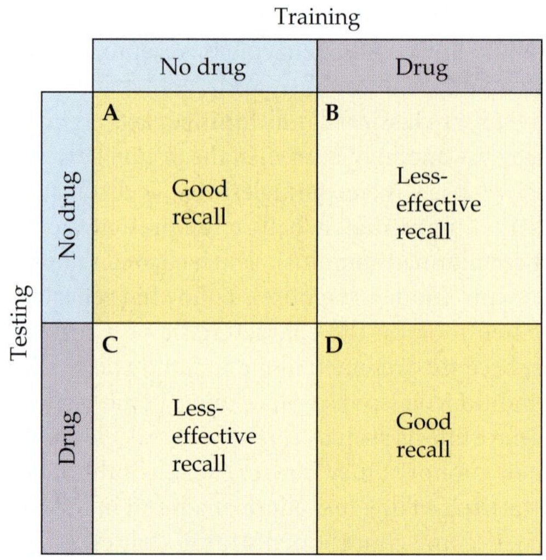

Figure 1.19 Experimental design to test state-dependent learning Four different conditions demonstrate the difficulties in transferring learning from one drug state to another. Individuals trained without drug and tested without drug (A) show maximum performance that is not much different than those trained and tested under the influence of the drug (D). However, subjects asked to perform in a state different from the training condition (B and C) showed less-efficient recall.

ing, it is argued, drug-induced cues. Thus in the absence of drug-induced cues, performance deteriorates much the same as if the test apparatus was altered. It has been shown in animal studies that the decrease in performance is very much related to the change in environmental cues and that a particular drug state does provide readily discriminable stimuli (Overton, 1984). Further discussion of the cueing properties of drugs follows in Chapter 4.

Chronic drug use can cause sensitization

Despite the fact that repeated drug administration produces tolerance for many drug effects, sensitization can occur for others. **Sensitization,** sometimes called reverse tolerance, is the enhancement of particular drug effects following repeated administration of the same dose of drug. For instance, prior administration of cocaine to animals significantly increases motor activity and stereotypy (continuous repetition of a simple action such as head bobbing) produced by subsequent stimulant administration. Chronic administration of higher doses of cocaine has also been shown to produce an increased susceptibility to cocaine-induced catalepsy, in which the animal remains in abnormal or distorted postures for prolonged intervals, as well as hyperthermia and convulsions (Post and Weiss, 1988). Cocaine and amphetamine are examples of drugs that induce tolerance for some effects (euphoria) and sensitization for others.

As is true for tolerance, the development of sensitization is dose-dependent and the interval between treatments is important. Further, cross-sensitization with other psychomotor stimulants has been documented. The augmentation of response to drug challenge tends to persist for long periods of abstinence, indicating that long-term physiological changes occur as a result of stimulant administration. However, conditioning also plays a significant role in the appearance of sensitization. Pretreatment with the stimulant and subsequent testing in dissimilar environments yields significantly less sensitization than that occurring in the identical environment. Further discussion of sensitization will be found in Chapter 3. Young and Goudie (1995) is an excellent source for more detail on the role of classical and operant conditioning in the development of tolerance to behavioral effects of drugs.

Section Summary

The concept of the receptor is vital to pharmacology, as drugs have biological effects only because they interact with receptors on target tissues. Drugs or ligands that bind and are capable of changing the shape of the receptor protein and subsequently alter cell function are called agonists. The ligands that attach most readily are said to have high affinity for the receptor. Antagonists, in contrast, are capable of binding and may have high affinity, but they produce no physiological change, that is, they have little or no efficacy. Antagonists also prevent agonists from binding to the receptor at the same moment, hence "blocking" agonist activity. Rather than being fixed, the number of receptors changes to compensate for either prolonged stimulation (causing down-regulation) or absence of receptor stimulation (up-regulation of receptors). Pharmacologists study the relationship between drug, receptor, and biobehavioral effect by analyzing dose–response curves. The curves show the threshold dose at which biobehavioral effects can first be measured. With increasing doses, the effect also increases in a linear fashion until the maximum effect is reached. The ED_{50} is the dose that produces a half-maximal (50%) effect and is used to compare the potency of drugs that produce similar biobehavioral effects. The more potent drug is the one that has the lower ED_{50}. Comparison of the ED_{50} with the TD_{50} (50% toxic dose) for a single drug helps us calculate the therapeutic index. A large therapeutic index suggests that the drug is effective at low doses but the toxic dose is high, making the drug relatively safe. A small TI suggests that there is not much difference between the effective and toxic doses, so the drug is potentially dangerous.

Receptor antagonists are competitive if they reduce the effects of an agonist by binding to the same receptor and reducing agonist–receptor interaction. This type of interaction reduces the potency of the agonist, as shown by a parallel shift of the dose–response curve to the right. However, the maximum effect is not altered, because raising the agonist concentration can overcome the action of the antagonist. Noncompetitive antagonists impair agonist function by altering the receptor at a modulatory site, by impeding the initiation of intracellular processes, or by disturbing the membrane surrounding the receptor. Drugs can also interact by altering the biological effects beyond the receptor's site of action. Drugs can produce physiological antagonism, additive effects, or potentiation. In potentiation, the two drugs produce effects greater than the sum of their individual effects.

When drugs are administered on more than one occasion, the magnitude of drug response often changes. Most often chronic drug use leads to tolerance, that is, a diminished effect, but in some circumstances drug effects increase with repeated use, a phenomenon called sensitization. Cross-tolerance may occur if repeated use of one drug reduces the effectiveness of a second drug. Although there are several types of tolerance, with distinct mechanisms, tolerance in general is a reversible condition. In addition, it is dependent on the dose and frequency of use, although some drugs induce tolerance rapidly while others require longer treatment or never cause tolerance at all. Further, not all effects of a drug undergo tolerance to the same extent or at the same rate. Drug-disposition tolerance occurs when drugs induce the formation of the liver's metabolizing enzymes. Increased enzyme action reduces the effective blood level of the drug more rapidly, so the biobehavioral effect is reduced. Pharmacodynamic tolerance depends on the compensation of the nervous system to the continued presence of the drug. Changes may include increases or decreases in receptor number or other compensatory intracellular processes. Behavioral tolerance occurs when learning processes and environmental cues contribute to the reduction in drug effectiveness. Habituation, Pavlovian conditioning, and operant conditioning can contribute to the change in drug response.

Recommended Readings

Hollinger, M. A. (1997). *Introduction to Pharmacology.* Taylor and Francis, Washington.

Swerdlow, J. L. (2000). Nature's Rx. *Natl. Geogr.* 197 (4). 98–117.

Zivin, J. A. (2000). Understanding clinical trials. *Sci. Am.* April, 69–75.

2 Structure and Function of the Nervous System

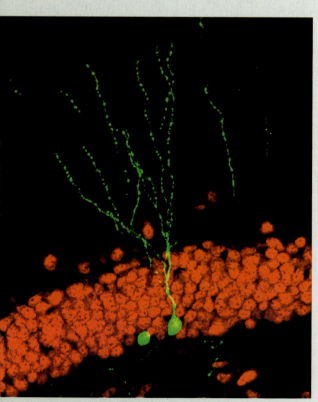

Neurogenesis in the adult mouse hippocampus is visualized by fluorescent microscopy.

Lou Gehrig was born in New York City in 1903 to German immigrant parents. After attending Columbia University he joined the Yankees as first baseman, where he earned the nickname "Iron Horse" for the strength and power of his game and his endurance even in the face of multiple injuries. His record, only recently broken, of playing 2130 consecutive games despite injuries, multiple bone breaks, and back spasms attests to his determination and fortitude. He was beloved among fans for his humility and character. Gehrig and his teammate Babe Ruth formed the core of the most incredible hitting team known to baseball. All of that ended in 1938 when it became evident that Gehrig was gradually losing the strength to swing the bat and his gait had deteriorated to a sliding of his feet along the ground. Not long after, he was diagnosed with amyotrophic lateral sclerosis (ALS), now most often called Lou Gehrig's disease.

This neurological disorder begins with muscle weakness, loss of muscle control, atrophy, and fatigue, and rapidly progresses so that all motor function is ultimately lost, leaving the individual unable to walk, speak, swallow, or breathe. Perhaps most devastating is that although both motor neurons from the spinal cord to skeletal muscles and descending motor neurons in the frontal lobe of the cerebral cortex degenerate, almost all other functions remain intact, including cognitive function, leaving the individual mentally alert and fully aware of his wasting away and ultimate total paralysis.

Symptoms of ALS do not show spontaneous remission, and no available treatment does more than slow the progression of the disease by a few months. At this time there is no known cause for ALS, nor is the cellular mechanism of nerve degeneration clear. However, both the cause and cure of ALS will be identified with further research into the fundamental functions of neurons and their interaction, which is the focus of Chapter 2.

As we already know, psychopharmacology is the study of how drugs affect emotion, memory, thinking, and behavior. Drugs can produce these widespread effects because they modify the function of the human brain, most often by altering the chemical nature of the nervous system. For an understanding of drug action we first need to know a bit about individual nerve cell structure and electrochemical function. Second, we need to have an essential understanding of how these individual cells form the complex circuits that represent the anatomical basis for behavior. We hope that for most readers, Chapter 2 will be a review of (1) the structure of nerve cells; (2) electrochemical properties of neurons; and (3) anatomy of the nervous system as we put the individual neurons together into functional units. Chapter 3 follows up with greater detail on the chemical nature of nerve cell function.

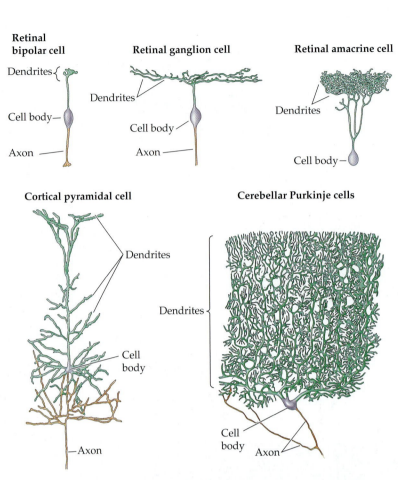

Figure 2.1 Varied shapes of neurons These drawings are from actual nerve cells stained by the Golgi technique. Neurons are drawn to different scales to show their varied structures.

Cells of the Nervous System

All tissues in the body are composed of cells, and the special characteristics of those cells determine the structure and function of the tissue or organ. In the nervous system there are two primary types of cells, nerve cells called **neurons** and supporting cells called **glial cells** that provide metabolic support, protection, and insulation for neurons (see the section on glial cells later in the chapter). The principal function of neurons is to transmit information in the form of electrical signaling over long distances. **Sensory neurons,** sensitive to environmental stimuli, convert the physical stimuli in the world around us and in our internal environment into an electrical signal and transmit that information to circuits of **interneurons,** which are nerve cells within the brain and spinal cord. Interneurons form complex interacting neural circuits and are responsible for conscious sensations, recognition, memory, decision making, and cognition. In turn, **motor neurons** direct a biobehavioral response appropriate for the situation. Although these neurons have common features, their structural arrangements and sizes vary according to their specific functions. Figure 2.1 provides some examples of the many possible shapes of neurons that were first described by the nineteenth-century histological studies of the Spanish neuroanatomist Ramón y Cajal. For much of the twentieth cen-

tury, neuroscientists relied on the same set of techniques developed by the early neuroanatomists to describe and categorize the diversity of cell types in the nervous system. However, from the late 1970s onward, remarkable new technologies (see Chapter 4) in cell biology and molecular biology provided investigators with many additional tools to identify minute differences in the structural features of neurons, trace their multiple connections, and evaluate physiological responses.

Neurons have three major external features

Although neurons come in a variety of shapes and sizes and utilize various neurochemicals, they have several principal external features in common (Figure 2.2). These features include (1) the cell body, or **soma,** containing the nucleus and other organelles that maintain cell metabolic function; (2) the **dendrites,** which are treelike projections from the soma that receive information from other cells; and (3) the **axon,** the single tubular extension that conducts the electrical signal from the cell body to the terminal buttons on the axon terminals. Like all other cells, neurons are enclosed by a

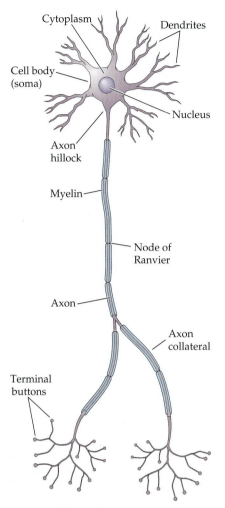

Figure 2.2 **Principal parts of neurons** Despite differences in size and shape, most neurons have numerous features in common.

semipermeable membrane and are filled with a salty, gelatinous fluid, the **cytoplasm.** Neurons are also surrounded by salty fluid (**extracellular fluid),** from which they take oxygen, nutrients, and drugs and into which they secrete metabolic waste products that ultimately reach the blood and then are filtered out by the kidneys (see Chapter 1). Like other cells, neurons have **mitochondria,** which are responsible for generating energy from glucose in the form of adenosine triphosphate (ATP). Mitochondria are found throughout the cell but particularly where energy needs are great. Since neurons use large quantities of ATP, mitochondrial function is critical for survival, and ATP is synthesized continually to support neuron function. The assumption that the rate of synthesis of ATP reflects neuron activity is an underlying premise of several neurobiological techniques that give us the opportunity to visualize the functioning of brain cells (see Chapter 4 for a discussion of positron emission tomography [PET] and functional magnetic resonance imaging [fMRI]).

Dendrites   The general pattern of neuron function involves the dendrites and soma receiving information from other cells across the gap between them, called the **synapse.** On the dendrites of a single neuron as well as on the soma there may be thousands of receptors, which respond to neurochemicals released by other neurons. Depending on the changes produced in the receiving cell, the overall effect may be either excitatory or inhibitory. Hence each neuron receives and integrates a vast amount of information from many cells, a function called **convergence.** The integrated information can in turn be transmitted to a few neurons or thousands of other neurons, a process known as **divergence.** If we look a bit more carefully using higher magnification, we see that the dendrites are usually covered with short **dendritic spines** (Figure 2.3A and B) that dramatically increase the receiving surface area.

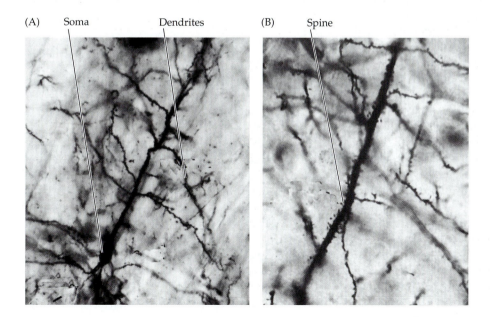

Figure 2.3 **Dendritic trees with spines** (A) A neuron with its dendrites is clearly apparent at 100× magnification. (B) Higher magnification (250×) shows multiple spines all along the dendrite. (From Jacobson, 1972.)

The dendrites and their spines exhibit the special feature of being constantly modified and can change shape rapidly in response to changes in synaptic transmission (Fischer et al., 1998). These changes occur throughout life and permit us to continue to learn new associations as we interact with our environment.

Axons and terminal buttons   The single long extension from the soma is the axon. Axons are tubular in structure and are filled with axoplasm (i.e., cytoplasm within the axon). Axons vary significantly in both length and diameter. Their function is to transmit the electrical signal (action potential) that is generated at the **axon hillock** down the length of the axon to the terminals. The axon hillock is that portion of the axon that is adjacent to the cell body.

Although there is usually only one axon for a given neuron, axons split or bifurcate into numerous branches called **axon collaterals,** providing the capacity to influence many more cells. At the end of the axons, there are small enlargements called **terminal buttons,** which are located near other cells' dendrites or somas. Terminal buttons are also called boutons or axon terminals. The terminal buttons contain small packets (**synaptic vesicles**) of neurochemicals (called **neurotransmitters**) that provide the capacity for chemical transmission of information across the synapse to the adjacent cells or target organ. Neurons are frequently named according to the neurotransmitter they synthesize and release. Hence cells that release dopamine are dopaminergic neurons, those that release serotonin are serotonergic, and so forth.

Most axons are wrapped with a fatty insulating coating, called **myelin,** created by concentric layers of glial cells (Figure 2.4A). Those glial cells that are responsible are of two types: Schwann cells, which myelinate peripheral nerves that serve muscles, organs, and glands; and oligodendroglia, which myelinate nerves within the brain and spinal cord. The myelin sheath provided by both types of glial cells is not continuous along the axon but has breaks in it where the axon is bare to the extracellular fluid. These bare spots are called **nodes of Ranvier** (Figure 2.4B) and are the sites where the action potential is regenerated during the conduction of the electrical signal along the length of the axon. The myelin sheath increases the speed of conduction along the axon; in fact, the thicker the myelin, the quicker the conduction. While a small number of neurons are unmyelinated and conduct slowly, others are thinly wrapped, and some rapidly conducting neurons may have a hundred or more wraps. Myelination also saves energy by reducing the effort required to restore the neuron to its resting state following the transmission of the electrical signal.

Soma   The cell body is responsible for the metabolic care of the neuron. Among its important functions is the synthesis of proteins that are needed throughout the cell for growth and maintenance. The proteins include such things as

enzymes, receptors, and components of the cell membrane. Within the nucleus are pairs of chromosomes that we inherited from our parents. **Chromosomes** are long strands of DNA, and **genes** are small portions of chromosomes that code for the manufacture of a specific protein molecule. Hence the **coding region** of a gene provides the "recipe" for a specific protein such as a receptor or enzyme. Although every cell in the body contains the full genetic library of information, each cell type manufactures only those proteins needed for its specific function. Hence liver cells manufacture enzymes to metabolize toxins, while neurons manufacture enzymes needed to synthesize neurotransmitters and carry out functions necessary for neural transmission. In addition, which specific genes are activated is also determined in part by our day-to-day experience. Neurobiologists are finding that experiences such as prolonged stress or chronic drug use may turn on or turn off the production of particular proteins by modifying transcription factors. **Transcription factors** are nuclear proteins that direct protein production. Transcription factors such as CREB bind to the **promotor region** of the gene adjacent to the coding region, modifying its rate of transcription.

Transcription occurs in the nucleus, where messenger RNA (mRNA) makes a complementary copy of the active gene. After moving from the nucleus to the cytoplasm, mRNA attaches to organelles called ribosomes, which decode the recipe and link the appropriate amino acids together to form the protein. This process is called **translation.** Some of the basic steps to protein synthesis are shown in Figure 2.5.

Having said that proteins are synthesized within the soma and knowing that the proteins are needed throughout the neuron, we must consider how the proteins are moved to the required destination. The process is called **axoplasmic transport** and it depends on structures of the cytoskeleton. The **cytoskeleton,** as the name suggests, is a matrix composed of tubular structures, which include microtubules and neurofila-

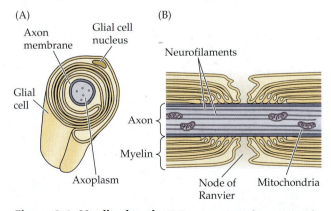

Figure 2.4 Myelin sheath (A) Cross section of an axon with multiple layers of glial cell wraps forming the myelin sheath. (B) Longitudinal drawing of a myelinated axon at a node of Ranvier.

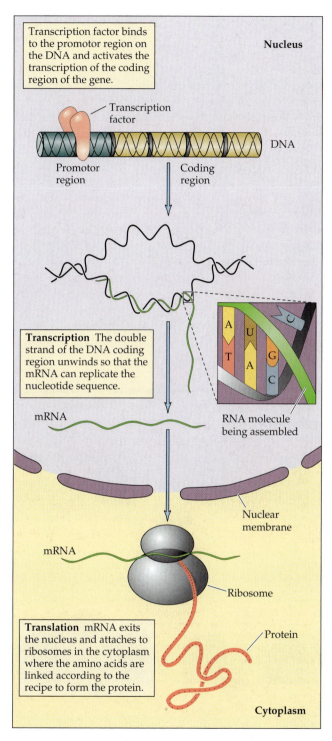

Transcription factor binds to the promotor region on the DNA and activates the transcription of the coding region of the gene.

Nucleus

Transcription factor

Promotor region

Coding region

DNA

Transcription The double strand of the DNA coding region unwinds so that the mRNA can replicate the nucleotide sequence.

mRNA

RNA molecule being assembled

Nuclear membrane

mRNA

Ribosome

Translation mRNA exits the nucleus and attaches to ribosomes in the cytoplasm where the amino acids are linked according to the recipe to form the protein.

Protein

Cytoplasm

Figure 2.5 Stages of protein synthesis Activation of a gene by a transcription factor initiates the formation of mRNA within the nucleus, followed by translation into a protein on the ribosomes in the cytoplasm.

ments that form a mesh-like mass that provides shape for the cell. In addition, the microtubules, which run longitudinally down the axon, provide a stationary track along which small packets of newly synthesized protein are carried by specialized motor proteins (Figure 2.6). The movement of materials occurs in both directions. Newly synthesized proteins are packaged in the soma and transported in an anterograde direction toward the axon terminals. At the terminals the contents are released, and retrograde axonal transport carries waste materials from the axon terminals back to the soma for recycling.

Characteristics of the cell membrane are critical for neuron function

One of the more important characteristics of neurons is the cell membrane. In Chapter 1 we learned that neuronal membranes are essentially a phospholipid bilayer that prevents most materials from freely passing (see Figure 1.3) unless they are lipid soluble. In addition to the phospholipids, membranes also have proteins inserted into the bilayer. Many of these proteins are **receptors,** large molecules that are the initial sites of action of neurotransmitters, hormones, and drugs. Details of these receptors and their functions are described in Chapter 3. Other important proteins associated with the membrane are **enzymes** that catalyze biochemical reactions in the cell. The third important group of proteins are ion channels and transporters. Because the membrane is not readily permeable to charged molecules, special devices are needed to move molecules such as amino acids, glucose, and metabolic products across the membrane. Movement of these materials is achieved by **transporter proteins,** which are described further in Chapter 3. In addition, charged particles (ions), such as potassium (K^+), sodium (Na^+), chloride (Cl^-), and calcium (Ca^{2+}), that are needed for neuron function can be moved through the membrane only via **ion channels.** These channels are protein molecules that penetrate through the cell membrane and have a water-filled pore through which ions can pass.

Ion channels have several important characteristics. First, they are relatively specific for a particular ion, although some allow more than one type of ion to pass through. Second, most channels are not normally open to allow free passage of the ions, but are in a closed configuration that can be opened momentarily by specific stimuli. These channels are referred to as **gated channels.** The two types of channels of immediate interest to us are the **ligand-gated channels** and the **voltage-gated channels.** Looking at Figure 2.7A, you can see that when a drug, hormone, or neurotransmitter binds to a receptor that recognizes the ligand, the channel protein changes shape and opens the gate, allowing a flow of a specific ion to move either into or out of the cell. The direction in which an ion moves is determined by its relative concentration; it always travels from high to low concentration. Hence, given an open gate, Na^+, Cl^-, and Ca^{2+} will move into the cell, while K^+ moves out. A second type of channel, which will be of importance later in this chapter, is the type that is opened by voltage differences across the membrane. These

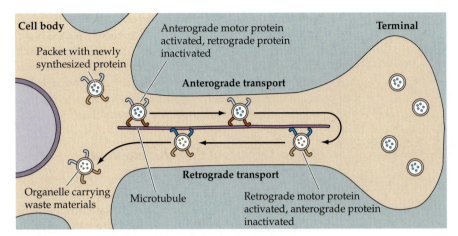

Figure 2.6 Axoplasmic transport The movement of newly synthesized proteins from the soma to the axon terminals (anterograde) is powered along the microtubules by a motor protein called kinesin. Old proteins are carried from the terminals to the soma (retrograde) by the motor protein dynein.

channels are opened not by ligands but by the application of a small electrical charge to the membrane surrounding the channel (Figure 2.7B). Other channels are modified by second messengers (Figure 2.7C), but discussion of these will have to wait until Chapter 3. Regardless of the stimulus opening the channel, it opens only briefly and then closes again, limiting the total amount of ion flux.

Glial cells provide vital support for neurons

Glial cells have a significant role in neuron function because they provide physical support to neurons, maintain the chemical environment of neurons, and provide immunological function. The four principal types include the oligodendroglia, Schwann cells, astrocytes, and microglia. **Schwann cells** and **oligodendroglia,** described earlier, produce the myelin sheath on axons of the peripheral nervous system (PNS) nerves and central nervous system (CNS) nerves, respectively (Figure 2.8A and B). Schwann cells and oligodendroglia differ in several ways in addition to their location in the nervous system. Schwann cells are dedicated to a single neuron, and these PNS axons, when damaged, are prompted

(A)

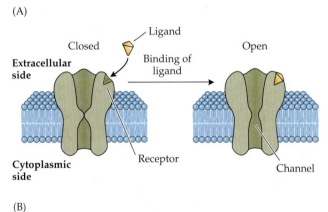

(B)

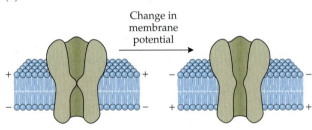

(C)

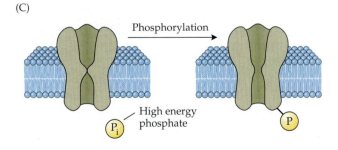

Figure 2.7 Ion channels (A) When a ligand (neurotransmitter, hormone, or drug) binds to a receptor on the channel, the ligand-gated channel protein changes shape and opens the gate, allowing passage of a specific ion. (B) A voltage-gated channel is opened when the electrical potential across the membrane near the channel is altered. (C) Modification of a channel by a second messenger which produces intracellular phosphorylation (addition of a phosphate group) and regulates the state of the channel. (After Siegelbaum and Koester, 1991.)

to regenerate axons because of Schwann cell response. First, the Schwann cells release growth factors, and second, they provide a pathway for the regrowth of the axon toward the target tissue. Oligodendroglia, in contrast, send out multiple paddle-shaped "arms," which wrap many different axons to produce segments of the myelin sheath. In addition, they do not provide nerve growth factors when an axon is damaged, nor do they provide a path for growth.

Two other significant types of glial cells are the astrocytes and microglia. **Astrocytes** are large, star-shaped cells having numerous extensions. They intertwine with neurons and provide structural support; in addition, they help to maintain the ionic environment around neurons and modulate the chemical environment as well by taking up excess neurochemicals that might otherwise damage cells. Because astrocytes have a close relationship with both blood vessels and neurons, it is likely that they may aid the movement of necessary materials from the blood to nerve cells. **Microglia** are far smaller than astrocytes and act as scavengers that collect at sites of neuron damage to remove the dying cells. In addition to this phagocytosis, microglia are the primary source of immune response in the CNS and are responsible for the inflammation reaction that occurs following brain damage. Table 2.1 summarizes the functions of glial cells.

TABLE 2.1 Functions of Glial Cells

Cell	Function
Astrocytes	Provide structural support
	Maintain ionic and chemical environment
	Store nutrients to provide energy for neurons
	Perform phagocytosis
Microglia	Perform phagocytosis
	Provide immune system function
Schwann cells	Form myelin sheath on a single axon in the PNS
	Release growth factors following neuron damage
	Provide a channel to guide axons to targets
Oligodendroglia	Form myelin sheath on multiple axons in the CNS
	Inhibit regrowth of axons following neuron damage

Section Summary

The nerve cells in the nervous system, called neurons, are surrounded by a cell membrane and filled with cytoplasm and the organelles needed for optimal functioning. Among the most important organelles are the mitochondria, which provide the energy for the metabolic work of the cell. The principal external features of a neuron reflect the special function of transmitting electrochemical messages over long distances. These cells have a soma, treelike dendrites, and a single axon extending from the soma that carries the electrical signal all the way to the axon terminals. The enlarged endings of the terminals contain vesicles filled with neurotransmitter molecules that are released into the synapse between the cells when the action potential arrives.

The dendrites of a neuron are covered with minute spines that increase the receiving surface area of the cell. Thousands of receptors that respond to neurotransmitters released by other neurons are found on the dendrites, dendritic spines, and soma of the cell. The axon hillock, which is located at the juncture of soma and axon, is responsible for summation (or integration) of the multiple signals to generate an action potential. Conduction of the action potential along the axon is enhanced by the insulating property of the myelin created by nearby glial cells.

The nucleus of the cell is located in the soma, and protein synthesis occurs there. The transcription of the genetic code for a specific protein by mRNA occurs within the nucleus, and the translation of the "recipe," carried by the mRNA, occurs on the ribosomes in the cytoplasm. The ribosomes are ultimately responsible for linking the appropriate amino acids together to

(A)

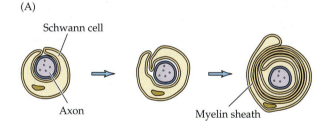

Schwann cell

Axon

Myelin sheath

(B)

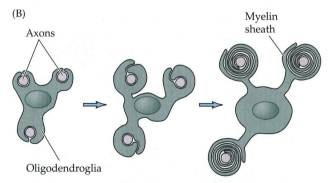

Axons

Oligodendroglia

Myelin sheath

Figure 2.8 Glial cells forming myelin (A) Schwann cells in the PNS dedicate themselves to a single axon and wrap many times to form the myelin for one segment. (B) Each oligodendroglia in the CNS sends out multiple sheetlike arms that wrap around segments of multiple nearby axons to form the myelin sheath.

create the protein. Which genes are activated depends on various transcription factors that are activated by changes in synaptic activity.

The newly manufactured proteins are moved by axoplasmic transport within the cell to where they are needed. Packets of protein are moved by motor proteins that slide along the neuron's microtubules (part of the cytoskeleton) to the terminals (anterograde transport). In a similar manner, protein waste and cell debris is transported from the terminals back to the soma (retrograde transport) for recycling.

The cell membrane is a phospholipid bilayer that prevents most materials from passing through, unless the material is lipid soluble. Special transporters into the cell carry other essential materials, such as glucose, amino acids, and neurotransmitters. Ion channels also penetrate the membrane and selectively allow ions such as Na^+, K^+, Cl^-, and Ca^{2+} to move across the membrane. In addition to transporters and ion channels, proteins associated with the membrane include receptors and enzymes.

The second type of cell in the nervous system is the glial cell. The four types described in this section are the Schwann cells and oligodendroglia, which are responsible for producing the myelin sheath on peripheral and central nervous system neurons, respectively, and the astrocytes and microglia. Astrocytes regulate the extracellular environment of the neurons and provide physical support and nutritional assistance. Microglia act-

ing as phagocytes remove cellular debris and provide immune function.

Electrical Transmission within a Neuron

The transmission of information within a single neuron is an electrical process and depends on the semipermeable nature of the cell membrane. When the normal resting electrical charge of a neuron is disturbed sufficiently by incoming signals from other cells, a threshold is reached that initiates the electrical signal (action potential) that conveys the message along the entire length of the axon to the axon terminals. This section of the chapter looks at each of the stages: resting membrane potential, local potentials, threshold, and action potential.

Ion distribution is responsible for the cell's resting potential

All neurons have a difference in electrical charge inside the cell compared to outside the cell, called the **resting membrane potential.** It can be measured by placing an electrode on the exterior of the cell in the extracellular fluid and a second, much finer microelectrode into the intracellular fluid inside the cell (Figure 2.9A and B). The inside of the neuron is more negative than the outside, and a voltmeter would tell us that the difference is approximately −70 millivolts (mV), making the neuron **polarized** in its resting state.

The selective permeability of the membrane and uneven distribution of ions inside and outside the cell is responsible for the membrane potential. This means that when the cell is at rest, there are more negatively charged particles (ions) inside the cell and more positively charged ions outside the cell. Figure 2.10 shows the relative concentration of different ions on either side of the membrane. Inside we find many large, negatively charged molecules, such as proteins and amino acids, that cannot leave the cell. Potassium is also in much higher concentration (perhaps 20 times higher) inside than

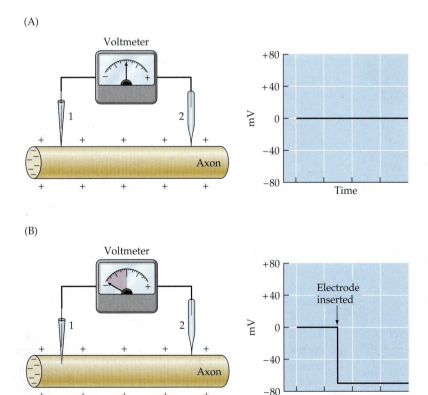

(A)

(B)

Figure 2.9 Membrane potential recording from a squid axon (A) When both electrodes are applied to the outside of the membrane, no difference in potential is recorded. (B) When the microelectrode is inserted into the axoplasm, a voltage difference between inside and outside is recorded. The graphs show the voltage change when one electrode penetrates the cell.

Units of concentration				
	● Na⁺	● K⁺	● Cl⁻	○ Ca²⁺	● ⁻ Protein
Outside cell	440	20	560	10	few
Inside cell	50	400	40–150	0.0001	many

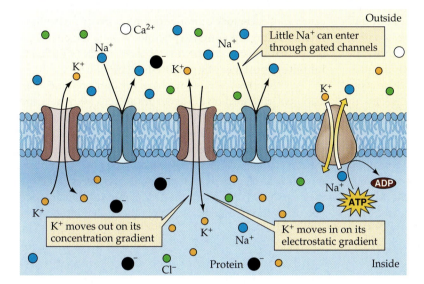

Figure 2.10 Distribution of ions inside and outside a neuron at resting potential Na⁺ and Cl⁻ are more concentrated outside the cell and cannot move in freely through their gated channels. Some K⁺ channels are not gated, allowing the concentration of the ion to force it outward while electrostatically it is pulled in. At –70 mV, equilibrium between the two forces is reached. The Na⁺–K⁺ pump helps to maintain the ion distribution. It requires significant energy (ATP) to move ions against their concentration gradients.

out. In contrast, Na⁺ and Cl⁻ are in greater concentration outside the cell than inside.

Several forces are responsible for this ion distribution and membrane potential. The concentration gradient and electrostatic pressure for the K⁺ ion is particularly important, because K⁺ moves more freely through the membrane than other ions since some of its channels are not gated at the resting potential. Recall that ions move through relatively specific channels and that most are gated, meaning that they are normally held closed until opened by a stimulus. Since the inside of the cell normally has numerous large, negatively charged materials that do not move through the membrane, the positively charged K⁺ ion is pulled into the cell because it is attracted to the internal negative charge (**electrostatic pressure**) (see Figure 2.10). However, as the concentration of K⁺ inside rises, K⁺ responds to the concentration gradient by moving out of the cell. The **concentration gradient** is a force to equalize the amount or concentration of material across a biological barrier. When the two forces on K⁺ (inward electrostatic force and outward concentration gradient) are balanced (called the **equilibrium potential** for potassium), the membrane potential is still more negative inside (–70 mV). In addition, because small amounts of Na⁺ leak into the cell, an energy-dependent pump (the **Na⁺–K⁺ pump**) contributes to the resting potential by exchanging Na⁺ for K⁺ across the membrane. For every three ions of Na⁺ pumped out, two K⁺ ions are pumped in, keeping the inside of the cell negative.

In summary, all cells are polarized at rest, having a difference in charge across their membranes. The potential is due to the uneven distribution of ions across the membrane that occurs because ions move through relatively specific channels that are normally not open. K⁺ has greater ability to move freely through ungated channels. Although all cells are polarized, what makes neurons different is that rapid changes in the membrane potential provide the means for neurons to conduct information, which in turn influences hundreds of other cells in the nervous system. This rapid change in membrane potential that is propagated down the length of the axon is called the **action potential.** In order for a cell to generate an action potential, the membrane potential must be changed from resting (–70 mV) to the **threshold** for firing (–50 mV). At –50 mV, voltage-gated Na⁺ channels open, generating a rapid change in membrane potential. Before we look closely at the action potential, let's see what happens to a neuron to cause the membrane potential to change from resting to threshold.

Local potentials are small, transient changes in membrane potential

While the membrane potential at rest is –70 mV, various types of stimuli that disturb the membrane can open ion channels momentarily, causing small, local changes in ion distribution and hence electrical potential differences called **local potentials.** To visualize the small changes in membrane potential, we attach our electrodes to an amplifier and to a computer that measures and records the changing voltage over time (Figure 2.11A and B). For instance, applying a small, positive electrical current or momentarily opening gated Na⁺ channels allows a relatively small number of Na⁺ ions to enter the cell. The ions enter because Na⁺ is more concentrated outside than inside, so the concentration gradient drives the ions in. The oscilloscope shows that the positively charged ions make the inside of the cell slightly more positive in a small, localized area of the membrane, bringing the membrane potential a tiny bit closer to the threshold for firing. This change is called a local **depolarization** and is excitatory. Other stimuli may open Cl⁻ channels, which allow Cl⁻ into the cell because the ion's concentration is greater on the outside of the cell. The local increase in the negatively charged ion makes the cell slightly more negative inside and brings the resting potential farther away from threshold. This **hyperpolarization** of the membrane is inhibitory. Finally, if gated K⁺ channels are opened by a stimulus, K⁺ is driven outward locally based on its concentration gradient. Because positively charged ions leave the cell, it becomes just slightly

more negative inside, making the membrane potential farther from threshold and causing a local hyperpolarization. These local potentials are of significance to psychopharmacology because when drugs or neurotransmitters bind to particular receptors in the nervous system, they may momentarily open specific ion channels (see Figure 2.7), causing an excitatory or inhibitory effect. Since neurotransmitters act on the postsynaptic membrane, the effects are called **excitatory postsynaptic potentials (EPSPs)** or **inhibitory postsynaptic potentials (IPSPs).**

These local potentials (hyperpolarizations and depolarizations), generated on the dendrites and cell body, have several significant characteristics. First, they are graded, meaning that the larger the stimulus, the greater the magnitude of the hyper- or depolarization. As soon as the stimulus stops, the ion channels close and the membrane potential returns to resting levels. These local potentials also decay rapidly as they passively travel along the cell membrane. Finally, local potentials show **summation,** sometimes called **integration,**

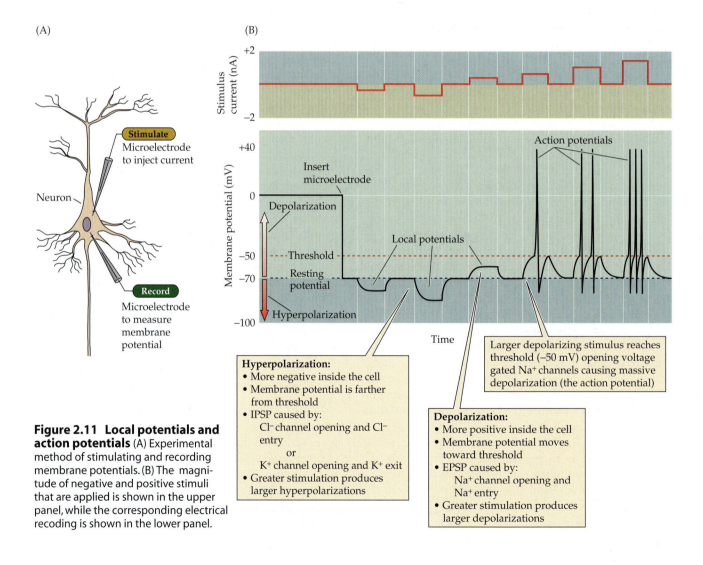

Figure 2.11 Local potentials and action potentials (A) Experimental method of stimulating and recording membrane potentials. (B) The magnitude of negative and positive stimuli that are applied is shown in the upper panel, while the corresponding electrical recoding is shown in the lower panel.

Hyperpolarization:
- More negative inside the cell
- Membrane potential is farther from threshold
- IPSP caused by:
  Cl⁻ channel opening and Cl⁻ entry
    or
  K⁺ channel opening and K⁺ exit
- Greater stimulation produces larger hyperpolarizations

Depolarization:
- More positive inside the cell
- Membrane potential moves toward threshold
- EPSP caused by:
  Na⁺ channel opening and Na⁺ entry
- Greater stimulation produces larger depolarizations

Larger depolarizing stimulus reaches threshold (−50 mV) opening voltage gated Na⁺ channels causing massive depolarization (the action potential) meaning that several small depolarizations can add up to larger changes in membrane potential, as several hyperpolarizations can produce larger inhibitory changes. When hyperpolarizations and depolarizations occur at the same time, they cancel each other out. The receptor areas of a neuron involved in local potential generation receive information from thousands of synaptic connections from other neurons that at any given instant produce IPSPs or EPSPs (as well as other biochemical changes to be described in Chapter 3). The integration of EPSPs and IPSPs occurs in the axon hillock (Figure 2.12) and is responsible for the generation of the action potential if the threshold for activation is reached.

Sufficient depolarization at the axon hillock opens voltage-gated Na+ channels, producing an action potential

The summation of local potentials at the axon hillock is responsible for the generation of the action potential. The −50mV membrane potential (threshold) is responsible for opening large numbers of Na^+ channels that are voltage gated; that is, the change in voltage across the membrane near these channels is responsible for opening them (Figure 2.13). Since Na^+ is much more concentrated outside the cell, its concentration gradient moves it inward; in addition, since the cell at threshold is still negative inside, Na^+ is also driven in by the

electrostatic gradient. These two forces move large numbers of Na^+ ions into the cell very quickly, causing the rapid change in membrane potential from −50 mV to +40 mV (called the rising phase of the action potential) before the Na^+ channels close and remain closed for a fixed period of time while they reset. The time during which the Na^+ channels are closed and cannot be opened, regardless of the amount of excitation, prevents the occurrence of another action potential and is called the **absolute refractory period.** The closing of Na^+ channels explains why the maximum number of action potentials that can occur is about 1200 impulses per second. The action potential is a rapid change in membrane potential lasting only about 1 millisecond. When the membrane potential approaches resting levels, the Na^+ channels are reset and ready to open.

Meanwhile, during the rising phase, the changing membrane potential due to Na^+ entry causes voltage-gated K^+ channels to open, and K^+ moves out of the cell. K^+ channels remain open after Na^+ channels have closed, causing the membrane potential to return to resting levels. The membrane potential actually overshoots the resting potential, so the membrane remains hyperpolarized for a short amount of time until the excess K^+ diffuses away or is exchanged for Na^+ by the Na^+–K^+ pump. Because the membrane is more polarized than normal, it is more difficult to generate an action potential. The brief hyperpolarizing phase is call the **relative**

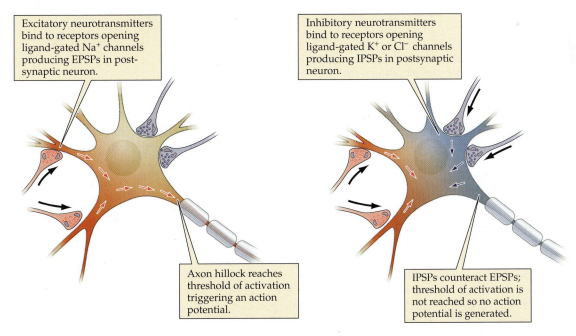

Excitatory neurotransmitters bind to receptors opening ligand-gated Na+ channels producing EPSPs in post-synaptic neuron.

Inhibitory neurotransmitters bind to receptors opening ligand-gated K+ or Cl− channels producing IPSPs in postsynaptic neuron.

Axon hillock reaches threshold of activation triggering an action potential.

IPSPs counteract EPSPs; threshold of activation is not reached so no action potential is generated.

Figure 2.12 Summation of local potentials Many inhibitory and excitatory synapses influence each neuron, causing local electrical potentials (IPSPs and EPSPs) as well as biochemical changes. At each instant in time the electrical potentials summate and may reach the threshold for firing. The integration of the electrical events occurs at the axon hillock where the action potential is first generated. The action potential is then conducted along the axon to the axon terminals.

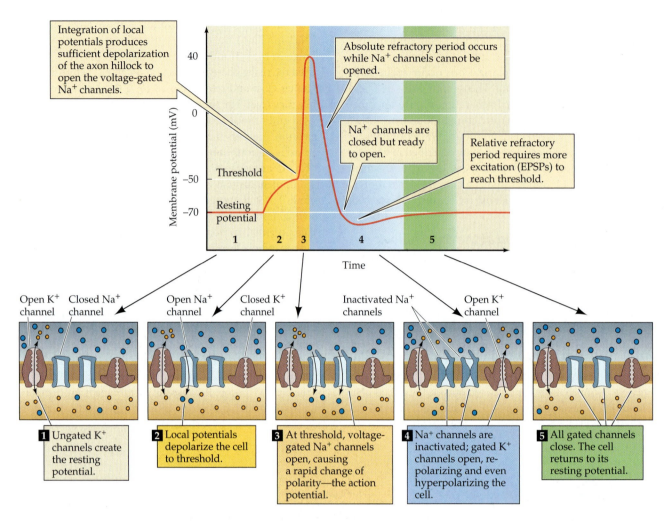

Integration of local potentials produces sufficient depolarization of the axon hillock to open the voltage-gated Na⁺ channels.

Absolute refractory period occurs while Na⁺ channels cannot be opened.

Na⁺ channels are closed but ready to open.

Relative refractory period requires more excitation (EPSPs) to reach threshold.

Threshold

Resting potential

1 Ungated K⁺ channels create the resting potential.

2 Local potentials depolarize the cell to threshold.

3 At threshold, voltage-gated Na⁺ channels open, causing a rapid change of polarity—the action potential.

4 Na⁺ channels are inactivated; gated K⁺ channels open, re-polarizing and even hyperpolarizing the cell.

5 All gated channels close. The cell returns to its resting potential.

Open K⁺ channel   Closed Na⁺ channel

Open Na⁺ channel   Closed K⁺ channel

Inactivated Na⁺ channels

Open K⁺ channel

Figure 2.13 Stages of the action potential The opening and closing of Na⁺ and K⁺ channels is responsible for the characteristic shape of the action potential.

refractory period because it takes more excitation to first reach resting potential and further depolarization to reach threshold. The relative refractory period explains why the intensity of stimulation determines rate of firing. Low levels of excitation cannot overcome the relative refractory period, but with an increasing amount of excitation, the neuron will fire again as soon as the absolute refractory period has ended.

If the threshold is reached, an action potential occurs (first at the hillock). Its size is unrelated to the amount of stimulation; hence it is considered all-or-none. Reaching the threshold will generate the action potential, but more excitatory events (EPSPs) will not make it larger; fewer excitatory events will not generate an action potential at all. The action potential moves along the axon because the positively charged Na⁺ ions spread passively to nearby regions of the axon, which by changing the membrane potential to threshold causes the opening of other voltage-gated Na⁺ channels (Figure 2.14). The regeneration process of the axon poten-

tial continues sequentially along the entire axon and does not decrease in size; hence it is called nondecremental (i.e., it does not decay). In myelinated axons the speed of conduction is as much as 15 times quicker than in nonmyelinated axons because the regeneration of the action potential occurs only at the nodes of Ranvier. This characteristic makes the conduction seem to jump along the axon, so it is called **saltatory conduction.** In addition, myelinated axons use less energy because the Na⁺–K⁺ pump, which uses large amounts of ATP, only has to work at the nodes rather than all along the axon. Now that we understand normal neuron firing, it is time to look at Box 2.1, which describes the abnormal firing during epileptic seizures.

Drugs and poisons alter axon conduction

As we will learn, most drugs act at synapses to modify chemical transmission. However, a few alter action potential con-

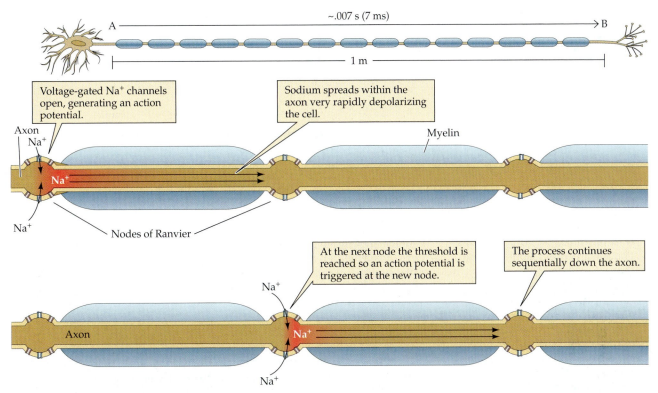

Figure 2.14 Conduction along myelinated axons The generation of the action potential at one node spreads depolarization along the axon, which in turn changes the membrane potential to threshold and opens voltage-gated Na⁺ channels at the next node of Ranvier.

ductance along the axon. Drugs that act as local anesthetics, such as procaine (Novocaine), lidocaine (Xylocaine), and benzocaine (Anesthesin), all impair axonal conduction by blocking voltage-gated Na⁺ channels. It should be apparent that if voltage-gated Na⁺ channels cannot open, then an action potential cannot occur and transmission of the pain signal cannot reach the brain. Hence the individual is not aware of the damaging stimulus. Local anesthetics are injected into specific sites between the tissue damage and the CNS to prevent conduction, but saxitoxin is a poison that blocks voltage-gated Na⁺ channels throughout the nervous system because it is ingested. (Saxotoxin is found in shellfish exposed to the "red tide" [caused by the organism *Gonyaulax*]). Oral ingestion circulates the toxin throughout the body and causes conduction failure and subsequent death due to suffocation.

Section Summary

All cells are polarized at rest, meaning that they have a difference in the electrical charge across the cell membrane. For neurons, the difference is usually about −70 mV, with the

inside being more negative than the outside. The action potential is an electrical event that is generated at the axon hillock and conducted down the full length of the axon to the terminals. The action potential can occur only if small, local electrical potentials, occurring on the soma and dendrites of the cell, summate and change the resting potential (−70 mV) to the threshold for firing (−50 mV).

The resting membrane potential exists because the semipermeable membrane causes ions to be unevenly distributed on each side of the membrane. In particular, because large, negatively charged molecules are trapped inside the cell, K⁺ ions are forced into the neuron through nongated channels by electrostatic pressure. As the internal concentration of K⁺ ions increases, the concentration gradient for K⁺ pushes the ions out of the cell. At the point when the inward pressure and outward pressure are balanced (equilibrium potential), the cell is still negative inside, with a −70-mV difference. Because there is some leakage of Na⁺ into the cell, the Na⁺–K⁺ pump also helps to maintain the negative membrane potential by exchanging three Na⁺ ions (moved out of the cell) for two K⁺ ions (taken in).

Local potentials are small, short-lived changes in membrane potential following the opening of ligand-gated chan-

Clinical Applications

Epilepsy

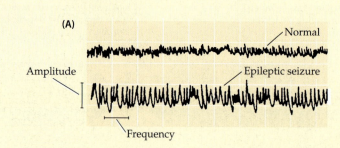

(A)

Amplitude

Normal

Epileptic seizure

Frequency

Epilepsy is a common neurological disorder that consists of recurrent disturbances of electrical activity in the brain involving large ensembles of neurons. These cells fire synchronously (at the same time), producing distinct electroencephalograms (EEGs) that vary with the type of seizure. The EEG reflects the summation of electrical activity of tens of thousands of neurons in the cerebral cortex beneath the electrodes pasted to the outside of the skull. EEG recordings show that in healthy individuals, neurons fire at different times, so the wave looks rapid and choppy and low in amplitude (Figure A). During a seizure, clusters of neurons fire at the same time, so the record appears with slow and rhythmic frequency but high amplitude. Although there are many events that can initiate a seizure, once the abnormal bursts of action potentials begin it spreads

from the origin (called the focus) to surrounding neurons and via synaptic pathways that are connected to the original site. Generalized seizures appear to start in multiple brain areas all at once and involve large areas of the cerebral cortex. The physical signs of the seizure depend upon which brain areas are involved in the uncontrolled electrical activity. Although none of the individual neurons are abnormal, the regulation of their firing is atypical.

An additional characteristic of seizures is that they spontaneously end in 15 seconds to 5 minutes because neurons become depleted of ATP. Vast amounts of energy are required to maintain the high rate of

firing, because the Na+–K+ pump utilizes ATP to restore the balance of ions that is needed to generate further action potentials. However, some abnormalities in the EEG are still apparent between seizures, and the subtle differences are useful in diagnosing the particular type of seizure.

While the precipitating factor for the onset of epilepsy is not known in some cases and is apparently developmental, in other cases the origin of the recurrent seizures is linked to a brain injury that makes neuronal circuits hyperexcitable, leading to spontaneous recurrent seizures. The types of brain injury are varied and include intrauterine and neonatal damage, stroke, damage caused by environ-

nels. These channels are found largely on the soma and dendrites and are opened when a neurotransmitter or drug binds to the receptor associated with the channel. Opening ligand-gated Na+ channels allows a relatively small amount of Na+ to enter the cell, making it slightly more positive in the local area near the channels. When the cell is more positive inside, the cell membrane potential is closer to the threshold for firing, so it is called an excitatory postsynaptic potential (EPSP). Other ligands may open Cl− channels, allowing Cl− to enter on its concentration gradient and making the cell more negative. Increased negative charge inside the cell moves the membrane potential farther from the threshold; hence it causes inhibitory postsynaptic potentials (IPSPs). The third type of channel involved in creating local potentials is the ligand-gated K+ channel. When it is opened, K+ exits according to its concentration gradient, leaving the cell more negative inside and farther from the threshold (IPSP).

The summation of all the EPSPs and IPSPs occurring at any single moment in time occurs at the axon hillock. If the

threshold (−50 mV) is reached, the great number of voltage-gated Na+ channels found in that region suddenly open, allowing large amounts of Na+ to enter the cell to produce the massive depolarization known as the action potential. When the inside of the cell becomes positive (+40 mV), voltage-gated Na+ channels close and cannot be opened until they reset at the resting potential. During the time when the channels are closed, called the absolute refractory period, no action potential can occur.

In addition, as the cell becomes more positive inside, voltage-gated K+ channels open and K+ exits from the cell, bringing the membrane potential back toward resting levels. The overshoot typically seen is a state in which the cell is more polarized than normal, so it is more difficult to reach the threshold to generate another action potential.

Once the action potential is generated at the axon hillock in an all-or-none fashion, it moves down the length of the axon by sequential opening of voltage-gated Na+ channels. In myelinated axons, the regeneration of the action potential occurs only at the nodes of Ranvier, producing a rapid, salta-

BOX 2.1 (continued)

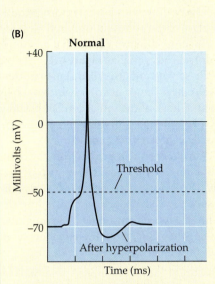

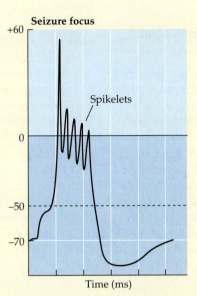

mental toxins or drug use, brain trauma such as occurs during an auto accident, and so forth.

Although diagnosis depends on evaluating the EEG records, intracellular recording with microelectrodes is needed to examine the cell function of individual neurons within the seizure focus. The normal action potential of a neuron (Figure B) involves the gradual change in membrane potential to the threshold, rapid

depolarization (the spike) caused by the opening of voltage-gated Na^+ channels, rapid repolarization (a return toward resting potential during the absolute refractory period), and characteristic hyperpolarization. Neurons within the seizure focus appear to differ in several respects. First, the depolarization is higher voltage and continues for a longer period of time, during which mini-spikes are evident. The occurrence of the mini-spikes is

the likely explanation for the recruitment of adjacent neurons during the seizure. Second, the hyperpolarization (relative refractory period) that occurs is both greater in magnitude and also extends for a longer period of time.

Among the pharmacological treatments for seizures is the drug phenytoin (Dilantin). Phenytoin, which represents one strategy for seizure control, acts by changing the normal cycling of the voltage-gated Na^+ channels that are responsible for the massive depolarization (spike) of the action potential. Phenytoin binds to the channel during the absolute refractory period, when it is closed and cannot be opened, holding it in that state. By preventing the mini-spikes, the drug prevents the spread of electrical activity to adjacent cells.

A second strategy is to enhance neurochemical inhibition. Increasing inhibition may keep cells in the focus from reaching the threshold for firing or prevent the recruitment of associated neurons. Drugs that increase the inhibitory effects of the neurotransmitter GABA (α-aminobutyric acid) are discussed in Chapter 17.

---

tory conduction that is also more energy efficient because the $Na^+–K^+$ pump needs to exchange ions only at the nodes. Regardless of the extent of myelination, all action potentials are nondecremental. The characteristics of local and action potentials are summarized in Table 2.2.

Organization of the Nervous System

Thus far we have described the structure of individual neurons and their ability to conduct electrical signals. Clearly, neurons never function individually but form interacting circuits referred to as neural networks. Such complexity allows us to make coordinated responses to changes in the environment. For example, as we perceive a potential danger, we suddenly become vigilant and more acutely aware of our surroundings. Meanwhile, internal organs

prepare us for action by elevating heart rate, blood pressure, available energy sources, and so forth. Most of us will also calculate the probable outcome of either fighting or running before taking a defensive or aggressive stance. Even simple responses require a complex coordination of multiple nuclei in the brain and spinal cord. The following section describes the organization of neurons into brain regions that serve specific functions. This section provides only the highlights of functional neuroanatomy and emphasizes those brain structures that receive more attention in subsequent chap-

TABLE 2.2 Characteristics of Local Potentials and Action Potentials

Local potentials	Action potentials
Graded	All-or-none
Decremental	Nondecremental
Spatial and temporal summation	Intensity of stimulus coded by rate of firing
Produced by opening of ligand-gated channels	Produced by opening of voltage-gated channels

ters. Box 2.2 provides a quick review of the terms used to describe the location of structures in the nervous system.

The nervous system comprises the central and peripheral divisions

The nervous system includes the central nervous system or CNS (the brain and spinal cord) and the peripheral nervous system or PNS (all nerves outside the CNS) (Figure 2.15A). The PNS in turn can be further divided into the somatic system, which controls voluntary muscles with both spinal nerves and cranial nerves, and the autonomic nervous system, consisting of autonomic nerves and some cranial nerves that control the function of organs and glands. The autonomic nervous system has both sympathetic and parasympathetic divisions, which help the organism to respond to changing energy demands. Figure 2.15B provides an overall view of the divisions of the nervous system. We begin by looking more closely at the peripheral nervous system.

Somatic nervous system   Each spinal nerve consists of many neurons, some of which carry sensory information and others motor information; hence they are called mixed nerves. Within each mixed nerve, sensory information is carried from the surface of the body and from muscles into the dorsal horn of the spinal cord by neurons that have their cell bodies in the dorsal root ganglia (Figure 2.16). These signals going into the spinal cord are called **sensory afferents.** Mixed nerves also have motor neurons, which are cells beginning in the ventral horn of the spinal cord and ending on skeletal muscles. These are called **motor efferents** and are responsible for making voluntary movements.

The 12 pairs of cranial nerves that project from the brain provide similar functions as the spinal nerves except that they serve primarily the head and neck; hence they carry sensory information such as vision, touch, and taste into the brain and control muscle movement needed for things like chewing and laughing. They differ from the spinal nerves in that they are not all mixed nerves; several are dedicated to

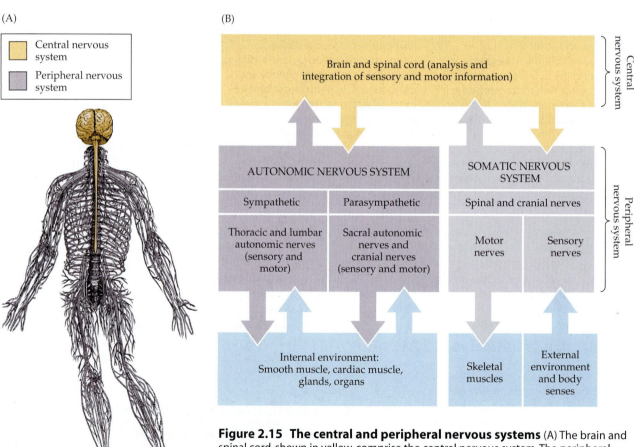

Figure 2.15 The central and peripheral nervous systems (A) The brain and spinal cord, shown in yellow, comprise the central nervous system. The peripheral nervous system, shown in purple, connects all parts of the body to the central nervous system. (B) Organization of the nervous system: The internal and external environments send sensory information by way of peripheral nerves to the CNS, where neural circuits analyze and integrate the information before sending signals to regulate muscle and internal organ function.

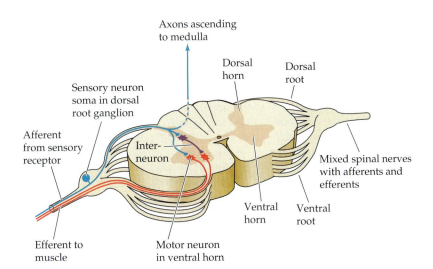

Figure 2.16 Spinal nerves of the peripheral nervous system Cross section of the spinal cord showing mixed spinal nerves with sensory afferents entering the dorsal horn and motor efferents leaving the ventral horn to innervate skeletal muscles. Notice that the soma for the afferent neuron is in the dorsal root ganglion.

BOX 2.2

The Cutting Edge

Finding Your Way in the Nervous System

In order to discuss anatomical relationships, a systematic method to describe location in three dimensions is needed. The directions are based on the **neuraxis,** an imaginary line beginning at the base of the spinal cord and ending at the front of the brain. For most animals the neuraxis is a straight line; however, because humans walk upright, the neuraxis bends, changing the relationship of the brain to the spinal cord (Figure A). For this reason, both the top of the head and the back of the body are called **dorsal,** while **ventral** refers to the underside of the brain and the front surface of the body. To avoid confusion, sometimes the top of the human brain is described as **superior** and the bottom, **inferior.** In addition, the head end of the nervous system is **anterior** or **rostral** and the tail end is **posterior** or **caudal.** Finally, **medial** means toward the center or midline of the body and **lateral** means toward the side. We can describe the location of any brain area using these three pairs of dimensional descriptors.

Much of our knowledge about the structure of the nervous system comes from examining two-dimensional slices (Figure B). The orientation of the slice (or **section**) is typically in any one of three different planes:

- **Horizontal** sections are slices parallel to the horizon.
- **Sagittal** sections are cut on the plane that bisects the nervous sys-

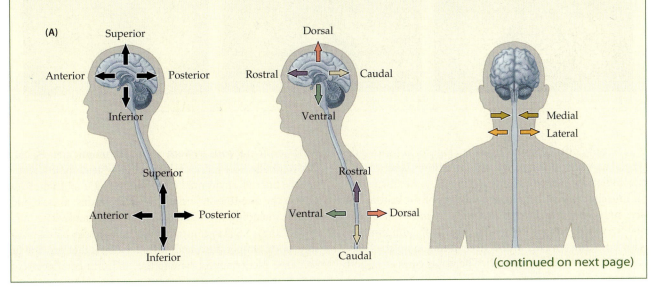

(continued on next page)

BOX 2.2 (continued)

tem into right and left halves. The **midsagittal** section is the slice that divides the brain into left and right symmetrical pieces.

• **Coronal** (or **frontal**) sections are cut parallel to the face.

Identifying specific structures in these different views takes a good deal of experience. However, computer-assisted evaluation allows us to visualize the brain of a living human in far greater detail than was previously possible. MRI and computerized tomography not only provide detailed anatomical images of brain slices but also reconstruct three-dimensional images of the brain using mathematical techniques. PET and fMRI provide a view of the functioning brain by mapping blood flow or glucose utilization in various disease states, following drug administration, or during other experimental manipulations.

(B)

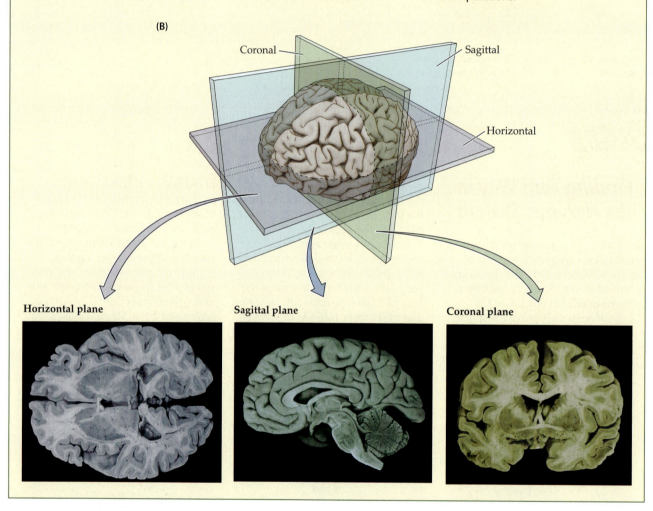

Coronal — Sagittal

Horizontal

Horizontal plane   **Sagittal plane**   **Coronal plane**

only sensory or only motor function. Figure 2.17 shows the cranial nerves and their functions. In addition, several of the cranial nerves innervate glands and organs rather than skeletal muscles, which means they are part of the autonomic nervous system (see the next section). The most unique cranial nerve is the vagus (nerve X), because it communicates with numerous organs in the viscera, including the heart, lungs, and gastrointestinal tract. The vagus consists of both sensory and motor neurons.

Autonomic nervous system   The autonomic nerves, collectively called the autonomic nervous system (ANS), regulate the internal environment by innervating smooth muscles such as the intestine and urinary bladder, cardiac muscle, and glands, including the adrenal and salivary glands. The purpose of the ANS is to control digestive processes, blood pressure, body temperature, and other functions that provide or conserve energy appropriate to the environmental needs of the organism. The ANS is divided into two components, the

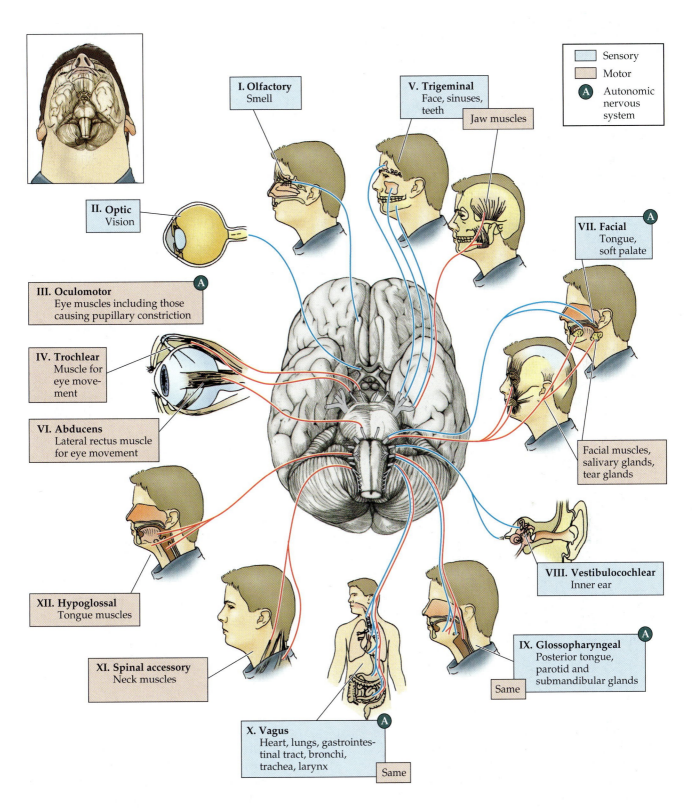

Figure 2.17 Cranial nerves This ventral surface view of the brain shows the 12 cranial nerves (numbered I through XII) and their functions. Some nerves consist of neurons that are only sensory (nerves I, II, and VIII), some are solely motor in function (nerves III, IV, VI, XI, and XII), and others are mixed, having both sensory afferents and motor efferents (nerves V, VII, IX, and X). In addition, several are considered part of the autonomic nervous system since they serve organs and glands (nerves III, VII, IX, and X).

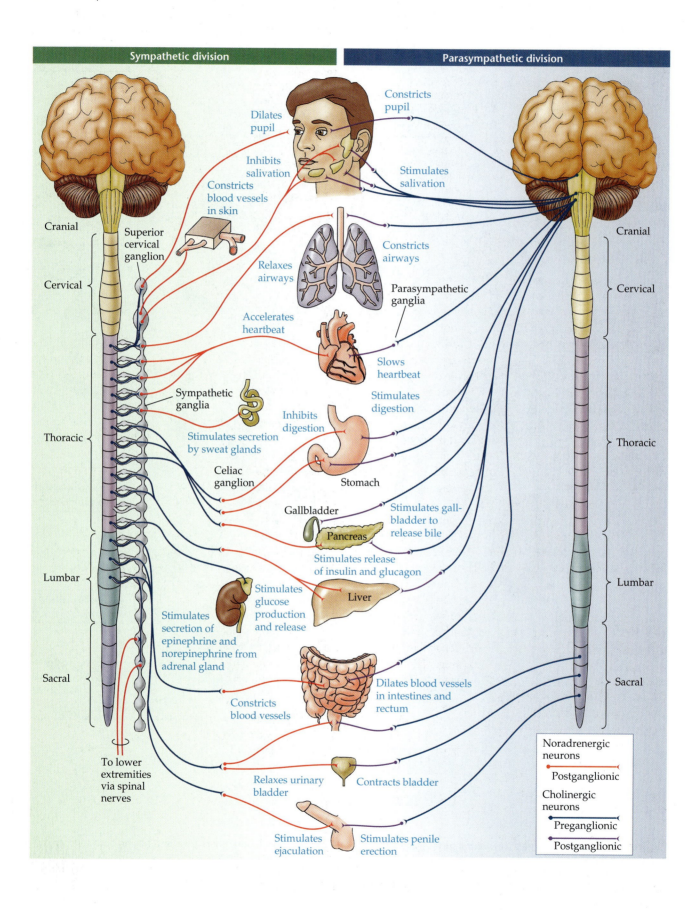

Sympathetic division

Parasympathetic division

Cranial

Superior
cervical
ganglion

Cervical

Dilates
pupil

Inhibits
salivation

Constricts
blood vessels
in skin

Constricts
pupil

Stimulates
salivation

Relaxes
airways

Constricts
airways

Accelerates
heartbeat

Parasympathetic
ganglia

Sympathetic
ganglia

Slows
heartbeat

Thoracic

Inhibits
digestion

Stimulates
digestion

Stimulates secretion
by sweat glands

Celiac
ganglion

Stomach

Gallbladder

Stimulates gall-
bladder to
release bile

Pancreas

Stimulates release
of insulin and glucagon

Lumbar

Stimulates
glucose
production
and release

Liver

Stimulates
secretion of
epinephrine and
norepinephrine from
adrenal gland

Sacral

Dilates blood vessels
in intestines and
rectum

Constricts
blood vessels

To lower
extremities
via spinal
nerves

Relaxes urinary
bladder

Contracts bladder

Stimulates
ejaculation

Stimulates penile
erection

Cranial

Cervical

Thoracic

Lumbar

Sacral

Noradrenergic
neurons

Postganglionic

Cholinergic
neurons

Preganglionic

Postganglionic

Figure 2.18 Autonomic nervous system (ANS) The internal organs, smooth muscles, and glands served by the ANS have both sympathetic and parasympathetic regulation. The two divisions have opposing effects on the organs; the sympathetic effects prepare the individual for action, while the parasympathetic effects serve to generate and store energy and reduce energy expenditure. Acetylcholine is the neurotransmitter released in all autonomic ganglia because preganglionic fibers are cholinergic neurons. At the target organs, the parasympathetic neurons release acetylcholine once again, while sympathetic neurons release norepinephrine (noradrenergic neurons). Their anatomical and neurotransmitter differences are described in the text and summarized in Table 2.3.

sympathetic and parasympathetic divisions, and both divisions serve most organs of the body (Figure 2.18). Although their functions usually work in opposition to one another, control of our internal environment is not an all-or-none affair. Instead, activity of the **sympathetic** division predominates when energy expenditure is necessary, such as during times of stress or excitement; hence its nickname is the "fight-or-flight" system. This system increases heart rate and blood pressure, stimulates secretion of adrenaline, and increases blood flow to skeletal muscles, among other effects. The **parasympathetic** division predominates at times when energy reserves can be conserved and stored for later use; hence this system increases salivation, digestion, and storage of glucose and other nutrients, as well as slowing heart rate and decreasing respiration.

In addition to contrasting functions, the two branches of the ANS have anatomical differences, including points of origin in the CNS. The cell bodies of the efferent sympathetic neurons are in the ventral horn of the spinal cord at the thoracic and lumbar regions (see Figure 2.18). Their axons project for a relatively short distance before they synapse with a cluster of cell bodies called sympathetic ganglia. Some of these ganglia are lined up very close to the spinal cord, while others such as the celiac ganglion are located somewhat farther away. These preganglionic fibers release the neurotransmitter acetylcholine onto the cell bodies in the ganglia. The postganglionic cells project their axons for a relatively long distance to the target tissues, where they release the neurotransmitter norepinephrine.

In contrast, the cell bodies of the efferent parasympathetic neurons are located either in the brain (cranial nerves III, VII, IX, and X) or in the ventral horn of the spinal cord at the sacral region. The preganglionic neurons travel long distances to synapse on cells in the parasympathetic ganglia that are not

neatly lined up along the spinal cord but are close to individual target organs. The preganglionic fibers release acetylcholine, just as the sympathetic preganglionics do. However, the parasympathetic postganglionic neurons, which are quite short, also release acetylcholine. Understanding the autonomic nervous system is especially important to psychopharmacologists because many psychotherapeutic drugs alter either norepinephrine or acetylcholine in the brain to relieve symptoms, but by altering those same neurotransmitters in the peripheral nerves, the drugs often produce annoying or dangerous side effects such as elevated blood pressure, dry mouth, or urinary problems (all related to autonomic function). Table 2.3 summarizes the differences between the two divisions of the ANS.

CNS functioning is dependent on structural features

The tough bone of the skull and vertebrae maintains the integrity of the delicate tissue of the brain and spinal cord. Additionally, three layers of tissue called **meninges** lie just within the bony covering and provide additional protection. The outermost layer, which is also the toughest, is the **dura mater.** The **arachnoid,** just below the dura, is a membrane with a weblike sublayer (subarachnoid space) filled with cerebrospinal fluid (CSF). The brain essentially floats in CSF, so the CSF cushions the organ from trauma and reduces the pressure on the base of the brain (see Figure 1.5B). Finally, the **pia mater** is a thin layer of tissue that sits directly on the nervous tissue.

The CSF not only surrounds the brain but also fills the irregularly shaped cavities within the brain, called **cerebral ventricles,** and the channel that runs the length of the spinal cord, called the **central canal.** The CSF is formed by the choroid plexus within the lateral ventricle of each hemisphere and flows to the third and fourth ventricles before moving into the subarachnoid space to bathe the exterior of the brain and spinal cord (see Figure 1.5A). CSF not only protects the brain but also helps in the exchange of nutrients and waste products between the brain and the blood. This

TABLE 2.3 Characteristics of the Sympathetic and Parasympathetic Divisions of the Autonomic Nervous System

Sympathetic	Parasympathetic
Energy mobilization	Energy conservation and storage
Origin in thoracic and lumbar spinal cord	Origin in cranial nerves and sacral spinal cord
Relatively short preganglionic fibers; long postganglionics	Long preganglionic fibers ending near organs; short postganglionics
Releases acetylcholine in ganglia and norepinephrine at target	Releases acetylcholine at both ganglia and target

exchange is possible because the capillaries found in the choroid plexus do not have the tight junctions typical of capillaries in the brain. These tight junctions constitute the blood–brain barrier, a vital mechanism to protect the delicate chemical balance in the CNS. Refer to Chapter 1 for a discussion of the blood–brain barrier.

The CNS has six distinct regions reflecting embryological development

The six anatomical divisions of the adult CNS are evident in the developing embryo. The CNS starts out as a fluid-filled tube that soon develops three enlargements at one end that become the adult hindbrain, midbrain, and forebrain, while the remainder of the neural tube becomes the spinal cord (Figure 2.19A). The fluid-filled chamber itself becomes the ventricular system in the brain and the central canal in the spinal cord. Within 2 months of conception, further subdivisions occur: the hindbrain enlargement develops two swellings, as does the forebrain. These divisions, in ascending order, are the

spinal cord, myelencephalon, metencephalon, mesencephalon, diencephalon, and telencephalon. Each region can be further subdivided into clusters of cell bodies, called **nuclei,** and their associated bundles of axons, called **tracts.** (In the PNS they are called **ganglia** and **nerves,** respectively.) These interconnecting networks of cells will be the focus in much of the remainder of this book, because drugs that alter brain function, that is, psychotropic drugs, modify the interactions of these neurons. The principal divisions of the CNS are summarized in Figure 2.19B and C.

Spinal cord   The spinal cord is made up of gray and white matter. The former appears butterfly shaped in cross section (Figure 2.20A) and is called gray matter because the large number of cell bodies in this region appear dark on histological examination. The cell bodies include cell groups that receive information from sensory afferent neurons entering the dorsal horn and cell bodies of motor neurons in the ventral horn that send efferents to skeletal muscles. The white matter surrounding the butterfly-shaped gray matter is made

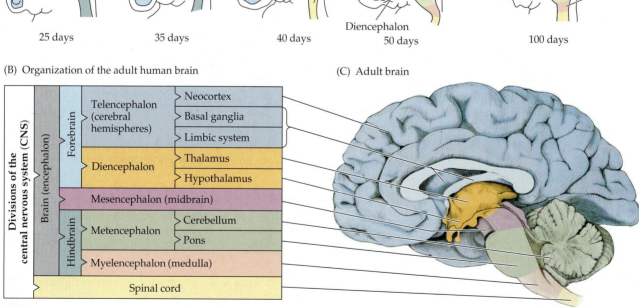

Figure 2.19 Divisions of the central nervous system (A) Beginning with the primitive neural tube in the human embryo, the CNS develops rapidly, and by day 50 of gestation the six divisions of the adult CNS are apparent in the fetus. (B) The organization of the CNS (brain and spinal cord) is presented in the table and color coded to match the divisions shown in the adult brain (sagittal section) (C).

(A)

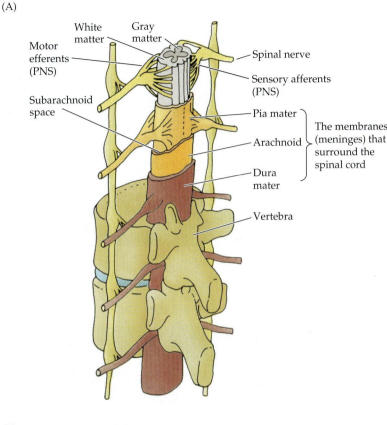

(B)

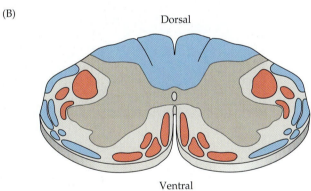

Figure 2.20 Spinal cord (A) A view of the spinal cord showing its relationship to the protective layers of meninges and the bony vertebra. Notice the clearly defined gray matter and white matter in cross section. (B) Schematic diagram of the ascending sensory tracts shown in blue and the descending motor tracts in red.

up of myelinated axons of ascending pathways that conduct sensory information to the brain and of descending pathways from higher centers to the motor neurons that initiate muscle contraction (Figure 2.20B).

As we move up the spinal cord and enter the skull, the spinal cord enlarges and becomes the **brain stem.** If you

examine the ventral surface of the brain (Figure 2.21A), the brain stem with its three principal parts, the medulla, pons, and midbrain, is clearly visible. The brain stem contains the reticular formation, a large network of cells and interconnecting fibers that extends up the core of the brain stem for most of its length (described later in the section on the metencephalon). Additionally, the brain stem is the origin of numerous cranial nerves that receive sensory information from the skin and joints of the face, head, and neck as well as serving motor control to the muscles in that region (see Figure 2.17). Finally, a significant volume of the brain stem is made up of ascending and descending axons coursing between the spinal cord and higher brain regions. The relationship of the structures of the brain stem is also apparent in the midsagittal view (Figure 2.21B).

Myelencephalon   The first major structure of the brain stem we encounter is the myelencephalon, or medulla. Within the **medulla,** multiple cell groups regulate vital functions including heart rate, digestion, respiration, blood pressure, coughing, and vomiting. When an individual dies from a drug overdose, the cause is most often depression of the respiratory center in the medulla. Also located in the medulla is the **area postrema,** or vomiting center described in Chapter 1 as a cluster of cells with a reduced blood–brain barrier that initiates vomiting in response to toxins in the blood. Drugs in the opiate class such as morphine act on the area postrema and produce vomiting, a common unpleasant side effect of treatment for pain. The nuclei for cranial nerves XI and XII that control the muscles of the neck and tongue are also located in the medulla.

Metencephalon   Two large structures within the metencephalon are the pons and cerebellum (see Figure 2.21). Within the central core of the pons and extending rostrally into the midbrain and caudally into the medulla is the **reticular formation.** The reticular formation is not really a structure but a collection of perhaps 100 small nuclei forming a network that plays an important role in arousal, attention, sleep, and muscle tone, as well as some cardiac and respiratory reflexes. One nucleus called the **locus coeruleus** is of particular importance to psychopharmacology because

(A) **Ventral view**

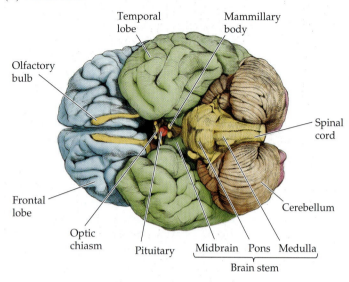

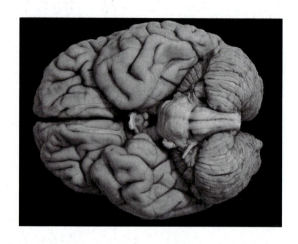

(B) **Midsagittal view**

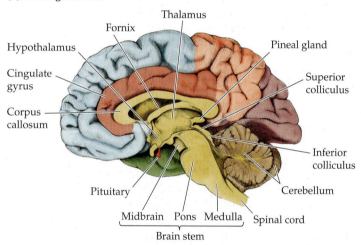

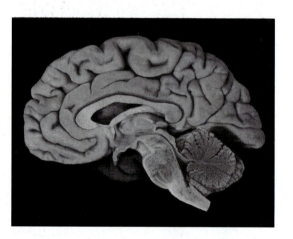

Figure 2.21 Two views of the human brain The drawings on the left in each panel label the structural features that are visible on the ventral external surface (A) and midsagittal (midline) section (B). The right side of each panel is the same view of a human postmortem brain specimen. (Courtesy of Mark Williams and Dale Purves, Duke University Medical Center.)

it is a cluster of cell bodies that distribute their axons to many areas of the forebrain. These cells are the principal source of all the neurons utilizing the neurotransmitter norepinephrine. When active, these cells cause arousal, increased vigilance, and attention. Drugs like amphetamine enhance their function, causing sleeplessness and enhanced alertness.

Other cell groups within the pons that also belong to the reticular formation are the **dorsal** and **median raphe nuclei.** These two clusters of cells are the source of most of the neurons in the CNS that utilize serotonin as their neurotransmit-

ter. Together, the cell bodies in the dorsal and median raphe send axons releasing serotonin to virtually all forebrain areas and function in the regulation of diverse processes including sleep, aggression and impulsiveness, neuroendocrine functions, and emotion. Having a generally inhibitory effect on CNS function, serotonin may maintain behaviors within specific limits. Drugs such as LSD produce their dramatic hallucinogenic effects by inhibiting the inhibitory functions of the raphe nuclei (see Chapters 6 and 14).

The **cerebellum** is a large foliated structure on the dorsal surface of the brain that connects to the pons by several large bundles of axons called **cerebellar peduncles.** The cerebellum is a significant sensorimotor center and receives visual, auditory, and somatosensory input as well as information about body position and balance from the vestibular system. By coordinating the sensory information with motor information received from the cerebral cortex, the cerebellum coordinates and smoothes out movements by timing and patterning skeletal muscle contractions. In addition, the cerebellum allows us to make corrective movements to maintain our balance and posture. Damage to the cerebellum produces poor coordination and jerky movements. Drugs such as alcohol at moderate doses inhibit the function of the cerebellum and cause slurred speech and staggering.

Mesencephalon   The midbrain has two divisions: the tectum and the tegmentum. The **tectum** is the dorsalmost structure and consists of the superior colliculi, which are part of the visual system, and the inferior colliculi, which are part of the auditory system (see Figure 2.21B). These nuclei are involved in reflexes including the pupillary reflex to light, eye movement, and reactions to moving stimuli.

Within the **tegmentum** are several structures that are particularly important to psychopharmacologists. The first is the **periaqueductal gray (PAG),** which surrounds the cerebral aqueduct that connects the third and fourth ventricles. The PAG is one of the areas important for the modulation of pain. Local electrical stimulation of these cells produces analgesia but no change in the ability to detect temperature, touch, or pressure. The PAG is rich in opioid receptors, making it an important site for morphine-induced analgesia. Chapter 9 describes the importance of natural opioid neuropeptides and the PAG in pain regulation. The PAG is also important in sequencing species-specific actions, such as defensive rage and predation.

The **substantia nigra** is a cluster of cell bodies whose relatively long axons innervate the striatum, a component of the basal ganglia (Figure 2.22). These cells constitute one of several important neural pathways that utilize dopamine as their neurotransmitter. This pathway is called the nigrostriatal tract. (The names of neural pathways often combine the site of origin of the fibers with their termination site, hence nigrostriatal, meaning substantia nigra to striatum.) This neural circuit is critical for the initiation and modulation of movement. Cell death in the substantia nigra is the cause of Parkinson's disease, a disorder characterized by tremor, rigidity, and inability to initiate movements. An adjacent cluster of dopaminergic cells in the midbrain is the **ventral tegmental area (VTA).** Some of these cells project axons to the septum, olfactory tubercle, nucleus accumbens, amygdala, and other limbic structures in the forebrain (see the section on the telencephalon). Hence these cells form the mesolimbic tract (note that "meso" refers to midbrain). Other cells in the VTA project to structures in the prefrontal cortex, cingulate cortex, and entorhinal areas and are considered the mesocortical tract. All three of these dopamine pathways are of significance in our discussions of Parkinson's disease (Chapter 5), drug addiction (Chapter 8), and schizophrenia (Chapter 18).

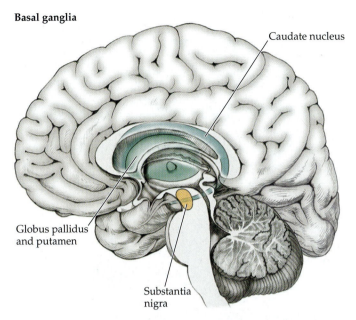

Basal ganglia

Caudate nucleus

Globus pallidus and putamen

Substantia nigra

Figure 2.22 The basal ganglia These four structures form neural pathways that utilize dopamine as their neurotransmitter. These neural circuits comprise a system for motor control.

Diencephalon   The two major structures in the diencephalon are the thalamus and hypothalamus. The **thalamus** is a cluster of nuclei that first process and then distribute sensory and motor information to the appropriate portion of the cerebral cortex. For example, the lateral geniculate nucleus of the thalamus receives visual information from the eyes before projecting it to the primary visual cortex. Most of the incoming signals are integrated and modified before being sent on to the cortex. The functioning of the thalamus helps the cortex to direct its attention to selectively important sensory messages while diminishing the significance of others; hence the thalamus helps to regulate levels of awareness.

The second diencephalic structure, the **hypothalamus,** lies ventral to the thalamus at the base of the brain. Although it is much smaller than the thalamus, it is made up of many small nuclei that perform functions critical to survival (Figure 2.23). The hypothalamus receives a wide variety of information about the internal environment and, in coordination with closely related structures in the limbic system (see the section on the telencephalon), initiates various mechanisms important for limiting the variability of the body's internal states (i.e., they are responsible for homeostasis). Several nuclei are involved in maintaining body temperature and salt–water balance. Other nuclei modulate hunger, thirst,

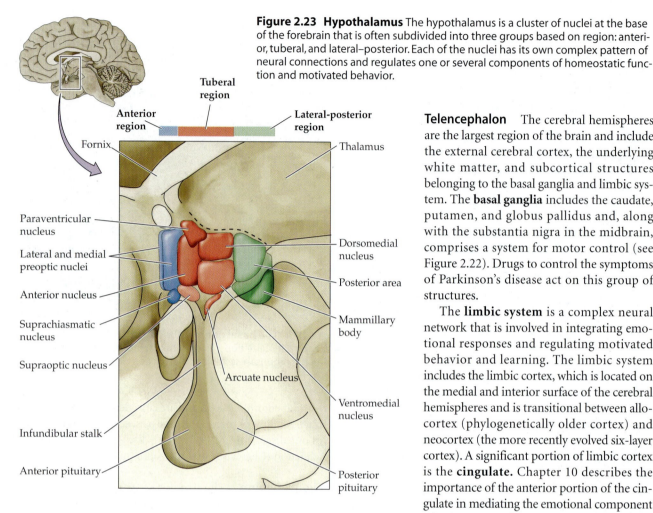

Figure 2.23 Hypothalamus The hypothalamus is a cluster of nuclei at the base of the forebrain that is often subdivided into three groups based on region: anterior, tuberal, and lateral–posterior. Each of the nuclei has its own complex pattern of neural connections and regulates one or several components of homeostatic function and motivated behavior.

Telencephalon The cerebral hemispheres are the largest region of the brain and include the external cerebral cortex, the underlying white matter, and subcortical structures belonging to the basal ganglia and limbic system. The **basal ganglia** includes the caudate, putamen, and globus pallidus and, along with the substantia nigra in the midbrain, comprises a system for motor control (see Figure 2.22). Drugs to control the symptoms of Parkinson's disease act on this group of structures.

The **limbic system** is a complex neural network that is involved in integrating emotional responses and regulating motivated behavior and learning. The limbic system includes the limbic cortex, which is located on the medial and interior surface of the cerebral hemispheres and is transitional between allocortex (phylogenetically older cortex) and neocortex (the more recently evolved six-layer cortex). A significant portion of limbic cortex is the **cingulate.** Chapter 10 describes the importance of the anterior portion of the cingulate in mediating the emotional component of pain. Some of the significant subcortical limbic structures are the amygdala, nucleus accumbens, and hippocampus, which is connected to the mammillary bodies and the septal nuclei by the fornix, the major tract of the limbic system (Figure 2.24). The **hippocampus** is most closely associated with the establishment of new long-term memories and spatial memory and has been the focus of research into Alzheimer's disease and its treatment (see Chapter 6). Additionally, the vulnerability of the hippocampus to high levels of stress hormones suggests its involvement in clinical depression and antidepressant drug treatment (see Chapter 16). The **amygdala** plays a central role in coordinating the various components of emotional responses, through its profuse connections with the olfactory system, hypothalamus (which is sometimes included in the limbic system even though it is a diencephalic structure), thalamus, hippocampus, striatum, and brain stem nuclei, as well as portions of the neocortex, such as the orbitofrontal cortex. The amygdala and associated limbic areas play a prominent role in our discussions of antidepressants, alcohol, and antianxiety drugs. In addition, chapters describing the reinforcing value of abused substances also focus on limbic structures, notably the **nucleus accumbens.**

energy metabolism, reproductive behaviors, and emotional responses such as aggression. The hypothalamus directs behaviors for adjusting to these changing needs by controlling both the autonomic nervous system and the endocrine system and organizing behaviors in coordination with other brain areas. Axons from nuclei in the hypothalamus descend into the brain stem to the nuclei of the cranial nerves that provide parasympathetic control. Additionally, other axons descend farther into the spinal cord to influence sympathetic nervous system function. Other hypothalamic nuclei communicate with the contiguous pituitary gland by two methods: neural control of the posterior pituitary and hormonal control of the anterior pituitary. By regulating the endocrine hormones, the hypothalamus has widespread and prolonged effects on body physiology. Of particular significance to psychopharmacology is the role of the paraventricular nucleus in regulating the hormonal response to stress, which is involved in clinical depression and anxiety disorders. The details of hypothalamic–pituitary relations are described in more detail in Chapter 3.

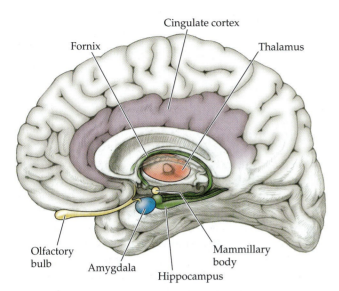

Figure 2.24 **Limbic system** Multiple subcortical structures interconnect to form the limbic system, which is critical to learning, memory, and emotional responses. Rich connection with areas of association cortex contribute to decision making and planning.

The cerebral cortex is divided into four lobes, each having primary, secondary, and tertiary areas

The cerebral cortex is a layer of tissue covering the cerebral hemispheres. In humans, the cortex (or "bark") is heavily convoluted, having deep grooves called **fissures,** smaller grooves called **sulci,** and bulges of tissue between called **gyri.** Thus the bulge of tissues immediately posterior to the central sulcus is the postcentral gyrus. The convolutions of the cortex greatly enlarge its surface area, to approximately 2.5 square feet. Only about one-third of the surface of the cortex is visible externally, with the remaining two-thirds hidden in the sulci and fissures. Figure 2.25 shows some of the external features of the cerebral cortex. There may be as many as 50 to 100 billion cells in the cortex, arranged in six layers horizontal to the surface. Since these layers have large numbers of cell bodies, they appear gray in color; hence they are the gray matter of the cerebral cortex. Each layer can be identified by cell type, size, density, and arrangement. Beneath the six layers, the white matter of the cortex consists of millions of axons that connect one part of the cortex with another or connect cortical cells to other brain structures. One of the largest of these pathways is the **corpus callosum** (see Figure 2.21B), which connects corresponding areas in the two hemispheres. In addition to the horizontal layers, the cortex also has a vertical arrangement of cells that form slender vertical columns running through the entire thickness of the cortex. These vertically oriented cells and their synaptic connections apparently provide the functional units for integration of information between various cortical regions.

The central sulcus and lateral fissure (see Figure 2.25) visually divide the cortex into four distinct lobes in each hemisphere: the **parietal lobe, occipital lobe,** and **temporal lobe,** all of which are sensory in function, and the **frontal lobe,** which is responsible for movement and executive planning. Within each lobe is a small primary area, adjacent secondary cortex, and tertiary areas called association cortex. Within the occipital lobe is the primary visual cortex, which receives visual information from the thalamus that originated in the retina of the eye. The primary auditory cortex receives auditory information and is located in the temporal lobe, and the primary somatosensory cortex, which receives information about body senses such as touch, temperature, and pain, is found in the parietal lobe just posterior to the

Figure 2.25 **Lateral view of the exterior cerebral cortex** The four lobes of the cerebral cortex are shown with distinct colors. Within each lobe is a primary area (darker in color) and secondary and tertiary association cortices. The caudal-most three lobes carry out sensory functions: vision (occipital), auditory (temporal), and somatosensory (parietal). The frontal lobe provides the executive mechanism that plans and organizes behavior and initiates the appropriate sequence of actions.

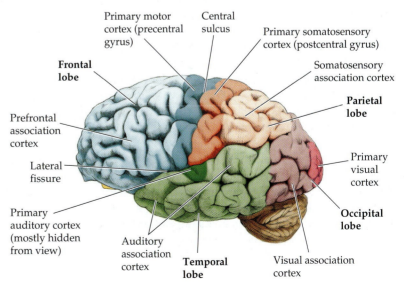

central sulcus. Neither the gustatory cortex, involving taste sensations, nor the primary olfactory area, receiving information regarding the sense of smell, are visible on the surface but lie within the folds of the cortex. The **primary cortex** of each lobe provides conscious awareness of sensory experience and the initial cortical processing of sensory qualities. Except for olfaction, all sensory information arrives in the appropriate primary cortex via projection neurons from the thalamus. In addition, except for olfaction, sensory information from the left side of the body goes to the right cerebral hemisphere first, and information from the right side goes to the left hemisphere. Visual information is somewhat different in that the left half of the visual field of each eye goes to the right occipital lobe and the right half of the visual field of each eye goes to the left occipital lobe.

Adjacent to each primary area is **secondary cortex** that consists of neuronal circuits responsible for analyzing the information transmitted from the primary area and providing recognition (or perception) of the stimulus. These areas also are the regions where memories are stored. Farther from the primary areas are association areas that lay down more-complex memories that involve multiple sensory systems such that our memories are not confined to a single sensory system but integrate multiple characteristics of the event. For example, many of us remember pieces of music from the past that automatically evoke visual memories of the person we shared it with or the time in our lives when it was popular. These **tertiary association areas** are often called the parietal–temporal–occipital association cortex because they represent the interface of the three sensory lobes and provide the higher-order perceptual functions needed for purposeful action.

Within the frontal lobe, the primary motor cortex mediates voluntary movements of the muscles of the limbs and trunk. Neurons originating in primary motor cortex directly, or in several steps, project to the spinal cord to act on spinal motor neurons that end on muscle fibers. As was true for the sensory systems, the motor neurons beginning in the frontal cortex are crossed, meaning that areas of the right primary motor cortex control movements of limbs on the left side of the body and vice versa. Adjacent to the primary motor cortex is the secondary motor cortex, where memories for well-learned motor sequences are stored. Neurons in this area connect directly to the primary motor cortex to direct movement. The rest of the frontal lobe comprises the prefrontal cortex, which receives sensory information from the other cortices via the large bundles of white matter running below the gray matter. Emotional and motivational input is contributed to the prefrontal cortex by limbic and other subcortical structures. The prefrontal cortex is critical for making decisions, planning actions, and evaluating optional strategies. Impaired prefrontal function is characteristic of several psychiatric disorders including borderline personality disorder, memory loss following traumatic brain injury, attention deficit disorder, and others. The significance of this brain region to the symptoms and treatment of schizophrenia is discussed in Chapter 18.

Section Summary

The nervous system is made up of the central and peripheral divisions. The CNS includes the brain and spinal cord, and the PNS is made up of the remaining nerves, both spinal and cranial. The PNS is further divided into the somatic nervous system, which includes the mixed spinal nerves that transmit both sensory and motor information to skeletal muscles, and the autonomic nervous system, which serves smooth muscles, glands, and visceral organs. The autonomic nervous system also has two divisions: the sympathetic, which serves to mobilize energy for times of "fight or flight"; and the parasympathetic, which reduces energy utilization and stores reserves. The 12 pairs of cranial nerves perform similar functions for the head and neck.

The CNS can be divided into six regions reflecting embryological development. Within each region are multiple nuclei and their associated axons, which form interconnecting neural circuits that elicit behaviors appropriate to changing conditions. The spinal cord is the first division and has clearly defined regions of gray and white matter when examined in cross section. The gray matter is the cell bodies that receive sensory information and the cell bodies of motor neurons that serve muscles. The white matter is tracts of axons that carry signals in the ascending direction to the brain and descending tracts for cortical control of the spinal cord. Moving rostrally, the spinal cord passes through an opening in the skull and becomes the brain stem. Much of the brain stem also contains the continuation of the axon bundles to and from the spinal cord and, in addition, has clusters of nuclei that can be described on a functional basis.

Continuous with the spinal cord is the myelencephalon, which contains the medulla. This region is populated by multiple nuclei that serve some of the vital functions for survival, such as respiration. The metencephalon includes the cerebellum, which functions to maintain posture and balance and provide fine motor control and coordination. The pons, also part of the metencephalon, contains several nuclei that represent the origins of most of the tracts utilizing the neurotransmitters norepinephrine (the locus coeruleus) and serotonin (the raphe nuclei) in the brain. Beginning in the medulla, running through the pons, and extending into the midbrain is the reticular formation, a network of interconnected nuclei that control arousal, attention, and survival functions. The upper end of the brain stem is the mesencephalon, or midbrain, which contains not only centers that control sensory reflexes such as pupillary constriction but also important sources of neurons (substantia nigra and ventral tegmental area) forming three major dopaminergic tracts. In addition, the periaqueductal gray organizes behaviors such as defensive rage and predation and serves as an important pain-modulating center.

The fifth region is the diencephalon, containing the thalamus, which relays information to the cerebral cortex, and the hypothalamus, which is important for maintaining homeostasis of physiological functions and for modulating motivated behaviors including eating, aggression, reproduction, and so forth. The many nuclei that constitute the hypothalamus control both the autonomic nervous system and the endocrine system.

The telencephalon includes both the cerebral cortex and multiple subcortical structures including the basal ganglia and the limbic system. The basal ganglia modulates movement. The limbic system is made up of several brain struc-tures with perfuse interconnections that modulate emotion, motivation, and learning. Some of the prominent limbic structures are the amygdala, hippocampus, nucleus accumbens, and limbic cortex.

The six-layered cerebral cortex is organized into four lobes: the occipital, temporal, and parietal, which are the sensory lobes involved in perception and memories, and the frontal, which regulates motor movements and contains the "executive mechanism" for planning, evaluating, and making strategies.

Recommended Readings

Rosenzweig, M. R., Breedlove, S. M., and Watson, N. V. (2004). *Biological Psychology* (4th Ed.). Sinauer Associates, Inc., Sunderland, Massachusetts.

Swerdlow, J. L. (1995). Quiet miracles of the brain. *Nat'l Geogr.*, 187, 2–41.

3 *Chemical Signaling by Neurotransmitters and Hormones*

*I*n the early twentieth century, physiologists were still unsure how nerve cells communicated with one another. Some thought electrical impulses "jumped the gap" from one neuron to another or from neurons to the cells of a target organ such as a muscle. Alternatively, the terminal might release a chemical substance that acted on the receiving cell. Some indirect evidence supported this chemical hypothesis of nerve cell communication, but no one had yet performed a definitive experiment testing the hypothesis.

This brings us to Otto Loewi, a German pharmacologist who carried out the long-awaited experiment in 1920. Loewi later recounted that the idea of chemical transmission had occurred to him as early as 1903, but at that time he had no way of testing the idea and thus forgot about it for many years. Meanwhile, he had begun studying the control of the frog heart by the vagus nerve, a parasympathetic nerve that reduces heart rate. In Loewi's own words:

> The night before Easter Sunday of that year (1920) I awoke, turned on the light, and jotted down a few notes on a tiny slip of thin paper. Then I fell asleep again. It occurred to me at six o'clock in the morning that during the night I had written down something most important, but I was unable to decipher the scrawl. The next night, at three o'clock, the idea returned. It was the design of an experiment to determine whether or not the hypothesis of chemical transmission I had uttered seventeen years ago was correct. I got up immediately, went to the laboratory, and performed a simple experiment on a frog heart according to the nocturnal design. (Loewi, 1960, p. 17)

In his "simple experiment," Loewi first removed the hearts of two frogs, only one of which still had the vagus nerve attached, and bathed the organs in a solution that would keep them functioning for a while. The vagus nerve of the first heart was electrically stimulated, which caused the heart to slow down as expected. The fluid that had been bathing the first heart was then transferred to the second heart, and, amazingly, the second heart slowed down as well. This meant that stimulation of the vagus nerve released a chemical substance that was responsible for the decrease in heart rate. Loewi named this unknown

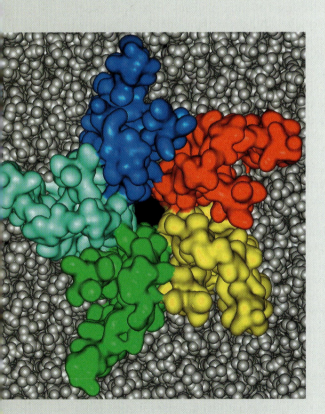

A model of the nicotinic acetylcholine receptor. This ionotropic receptor consists of five subunits that form a central pore through which ions can flow.

chemical Vagusstoff ("vagus material"), and within a few years it was identified as the substance acetylcholine (ACh). Interestingly, Loewi admitted that if he had carefully considered this experiment in the daytime instead of rushing to the lab in the middle of the night, he would have rejected it as being unlikely to succeed. For example, even if a chemical is released from the nerve, it might be in quantities too small to affect the recipient heart. Fortunately, Loewi had some luck on his side (in addition to his insight): not only did the vagus nerve liberate enough ACh to affect the recipient heart, but the neurotransmitter was able to persist in the transferred fluid because the frog heart has a lower capacity to break down ACh than the hearts of many other species.

Loewi's experiment introduces one of the body's great systems, cellular communication, the system of synaptic transmission. In the rest of this chapter, you will learn more about synapses, neurotransmitters, and the mechanisms of neurotransmitter action. The final section is devoted to a second important communication system, the endocrine system, which is responsible for secretion of hormones into the bloodstream.*

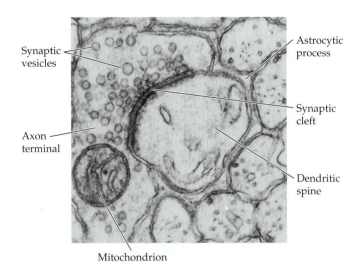

Figure 3.1 An electron micrograph of an axodendritic synapse illustrating the major features of a typical connection between an axon terminal of the presynaptic cell and a dendritic spine of the postsynaptic cell. (From Peters et al., 1991.)

Chemical Signaling between Nerve Cells

The word *synapse* was coined in 1897 by the British physiologist Sir Charles Sherrington. He derived the term from the Greek word *synapto*, which means "to clasp." Using only a light microscope, Sherrington could not see the actual point of communication between neurons, but physiological experiments had shown that transmission only occurs in one direction (from what we now call the **presynaptic cell** to the **postsynaptic cell**). The synapse was considered to be the specialized mechanism underlying this neuronal communication. Sherrington even correctly inferred that the sending (presynaptic) and receiving (postsynaptic) cells do not actually touch each other. Of course, the concept of chemical transmitter substances had not yet been conceived, since Loewi's frog heart experiment was still more than 20 years away and other critical studies had also not yet been performed.

Our current knowledge of synaptic structure comes from the electron microscope, which gives us much greater magnification than standard light microscopes. The most common synapses in the brain are **axodendritic synapses.** These are synapses in which an axon terminal from the presynaptic neuron communicates with a dendrite of the postsynaptic cell. An electron micrograph displaying this kind of synapse is shown in Figure 3.1 (see also Figure

3.2A). The dendrites of some neurons have short spines along their length, which are reminiscent of thorns growing out from a rosebush. When spines are present, they are important locations for synapses to form, and this is the case for the synapse shown in Figure 3.1. There is an exceedingly small (about 20 nm, which is 20×10^{-9} m) gap between the pre- and postsynaptic cells that must be traversed by neurotransmitter molecules after their release. This gap is called the **synaptic cleft.** In the axon terminal, we can see many small sac-like objects, termed **synaptic vesicles,** each of which is filled with several thousand molecules of a neurotransmitter. As we shall see, the vesicles are normally the source of transmitter release. The electron micrograph also shows a profile of a **mitochondrion** in the axon terminal. Mitochondria are the cellular organelles responsible for energy (adenosine triphosphate, or ATP) production, and they are needed in large amounts in the terminals for various functions such as ion pumping and transmitter release. Finally, we see that the synapse is surrounded by processes (fibers) from astrocytes. In Chapter 7, we discuss an important role for these glial cells in regulating transmission by amino acid transmitters.

Other types of synapses are also present in the brain. For example, **axosomatic synapses** are synapses between a nerve terminal and a nerve cell body (Figure 3.2B). They function in a manner similar to axodendritic synapses. **Axoaxonic synapses** involve one axon synapsing on the terminal of another axon (Figure 3.2C). This unusual arrangement permits the presynaptic cell to alter neurotransmitter release

---

*The third great signaling system is the immune system, discussion of which is beyond the scope of this text.

(A) Axodendritic   (B) Axosomatic   (C) Axoaxonic

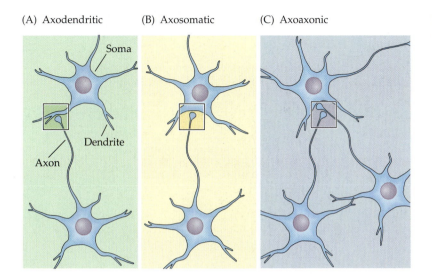

Figure 3.2 The three types of synaptic connections between neurons

from the postsynaptic cell directly at the terminals. For example, activity at an axoaxonic synapse may reduce transmitter release from the terminal. This is called **presynaptic inhibition** of release. Enhanced release of transmitter, on the other hand, is called **presynaptic facilitation.**

In neuronal communication, the receiving cell may be another neuron, but it may also be a muscle cell or a cell specialized to release a hormone or other secretory product. The connection point between a neuron and a muscle is called a **neuromuscular junction** instead of a synapse. A neuromuscular junction has many structural and functional similarities to a conventional synapse, and much has been learned about synaptic transmission by studying neuromuscular junctions.

Neurotransmitter Synthesis, Release, and Inactivation

As previously mentioned, **neurotransmitters** are chemical substances released by neurons to communicate with other cells. Scientists first thought that only a few chemicals were involved in neurotransmission, but well over 100 chemicals have now been identified. As there are many thousands of chemicals present in any cell, how do we know whether a particular substance qualifies as a neurotransmitter? Verifying a chemical's status as a neurotransmitter can be a difficult process, but here are some of the important criteria:

1. The presynaptic cell should contain the proposed substance along with a mechanism for manufacturing it.

2. A mechanism for inactivating the substance should also be present.

3. The substance should be released from the axon terminal upon stimulation of the neuron.

4. There should be receptors for the proposed substance on the postsynaptic cell. (Receptors are discussed in greater detail later in the chapter.)

5. Direct application of the proposed substance or an agonist drug that acts on its receptors should have the same effect on the postsynaptic cell as stimulating the presynaptic neuron (which presumably would release the substance from the axon terminals).

6. Applying an antagonist drug that blocks the receptors should inhibit both the action of the applied substance and the effect of stimulating the presynaptic neuron.

Even if all criteria have not yet been met for a suspected neurotransmitter, there is often sufficient evidence to make a strong case for transmitter candidacy.

Neurotransmitters encompass several different kinds of chemical substances

Despite the great number of neurotransmitters, most of them conveniently fall into several chemical classes. The major types of transmitters and some examples of each are shown in Table 3.1. A few neurotransmitters are categorized as **amino acids.*** Amino acids serve numerous functions: they are the individual building blocks contained within proteins, they also play other metabolic roles, including their role as neurotransmitters. In Chapter 7, we cover the two most important amino acid neurotransmitters, glutamate

---

*Amino acids are so named because they contain both an amino group ($-NH_2$) and a carboxyl group ($-COOH$), the latter of which gives off a hydrogen ion (H^+) and thus acts like an acid.

TABLE 3.1 Major Categories of Neurotransmitters[a]

Classical neurotransmitters	Non-classical neurotransmitters
Amino acids	**Neuropeptides**
Glutamate	Endorphins and enkephalins
γ-aminobutyric acid (GABA)	Corticotropin-releasing factor (CRF)
Glycine	Many others
Monoamines	**Lipids**
Dopamine (DA)	Anandamide
Norepinephrine (NE)	**Gases**
Serotonin (5-HT)	Nitric oxide (NO)
Acetylcholine	

[a]It should be noted that this is only a small sample of the more than 100 substances known or suspected to be neurotransmitters in the brain.

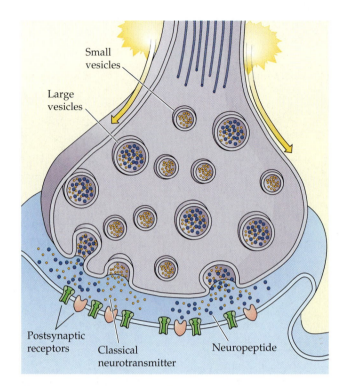

Figure 3.3 Axon terminal of a neuron that synthesizes both a classical neurotransmitter and a neuropeptide The small vesicles contain only the classical transmitter, whereas the large vesicles contain the neuropeptide and the classical neurotransmitter, which are stored and released together.

and γ-aminobutyric acid (GABA). Several other transmitters are **monoamines,** which are grouped together because each possesses a single (hence "mono") amine group. Monoamine transmitters are derived from amino acids by a series of biochemical reactions that include removal of the acidic part (–COOH) of the molecule. Consequently, we say that the original amino acid is a **precursor** because it precedes the amine in the biochemical pathway. In Chapters 5 and 6, we discuss the best-characterized monoamine transmitters: dopamine (DA), norepinephrine (NE), and serotonin (5-HT). One important neurotransmitter that is neither an amino acid nor a monoamine is ACh (see Chapter 6). Together with acetylcholine, the amino acid and monoamine neurotransmitters are sometimes called "classical" transmitters because they were generally discovered before the other categories.

Besides the classical transmitters, there are several other types of neurotransmitters. The largest group of "non-classical" neurotransmitters are the **neuropeptides,** whose name simply means peptides found in the nervous system. Peptides are small proteins, typically made up of 3 to 40 amino acids instead of the 100+ amino acids found in most proteins. Neuropharmacologists are very interested in the family of neuropeptides called endorphins and enkephalins, which stimulate the same opioid receptors that are activated by heroin and other abused opiate drugs (see Chapter 10). Another important neuropeptide is corticotropin-releasing factor (CRF), which is now believed to play a role in anxiety. A few transmitters are considered **lipids,** which is the scientific term for fatty substances. For example, in Chapter 13 we discuss a substance called anandamide, a lipid made in the brain that acts like marijuana (or, more specifically, Δ^9-tetrahydrocannabinol [THC], which is the major active

ingredient in marijuana). Finally, the most recently discovered and intriguing group of neurotransmitters are the **gaseous transmitters.** Later in this chapter we discuss nitric oxide, the best known of these unusual transmitters, and we will see that these substances break some of the normal rules followed by other transmitter molecules.

When scientists first discovered the existence of neurotransmitters, it was natural to assume that each neuron only made and released one transmitter substance, suggesting a simple chemical coding of cells in the nervous system. Much research over the past 20 years has shattered that initial assumption. We now know that many neurons make and release two, three, or occasionally even more, different transmitters. Some instances of transmitter coexistence within the same cell involve one or more neuropeptides along with a classical transmitter. In such cases, the neuron has two different types of synaptic vesicles: small vesicles that contain only the classical transmitter and large vesicles that contain the neuropeptide along with the classical transmitter (Figure 3.3).

Classical transmitters and neuropeptides are synthesized by different mechanisms

How and where in the nerve cell are neurotransmitters manufactured? Except for the neuropeptides, transmitters are synthesized by enzymatic reactions that can occur anywhere in the cell. Typically, the enzymes required for producing a

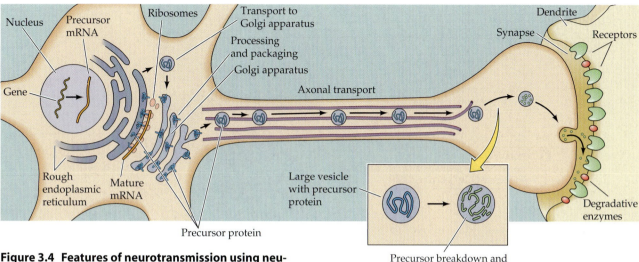

Figure 3.4 Features of neurotransmission using neuropeptides Neuropeptides are synthesized from larger precursor proteins, which are packaged into large vesicles by the Golgi apparatus. During transport from the cell body to the axon terminal, enzymes that have also been packaged within the vesicles break down the precursor protein to liberate the neuropeptide. After being released at the synapse and stimulating postsynaptic receptors, the neuropeptide is inactivated by degradative enzymes.

neurotransmitter are shipped out in large amounts to the axon terminals, so the terminals are an important site of transmitter synthesis. The neuropeptides are different, however. Their precursors are protein molecules, within which the peptides are embedded. The protein precursor for each type of peptide must be made in the cell body, which is the site of almost all protein synthesis in the neuron. The protein is then packaged into large vesicles along with enzymes that will break down the precursor and liberate the neuropeptide (Figure 3.4). These vesicles are transported to the axon terminals so that release occurs from the terminals, as with the classical transmitters. On the other hand, new neuropeptide molecules can only be generated in the cell body, not in the terminals. An important consequence of this difference is that replenishment of neuropeptides is slower than for small-molecule transmitters. When neurotransmitters are depleted by high levels of neuronal activity, small molecules can be resynthesized rapidly within the axon terminal. In contrast, neuropeptides cannot be replenished until large vesicles containing the peptide have been transported to the terminal from their site of origin within the cell body.

Chemicals that don't act like typical neurotransmitters are sometimes called neuromodulators

Some investigators use the term **neuromodulators** to describe substances that don't act exactly like typical neurotransmitters. For example, a neuromodulator might not have a direct effect itself on the postsynaptic cell. Instead, it might alter the action of a standard neurotransmitter by enhancing, reducing, or prolonging the transmitter's effectiveness. Peptides that are co-released with a classical transmitter sometimes exhibit this kind of modulatory effect. Neuromodulators are also sometimes characterized as diffusing beyond the synapse to influence cells farther away. No matter which criteria you use, though, the dividing line between neurotransmitters and neuromodulators is vague. For example, a particular chemical may sometimes act within the synapse, but in other circumstances it may act at a distance from its site of release. Therefore, we will refrain from talking about neuromodulators and instead use the term *neurotransmitter* throughout the remainder of the book.

Neurotransmitter release involves the exocytosis and recycling of synaptic vesicles

As shown in Figure 3.5, synaptic transmission involves a number of processes that occur within the axon terminal and the postsynaptic cell. We will begin our discussion of these processes with a consideration of neurotransmitter release from the terminal. When a neuron fires an action potential, the depolarizing current sweeps down the length of the axon and enters all of the axon terminals. This wave of depolarization has a very important effect within the terminals: it opens large numbers of voltage-sensitive calcium (Ca^{2+}) channels, causing a rapid influx of Ca^{2+} ions into the terminals. The resulting increase in Ca^{2+} concentration within the terminals is the direct trigger for neurotransmitter release.

Exocytosis   You already know that the neurotransmitter molecules destined to be released are stored within synaptic

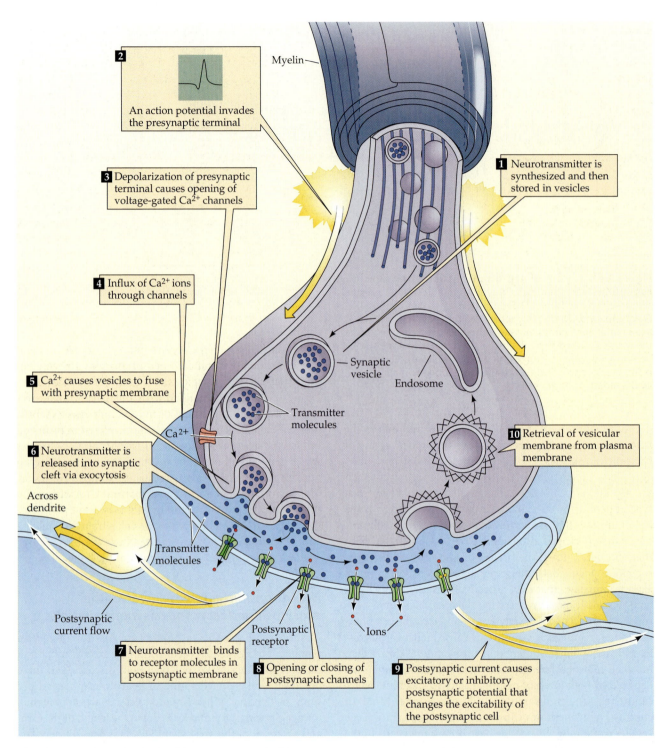

2 An action potential invades the presynaptic terminal

Myelin

1 Neurotransmitter is synthesized and then stored in vesicles

3 Depolarization of presynaptic terminal causes opening of voltage-gated Ca²⁺ channels

4 Influx of Ca²⁺ ions through channels

Synaptic vesicle

Endosome

5 Ca²⁺ causes vesicles to fuse with presynaptic membrane

Transmitter molecules

Ca²⁺

10 Retrieval of vesicular membrane from plasma membrane

6 Neurotransmitter is released into synaptic cleft via exocytosis

Across dendrite

Transmitter molecules

Postsynaptic current flow

Postsynaptic receptor

Ions

7 Neurotransmitter binds to receptor molecules in postsynaptic membrane

8 Opening or closing of postsynaptic channels

9 Postsynaptic current causes excitatory or inhibitory postsynaptic potential that changes the excitability of the postsynaptic cell

Figure 3.5 Processes involved in neurotransmission at a typical synapse using a classical neurotransmitter

vesicles, yet these molecules must somehow make their way past the membrane of the axon terminal and into the synaptic cleft. This occurs through a remarkable process known as **exocytosis.** Exocytosis is a fusion of the vesicle membrane with the membrane of the axon terminal, which exposes the inside of the vesicle to the outside of the cell. In this way, the vesicle is opened and its transmitter molecules are allowed to diffuse into the synaptic cleft. If you look back at the synapse shown in Figure 3.1, you can see that some vesicles are very close to the terminal membrane, whereas others are farther away. In fact, transmitter release doesn't occur just anywhere along the terminal, but only at specialized regions near the postsynaptic cell, which stain darkly in the electron micrograph. These release sites are called **active zones.** For exocytosis to take place, a vesicle must be transported to an active zone by a mechanism that isn't yet fully understood. There, the vesicle must "dock" at the active zone, much like a boat docking at a pier. This docking step is carried out by a cluster of proteins, some located in the vesicle membrane and others residing in the membrane of the axon terminal. Docking is followed by a step called "priming," which readies the vesicle for exocytosis once it receives the Ca^{2+} signal. Indeed, the Ca^{2+} channels that open in response to the membrane depolarization are concentrated in the active zones near the sites of vesicle docking, so the protein machinery is exposed to particularly high concentrations of Ca^{2+} when the channels open. One or more proteins that are sensitive to Ca^{2+} then cause the vesicle and terminal membranes to fuse, which allows the vesicle to open and the transmitter to be released. This process is illustrated in Figure 3.6.

Discussing the various proteins involved in vesicle docking and fusion is beyond the scope of this book, but it's nevertheless interesting to briefly consider how these proteins have been discovered. One method has been to analyze the effects of various drugs or naturally occurring toxins that affect the release process. For example, botulism poisoning results from a bacterial toxin (botulinum toxin) that blocks transmitter release at neuromuscular junctions, thus causing paralysis. Researchers have found that this blockade of release is due to enzymes within the toxin that attack some of the proteins that are required for the exocytosis process (see also Chapter 6). Another important method has been to use genetic mutants of the fruit fly *Drosophila melanogaster*. Using genetic engineering techniques, researchers knocked out the gene for a protein they suspected was important for exocytosis. The fruit fly larvae exhibited no transmitter release at the neuromuscular junction when their motor nerves were stimulated; consequently, the larvae were virtually paralyzed and couldn't even hatch from their egg cases (Deitcher et al., 1998).

Endocytosis   When a synaptic vesicle fuses with the axon terminal to release its transmitter contents, the vesicle membrane is temporarily added to the membrane of the terminal. If this process were never reversed, we can imagine that the terminal membrane would grow larger and larger as more and more vesicle membrane was added to it. In reality, a process called **endocytosis** quickly retrieves the vesicle membrane from the terminal membrane. New vesicles are then rapidly formed and refilled with neurotransmitter molecules so that they can participate again in transmitter release. This continu-

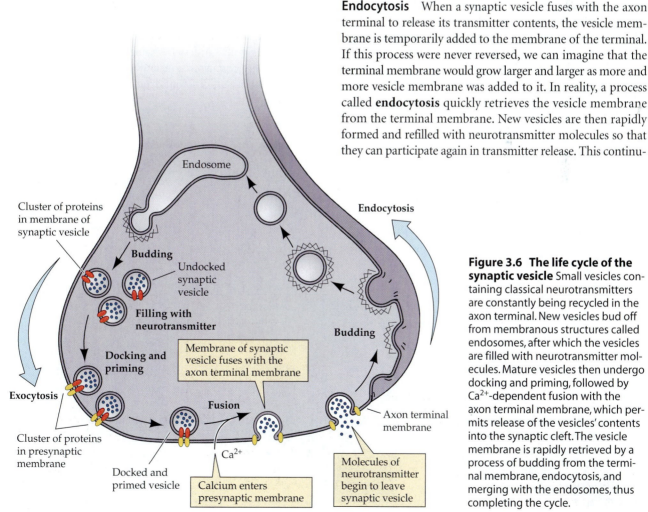

Figure 3.6 The life cycle of the synaptic vesicle Small vesicles containing classical neurotransmitters are constantly being recycled in the axon terminal. New vesicles bud off from membranous structures called endosomes, after which the vesicles are filled with neurotransmitter molecules. Mature vesicles then undergo docking and priming, followed by Ca^{2+}-dependent fusion with the axon terminal membrane, which permits release of the vesicles' contents into the synaptic cleft. The vesicle membrane is rapidly retrieved by a process of budding from the terminal membrane, endocytosis, and merging with the endosomes, thus completing the cycle.

ous release and re-formation of vesicles is termed **vesicle recycling** (see Figure 3.6). It is worth noting that recycling only occurs with the small vesicles containing classical transmitters, but not with the larger neuropeptide-containing vesicles. You'll recall that neuropeptide precursor proteins must be packaged into the large vesicles in the cell body; therefore, recycling of such vesicles cannot occur at the axon terminal.

Several mechanisms control the rate of neurotransmitter release by nerve cells

Neurotransmitter release is regulated by several different mechanisms. The most obvious is the rate of cell firing. When a neuron is rapidly firing action potentials, it will release much more transmitter than when it is firing at a slow rate. A second factor is the probability of transmitter release from the terminal. It might seem odd that an action potential could enter a terminal and open Ca^{2+} channels but not release any transmitter. Yet many studies have shown that synapses in different parts of the brain vary widely in the probability that even a single vesicle will undergo exocytosis in response to an action potential. Estimated probabilities range from less than 0.1 (10%) to 0.9 (90%) or greater for different populations of synapses. We don't yet know why these probabilities can vary so much, but it is clearly an important factor in the regulation of neurotransmitter release.

A third factor in the rate of transmitter release is the presence of **autoreceptors** on axon terminals or cell bodies and dendrites (Figure 3.7). An autoreceptor on a particular neuron is a receptor for the same neurotransmitter released by that neuron ("auto-" in this case means "self"). Neurons may possess two different kinds of autoreceptors: **terminal autoreceptors** and **somatodendritic autoreceptors.** Terminal autoreceptors are so named because they are located on axon terminals. When they are activated by the neurotransmitter, their main function is to inhibit further transmitter release. This function is particularly important when the cell is firing rapidly and there are high levels of neurotransmitter in the synaptic cleft. Think of the thermostat ("autoreceptor") in your house, which shuts off the furnace ("release mechanism") when the level of heat ("neurotransmitter") gets too high. Somatodendritic autoreceptors are also descriptively named, since they are autoreceptors found on the cell body (soma) or dendrites. When these autoreceptors are activated, they slow the rate of cell firing, which ultimately causes less neurotransmitter release, as fewer action potentials reach the axon terminals to stimulate exocytosis.

Researchers can use drugs to stimulate or block specific autoreceptors, thereby influencing the release of a particular neurotransmitter for experimental purposes. For example, administration of a low dose of the drug apomorphine to rats or mice selectively activates the terminal autoreceptors for DA. This results in less DA release, an overall reduction in dopaminergic transmission, and reduced locomotor activity in the animals. A different drug, whose name is abbrevi-

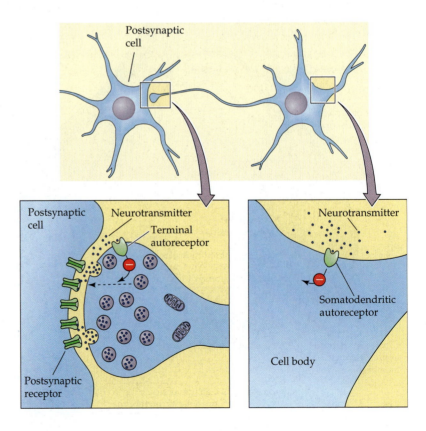

Figure 3.7 Terminal and somatodendritic autoreceptors Many neurons possess autoreceptors on their axon terminals and/or on their cell bodies and dendrites. Terminal autoreceptors inhibit neurotransmitter release, whereas somatodendritic autoreceptors reduce the rate of cell firing.

ated 8-OH-DPAT, activates the somatodendritic autoreceptors for 5-HT and powerfully inhibits the firing of serotonergic neurons. The behavioral effects of 8-OH-DPAT administration include increased appetite and altered responses on several tasks used to assess anxiety.

Finally, you'll recall from our earlier discussion that in addition to autoreceptors, axon terminals may also have receptors for other transmitters released at axoaxonal synapses. Such receptors have come to be known as **heteroreceptors,** to distinguish them from autoreceptors. Heteroreceptors also differ from autoreceptors in that they may either enhance or reduce the amount of transmitter being released from the axon terminal.

Neurotransmitters are inactivated by reuptake and by enzymatic breakdown

Any mechanical or biological process that can be turned on also must have a mechanism for termination (imagine the problem you would have with a car in which the ignition could not be turned off once the car had been started). Thus, it is necessary to terminate the synaptic signal produced by each instance of transmitter release so that the postsynaptic cell is free to respond to the next release. This termination is accomplished by removing neurotransmitter molecules from the synaptic cleft. How is this done?

Several different processes responsible for neurotransmitter removal are shown in Figure 3.8. One mechanism is enzymatic breakdown within or near the synaptic cleft. This mechanism is very important for the classical neurotransmitter ACh, for the lipid and gaseous transmitters, and also for the neuropeptide transmitters. An alternative mechanism

is for the neurotransmitter to be removed from the synaptic cleft by a transport process involving specialized proteins called **transporters** located on the cell membrane. This mechanism is important for amino acid transmitters like glutamate and GABA and also for amine transmitters such as DA, NE, and 5-HT. Transport out of the synaptic cleft is sometimes accomplished by the same cell that released the transmitter, in which case it is called **reuptake.** In other cases, the transmitter may be taken up either by the postsynaptic cell or by nearby glial cells (specifically astrocytes). Some important psychoactive drugs work by blocking neurotransmitter transporters. Cocaine, for example, blocks the transporters for DA, 5-HT, and NE. Many antidepressant drugs block the 5-HT transporter, the NE transporter, or both. Since these transporters are so important for clearing the neurotransmitter from the synaptic cleft, it follows that when the transporters are blocked, neurotransmitter molecules remain in the synaptic cleft for a longer period of time and neurotransmission is enhanced at those synapses.

When neurotransmitter transporters are active, some transmitter molecules removed from the synaptic cleft are reused by being packaged into recycled vesicles. However, other transmitter molecules are broken down by enzymes present within the cell. Thus, uptake and metabolic breakdown are not mutually exclusive processes. Many transmitter systems use both mechanisms. Finally, it is important to keep in mind the distinction between autoreceptors and transporters. Even though both may be present on axon terminals, they serve different functions. Terminal autoreceptors modulate transmitter release, but they don't transport the neurotransmitter. Transporters take up the transmitter from the synaptic cleft, but they are not autoreceptors.

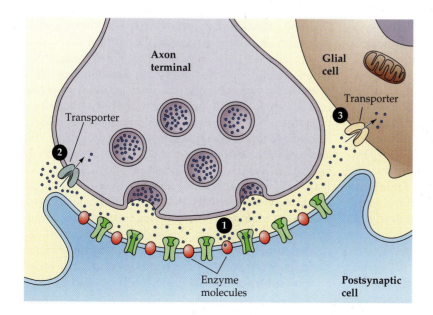

Figure 3.8 Neurotransmitter inactivation Neurotransmitter molecules can be inactivated by (1) enyzmatic breakdown; (2) reuptake by the axon terminal; or (3) uptake by nearby glial cells. Cellular uptake is mediated by specific membrane transporters for each neurotransmitter.

Section Summary

Synapses are specialized structures that mediate chemical communication between nerve cells. Synapses can be classified as axodendritic, axosomatic, or axoaxonic, depending on which part of the postsynaptic cell is receiving input from the presynaptic axon terminal. Axodendritic and axosomatic synapses affect the firing of the postsynaptic cell, whereas axoaxonic synapses either stimulate or inhibit neurotransmitter release from terminals of the postsynaptic cell. Connections between neurons and muscle cells are called neuromuscular junctions, and they have many features in common with ordinary synapses.

The chemical substances released at synapses and neuromuscular junctions are called neurotransmitters. The initial criteria for determining whether a substance qualifies as a neurotransmitter include (1) the presence of the substance in axon terminals, along with a mechanism for synthesis of the substance; (2) the presence of a mechanism for inactivating the substance; (3) release of the substance upon nerve stimulation; and (4) the presence of appropriate receptors on the postsynaptic cell. Pharmacologically, (5) application of the substance or an agonist drug to the postsynaptic cell should mimic the effect of nerve stimulation, whereas (6) applying an antagonist drug should block the effects of both nerve stimulation and the substance itself. Most neurotransmitters fall into one of several broad chemical categories: amino acid transmitters, monoamine transmitters, lipid transmitters, neuropeptide transmitters, and gaseous transmitters. Acetylcholine is an important neurotransmitter that doesn't fall into any of these categories. Many instances are known where two or more different neurotransmitters are synthesized and released from the same neuron.

Except for the neuropeptides, the axon terminals are the most critical site for the synthesis of most neurotransmitters. However, neuropeptides are formed from large precursor proteins that must be produced in the cell body and then transported down the axon to the terminals. Most neurotransmitters, including neuropeptides, are stored in synaptic vesicles. Within each axon terminal, a few vesicles are docked at specialized places called active zones. When an action potential invades the terminal, Ca^{2+} channels open in response to the membrane depolarization. This triggers a process known as exocytosis, which involves fusion of the vesicle membrane with the terminal membrane, followed by release of neurotransmitter molecules into the synaptic cleft. The vesicle membrane is subsequently removed from the axon terminal by the process of endocytosis, and new vesicles are generated. This continuous process of vesicle release and re-formation is called vesicle recycling.

Neurotransmitter release is controlled by several factors. First, faster firing by the neuron leads to increased release. Second, when an action potential reaches the axon terminal, it may or may not lead to vesicle exocytosis. The probability of release varies widely at different synapses throughout the brain. Third, transmitter release can be inhibited by the action of autoreceptors located either on the terminal (called terminal autoreceptors) or on the membrane of the cell body and dendrites (somatodendritic autoreceptors).

Finally, there are several mechanisms for terminating the action of neurotransmitters. One mechanism is enzymatic breakdown, which is important for ACh, lipid and gaseous transmitters, and neuropeptides. Another mechanism, which is used by amino acid and monoamine transmitters, is transport out of the synaptic cleft either by the axon terminal that released the transmitter (reuptake) or by nearby glial cells. Even when reuptake occurs, however, enzymatic metabolism within the cell is still needed to prevent the neurotransmitter from building up to excessive levels.

Neurotransmitter Receptors and Second-Messenger Systems

There are two major families of neurotransmitter receptors

In Chapter 1, you were introduced to the concept of a drug receptor. Many of the receptors for psychoactive drugs are actually receptors for various neurotransmitters. For this reason, it is very important to understand the characteristics of neurotransmitter receptors and how they function.

Virtually all neurotransmitter receptors are proteins, and in most cases these proteins are located on the plasma membrane of the cell. As we saw earlier, the cell possessing the receptor may be a neuron, a muscle cell, or a secretory cell. The neurotransmitter molecule binds to a specific site on the receptor molecule, which activates the receptor and produces a biochemical alteration in the receiving cell that may affect its excitability. For example, postsynaptic receptors on neurons usually influence the likelihood that the cell will generate an action potential. The effect of receptor activation may either be excitatory (increasing the probability of an action potential) or inhibitory (decreasing the probability of an action potential), depending on what the receptor does to the cell (see following sections). Recall that if a particular drug mimics the action of the neurotransmitter in activating the receptor, we say that the drug is an agonist at that receptor (see Chapter 1). If a drug blocks or inhibits the ability of the neurotransmitter to activate the receptor, then the drug is called an antagonist.

Two key concepts are necessary for understanding neurotransmitter receptors. First, almost all neurotransmitters discovered so far have more than one kind of receptor. Different varieties of receptors for the same transmitter are called **receptor subtypes** for that transmitter. The existence of sub-

TABLE 3.2 **Comparison of Ionotropic and Metabotropic Receptors**

Characteristics	Ionotropic receptors	Metabotropic receptors
Structure	4 or 5 subunits that assemble in the cell membrane	1 subunit
Mechanism of action	Contain an intrinsic ion channel that opens in response to neurotransmitter or drug binding	Activate G proteins in response to neurotransmitter or drug binding
Coupled to second messengers?	No	Yes
Speed of action	Fast	Slower

types adds complexity to the study of receptors, making the task of pharmacologists (as well as students!) more difficult. But this complexity has a positive aspect: If you can design a drug that stimulates or blocks just the subtype that you're interested in, you may be able to treat a disease more effectively and with fewer side effects. That is one of the central ideas that underlies modern drug design and the continuing search for new pharmaceutical agents.

The second key concept is that most neurotransmitter receptors fall into two broad categories: **ionotropic receptors** and **metabotropic receptors.** A particular transmitter may only use receptors that fit one or the other of these gen-

eral categories, or its receptor subtypes may fall into both categories. As shown in Table 3.2, ionotropic and metabotropic receptors differ in both their structure and function, so we will discuss them separately.

Ionotropic receptors   Ionotropic receptors work very rapidly, so they play a critical role in fast neurotransmission within the nervous system. Each ionotropic receptor is made up of several proteins called **subunits,** which come together in the cell membrane to form the complete receptor. Either four or five subunits are needed, depending on the receptor's overall structure (Figure 3.9A). At the center of the receptor

(A)

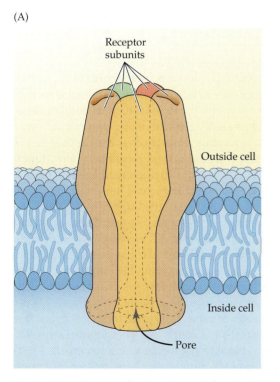

(B)

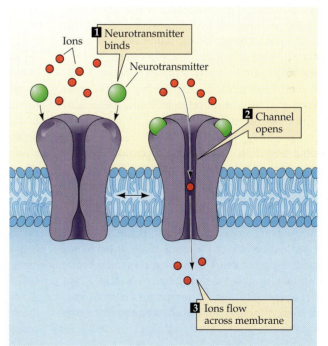

Figure 3.9 Structure and function of ionotropic receptors (A) Each receptor complex comprises either five (as shown) or four protein subunits that form a channel or pore in the cell mem-

brane. (B) Binding of the neurotransmitter to the receptor triggers channel opening and the flow of ions across the membrane.

is a channel or pore through which ions can flow. The receptor also possesses one or more binding sites for the neurotransmitter. In the resting state with no neurotransmitter present, the receptor channel is closed and no ions are moving. When the neurotransmitter binds to the receptor and activates it, the channel immediately opens and ions flow across the cell membrane (Figure 3.9B). When the neurotransmitter molecule leaves (dissociates from) the receptor, the channel quickly closes. Because of these features, a common alternative name for ionotropic receptors is **ligand-gated channel receptors.**[*]

Some ionotropic receptor channels allow sodium (Na^+) ions to flow into the cell from the extracellular fluid. Since these ions are positively charged, the cell membrane is depolarized, thereby producing an excitatory response of the postsynaptic cell. The best-known example of this kind of excitatory ionotropic receptor is the nicotinic receptor for ACh, which we discuss further in Chapter 6. A second type of ionotropic receptor channel permits the flow of Ca^{2+} as well as Na^+ ions across the cell membrane. As we will see shortly, Ca^{2+} can act as a **second messenger** to trigger many biochemical processes in the postsynaptic cell. One important ionotropic receptor that functions in this way is the *N*-methyl-D-aspartate (NMDA) receptor for the neurotransmitter glutamate (see Chapter 7). Finally, a third type of receptor channel is selective for chloride (Cl^-) ions to flow into the cell. These ions are negatively charged, thus leading to a hyperpolarization of the membrane and an inhibitory response of the postsynaptic cell. A good example of this kind of inhibitory ionotropic receptor is the $GABA_A$ receptor (see Chapter 7). From this discussion, you can see that the characteristics of the ion channel controlled by an ionotropic receptor are the key factor in determining whether that receptor excites the postsynaptic cell, inhibits the cell, or activates a second-messenger system.

Metabotropic receptors Metabotropic receptors act more slowly than ionotropic receptors. It takes longer for the postsynaptic cell to respond, but the response is also somewhat more long-lasting than in the case of ionotropic receptors. Metabotropic receptors comprise only a single protein subunit, which winds its way back and forth through the cell membrane seven times. Using the terminology of cell biology, we say that these receptors have seven **transmembrane domains;** in fact, they are sometimes abbreviated 7-TM receptors (Figure 3.10). It is important to note that metabotropic receptors do not possess a channel or pore. How, then, do these receptors work?

---

[*]This terminology distinguishes such channels from voltage-gated channels, which are controlled by the voltage across the cell membrane rather than the binding of a ligand such as a neurotransmitter or drug.

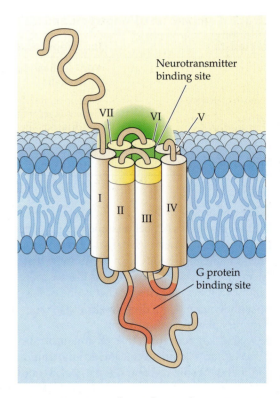

Figure 3.10 Structure of metabotropic receptors Each receptor comprises a single protein subunit with seven transmembrane domains (labeled here by Roman numerals).

Metabotropic receptors work by activating other proteins in the cell membrane called **G proteins.** Consequently, another name for this receptor family is **G protein–coupled receptors.** There are many different kinds of G proteins, and how a metabotropic receptor influences the postsynaptic cell depends on which G protein(s) the receptor activates. However, all G proteins operate by two major mechanisms. One is by stimulating or inhibiting the opening of ion channels in the cell membrane (Figure 3.11A). Potassium (K^+) channels, for example, are stimulated by specific G proteins at many synapses. When these channels open, K^+ ions flow out of the cell, the membrane is hyperpolarized, and consequently the cell firing is suppressed. This is a common mechanism of synaptic inhibition used by various receptors for ACh, DA, NE, 5-HT, GABA, and some neuropeptides like the endorphins. Note that the K^+ channels controlled by G proteins are not the same as the voltage-gated K^+ channels that work together with voltage-gated Na^+ channels to produce action potentials.

The second mechanism by which metabotropic receptors and G proteins operate is by stimulating or inhibiting certain enzymes in the cell membrane (Figure 3.11B). These enzymes are sometimes called **effector enzymes** because they produce biochemical and physiological effects in the postsynaptic cell.

(A)

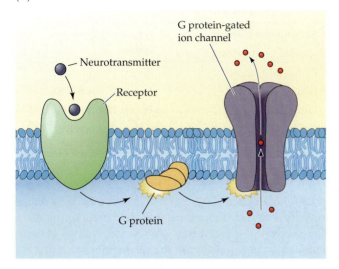

(B)

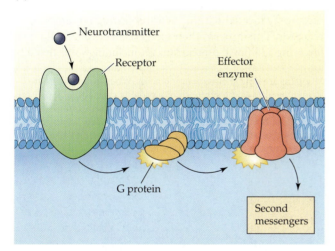

Figure 3.11 Functions of metabotropic receptors
Metabotropic receptors activate G proteins in the membrane, which may either (A) alter the opening of a G protein-gated ion channel or (B) stimulate an effector enzyme that either synthesizes or breaks down a second messenger.

Most of the effector enzymes controlled by G proteins are involved in either the synthesis or breakdown of small molecules called second messengers. Second messengers were first discovered in the 1960s and later found to play an important role in the chemical communication processes of both neurotransmitters and hormones. In these processes, the neurotransmitter or hormone was considered to be the "first messenger," and the "second messenger" within the receiving cell (the postsynaptic cell, in the case of a neurotransmitter) then carried out the biochemical change signaled by the first mes-

senger. Putting everything together, this mechanism of metabotropic receptor function involves (1) activation of a G protein, followed by (2) stimulation or inhibition of an effector enzyme in the membrane of the postsynaptic cell, followed by (3) increased synthesis or breakdown of a second messenger, followed by (4) biochemical or physiological changes in the postsynaptic cell due to the altered levels of the second messenger (see Figure 3.11B). This sequence of events is an example of a biochemical "cascade."

Second messengers work by activating specific protein kinases in a cell

Second-messenger systems are too complex to be completely covered in this text. We will therefore highlight a few of the most important systems and how they alter cellular function. One of the key ways in which second messengers work is by activating enzymes called **protein kinases** (Figure 3.12). Kinases are enzymes that **phosphorylate** another molecule; that is, they catalyze the addition of one or more phosphate groups ($-PO_4^{2-}$) to the molecule. As the name suggests, a protein kinase phosphorylates a protein. The substrate protein might be an ion channel, an enzyme involved in neurotransmitter synthesis, a neurotransmitter receptor or transporter, a

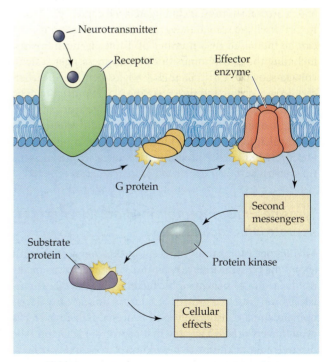

Figure 3.12 The mechanism of action of second messengers Second messengers work by activating protein kinases to cause phosphorylation of substrate proteins within the postsynaptic cell.

structural protein, or almost any other kind of protein. The phosphate group(s) added by the kinase then alters the functioning of the protein in some way. For example, an ion channel might open, a neurotransmitter-synthesizing enzyme might be activated, a receptor might become more sensitive to the neurotransmitter, and so forth. Furthermore, kinases can phosphorylate proteins in the cell nucleus that turn on or turn off specific genes in that cell. You can see that protein kinases activated by second messengers are capable of producing widespread and profound changes in the postsynaptic cell, even including long-lasting changes in gene expression.

Now let us consider a few specific second messengers and their protein kinases. The first second messenger to be discovered was **cyclic adenosine monophosphate (cAMP)**. Levels of cAMP are controlled by receptors for a number of different neurotransmitters, including DA, NE, 5-HT, and endorphins. Cyclic AMP stimulates a protein kinase called **protein kinase A (PKA)**. A related second messenger is **cyclic guanosine monophosphate (cGMP)**. One of the key regulators of cGMP is the novel gaseous messenger nitric oxide (Box 3.1). Cyclic GMP has its own kinase known as **protein kinase G (PKG)**. A third second-messenger system is sometimes termed the **phosphoinositide second-messenger system**. This complex system has several different effects, including activation of **protein kinase C (PKC)** and elevation of the level of Ca^{2+} ions within the postsynaptic cell. The phosphoinositide system is controlled by receptors for several neurotransmitters, including ACh, NE, and 5-HT. Finally, Ca^{2+} itself is a second messenger. Calcium levels in the cell can be increased by a number of different mechanisms, including the phosphoinositide second-messenger system, voltage-sensitive Ca^{2+} channels, and, as mentioned earlier, certain ionotropic receptors like the NMDA receptor. The protein kinase activated by Ca^{2+} requires the participation of an additional protein known as calmodulin. Hence, it is called **calcium/calmodulin kinase (CaMK)**. Ca^{2+} also helps to activate PKC. Table 3.3 summarizes these second-messenger systems and their associated protein kinases.

Tyrosine kinase receptors mediate the effects of neurotrophic factors

There is one more family of receptors that you need to learn about, the **tyrosine kinase receptors**. These receptors mediate the action of **neurotrophic factors**, proteins that stimulate the survival and growth of neurons during early development and are also involved in neuronal signaling. **Nerve growth factor (NGF)** was the first neurotrophic factor to be discovered, but there are now known to be many others, including **brain-derived neurotrophic factor (BDNF), neurotrophin-3 (NT-3),** and **NT-4.**

Three specific tyrosine kinase receptors are used by these neurotrophic factors: **trkA** (pronounced "track A") for NGF,

TABLE 3.3 Second-Messenger Systems and Protein Kinases

Second-messenger system	Associated protein kinase
Cyclic AMP (cAMP)	Protein kinase A (PKA)
Cyclic GMP (cGMP)	Protein kinase G (PKG)
Phosphoinositide	Protein kinase C (PKC)
Calcium (Ca^{2+})	Calcium/calmodulin kinase (CaMK)

trkB for BDNF and NT-4, and **trkC** for NT-3. The trk receptors are activated through the following mechanism. After the neurotrophic factor binds to its receptor, two of these complexes come together in the cell membrane, a process that is necessary for receptor activation (Figure 3.13). When the two trk receptors are activated, they phosphorylate each other on tyrosine residues* (hence the "tyrosine kinase receptor") located within the cytoplasmic region of each receptor. This process then triggers a complex sequence involving additional protein kinases, including some that dif-

---

*Proteins are long chains of amino acids. When amino acids are strung together in the synthesis of a protein, each adjacent pair of amino acids loses a water molecule (an H from one amino acid and an OH from the other). What remain are called "amino acid residues." Each residue is named for the specific amino acid it was derived from; in this case it is tyrosine.

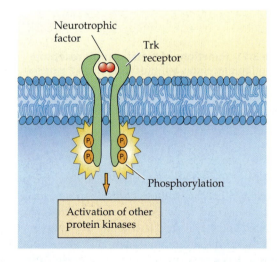

Figure 3.13 Activation of trk receptors Neurotrophic factors stimulate trk receptors by bringing two receptor molecules into close proximity in the cell membrane, which then leads to reciprocal phosphorylation of tyrosine residues and activation of other protein kinases.

BOX 3.1

The Cutting Edge

Just Say NO

A few neurotransmitters don't follow the rules outlined in this chapter. The most striking of these are two small molecules that are gases at room temperature: **nitric oxide** (**NO**) and **carbon monoxide** (**CO**). Yes, there is good evidence that the potentially deadly CO found in automobile exhaust and poorly ventilated furnaces is actually a signaling molecule in the brain. But we know much more about the workings of NO, so that will be the main focus of this discussion.

Nitric oxide is produced from the amino acid arginine in a simple biochemical reaction catalyzed by the enzyme **nitric oxide synthase** (**NOS**). There are several forms of NOS, one of which is found primarily in neurons and another that is present in endothelial cells (the cells that comprise the walls of blood vessels). The enzyme NOS, and therefore NO formation, is stimulated by increases in Ca^{2+} within the cell. The physiological role of NO has often been investigated using drugs that block NO synthesis by inhibiting NOS. Two such drugs are 7-nitroindazole (7-NI) and *N*-nitro-L-arginine methyl ester (L-NAME). After its release, NO is eventually inactivated by chemically reacting with oxygen (O_2) to yield NO_2 or NO_3.

There are several reasons why we say that NO breaks the normal rules for a neurotransmitter. First, as a gas, it readily passes through membranes. Thus it cannot be stored in synaptic vesicles like most transmitter substances. So nerve cells must make NO on demand when it is needed. Second, since NO is not in vesicles, it is not released by exocytosis but simply diffuses out of the nerve cell through the cell membrane. Third, once it reaches the extracellular fluid, NO is not con-

fined to the synapse but may travel some distance until it reaches target cells. Finally, in many cases NO is released by the postsynaptic rather than the presynaptic cell in the synapse. You'll recall that some neurotransmitter receptors can increase

Ca^{2+} levels within the postsynaptic cell. This may occur either through an ionotropic receptor such as the NMDA receptor or through a metabotropic receptor like certain of the receptors for ACh. If NOS is present and is activated by this rise in Ca^{2+}, then NO will

(continued on next page)

(A) Classical synaptic signaling

(B) Signaling by nitric oxide

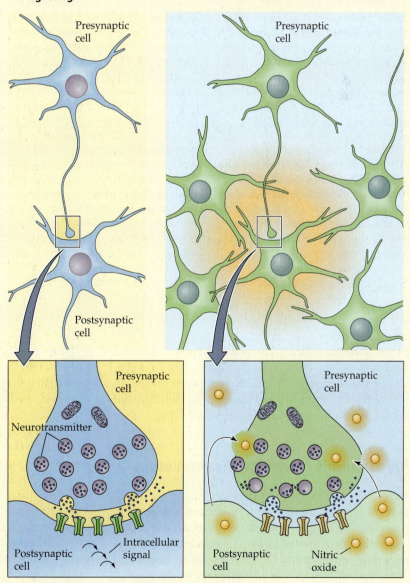

Presynaptic cell

Postsynaptic cell

Neurotransmitter

Presynaptic cell

Intracellular signal

Postsynaptic cell

Presynaptic cell

Postsynaptic cell

Presynaptic cell

Postsynaptic cell

Nitric oxide

BOX 3.1 (continued)

be produced by the postsynaptic cell, pass through the cell membrane, and travel to neighboring cells. One of the affected cells may even be the presynaptic cell, thus giving us an instance of neural transmission in reverse! Some of these features of NO signaling, and how they differ from the features of more typical synaptic signaling, are shown in Figure A.

The discovery of NO came about unexpectedly from the study of smooth muscle cells that surround the walls of arteries and that regulate the rate of arterial blood flow. A number of chemical substances, including the neurotransmitter ACh, were known to relax these smooth muscle cells, thus causing vasodilation (widening of the blood vessels) and increased blood flow. However, the mechanism by which this occurred was unclear until the early 1980s, when researchers showed that endothelial cells were necessary for the relaxant effect of ACh on the muscle. In addition, they showed that ACh stimulated the endothelial cells (by increasing intracellular Ca^{2+} levels) to produce a chemical factor that traveled to the nearby muscle cells and caused them to relax. This chemical factor was subsequently shown to be NO. One of the major mechanisms by which NO acts on its target cells is to activate an enzyme that synthesizes the second messenger cGMP. In smooth muscle, it is the rise in cGMP within the cells that leads to the relaxation response and the resulting dilation of the arteries.

Since the discovery of the relationship between NO and cGMP, this system has been the subject of many studies. One valuable outcome of this research concerns the effects of these agents on blood flow to the penis. An erection occurs when the penis is engorged with blood, which requires relaxation of the smooth muscles surrounding the penile arteries. As we have seen, smooth muscle relaxation is induced by cGMP. In turn, the amount of cGMP in the muscle cells depends on the rates of both its synthesis (due to NO) and breakdown. Cyclic GMP breakdown is catalyzed by the enzyme **cGMP phosphodiesterase.** A drug called sildenafil inhibits cGMP phosphodiesterase in the penis, thereby elevating cGMP levels and facilitating the erection. This compound, which is better known by its trade name Viagra, has helped many men overcome problems with erectile dysfunction.

Of course, the development of Viagra is not the only reason that pharmacologists are interested in NO. This messenger substance has also been implicated in the behavioral changes that occur in animals following repeated treatment with abused drugs. When rats or mice are chronically administered opioid drugs such as morphine, they develop a characteristic tolerance and physical dependence. These effects can be reduced by treatment of the animals with the NOS inhibitor L-NAME (Dambisya and Lee, 1996; Leza et al., 1996). If animals are injected once a day with cocaine, on the other hand, they show sensitization (the opposite of tolerance; see Chapter 1) to the behaviorally stimulating effects of the drug. Cocaine sensitization is likewise blocked both in genetically engineered mice that lack NOS (Itzhak et al., 1998) and in mice treated with the NOS inhibitor 7-NI (Itzhak, 1997). As tolerance, dependence, and sensitization have all been related to the addictive properties of abused drugs, it is possible that medications designed to alter NO levels may eventually be developed to help treat drug addicts. In addition, NOS inhibitors may have the additional therapeutic use of minimizing the development of tolerance in patients taking opiates for relief of chronic pain.

fer from those described in the previous section. Tyrosine kinase receptors and the neurotrophic factors they serve generally participate more in regulating long-term changes in gene expression and neuronal functioning than in rapid synaptic events that determine the rate of cell firing.

Pharmacology of Synaptic Transmission

Drugs can either enhance or interfere with virtually all aspects of synaptic transmission. Synaptic effects form the basis of almost all of the actions of psychoactive drugs, including drugs of abuse as well as those prescribed for the treatment of serious mental disorders such as depression and schizophrenia. Figure 3.14 illustrates the major ways in which such drugs can alter the neurotransmission process.

Drugs may either increase or decrease the rate of transmitter synthesis. If the drug is a chemical precursor to the transmitter, then the rate of transmitter formation may be increased. Two examples of this approach involve L-dihydroxyphenylalanine (L-DOPA), which is the precursor to DA, and 5-hydroxytryptophan (5-HTP), which is the precursor to 5-HT. Because patients suffering from Parkinson's disease are deficient in DA, the primary treatment for this neurological disorder is L-DOPA (see Chapter 5 for more information). Alternatively, a drug decreases levels of a neurotransmitter by inhibiting a key enzyme needed for transmitter synthesis. Alpha-methyl-para-tyrosine inhibits the enzyme tyrosine hydroxylase, which helps manufacture both DA and NE, whereas para-chlorophenylalanine inhibits the 5-HT-synthesizing enzyme tryptophan hydroxylase.

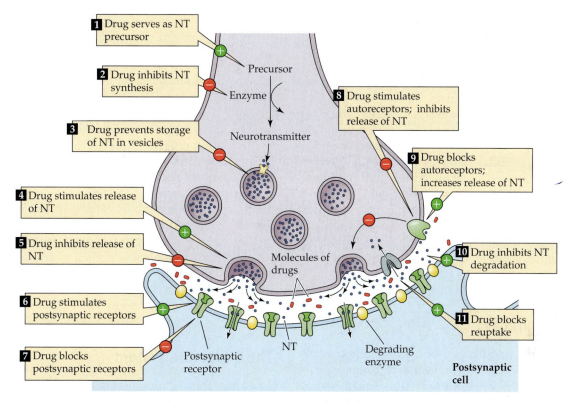

Figure 3.14 Summary of the mechanisms by which drugs can alter synaptic transmission NT = neurotransmitter; + denotes a mechanism that stimulates or facilitates transmission; – denotes a process that inhibits transmission.

Besides administering a precursor substance, you can also enhance the action of a neurotransmitter by reducing its inactivation. This can be accomplished in two ways. First, levels of the transmitter can be increased by blocking the enzyme involved in its breakdown. Physostigmine blocks the enzyme acetylcholinesterase, which breaks down ACh, whereas phenelzine blocks monoamine oxidase (MAO), an enzyme that is important in the breakdown of DA, NE, and 5-HT. As we will see in Chapter 16, phenelzine and other MAO-inhibiting drugs are sometimes used to treat patients with depression. For neurotransmitters that use transporters for reuptake out of the synaptic cleft, a second way to reduce neurotransmitter inactivation is to block those transporters. This increases the amount and prolongs the presence of the transmitter in the synaptic cleft, thereby enhancing its effects on the postsynaptic cell. As described previously, cocaine blocks the transporters for DA, NE, and 5-HT, and drugs that more selectively prevent reuptake of 5-HT are commonly used as antidepressant medications (see Chapters 11 and 16).

Other drugs affect neurotransmitter storage or release. For example, reserpine blocks the storage of DA, NE, and 5-HT in synaptic vesicles. Reserpine treatment initially causes a burst of neurotransmitter release as the vesicles empty out,

but this is followed by a period of extremely low transmitter levels, because storage in vesicles is necessary to prevent breakdown of transmitter molecules by enzymes present in the axon terminal. Amphetamine stimulates the release of DA and NE from the cytoplasm of the axon terminal, whereas a related substance called fenfluramine produces the same effect on 5-HT. These releasing agents work by reversing the effect of the neurotransmitter transporters. That is, instead of the transporters taking up transmitter molecules into the neuron from the synaptic cleft, they work in the reverse direction to carry the transmitter out of the neuron and into the synaptic cleft. As we saw earlier, some drugs alter neurotransmitter release in a different way, by stimulating or inhibiting autoreceptors that control the release process. Clonidine and 8-OH-DPAT stimulate autoreceptors for NE and 5-HT, respectively. In both cases, such stimulation reduces release of the related transmitter. Autoreceptor inhibition can be produced by yohimbine in the case of NE and pindolol in the case of 5-HT. Not surprisingly, administration of these compounds increases transmitter release.

One final mechanism of action can be seen in drugs that act on postsynaptic receptors for a specific neurotransmitter.

If the drug is an agonist for a particular receptor subtype, it will mimic the effect of the neurotransmitter on that receptor. If the drug is a receptor antagonist, it will inhibit the effect of the transmitter on the receptor. Many psychoactive drugs, both therapeutic and recreational, are receptor agonists. Examples include benzodiazepines, which are agonists at benzodiazepine receptors and are used clinically as sedative and anti-anxiety drugs (see Chapter 17); opiates like heroin and morphine, which are agonists at opioid receptors (see Chapter 10); nicotine, which is an agonist at the nicotinic receptor subtype for ACh (see Chapter 6); and THC, which is an agonist at cannabinoid receptors (see Chapter 13). Receptor antagonists are likewise important in pharmacology. Most drugs used to treat schizophrenic patients are antagonists at the D_2 receptor subtype for DA (see Chapter 18), while the widely ingested substance caffeine is an antagonist at receptors for the neurotransmitter adenosine (see Chapter 12).

Section Summary

Multiple receptor subtypes exist for almost all neurotransmitters. Despite this diversity, neurotransmitter receptors can be categorized as either ionotropic or metabotropic. Ionotropic receptors comprise multiple protein subunits that form an intrinsic ion channel in the center of the receptor complex. They are permeable either to cations such as Na^+ or Ca^{2+}, or anions such as Cl^-. Ionotropic receptors mediate fast excitatory and inhibitory neurotransmission, particularly involving amino acid transmitters like glutamate and GABA. Metabotropic receptors are each composed of only a single subunit. They function by coupling to G proteins in the membrane, which in turn regulate ion (for example, K^+) channel opening and also stimulate or inhibit effector enzymes involved in the synthesis or breakdown of second-messenger molecules. Metabotropic signaling is slower but longer-lasting than signaling via ionotropic receptors.

Second messengers typically work by activating specific protein kinases, enzymes that alter the functioning of other proteins by catalyzing the addition of one or more phosphate groups. Some key second-messenger systems involved in neurotransmission are the cAMP, cGMP, and phosphoinositide systems. These second messengers activate protein kinase A, protein kinase G, and protein kinase C, respectively. An additional component of the cGMP system is the novel gaseous messenger nitric oxide, which stimulates cGMP formation. Besides the substances already mentioned, Ca^{2+} can function as a second messenger and can activate calcium/calmodulin kinase.

Other receptors, called tyrosine kinase receptors, mediate signaling by neurotrophic factors such as NGF, BDNF, NT-3, and NT-4. Each neurotrophic factor molecule binds to two receptors in the cell membrane, thereby triggering reciprocal phosphorylation of tyrosine residues followed by a further signaling cascade. Neurotrophic factors generally regulate long-term changes in gene expression involved in neuronal survival, growth, and maintenance.

Psychoactive drugs exert their subjective and behavioral effects almost entirely by modifying one or more aspects of synaptic transmission. Drugs may increase or decrease the rate of transmitter synthesis, or they may reduce transmitter inactivation by inhibiting enzymatic breakdown or blocking reuptake. Other modes of drug action involve blockade of vesicular neurotransmitter storage, stimulation of transmitter release, or activation or inhibition of neurotransmitter autoreceptors. Finally, a key mechanism of action of many psychoactive drugs is direct stimulation (agonists) or blockade (antagonists) of neurotransmitter receptors.

The Endocrine System

As we have seen, neurotransmitters normally travel only a tiny distance before reaching their target at the other side of the synaptic cleft or sometimes a little farther away. Another method of cellular communication, however, involves the release of chemical substances called **hormones** into the bloodstream. Hormones are secreted by specialized organs called **endocrine glands.** Upon reaching the circulation, hormones can travel long distances before reaching target cells anywhere in the body. To respond to a given hormone, a target cell must possess specific receptors for that hormone, just as a postsynaptic cell must to respond to a neurotransmitter. Moreover, sometimes the same substances (for example, norepinephrine and epinephrine) are used both as neurotransmitters within the brain and as hormones within the

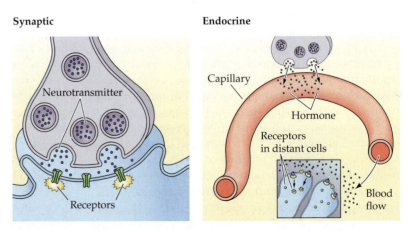

Figure 3.15 Comparison of synaptic versus endocrine communication

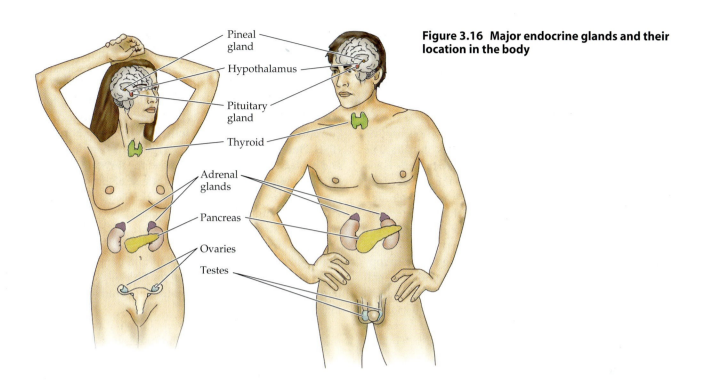

Figure 3.16 Major endocrine glands and their location in the body

endocrine system. Thus, synaptic and endocrine communication are similar in many respects, though they differ in the proximity of the cells involved and the anatomic features of synapses that were described earlier (Figure 3.15).

Endocrine glands can secrete multiple hormones

As shown in Figure 3.16, a number of endocrine glands are located throughout the body. Some of these glands secrete more than one type of hormone. We'll now give a brief description of each gland and its associated hormone(s), including the chemical classification and functions of that hormone.

The **adrenal glands** lie over each kidney. The adrenals are actually two separate glands that have come together during embryonic development (Figure 3.17). The inner part of the gland, which is called the **adrenal medulla,** is derived from nervous system tissue. Like a sympathetic ganglion, it receives input from the preganglionic fibers of the sympathetic nervous system (see Chapter 2). Cells of the adrenal medulla, which are called **chromaffin cells,** secrete the hormones **epinephrine (EPI)** and **norepinephrine (NE),** both of which are monoamines. Physical or psychological stressors stimulate the release of EPI and NE as part of the classic "fight-or-flight" response. Once in the bloodstream, these hormones mobilize glucose (sugar) from the liver to provide immediate energy, and they also divert blood from the internal organs (e.g., the organs of digestion) to the muscles in case physical action is needed. Some of their effects con-

tribute to the physical sensations that we experience when we're highly aroused or stressed (e.g., racing heart and cold, clammy hands).

The outer part of the adrenal gland, the **adrenal cortex,** secretes hormones called **glucocorticoids.** Which glucocorticoid is present depends on the species: humans and other primates make **cortisol** (sometimes called hydrocortisone), whereas rats and mice make **corticosterone.** Glucocorticoids belong to a class of molecules known as **steroids,** all of which are derived from the precursor cholesterol. One of the main functions of glucocorticoids is to maintain normal blood glucose levels and to help store excess glucose for future use.

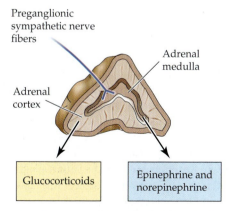

Figure 3.17 Structure of the adrenal gland, showing the outer cortex and the inner medulla

These hormones are also secreted in increased amounts during stress and normally help us cope with stressful experiences. However, there is substantial evidence that chronic stress may lead to serious consequences—possibly even damage to certain parts of the brain—if high glucocorticoid levels persist for long periods of time (Sapolsky, 1996).

Other glands that secrete steroid hormones are the **gonads:** the **ovaries** in females and the **testes** in males. The ovaries secrete female sex hormones called **estrogens** (such as **estradiol**) and **progesterone,** whereas the testes secrete male sex hormones called **androgens** (such as **testosterone**). These hormones determine some of the physical differences between males and females (the so-called secondary sex characteristics) that occur following puberty. Testosterone also has two other important roles. During early development, this hormone acts within the brain to produce neural changes important for determining later gender-based differences in behavior. Then, later on, it plays a significant role in stimulating sexual motivation in males and even in females (both genders possess some amount of each other's sex hormones).

Within the pancreas, there is an endocrine gland known as the **islets of Langerhans.** Cells within this tissue secrete two hormones, **insulin** and **glucagon.** Insulin release is stimulated by food intake, and together with glucagon, it plays an important role in regulating glucose and other sources of metabolic energy. Lack of insulin gives rise to the serious disorder diabetes. Both insulin and glucagon are peptide hormones, similar to the neuropeptides discussed earlier but somewhat larger in size.

Residing in the throat is the **thyroid gland,** which secretes **thyroxine (T4)** and **triiodothyronine (T3).** These hormones are also important for normal energy metabolism. Underactivity of the thyroid gland (hypothyroidism) causes feelings of weakness and lethargy, whereas thyroid overactivity (hyperthyroidism) leads to excessive energy and nervousness. The two thyroid hormones are made from the amino acid tyrosine, which is the same precursor used to make DA, NE, and EPI (see Chapter 5).

The **pineal gland** is situated just over the brain stem and is covered over by the cerebral hemispheres. This gland secretes the hormone **melatonin,** which is synthesized using the neurotransmitter 5-HT as a precursor. Melatonin has been implicated in the control of various rhythmic functions, which differ depending on the species. In humans and many other vertebrates, most melatonin secretion occurs during the night, which suggests a possible role in controlling sleep rhythms. Tablets containing small amounts of melatonin can be purchased over the counter in drug stores and supermarkets, and for some people, these tablets induce drowsiness and faster sleep onset.

The **pituitary gland** is sometimes called the "master gland," as it secretes several hormones that control other glands. The pituitary is found just under the hypothalamus and is connected to that brain structure by a thin stalk. Like the adrenals, the pituitary actually comprises two separate glands with different hormones that serve distinct functions. The **anterior pituitary** secretes **thyroid-stimulating hormone (TSH;** also known as thyrotropin), **adrenocorticotropic hormone (ACTH), follicle-stimulating hormone (FSH), luteinizing hormone (LH), growth hormone (GH),** and **prolactin (PRL).** TSH stimulates the thyroid gland and ACTH promotes the synthesis and release of glucocorticoids from the adrenal cortex. FSH and LH together control the growth and functioning of the gonads, whereas LH also stimulates estrogen and androgen secretion by the ovaries and testes, respectively. GH stimulates the production of insulin-like growth factor I (IGF-I) from peripheral organs such as the liver; IGF-I is critical for skeletal growth during development. Lastly, PRL promotes milk production by the mammary glands.

The pituitary stalk connecting the hypothalamus with the pituitary gland contains blood vessels that carry special **hypothalamic-releasing hormones** (Figure 3.18). These hormones are mainly neuropeptides manufactured by various groups of neurons in the hypothalamus. Instead of forming normal synapses, these neurons release the peptides into blood capillaries in a region called the **median eminence.** Blood vessels then carry the releasing hormones to the hormone-secreting cells of the anterior pituitary. For example, **thyrotropin-releasing hormone (TRH)** is a hypothalamic peptide that stimulates the release of TSH, **corticotropin-releasing hormone (CRH)** (alternatively called corticotropin-releasing factor, or CRF) stimulates ACTH release (corticotropin is another name for ACTH), and **gonadotropin-releasing hormone (GnRH)** stimulates both FSH and LH. We can thus see that the endocrine system sometimes functions through the interactions of several glands, with one gland controlling another until the final hormone is secreted. For example, stress does not directly cause increased glucocorticoid secretion from the adrenal cortex. Instead, stress leads to enhanced CRH release from the hypothalamus, which provokes ACTH release from the anterior pituitary; the ACTH travels through the bloodstream to the adrenal glands, where it stimulates the secretion of glucocorticoids. Because of this complicated control system, it may take a few minutes before the level of glucocorticoids in our blood is significantly increased. Thus the endocrine system works much more slowly than chemical communication by neurotransmitters.

In addition to blood vessels connecting the hypothalamus to the anterior pituitary, the pituitary stalk also contains the axons of specialized secretory neurons located in the hypothalamus. These axons reach the **posterior pituitary,** where, like the hypothalamic neurons mentioned earlier, they form endings on blood vessels instead of other

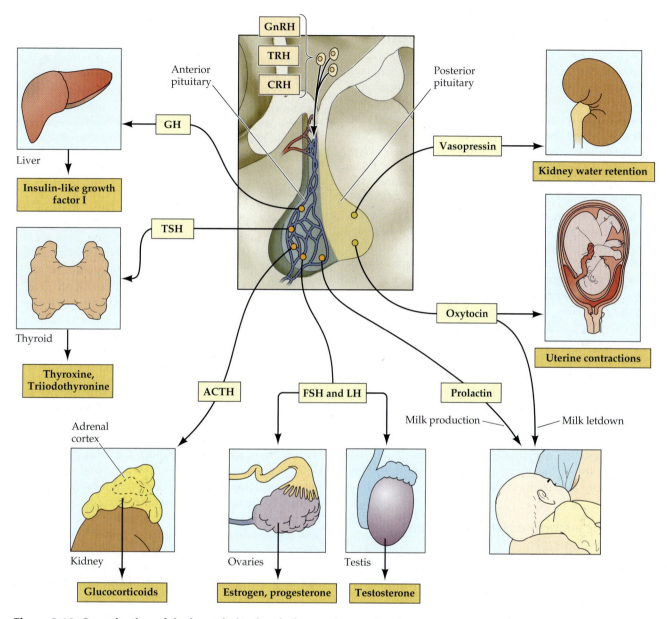

Figure 3.18 Organization of the hypothalamic–pituitary axis Note that the axon terminals of the hypothalamic-releasing hormone neurons are located near blood capillaries in the median eminence, whereas the oxytocin and vasopressin neurons send their axons all the way into the posterior lobe of the pituitary gland. For the purpose of simplicity, not all hypothalamic-releasing hormones are shown.

cells. The secretory neurons synthesize and release the peptide hormones **vasopressin** and **oxytocin** from the posterior pituitary into the bloodstream. Vasopressin (also called antidiuretic hormone) acts on the kidneys to increase water retention (that is, make the urine more concentrated). Alcohol inhibits vasopressin secretion, which is one of the reasons people urinate so frequently when they drink (it's not just the increased fluid consumption). Oxytocin is known mainly for two important physiological functions in female mammals: stimulation of uterine contractions during childbirth and triggering of milk letdown from the breasts during lactation. In recent years, there have also been interesting findings from animal studies suggesting that both oxytocin and vasopressin may play an important role in parenting and other kinds of affiliative behavior (Young et al., 2001).

Mechanisms of hormone action vary

As mentioned in Chapter 1, there are two broad types of receptors used in cellular communication: extracellular (membrane) receptors and intracellular receptors. Earlier in the present chapter we observed that most neurotransmitter receptors are located on the cell membrane. In contrast, hormones use a variety of different kinds of receptors, both extracellular and intracellular.

Peptide hormones function by means of membrane receptors (Figure 3.19A). Some of these are just like metabotropic neurotransmitter receptors, working through second-messenger systems. One example is the receptors for CRH, which stimulate formation of the second messenger cAMP. However, some hormones, such as insulin, use tyrosine kinase receptors similar to the trk receptors described earlier.

Steroid and thyroid hormones operate through intracellular receptors (Figure 3.19B). These receptors are proteins just like the membrane receptors for neurotransmitters or peptide hormones, but they are generally located within the cell nucleus, where they function as **transcription factors** to either turn on or turn off the expression of specific genes within the cell. Since gene expression determines which proteins are made by the cell, the ultimate effects of steroid and thyroid hormones are seen in the altered synthesis of particular proteins. This process takes much longer (many minutes to a few hours or more) than the rapid effects typically produced by membrane receptors. On the other hand, changes in gene expression and protein synthesis are also longer-lasting, thus allowing an animal or person to keep responding to a hormone long after it is released.

Why is the endocrine system important to pharmacologists?

By this time, you may be wondering why pharmacologists are concerned about hormones and the endocrine system.

Actually, there are a number of good reasons, four of which we'll briefly mention here:

1. Both therapeutic and abused drugs can alter the secretion of many hormones, causing physiological abnormalities. For example, chronic alcoholism can lead to reduced testosterone levels, testicular atrophy, and impotence in men. Alcoholic women may have menstrual disorders and at least temporarily become infertile (see Chapter 9).

2. Hormones may alter the behavioral responses to drugs. This is illustrated in the important role played by glucocorticoids in the effects of amphetamine and cocaine (Box 3.2).

3. Hormones themselves sometimes have psychoactive properties like those of certain drugs. We mentioned earlier that melatonin has a sedative effect on many people. In Chapter 16, we also discuss how thyroid hormones are occasionally given as antidepressant medications.

4. The secretion of pituitary hormones and other hormones dependent on the pituitary is controlled by neurotransmitter systems in the brain. This fact enables us to use the endocrine system as a "window to the brain" that tells us if a particular neurotransmitter system has been altered by disease (such as a psychiatric or neurological disorder), injury, or prior psychoactive drug use.

Let's look at an example of how this works. A drug known as fenfluramine stimulates the release of 5-HT from axon endings. Serotonin is one of several neurotransmitters that regulates secretion of the anterior pituitary hormone prolactin (PRL). Consequently, PRL levels in the blood are elevated following administration of fenfluramine in both humans or animals. Furthermore, deficient functioning of the 5-HT system shows up as a reduced PRL response to fenfluramine. This approach has recently been used to study the long-term effects of 3,4-methylenedioxymethamphetamine (MDMA, or "Ecstasy"), a drug that can cause damage to the 5-HT system. A group of Italian researchers gave fenfluramine to

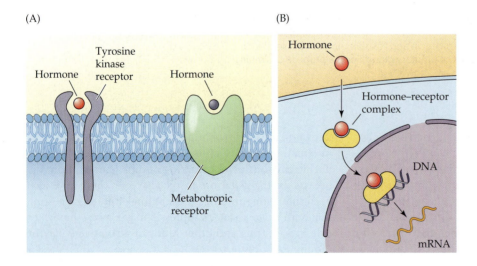

(A)   (B)

Figure 3.19 Hormonal signaling is mediated by a variety of extracellular and intracellular receptors

BOX 3.2 Pharmacology in Action

Stress, Glucocorticoids, and Psychostimulants

Among the most addictive drugs are cocaine and amphetamine, members of the general category called psychostimulants (see Chapter 11). In parallel with their high addiction potential, psychostimulants are very reinforcing to animals. For example, rats, mice, and even primates will self-administer these drugs by performing an operant response such as pressing a lever (see Chapter 4). Psychostimulants also produce increased locomotor activity when given to rats and mice in low doses.

There are clinical reports that abstinent human addicts sometimes relapse (return to their drug abuse) when confronted with stressful life events. These reports have led investigators to study how stress and stress hormones (glucocorticoids, for example) may affect drug responses in animals. The results show that stressors generally enhance the responsiveness of rats and mice to psychostimulants, as measured in several different ways (Piazza and Le Moal, 1996). First, prior stress increases the locomotor-stimulating effects of amphetamine or cocaine. Second, stress can enhance the initiation or increase the rate of psychostimulant self-administration under the appropriate conditions. Third, stress can enhance psychostimulant-seeking

behavior in animal models of drug relapse. In such studies, the animals are first conditioned to self-administer the drug (cocaine, for example) on a daily basis. Once the self-administration response has stabilized, the animals are subjected to a prolonged period of behavioral extinction in which no drug is given regardless of how many times the lever is pressed. At this point, there is usually very little behavioral responding by the subjects. However, several studies found that prior exposure of rats to a foot shock stress for just 10 or 15 minutes led to a large increase in lever pressing, even though there was still no cocaine available to the animals (Erb et al., 1996; Ahmed and Koob, 1997).

Based on these findings, it appears that stress increases the motivation for drug-seeking behavior in animals, just as it does in humans. It is important to note that this effect is selec-

tive, since it does not carry over to other motivational systems such as food reward. This difference is illustrated in the accompanying figure, which shows the influence of a social stressor on cocaine-reinforced but not food-reinforced responding in rats (Miczek and Mutschler, 1996).

Since we know that stress causes the release of glucocorticoids from the adrenal cortex, could these hormones be involved in the effects of stress on psychostimulant sensitivity? The answer appears to be yes. In one recent study, adrenalectomy (surgical removal of the adrenal glands) of rats prevented the ability of foot shock stress to reinstate lever pressing in a cocaine relapse model (Erb et al., 1998). However, when adrenalectomized rats were treated with corticosterone (the main glucocorticoid in rodents), foot shock had the same effect as in normal animals. There is also evidence that corticosterone mediates the effects of stress on the locomotor response to psychostimulants. Rats can be adrenalectomized

(continued on next page)

Selective effect of social stress on cocaine-reinforced responding Male rats were trained to press a lever for either cocaine reinforcement (A) 0.125 mg per infusion, (B) 0.063 mg per infusion, or food reinforcement using operant schedules that yielded comparable response rates. After three baseline sessions, three additional sessions were conducted in which each subject was placed for 60 minutes within the cage of a resident male rat (the "intruder" was protected from physical attack by a wire mesh enclosure) and then immediately tested for lever-pressing behavior. As shown in the right part of each graph, this social stress caused a large increase in cocaine self-administration but had no effect on responding for food. (After Miczek and Mutschler, 1996.)

(A)

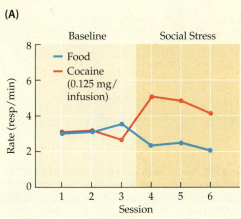

(B)

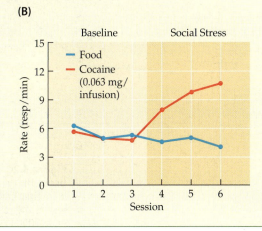

and then treated with corticosterone in a way that keeps the blood level constant. Under such conditions, stress did not enhance the locomotor response to amphetamine (Deroche et al., 1992).

People often think that "hard" drugs such as cocaine or heroin are instantly addicting if taken even once. As will be discussed in Chapter 8, this is a mistaken idea. Some individuals seem to be much more vulnerable than others to the potentially addicting qualities of abused drugs. Although we don't yet know why this is, Piazza and Le Moal (1996) hypothesize that stress reactivity may play a significant role in this individual variability. In an important study published in 1991, Piazza and his colleagues found that normal rats could be divided into two groups, "high responders" (HR) and "low responders" (LR), based on their behavioral and hormonal responses to the mild stress of being placed in a novel environment. The HR group moved around more in the novel environment

and showed a prolonged increase in plasma corticosterone levels compared to the LR group. When these same animals were given the opportunity to self-administer amphetamine, the HR group responded much more strongly for the drug. Furthermore, self-administration by the LR group could be increased by giving them corticosterone (Piazza et al., 1991). Thus, even in the absence of experimenter-induced stress, glucocorticoids alter the reinforcing effects of psychostimulants and may play a role in naturally occurring individual differences in drug sensitivity.

How do stress and glucocorticoids affect responsiveness to psychostimulants? In later chapters, you will learn that a neural pathway from a brain area called the ventral tegmental area to another area known as the nucleus accumbens is critical for behavioral responses to psychostimulant drugs. This pathway uses DA as its neurotransmitter. One group of investigators

found that prior stress enhances the ability of cocaine to increase DA in the nucleus accumbens and that this effect requires elevated levels of corticosterone produced by the stress (Rougé-Pont et al., 1995). This provides a possible mechanism for some of the findings presented above. According to this idea, stress causes secretion of glucocorticoids from the adrenal cortex. These hormones alter the responsiveness of the DA system so that when cocaine or amphetamine is given, more DA is released in the nucleus accumbens. In turn, this increase in DA leads to greater locomotor behavior by the animal, enhanced initiation of psychostimulant self-administration, or heightened drug-seeking behavior if the self-administration response had previously been extinguished. More research is needed to test this theoretical model relating stress and glucocorticoids to DA and psychostimulant sensitivity.

young men who had a history of repeated MDMA use and monitored the levels of PRL in the subjects' blood over the following 3 hours. Compared to control subjects, the MDMA users showed virtually no increase in PRL, even after 12 months of abstinence from the drug (Gerra et al., 2000; Figure 3.20). These results are consistent with brain imaging studies that also indicate abnormalities in the 5-HT system with MDMA use (see Chapter 11).

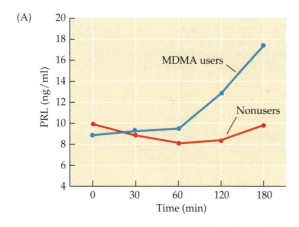

(A)

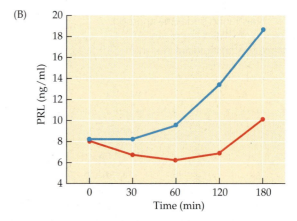

(B)

Figure 3.20 Plasma PRL responses to fenfluramine in MDMA users and nonusers Thirty milligrams of D-fenfluramine was given orally at time 0 and blood samples were then collected at 30-minute intervals for the next 3 hours. The MDMA users were tested after either (A) 3 weeks or (B) 12 months of abstinence from the drug. (After Gerra et al., 2000.)

Section Summary

Like neurotransmitters, hormones secreted by endocrine glands represent an important class of signaling molecules. Hormones are released into the bloodstream, where they may travel long distances before reaching their target cells in the body. Despite important differences between synaptic and endocrine communication, the same substance is sometimes used as both a neurotransmitter and a hormone.

The endocrine glands discussed in this chapter include the adrenal glands, the gonads, the thyroid gland, the pineal gland, and the pituitary gland. Each adrenal gland comprises an inner medulla and an outer cortex. The adrenal medulla is derived from nervous system tissue and receives input from the preganglionic fibers of the sympathetic nervous system. The chromaffin cells of the adrenal medulla secrete the hormones epinephrine and norepinephrine, both of which are released in response to stressful stimuli. The adrenal cortex secretes gluococorticoids such as cortisol and corticosterone. These steroid hormones serve important metabolic functions, but they also respond to stress like epinephrine and norepinephrine.

Other steroid hormones are synthesized and released by the gonads. In females, ovaries secrete estrogens and progesterone, whereas in males, testes secrete androgens such as testosterone. These gonadal steroids are responsible for many of the secondary sex characteristics that appear following puberty. During early development, testosterone produces structural changes in the brain that differentiate males from females, and then later in life it is involved in stimulating sexual motivation.

The islets of Langerhans and the thyroid gland secrete hormones important in energy metabolism. Insulin and glucagon are released from separate populations of cells within the islets of Langerhans. Together, these two peptide hormones regulate blood levels and storage of glucose and other sources of metabolic energy. The hormones of the thyroid gland, thyroxine and triiodothyronine, are both made from the amino acid tyrosine. Hypo- or hyperthyroidism leads to characteristic symptoms of either lethargy or excessive energy, respectively.

Two endocrine glands located close to the brain are the pineal gland and the pituitary gland. The pineal gland, situated just over the brain stem, synthesizes the hormone melatonin using 5-HT as a precursor. Melatonin has been implicated in the regulation of various types of rhythmic activity, including sleep. The pituitary gland is found just under the hypothalamus and is connected to it. The pituitary is divided into two separate glands, the anterior and posterior pituitary glands, which serve different functions.

The anterior pituitary secretes TSH, ACTH, FSH, LH, GH, and PRL. TSH and ACTH stimulate the thyroid and adrenal glands (cortex), respectively, whereas FSH and LH together control the growth and functioning of the gonads. GH stimulates skeletal growth during development, and PRL plays an important role in promoting milk production during lactation. The hypothalamic-releasing hormones TRH, CRH, and GnRH are neuropeptides synthesized within the hypothalamus that trigger the release of TSH, ACTH, and the gonadotrophins FSH and LH. Because of this organizational structure, in which several glands must stimulate each other until the final hormone product is secreted, the endocrine system works much more slowly than chemical communication by neurotransmitters.

The posterior pituitary secretes two small peptide hormones, vasopressin and oxytocin. Vasopressin enhances water retention by the kidneys, whereas oxytocin stimulates uterine contractions during childbirth and also triggers milk letdown from the breasts during lactation. There is also evidence that these hormones promote affiliative behaviors in some species.

The actions of hormones are mediated by several different kinds of receptors. Some are metabotropic receptors similar to those discussed for various neurotransmitters. Others are intracellular receptors that function as transcription factors that control gene expression. Still others are tyrosine kinase receptors.

The endocrine system is important to pharmacologists for several reasons. These include the fact that (1) drugs can adversely alter endocrine function; (2) hormones may alter the behavioral responses to drugs; (3) hormones themselves sometimes have psychoactive properties; and (4) the endocrine system can be used as a window to the brain to help us determine the functioning of a specific neurotransmitter system by measuring changes in hormone secretion under the appropriate conditions.

Recommended Readings

Cousin, M. A., and Robinson, P. J. (1999). Mechanisms of synaptic vesicle recycling illuminated by fluorescent dyes. *J. Neurochem.*, 73, 2227–2239.

Greengard, P. (2001). The neurobiology of slow synaptic transmission. *Science*, 294, 1024–1030.

Miller, R. J. (1998). Presynaptic receptors. *Annu. Rev. Pharmacol. Toxicol.*, 38, 201–227.

Schulklin, J., (1999). *The Neuroendocrine Regulation of Behavior.* Cambridge University Press, Cambridge.

Walmsley, B., Alvarez, F. J., and Fyffe, R. E. W. (1998). Diversity of structure and function at mammalian central synapses. *Trends Neurosci.*, 21, 81–88.

Webster, R. (ed.) (2001). *Neurotransmitters, Drugs, and Brain Function.* John Wiley & Sons, Hoboken, NJ.

Zoli, M., Jansson, A., Syková, E., Agnati, L. F., and Fuxe, K. (1999). Volume transmission in the CNS and its relevance for neuropsychopharmacology. *Trends Pharmacol. Sci.*, 20, 142–150.

4 Methods of Research in Neurobehavioral Pharmacology

How would you feel with an electrode implanted deep within your brain that delivered mild electrical pulses to change your neural activity? If you happen to be one of the thousands of people suffering from chronic disabling disorders like Parkinson's disease, chronic pain, or epilepsy, the answer is that you might feel dramatic relief.

Deep brain stimulation therapy is one of the newest techniques to treat debilitating neurological disorders in patients who fail to respond to currently available medications. The treatment involves applying minute amounts of electrical current to precise brain sites to modify the brain signals that cause undesirable symptoms. It involves surgically implanting a fine wire deep into the individual's brain that is connected by an extension wire placed under the skin to a pacemaker-type electrical generator. The battery-powered generator is surgically placed under the skin near the collarbone and can be programmed by the neurophysiologist to deliver the precise stimulation needed by an individual patient for greatest relief and fewest side effects. Patients can also control the stimulation delivered by using a magnet to increase or decrease the "dosage" as required. This method, recently tested at medical facilities all around the world, demonstrates the creative and practical application of years of basic animal research into neurobiological methods. Chapter 4 describes a number of these research techniques in greater detail.

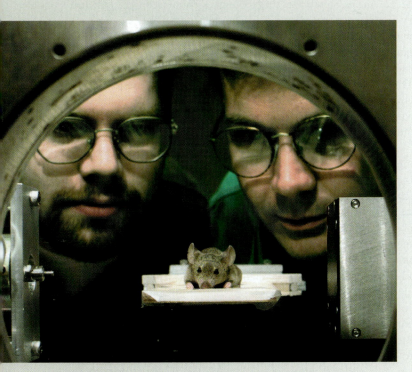

This miniature CT scanner provides extraordinary detail of brain structure with minimal discomfort to animal subjects.

Techniques in Neuropharmacology

Multiple Neurobiological Techniques for Assessing the CNS

The discovery of chemical transmission of information between nerve cells paved the way for the birth of neuropharmacology. Since then, there has been an explosion of research directed toward understanding the nature of brain function and the biology of what makes us human. With the variety and power of new analytical tools and techniques we can look inside the brain to find answers to questions that touch individual lives. Even nonscientists can appreciate the advances in neuroscience research that bring us ever closer to understanding the essence of human behavior as well as some of the most troubling problems of mankind: dementia, depression, autism, and neurodegenerative disorders.

The new tools provide the means to explore the brain to answer our questions, but it takes disciplined and creative scientific minds and teamwork to pose the right questions and use available tools optimally. The scientific method, utilizing rigorous hypothesis testing under controlled conditions, is the only real method we have to investigate how molecules responsible for nerve cell activity relate to complex human behaviors and thinking. Analysis spans the entire range from molecular genetics to cell function to integrated systems of neuronal networks and finally to observable behavior. To understand the brain requires a convergence of efforts from multiple disciplines that together form the basis of neuroscience: psychology, biochemistry, neuropharmacology, neuroanatomy, endocrinology, computer science, neuropsychology, and molecular biology. Ultimately, the knowledge we acquire depends on integrating information derived from a wide variety of research techniques from all of these fields.

As you might expect, the list of techniques is very long and increases every day. Chapter 4 focuses on a few of the more common methods and helps you to understand each method's purpose as well as some of its potential weaknesses. Perhaps the most important goal of this chapter is to encourage you, when you read scientific papers, to critically evaluate the methods and the controls used, because the conclusions we draw from experiments are only as good as the methodology used to collect the data.

The essence of neuropsychopharmacology is the use of drugs as a means to modify synaptic activity and subsequent behavior. Chapter 3 describes some of the chemical agents used to alter the synthesis, packaging, and release of neurotransmitters as well as prolong or shorten neurotransmitter action by altering metabolism or reuptake. Most important is the use of agonists to mimic and antagonists to reduce normal neurotransmitter action at the receptor.

Because synaptic activity is so important, the first part of Chapter 4 emphasizes techniques that look at the location and function of neurotransmitters and neurotransmitter receptors. The methods are both **in vivo,** meaning observed in the living organism, and **in vitro,** which is measurement outside the living body (traditionally in a test tube). We also look at a variety of rather remarkable imaging techniques that permit us to visualize the activity of the living human brain. Since genetic engineering is an increasingly powerful tool, we will describe its use in neuropharmacology. The second part of the chapter focuses on behavioral pharmacology. Behavior, mood, and thinking represent the focus of neuropsychopharmacology, so it is of equal importance to understand and critically evaluate the techniques used to quantify behavioral changes. Both the biochemical and the behavioral techniques selected will be used in subsequent chapters. Feel free to return to this chapter to review a method when you encounter it later.

Stereotaxic surgery is needed for accurate in vivo measures of brain function

The classic techniques of physiological psychology (lesioning, microinjection, and electrical recording) are equally important in understanding the action of psychoactive drugs. Stereotaxic surgery is an essential technique in neuroscience that permits a researcher to implant one of several devices into the brain of an anesthetized animal with significant precision. The stereotaxic device itself (shown in Figure 4.1A) is essentially a means to stabilize the animal's head in a fixed orientation so that the carrier portion can be moved precisely in three dimensions to place the tip of an electrode or drug delivery tube in a predetermined brain site. The brain site coordinates are calculated using a brain atlas, which is a collection of frontal sections of brain of the appropriate species in which distances are measured from skull surface features (Figure 4.1B). Accuracy of placement is determined histologically after the experiment is complete. The halo bracket (Figure 4.1C) is the equivalent apparatus used in human neurosurgery, and the target site is identified with a computerized imaging technique like magnetic resonance imaging (MRI) or computerized tomography (CT) (see the section on imaging techniques later in the chapter).

Lesioning and microinjection Experimental ablation, or **lesioning,** uses a stereotaxic device to position a delicate electrode, insulated along its length except for the exposed tip, deep within the brain. The tissue at the tip is destroyed when a very-high-frequency radio current is passed through the electrode to heat the cells. The rationale of the experiment is

(A)

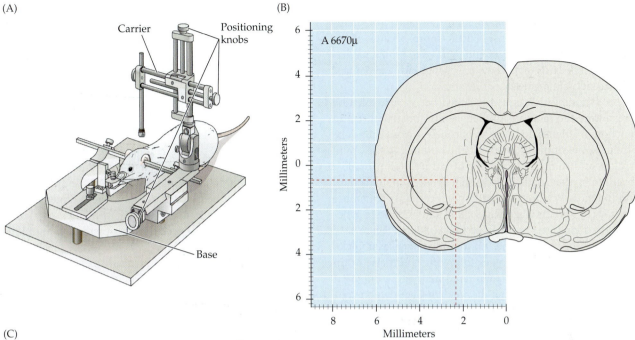

(B)

Figure 4.1 Stereotaxic surgery (A) A stereotaxic device used for precise placement of electrodes during brain surgery on animals. The base holds the anesthetized animal's head and neck in a stationary position. The carrier portion places the electrode or cannula in a precise location based on the coordinates of the target area identified with the brain atlas (B). (C) A similar apparatus is used for human brain surgery. Location of the procedure is determined by CT or MRI.

(C)

that a comparison of the animal's behavior before and after the lesion will tell us something about the function of that brain area.

Electrolytic lesions destroy all tissue at the tip of the electrode, including cell bodies, dendrites, and axons. Alternatively, a **neurotoxin** (a chemical damaging to nerve cells) can be injected via a cannula (a hollow tube inserted like an electrode) to destroy cells. Of course, the same type of cannula can be used to administer drugs or neurotransmitters that stimulate cells in the central nervous system (CNS) before

evaluating behavior (see the discussion of intracerebroventricular administration in Chapter 1). Chemical lesions have the advantage of being significantly more specific because neurotoxic chemicals, such as kainic acid or ibotenic acid, kill the cell bodies in the vicinity of the cannula tip but spare the axons passing through the same area. In either case, this procedure can be used to identify the brain area responsible for a drug-induced change in behavior. For instance, we might wonder which brain area is responsible for the reinforcing effects of a drug like amphetamine. Suppose that after lesioning the nucleus accumbens in the diencephalon, we find that rats no longer will self-administer amphetamine by pressing a lever in an operant chamber (see the section on operant behavior later in the chapter). We may want to conclude that the nucleus accumbens is responsible for reinforcement, but lesion studies must always be evaluated cautiously. Even when a lesion changes behavior, we still don't know what specific function that brain area served. In our example, further investigation would be needed to determine *how* the lesion interfered with the self-administration. Does the nucleus accumbens modulate reinforcement? Or is it possible that the animal lost motor control or failed to remember the appropriate response? Furthermore, because of the small size of brain structures and their overlapping nature, the possibility exists that behavioral change is due to damage to adjacent brain regions.

The lesioning technique has always been a valuable tool to examine the relationship between brain structure and function in animals. In humans, of course, lesions cannot be produced intentionally, but accidents, trauma to the brain, strokes, and tumors ("accidents of nature") all provide a means to investigate the relationship between brain damage and function. Psychology students will certainly remember the story of Phineas Gage, whose skull and brain were penetrated by a long steel rod in a blasting accident (Figure 4.2). His case history has become famous for being an example of profound behavioral changes following traumatic brain injury. Previously a mild-mannered man and competent foreman of a work crew, after the accident Gage demonstrated childish behavior and an inability to organize his daily activities, displaying frequent uncontrolled outbursts and episodes of violence. However, several significant problems exist in evaluating such case studies. First, although behavioral measures and neuropsychological testing after injury can identify deficits in function, it is rare that skills were evaluated prior to the injury. For this reason it is difficult to know to what extent the functioning changed as a result of the injury. Second, until very recently, there was no way to know specifically where the brain damage occurred. The development of scanning techniques like CT and MRI have greatly improved the ability to identify quite specifically the locus of damage. Third, "accidents of nature" produce unique damage to brain structures in each individual, so generalizations to a larger population are unwarranted.

Because neuropharmacology is interested in neurochemical regulation of behavior, the lesioning techniques used are often specific for a neural pathway utilizing a particular neurotransmitter. These **specific neurotoxins** are most often injected directly into the brain, where they are taken up by the neurons' normal reuptake mechanism. Once inside the cell, the toxin destroys the cell terminal. In this way, behavioral measures made before and after a neurotoxic lesion tell us about the role of the neurotransmitter in a particular behavior. For example, intracerebroventricular administration of 6-hydroxydopamine produces nerve terminal degeneration in both noradrenergic and dopaminergic cells and profound neurotransmitter depletion. More selective effects are achieved when the neurotoxin is injected directly into a target area. Earlier we suggested that lesioning the nucleus accumbens reduced self-administration of amphetamine in rats. We might further test our understanding of the role of the nucleus accumbens in reinforcement by selectively destroying the large number of dopamine cell terminals in that area using the neurotoxin 6-hydroxydopamine before evaluating the drug-taking behavior.

Microdialysis   A different technique that uses stereotaxic surgery is **microdialysis.** Although researchers have been able to measure neurotransmitters released from brain slices in vitro for many years, microdialysis lets us measure neurotransmitters released in a specific brain region while the subject is actively engaged in behavior (Figure 4.3A).

The technique requires a specialized cannula made of fine, flexible tubing that is implanted stereotaxically (Figure 4.3B). The cannula is sealed along its length except at the tip, allowing investigators to collect material in extracellular fluid at nerve terminals at precise sites even deep within the brain. Artificial cerebrospinal fluid (CSF) is gently moved into the microdialysis cannula by a pump. The CSF in the cannula and in the extracellular fluid are identical except for the material to be collected. Based on the difference in concentration, the chemicals of interest move across the membrane from the synaptic space into the cannula. A second pump removes the CSF from the cannula into a series of tubes, to be analyzed by high-performance liquid chromatography (HPLC) or another method.

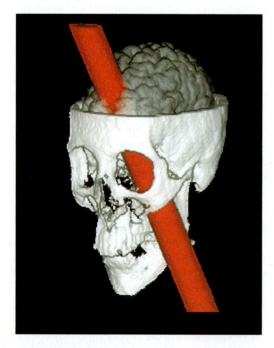

Figure 4.2 Computer reconstruction of the trajectory of the steel rod that penetrated Phineas Gage's skull during a nineteenth century blasting accident. The massive damage to the frontal part of the brain and the behavioral deficits he demonstrated after the accident stimulated thinking about the role of the frontal cortex in complex brain functions. Gage's skull is presently housed in the Warren Museum at Harvard Medical School. (From H. Damasio et al., 1994; courtesy of Hanna Damasio.)

(A)

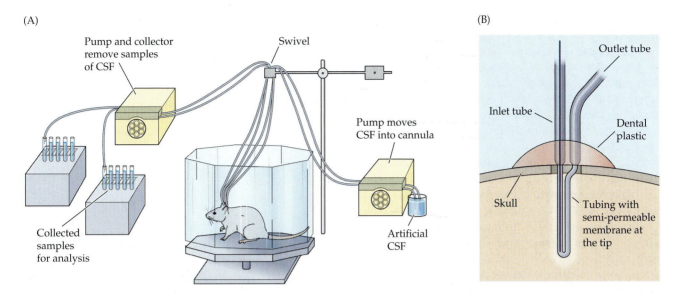

Pump and collector remove samples of CSF

Swivel

(B)

Outlet tube

Inlet tube

Dental plastic

Skull

Tubing with semi-permeable membrane at the tip

Pump moves CSF into cannula

Artificial CSF

Collected samples for analysis

Figure 4.3 Collection of extracellular fluid with microdialysis (A) Microdialysis allows the collection of samples from deep within the brain in unanesthetized and freely moving animals under relatively normal conditions. The collected samples are identified and measured by one of several analytic techniques, such as HPLC. (B) Typical microdialysis probe, which uses flexible tubing that is sealed except at the tip, where it is semipermeable. It is held in place by dental plastic on the animal's skull. (A after Philippu, 1984; B after Ungerstedt, 1984.)

A major improvement over older collection methods is that only tiny amounts of material need to be collected for accurate measurement. The improved accuracy is due to the development of highly sensitive analytic techniques (such as HPLC), which can be combined with microdialysis collection.

HPLC, like other types of chromatography, serves two purposes. First, chromatography separates the sample into component parts depending on characteristics of the sample, such as molecular size or ionic charge. Second, the concentration of the molecules of interest can be determined (Figure 4.4).

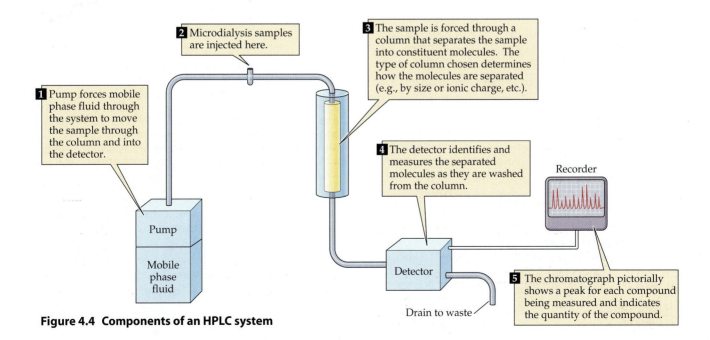

2 Microdialysis samples are injected here.

3 The sample is forced through a column that separates the sample into constituent molecules. The type of column chosen determines how the molecules are separated (e.g., by size or ionic charge, etc.).

1 Pump forces mobile phase fluid through the system to move the sample through the column and into the detector.

4 The detector identifies and measures the separated molecules as they are washed from the column.

Recorder

Pump

Mobile phase fluid

Detector

Drain to waste

5 The chromatograph pictorially shows a peak for each compound being measured and indicates the quantity of the compound.

Figure 4.4 Components of an HPLC system

Microdialysis is important to neuropsychopharmacology because it can be used in several types of experiments combining biochemical and behavioral analyses. For example, we might evaluate the released neurochemicals during ongoing behaviors such as sleep and waking, feeding, or operant tasks to provide a window into the functioning CNS. Second, we might investigate the effects of drugs on extracellular concentrations of neurotransmitters in selected brain areas. Since the sample collection can be made in freely moving animals, correlated changes in behavior can be monitored simultaneously. Finally, the collection of extracellular materials at nerve terminals following discrete electrical or chemical stimulation of neural pathways is another valuable role.

A second method used to measure neurotransmitter release is **in vivo voltammetry.** Whereas microdialysis collects samples of extracellular fluid for subsequent analysis, in vivo voltammetry uses stereotaxically implanted microelectrodes to measure neurochemicals in the extracellular fluid of freely moving animals. In voltammetry a very fine electrode is implanted and a small electrical potential is applied. Changes in the current flow at the electrode tip reflect changes in the concentration of electroactive substances such as neurotransmitters or their metabolites. A major advantage is that because the measurements are made continuously and require as little as 15 milliseconds to complete, researchers can evaluate neurotransmitter release as it is occurring in real time.

Electrophysiological stimulation and recording   In a similar fashion, implanted **macroelectrodes** (Figure 4.5A) can be used to activate cells at the tip while evaluating the change in animal behavior during stimulation. The minute amount of electric current applied changes the membrane potential of those cells and generates action potentials. The action potentials in turn cause the release of neurotransmitter at the cell terminals to mimic normal synaptic transmission. Hence the electrical stimulation should produce biobehavioral effects that are similar to those seen upon injection of the natural neurotransmitter or neurotransmitter agonists into the brain. In addition, one would expect that stimulation of a given cell group should produce effects opposite those of a lesion at the same site. Macroelectrodes can also be used to record the summated electrical response of thousands of neurons in a specific brain region following drug treatment or other experimental manipulation in a freely moving animal. If we had found, for example, that lesioning the periaqueductal gray (PAG) in the midbrain prevented the pain-reducing effects of morphine, we might want to find out what effect activating those PAG neurons has. What we would find is that if electrodes implanted in the PAG are activated, the animal fails to respond to painful stimuli. Likewise, if pain-killing opioids like morphine or

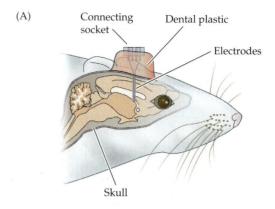

(A) Connecting socket — Dental plastic — Electrodes — Skull

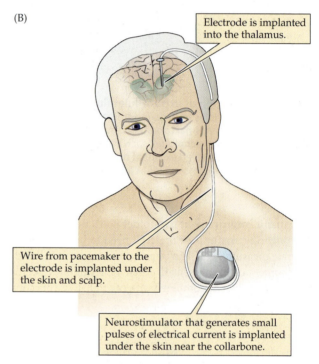

(B) Electrode is implanted into the thalamus.

Wire from pacemaker to the electrode is implanted under the skin and scalp.

Neurostimulator that generates small pulses of electrical current is implanted under the skin near the collarbone.

Figure 4.5 Electrical brain stimulation and recording
(A) Stereotaxically implanted electrodes held in place on the skull with dental plastic. After recovery, the animal can be plugged into a device that can electrically stimulate the cells at the tip or monitor and record changes in electrical activity. (B) Diagram of the Tremor Control System, which consists of an insulated wire electrode surgically implanted deep in the brain. The electrode is connected to a pulse generator implanted under the skin near the collarbone. The generator is programmed to deliver the amount of electric current needed to reduce the tremor on the opposite side of the body. Patients also have individual control by passing a hand-held magnet over the skin above the pulse generator.

codeine are microinjected into that brain area via an indwelling cannula, the animal also demonstrates profound analgesia.

In the opening paragraphs of this chapter, you read about patients who have benefited from the many years of animal research into the stereotaxic implantation of electrodes into the brain and electrical stimulation. Figure 4.5B shows the adaptation of the technique to humans being treated for Parkinson's disease. Small pulses of electric current applied to the thalamus cause the cells to fire and release neurotransmitter, which reduces the tremor on the opposite side of the body.

An alternative to macroelectrode recording, which is a summation of electrical activity in a brain region, is single-unit recording, which uses **microelectrodes.** Stereotaxically implanting a fine-tipped electrode either into a single cell (**intracellular recording**) or into the extracellular fluid near a single cell (**extracellular recording**) monitors the response of individual cells under various conditions. Intracellular recording must utilize an anesthetized animal, because the electrode must remain in a precise position in order to record the membrane potential of the cell. An advantage of extracellular single-cell recording is that it can be done in a mobile animal (Figure 4.6). The downside to extracellular recording is that the electrode records only the occurrence of action potentials in the nearby neuron and cannot monitor the change in the cell's membrane potential. Returning to

our earlier example of morphine action, we find that the drug produces strong selective inhibition of neurons in the spinal cord, which prevents the projection of pain information to higher brain centers, thereby contributing to the analgesic effect.

In addition to measuring membrane potentials of groups of cells and single cells, thanks to the Nobel Prize-winning research of Neher and Sakmann conducted in the 1970s neuroscientists can also study the function of *individual* ion channels, which collectively are responsible for the membrane potential. The technique, known as **patch clamp electrophysiology,** works best with individual cells in culture but can also be used on exposed cells in slices of brain. The method involves attaching a recording micropipette to a piece of cell membrane by suction. When the pipette is pulled away, a small membrane patch containing one or more ion channels remains attached. The subsequent electrical recording through the pipette represents in real time the channel opening, the flow of ions (electrical current) during the brief period when it is open, and the channel closing.

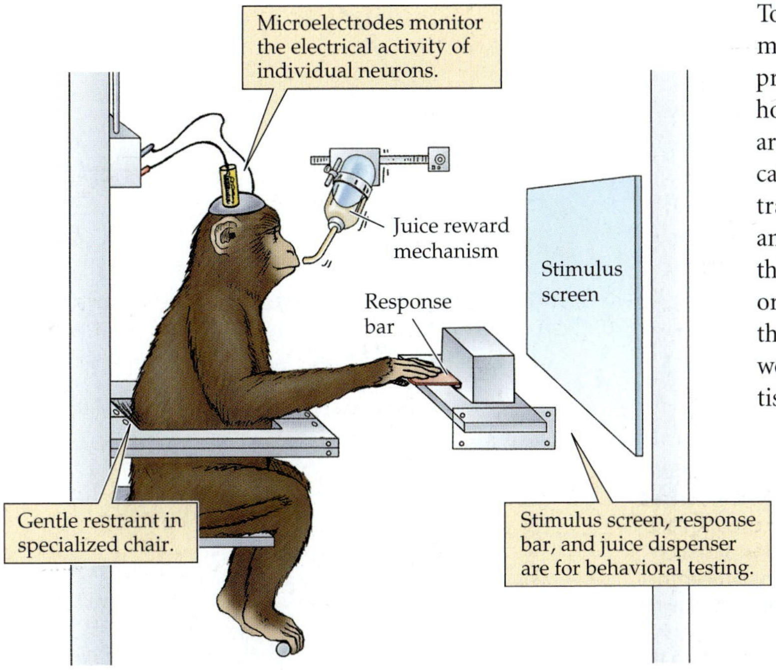

Neurotransmitters, receptors, and other proteins can be quantified and visually located in the CNS

To both quantify and locate neurotransmitters and receptors in the CNS, several methods are required. To count or measure a particular molecule, a "soup" method is often used, in which a tissue sample is precisely dissected out and ground up, creating a homogenate before being evaluated. Homogenates are used in any one of many possible neurochemical analyses which are referred to as assays. In contrast, for localization, the landmarks of the tissue and relationship of structures must be preserved, so the visualization method is done on an intact piece or slice of tissue. Hence, when we want to measure the number of receptors in a particular brain area we are likely to use a radioligand binding assay in a tissue homogenate, but if we want to see where in the brain particular receptors are located (as well as measure them) we are more likely to use a slice preparation with autoradiography. Table 4.1 summarizes the "soup" and "slice" techniques described in the following section of the chapter.

Radioligand binding   To study the number of receptors in a given brain region and their affinity for drugs, the **radioligand binding** method was developed. Once the brain region we are interested in is dissected out,

Figure 4.6 **Extracellular microelectrode recording** from single neurons in the brain of an awake, responding rhesus monkey. This experimental setup might be used to evaluate the effects of a previously administered drug on the animal's response to visual stimuli and on the electrical activity of a single cell.

TABLE 4.1 Methods Used to Quantify and Visualize Target Molecules in the Nervous System

Target molecule	Tissue extract assay to quantify	Brain slice preparation to visualize
Receptor site	Radioligand binding	Receptor autoradiography
Receptors and other proteins	Radioimmunoassay (RIA)	Immunocytochemistry(ICC)
mRNA	Dot blot or Northern blot	In situ hybridization (ISH)

it is ground up to make a homogenate. A ligand (usually a drug or chemical) that is radioactively labeled (now called the radioligand) is incubated with the tissue under conditions that optimize its binding. After a brief time, any radioligand that has not bound is removed, often by washing and filtering. The amount of radioligand bound to the tissue is then measured with a scintillation (or gamma) counter and reflects the number of receptors in the tissue.

Although the binding procedure is quite simple, interpretation of the results is more complex. How can we be sure that the radioligand is actually binding to the specific biological receptors of interest, rather than to other sites based on artifacts of the procedure? Several criteria that must be met include (1) specificity; (2) saturability; (3) reversibility and high affinity; and (4) biological relevance. Specificity means that the ligand is binding only to the receptor we are concerned with in this tissue and to nothing else. Of course, drugs often bind to several receptor subtypes, but they may also attach to other cell components that produce no biological effects. To measure the amount of a ligand that binds to the site that we are concerned with, we add very high concentrations of a nonradioactive competing ligand to some tubes to show that most of the radioactive binding is displaced. That which remains is likely to be nonspecifically bound to sites such as assay additives (e.g., albumin) or cellular sites (e.g., enzymes) that we are less interested in at the moment. Nonspecific binding is subtracted when the data are calculated for specific binding. When binding to specific subtypes of

receptors is necessary, ligands must be designed to distinguish between the receptor proteins.

Saturability means that there are a finite number of receptors in a given amount of tissue. By adding increasing amounts of radioligand to a fixed amount of tissue, one would expect to see gradual increases in binding until all sites are filled (Figure 4.7A). Binding in the assay must also be reversible, because a neurotransmitter in vivo will bind and release many times to initiate repeated activation of the cellular action. This reversibility is demonstrated in binding assays because the radioactive ligand can be displaced by the same drug that is not radiolabeled (Figure 4.7B). The unbinding (dissociation) of the ligand from the receptor must also be consistent with the reversal of physiological effects of the ligand.

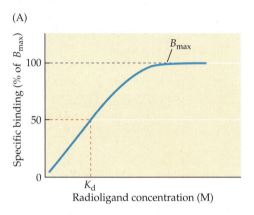

(A)

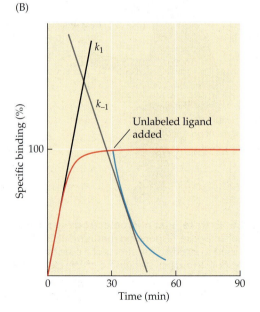

(B)

Figure 4.7 Radioligand binding to receptors (A) A hypothetical saturation curve shows that as radioligand concentration increases, specific binding to the receptor also increases until all the sites are filled (B_{max}). The K_d is defined as the ligand concentration at which 50% of the receptors are occupied and is an indication of receptor affinity. (B) Hypothetical association and dissociation curves. The red line represents the association of a radioligand with its receptors over time. The rate of association (k_1) is estimated by calculating the slope of the straight line that best fits the curvilinear data. After maximum binding has occurred (association and dissociation are in equilibrium), excess unlabeled ligand is added. The blue line represents the dissociation of the radioligand from its receptors in the presence of large amounts of unlabeled ligand. The slope of the straight line that best fits that portion of the curve provides an estimate of the rate of dissociation (k_{-1}).

Ideally, the binding of chemically similar drugs should correlate with some measurable biochemical or behavioral effect. For example, the classic antipsychotic drugs all bind to a particular subtype of receptor (D_2) for the neurotransmitter dopamine. Not only do the drugs in this class bind to the D_2 receptor, but their affinity for the receptor correlates with the effectiveness of the drugs in reducing the symptoms of schizophrenia (see Chapter 17). Unfortunately, experiments of this type rarely produce perfectly correlated results in binding affinity and functional potency because drug effects in the intact organism are dependent on many factors in addition to drug–receptor interaction, for example, absorption and distribution.

Receptor autoradiography   Receptor binding is a classic tool in neuropharmacology that tells us about receptor number and affinity for a particular drug in a specific piece of brain tissue. When we want to visualize the distribution of receptors within the brain, we use receptor autoradiography. The process begins with standard radioligand binding as described above except that slide-mounted tissue slices rather than ground-up tissue are used. After the unbound radioactively labeled drug is washed away, the slices are processed by **autoradiography.** The slides are put into cassettes, a specialized autoradiographic film is placed on top of the slides so that it is in physical contact with the tissue sections, and the cassettes are stored in the dark to allow the radioactive material that is bound to receptors to act on the film. The particles that are constantly emitted from the radioactive material in the tissue expose the film and show not only the amount of radioligand bound but also its location. This method is especially good for studying the effects of brain lesions on receptor binding because each lesioned animal can be evaluated independently by comparing the lesioned and nonlesioned sides of the brain. This method might also give us clues about how various psychoactive drugs produce their behavioral effects. For instance, mapping the binding of cocaine in monkey brain shows a distinct pattern of localization and density in selected brain areas (Figure 4.8). With a clear understanding of anatomical distribution, we can begin to test specific hypotheses regarding the behavioral consequences of activating these receptors using microinjections of receptor-selective agonists and antagonists.

In vivo receptor binding   The same autoradiographic processing can be done on brain slices of an animal that had previously been injected in vivo with a radiolabeled drug. The drug enters the general circulation, diffuses into the brain, and binds to receptors. The animal is then killed and the brain is sliced and processed by autoradiography. The technique shows the researcher where a particular drug or neurotransmitter binds in an intact animal. Unfortunately, results with this technique are more difficult to interpret because of the complexities of bioavailability and distribu-

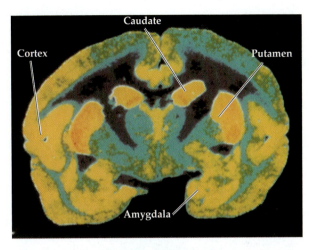

Figure 4.8 Autoradiogram of the distribution of cocaine binding in monkey brain The highest levels of cocaine binding are in areas colored yellow and orange. (Courtesy of Bertha Madras and Marc J. Kaufman.)

tion, diffusion through the blood–brain barrier, and metabolism of the drug. Nevertheless, its potential is tremendous because in vivo binding can be assessed in living human subjects using positron emission tomography (PET) (see the section on brain imaging) to map the pattern of drug–receptor binding and correlate it with clinical effects.

Assays of enzyme activity   Enzymes are proteins that act as biological catalysts to speed up reaction rates, but they are not used up in the process. We find many different enzymes in every cell, and each has a role in a relatively specific reaction. The enzymes that are particularly interesting to neuropharmacologists are those involved in the synthesis or metabolism of neurotransmitters, neuromodulators, and second messengers. In addition, neuropharmacologists are interested in identifying the conditions that regulate the rate of activity of the enzyme. For example, acute morphine treatment inhibits adenylyl cyclase activity. Adenylyl cyclase is the enzyme that synthesizes the second messenger cyclic adenosine monophosphate (cAMP). However, chronic exposure to morphine produces a gradual but dramatic up-regulation of the cAMP system, suggesting that the second-messenger system acts to compensate for the acute effect of opioid inhibition. It is perhaps one of the best-studied biochemical models of opioid tolerance and is discussed further in Chapter 10.

Sometimes the mere presence of an enzyme in a cell cluster is important since it can be used to identify those cells that manufacture a specific neurotransmitter. The next section describes the use of antibodies and immunocytochemistry to locate enzymes in the brain.

Antibody production   Some of the newest methods for identifying and measuring receptors and other proteins are far more specific and sensitive than ever before because they

(A)

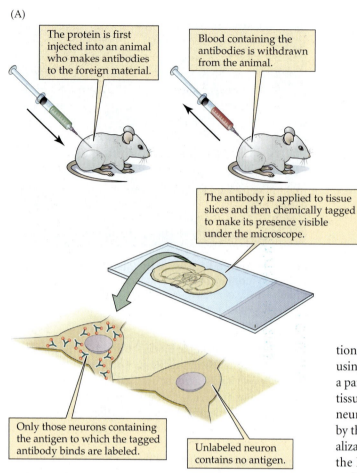

The protein is first injected into an animal who makes antibodies to the foreign material.

Blood containing the antibodies is withdrawn from the animal.

The antibody is applied to tissue slices and then chemically tagged to make its presence visible under the microscope.

Only those neurons containing the antigen to which the tagged antibody binds are labeled.

Unlabeled neuron contains no antigen.

(B)

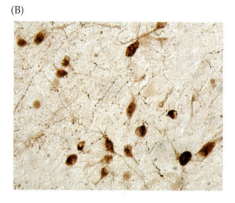

Figure 4.9 Immunocytochemistry uses tagged antibodies to locate molecules within cells. (A) Steps in ICC localization. (B) Immunocytochemical identification of cells containing the neuropeptide hypocretin in the human lateral hypothalamus. (A after Bear et al., 2001; B courtesy of Jerome Siegel.)

use an antibody. An **antibody** is a protein produced by the white blood cells of the immune system to recognize, attack, and destroy a specific foreign substance (the antigen). Researchers use this immune response to create supplies of antibodies that bind to specific proteins (receptors, neuropeptides, or enzymes) they want to locate in the brain (Figure 4.9A). The first step is to create an antibody by injecting the antigen (for example, the neuropeptide hypocretin) into a host animal and at various times taking blood samples to collect antibodies. With the antibody prepared, we are ready to look for the peptide in tissue slices using immunocytochemistry. Antibodies can also be used to quantify very small amounts of material using radioimmunoassays (see below).

Immunocytochemistry For **immunocytochemistry (ICC),** the brain is first fixed (hardened) using a preservative such as formaldehyde. Tissue slices are then cut and incubated with the antibody in solution. The antibody attaches to the antigen wherever cells are present that contain that antigen. In the final step, the antibody is tagged so that the antigen-containing cells can be visualized (see Figure 4.9A). This is usually accomplished either by means of a chemical reac-

tion that creates a colored precipitate within the cells or by using a fluorescent dye that glows when exposed to light of a particular wavelength. The researcher can then examine the tissue slices under a microscope and see which brain areas or neurons contain the antigen. The technique is limited only by the ability to raise antibodies. Figure 4.9B shows the visualization of cells that contain the neuropeptide hypocretin in the lateral hypothalamus of a healthy human subject. In patients with the sleep disorder narcolepsy, the number of hypocretin neurons is reduced by about 90% (Thannicakal et al., 2000). These results, along with animal experiments using neurotoxin lesioning and genetic modification, suggest that hypocretin in the hypothalamus may regulate the onset of sleep stages. ICC is similar to autoradiography in principle, but it is far more selective because of the use of the antibody (which recognizes only a very specific protein) and much quicker because it does not require the development time of the autoradiographic film.

Radioimmunoassay Antibodies are also useful in quantifying physiologically important molecules in body fluids such as blood, saliva, or CSF, as well as in tissue extracts. **Radioimmunoassay (RIA)** is based on competitive binding of an antibody to its antigen (the molecule being measured). The use of antibodies makes the procedure highly specific for the molecule of interest and very sensitive (Figure 4.10).

RIA involves preparing a standard curve of known antigen concentrations against which unknown samples can be compared. The standard curve is created by first combining a preset amount of antibody with a known concentration of radioactively labeled antigen in all the assay tubes. At this point all the tubes are identical, that is, all the antibody would be reversibly attached to radioactive antigen. However, the experimenter then adds different, known concentra-

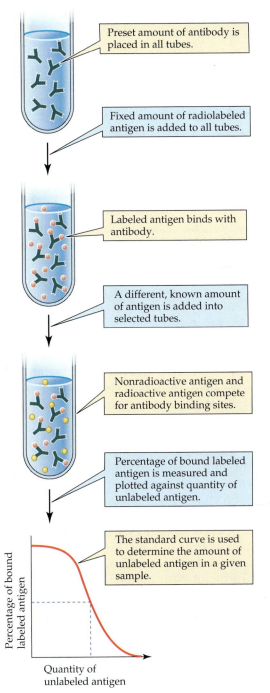

Preset amount of antibody is placed in all tubes.

Fixed amount of radiolabeled antigen is added to all tubes.

Labeled antigen binds with antibody.

A different, known amount of antigen is added into selected tubes.

Nonradioactive antigen and radioactive antigen compete for antibody binding sites.

Percentage of bound labeled antigen is measured and plotted against quantity of unlabeled antigen.

The standard curve is used to determine the amount of unlabeled antigen in a given sample.

Percentage of bound labeled antigen

Quantity of unlabeled antigen

Figure 4.10 Radioimmunoassay The steps in the RIA procedure that produce a typical standard curve. The curve in turn is used to calculate the amount of unknown antigen in a given sample.

tions of unlabeled antigen, which compete with the radioactively labeled antigen. The higher the concentration of unlabeled competitor antigen added, the lower the amount of radioactive antigen bound after the mixture has been incubated. The values are plotted as a standard curve and analyzed using appropriate computer software.

To determine how much of the antigen is in any experimental sample, other test tubes are prepared in just the same way except that the samples containing unknown amounts of antigen are added instead of the known antigen. By measuring the amount of radioactive antigen bound in the sample tubes compared to the standard curve, the amount of antigen in the sample can be calculated.

In situ hybridization **In situ hybridization (ISH)** makes it possible to locate cells in tissue slices that are *manufacturing* a particular protein or peptide in much the same manner that ICC identifies cells *containing* a particular protein. ISH is particularly useful in neuropharmacology for detecting the specific messenger RNA (mRNA) molecules responsible for directing the manufacture of the wide variety of proteins essential to neuron function, such as enzymes, structural proteins, receptors, ion channels, and peptides. For example, Figure 4.11A shows the location of the mRNA for enkephalin, one of several opioid peptides in the adult rat brain (see Chapter 10). Because the method detects cells with a precise RNA sequence, it is exceptionally specific and extremely sensitive. Besides *locating* cells containing specific mRNA, ISH is also used to study *changes* in regional mRNA levels after experimental manipulations. The amount of mRNA provides an estimate of the rate of synthesis of the particular protein. This means that if chronic drug treatment caused a decrease in enkephalin mRNA that we visualized in Figure 4.11A, we could conclude that the protein the mRNA codes for has been down-regulated, that is, less of that protein is being synthesized.

As you recall from Chapter 2, the double strands of DNA and corresponding mRNA (Figure 4.11B and C) have unique base-pair sequences responsible for directing the synthesis of a particular protein with its unique amino acid sequence. ISH depends on the ability to create probes by labeling single-stranded fragments of RNA made up of base-pair sequences complementary to those of the mRNA of interest (Figure 4.11D). After the single strands are prepared, they are labeled radioactively or with dyes. When the tissue slices or cells are exposed to the labeled probe, the probe attaches (binds, or hybridizes) to the complementary base-pair sequences. After incubation, the tissue is washed and dehydrated before being placed in contact with X-ray film or being processed in other ways for visualization of cells containing the specific mRNA. The technique is extremely sensitive and can detect a very small number of cells that express a particular gene. If the researcher is interested only in measuring the amount of mRNA rather than visualizing its location, hybridization can be done using a tissue homogenate rather than a tissue slice. Two available methods of ISH that use homogenates are called Northern blot and dot blot.

DNA microarrays Microarrays, also called DNA chips or gene chips, provide the newest and most dramatic improvement in gene technology. Because the nervous system exhibits

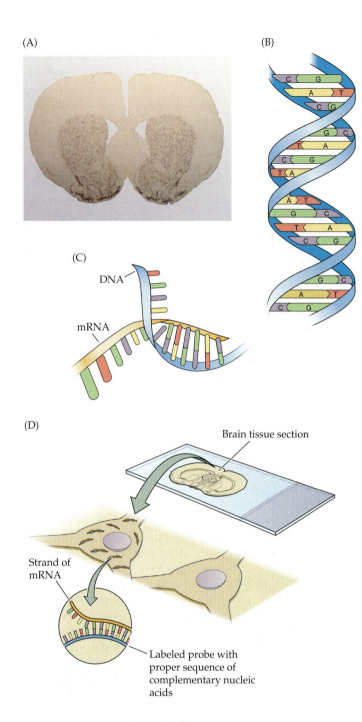

(A)

(B)

(C)

DNA

mRNA

(D)

Brain tissue section

Strand of mRNA

Labeled probe with proper sequence of complementary nucleic acids

Figure 4.11 In situ hybridization (A) Localization of enkephalin mRNA in a slice from rat brain. (B) Structure of a DNA molecule. The nucleotide bases always bind in a complementary fashion: thymine to adenine and guanine to cytosine. (C) A strand of mRNA has copied the code from a partially unraveled DNA molecule in the nucleus and will carry the genetic code to the ribosomes in the cytoplasm, where the protein will be created. (D) In ISH, a labeled probe has been created with the correct sequence of complementary bases. When the strand of mRNA in the cell and the labeled probe hybridize, or bond to one another, the product labels the cell that contains the genetic code for the protein of interest. (A courtesy of Brian Sauer and Suzanne Pham.)

the greatest complexity of gene expression of all tissues, being able to examine all of the genes simultaneously can tell researchers which genes switch on and off together in response to a disease state, drug treatment, or environmental condition. One would assume that genes that increase or decrease their expression under the same condition probably work together to induce a cellular response. In addition, measuring the amount of various RNAs in a sample tells us both the types and amounts of proteins present. A study by Mirnics and colleagues (2000) demonstrated the technical elegance of microarray by identifying multiple presynaptic proteins that are underexpressed in the frontal lobes of schizophrenic individuals. Their results provide a predictive and testable model of the disorder.

The method is similar to that described for ISH, but rather than measuring a single mRNA, microarrays consist of between 1000 and 20,000 distinct complementary DNA sequences on a single chip (a structural support) of approximately thumbnail size. Each spot is only about 50 to 150 μm in diameter. This makes it possible to screen the expression of the entire genome of an organism in a single experiment on just a few chips. The tissue to be evaluated (for example, the frontal lobe from a schizophrenic individual compared to a normal frontal lobe) is dissected, and the mRNAs are isolated and labeled, then hybridized to the large number of immobilized DNA molecules on the chip. A scanner automatically evaluates the amount of hybridization of each of the thousands of spots on the chip, and computer analysis is used to identify the patterns of gene activity. Several excellent reviews of the microarray procedure and its application in areas such as aging, neuropharmacology, and psychiatric disorders are available (Luo and Geschwind, 2001; Marcotte et al. 2001).

New tools are used for imaging the structure and function of the brain

Most conventional neurobiological techniques are designed to quantify or to localize significant substances in the nervous system. One of the greatest challenges in psychopharmacology has been to evaluate the functioning of the brain under varying conditions, particularly in the living human being. Advances in technology not only make the visualization of the CNS far more precise, but also provide the opportunity to visualize the functioning brain.

Autoradiography of dynamic cell processes   You are already familiar with the technique of autoradiography for mapping cell components such as neurotransmitter receptors that have been radioactively labeled. Another important application of autoradiography is the tracing of active processes in the brain such as cerebral blood flow, oxygen consumption, local glucose utilization, or local rates of cerebral protein synthesis. **2-Deoxyglucose autoradiography** is based on the assumption that when nerve cell firing increases, the metabolic rate, that is, the utilization of glucose and oxygen, also increases. By identifying cells that take up more glucose under experimental conditions such as drug treatment, we can tell which brain regions are most active. 2-Deoxyglucose (2-DG) is a modified form of the glucose molecule that is taken up by active nerve cells but is not processed in the same manner as glucose and remains trapped in the cell. If the 2-DG has been labeled in some way, the most active cells can be identified. The method involves injecting an animal with radioactive 2-DG before evaluating its behavior in a test situation. The experimenter then kills the animal, removes the brain, and slices it in preparation for autoradiography (described earlier). A similar (but nonlethal) technique can be performed with human subjects, using PET as described below.

A second way of identifying which brain cells are active is to locate cells that show increases in nuclear proteins involved in protein synthesis. The assumption is that when cells are activated, selected proteins called transcription factors (such as c-fos) dramatically increase in concentration over 30 to 60 minutes. The c-fos protein subsequently activates the expression of other genes that regulate protein synthesis. c-Fos can be located in the brain using ICC to stain cells with increased levels of the fos protein and hence increased cell activity.

Imaging techniques   Since our ultimate goal is to understand how drugs affect the human brain and behavior, the most exciting advance in recent years has been the ability to visualize the living human brain. Although we can learn a lot by studying individuals with brain damage, until recently we could only guess at where the damage was located because the brain was not accessible until the individual died, often many years later. It was virtually impossible to know which specific brain area was responsible for the lost function. The human brain remained a bit of a "black box," and our understanding of the neural processes responsible for human thinking and behavior were advanced primarily due to animal experiments. Because of recent advances in X-ray and computer technology, neuroscience can now not only safely visualize the detailed anatomy of the human brain but also identify the neural processes responsible for a particular mental activity. CT and MRI are techniques that create pictures of the human nervous system in far greater detail than previously possible with standard X-ray. Other techniques are designed to see functional activity in the human brain. These include PET, functional MRI, and computer-assisted electrical recording.

When standard X-rays are passed through the body, they are differentially absorbed depending on the density of the various tissues. Rays that are not absorbed strike a photographic plate, forming light and dark images. Unfortunately, the brain is made up of many overlapping parts that do not differ dramatically in their ability to absorb X-rays, so it is very difficult to distinguish the individual shapes of brain structures. **Computerized tomography (CT)** not only increases the resolution (sharpness of detail) of the image but also provides an image in three dimensions.

The individual undergoing a CT scan (sometimes called CAT scan, for computerized axial tomography) lies with his head placed in a cylindrical X-ray tube (Figure 4.12A). A

(A) Computerized tomography (CT)

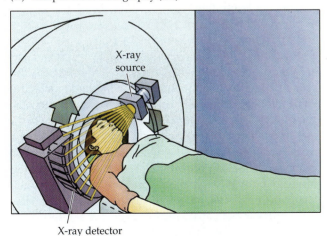

(B)

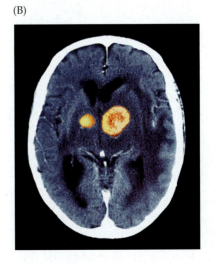

Figure 4.12 Computerized tomography (A) The cylindrical CT scanner rotates around the head, sending parallel X-ray beams through the tissue to be detected on the opposite side. A computerized image in the form of a brain slice is constructed from the data. (B) Horizontal CT scan showing a tumor (orange) at the level of the basal ganglia. Anterior is toward the top of the scan.

series of narrow, parallel beams of radiation are aimed through the tissue and toward the X-ray detectors. The X-ray source is rotated around the head while the detectors move on the opposite side in parallel. At each point of rotation, the source and detectors also move linearly. In this manner they make a series of radiation transmission readings, which is calculated by a computer and visually displayed as a "slice" through the brain (Figure 4.12B). The slices can be reconstructed by the computer into three-dimensional images for a better understanding of brain structure.

Magnetic resonance imaging (MRI) further refines the ability to view the living brain by using computerized measurements of the distinct waves that different atoms emit when placed in a strong magnetic field and activated by radio-frequency waves. This method distinguishes different body tissues based on their individual chemical composition. Because tissues contain different amounts of water, they can be distinguished by scanning the magnetic-induced resonance of hydrogen. The image provides exquisite detail and, as is true for CT, sequential slices can be reconstructed to provide three-dimensional images (Figure 4.13).

It did not take long for scientists to realize the power of their new tool, and they proceeded to use the computerized scanning technique to view the localization of radioactively labeled materials injected into a living human. **Positron emission tomography (PET)** does not create images of the brain but maps the distribution of a radioactively labeled substance that has been injected into an individual. To do this safely with human subjects, we must use radioisotopes

that decay quickly rather than accumulate. While radioactive isotopes used in many laboratory experiments have relatively long half-lives, on the order of 1200 years for ^{3}H or 5700 years for ^{14}C, those used for PET have half-lives of 2 minutes (^{15}O), 20 minutes (^{11}C), or 110 minutes (^{18}F). Isotopes that decay and lose their radioactivity quickly (i.e., have a short half-life) emit positrons, which are like electrons but have a positive charge. When a positron expelled from the nucleus collides with an electron, both particles are annihilated and emit two gamma rays traveling in opposite directions. In a PET scanning device (Figure 4.14A), detectors surround the head to track these gamma rays and locate their origin. The information is analyzed by computer and visualized as an image on the monitor.

PET is useful to neuropharmacology in several ways (Farde, 1996). First, a radioactively labeled drug or ligand can be administered and the location of binding in brain tissue can be seen. The technique has been used successfully to localize neurotransmitter receptors and identify where drugs bind. Perhaps even more exciting is the use of PET to determine which parts of the brain are active during the performance of particular tasks or cognitive problem solving (Figure 4.14B). PET allows us to visualize brain activity, which is reflected in increases in glucose utilization, oxygen use, and blood flow, depending on which reagent has been labeled. Very much like autoradiography in living humans, PET can be used along with 2-DG to map brain areas that utilize increased glucose or demonstrate increased blood flow, both indicative of heightened neural activity.

Single-photon emission computerized tomography (SPECT) is very similar to PET imaging, but it is much simpler and less expensive since the radiolabeled probes do not have to be synthesized but are commercially available. When scanned, the radioactive compounds, either inhaled or injected, show the changes in regional blood flow. Although resolution is less accurate than with PET, the SPECT data can be combined with CT or MRI scans to localize the active areas more precisely than with SPECT alone.

Functional MRI (fMRI) has become the newest and perhaps most powerful tool in the neuroscientist's arsenal for visualizing brain activity. To meet the increased metabolic demand of active neurons, the flow of blood carrying oxygen to these cells increases. Functional MRI can detect the increases in blood oxygenation caused by cell firing because oxygenated hemoglobin (the molecule that carries the oxygen in the blood and provides the red color) has a different magnetic resonance signal than oxygen-depleted hemoglobin. Functional MRI has several advantages over PET. First, fMRI provides both anatomical and functional information in each subject and the detail of the image is far superior. Second, since the individual does not have to be injected with radioactive material, the measures can be made repeatedly to show changes over time. For the same reason, the procedure is essentially risk free, except for the occasional case of claus-

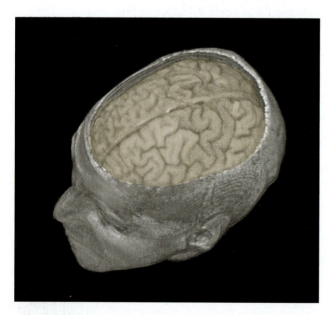

Figure 4.13   A three-dimensional image formed with MRI Computer technology provides the opportunity to create three-dimensional representations of the brain from sequential slices.

(A) Positron emission tomography (PET)

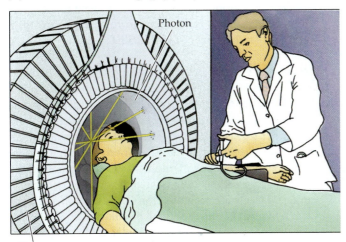

Photon

Photon
detectors

(B)

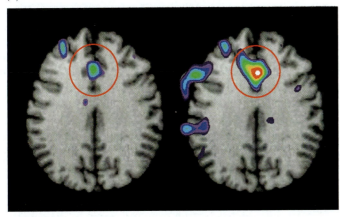

Figure 4.14 Positron emission tomography
(A) A typical scanning device for PET. Notice the photode-tectors that surround the head to track the gamma rays produced when a positron expelled from the nucleus col-lides with an electron. (B) PET scan image showing active brain areas by measuring regional cerebral blood flow under two conditions. The subject on the left, who was told to expect only mild discomfort from putting a hand into 47°C water, showed less neuronal activity (correlated with less blood flow) in the anterior cingulate cortex than the subject on the right, who expected more pain. Highly active areas are colored orange, red, and white. Further experiments might assess how certain drugs change the pattern of activation. (From Rainville et al., 1997; courtesy of Pierre Rainville.)

trophobia caused by the scanner. Third, the process is so rapid that brain activity can be monitored in real time (i.e., as it is occurring). In combination with recording electrical activity with electroencephalography (see the following paragraph), fMRI can produce three-dimensional images showing neural activity in interconnecting networks of brain centers. Temporal sequencing of information processing becomes possible, so one can see the changing locations of brain activity during tasks and cognitive processes. For an excellent introduction to brain imaging and its relationship to cognitive processes, refer to Posner and Raichle (1994).

Electroencephalography (EEG) In addition to improved visualization techniques and methods of mapping metabolic function in the human brain, a third non-invasive method of investigating human brain activity is now used often in neuropharmacology: electrical recording with **electroencephalography (EEG).** Electrodes are taped to the scalp in several locations (Figure 4.15A), and the electrical activity that is recorded reflects the sum of electrical events of populations of neurons. Multiple elec-

(A) Multichannel EEG recording

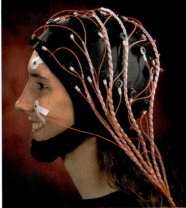

(B)

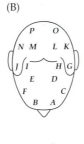

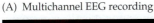

200 mV

1 s

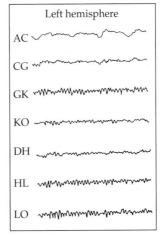

Left hemisphere

AC

CG

GK

KO

DH

HL

LO

Figure 4.15 Electroen-cephalography (A) In humans, changes in electrical activity of the brain are detected by record-ing electrodes that are attached to the surface of the individual's scalp. The electrodes record the activity of thousands of cells simultaneously. (B) Examples of a typical electroencephalogram showing the differences in electri-cal potential between specific locations on the scalp.

trodes are used because a comparison of the signals from various locations can identify the origin of some waves. Although the method cannot identify specific cells that are active, it has been useful in studies of consciousness, sleep, and dreaming, as well as studies of seizure activity Figure 4.15B shows typical EEG records. Computer analysis of EEG signals can produce a color-coded map of brain electrical activity, which allows a visualization of electrical response to changing stimuli. Brain electrical activity mapping (BEAM) is one of the available display systems. Because EEG can detect electrical events in real time, it is very useful in recording electrical changes in response to momentary sensory stimulation; these changes are called **event-related potentials** or sensory evoked potentials. Evaluation of electrical responses in various clinical populations has led to improved understanding of attention deficits and processing differences in individuals with schizophrenia, Huntington's disease, attention deficit disorder, and so forth.

Genetic engineering helps neuroscientists to ask and answer new questions

The excitement surrounding the completion of the Human Genome Project, in which all of the human genetic material has been mapped, has permeated both the scientific and the popular press. Although the term *genetic engineering* evokes both excitement and some trepidation in most people, the technology has at the very least provided amazing opportunities for neuroscience. Genetic engineering involves chemically modifying precise sites in the molecular structure of a gene in order to change the structure of the product produced by normal gene expression.

Targeted mutations, or knockout techniques   This new method, based on advances in molecular biology, may represent the most sophisticated of all lesioning techniques yet described. With the ability to identify which piece of the chromosomal DNA (i.e., the gene) is responsible for directing the synthesis of a particular protein, neuroscience has the opportunity to alter that gene, causing a change in the expression of the protein. In essence, we are producing an animal model that lacks a particular protein (e.g., an enzyme, ion channel, or receptor) so that we can evaluate the post-lesioning behavior. We can also use these animals to identify the importance of that protein to specific drug effects.

The procedure requires elimination of the gene in isolated embryonic cells by destroying the base sequence on the chromosome that codes for a particular protein. The altered genes are then inserted into fertilized eggs of a foster mother. After birth, the pups are examined for incorporation of the altered DNA into their genes and for the possible expression of the mutation (e.g., altered behavior). As adults they are bred to create homozygous mice that lack the gene completely (**knockout mice**). Comparing the behavior and drug response of the altered mice with those of unaltered animals

will tell us about the function of the protein that has been deleted. For neuropharmacologists, the protein of interest is often a receptor subtype or an enzyme that controls an important synthesizing or metabolizing process.

Gene replacement   A second strategy involves the replacement of one gene for another, producing **transgenic mice.** As we learn more about the pathological genes responsible for neuropsychiatric diseases such as Huntington's and Alzheimer's diseases, it is possible to remove the human genes and insert them into mice to produce true animal models of the disorders. For an example, see the work by Carter and coworkers (1999), which measures motor deficits in mice transgenic for Huntington's disease. With authentic animal models, neuroscience will be able to identify the cellular processes responsible for a disorder and develop appropriate treatments.

As is true for any revolutionary new technique, caution in interpreting the results is warranted. First, because behaviors are not regulated by single genes but by multiple interacting genes, changing or eliminating only one alters only a small part of the overall behavioral trait. Second, compensation by other genes for the missing or overexpressed gene may mask the functional effect of the mutation. Third, since the altered gene function occurs in all tissues at all stages of development, it is possible that changes in other organs or other brain areas are responsible for the behavioral changes. Finally, since these animals are developing organisms, environmental factors also have a significant effect on the ultimate gene expression. Several articles provide greater detail on the potential pitfalls of gene-targeting studies (Crawley, 1996; Gerlai, 1996; Lathe, 1996).

In addition to creating "mutant" animals, the genetic material can be inserted into cells (maintained in cell culture) that do not normally have a particular protein (e.g., receptor). The normal cell division process produces large numbers of identically altered cells, which we call **cloning.** These cells can then be used to screen new drugs using conventional pharmacological techniques for identifying agonists and antagonists.

A variation of gene modification uses short-term manipulations of the genetic material by intraventricular injection of **antisense nucleotides** that bind to targeted mRNAs, delay their translation, and increase their degradation. Such treatment produces a reversible "mutant" animal whose behavior or drug responsiveness can be evaluated. For instance, earlier research suggested that a decrease in the function of the neuropeptide called vasoactive intestinal peptide (VIP) in the hypothalamus (specifically the suprachiasmatic nucleus) may be responsible for the disturbances in circadian rhythms that occur during aging. To test this hypothesis, Harney et al. (1996) used antisense oligonucleotides that targeted VIP-containing neurons in the suprachiasmatic nucleus. Figure 4.16 shows the reduction in VIP concentration in the suprachias-

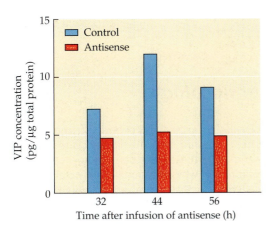

Figure 4.16 Effect of antisense on protein synthesis
Vasoactive intestinal peptide (VIP) concentrations in the suprachiasmatic nucleus of the hypothalamus are significantly reduced in animals treated with antisense oligonucleotides directed at VIP mRNA as compared to control animals. The decrease in VIP is apparent at each of the times measured. (After Harney et al., 1996.)

matic nucleus at different times after antisense administration. What the investigators found was that suppressing the synthesis of VIP in this brain region does indeed mimic the effect of age on cyclic hormone secretion. This technique is well suited to study the biological rhythm of reproductive hormones and their effects on behavior.

Section Summary

The goals of neuropsychopharmacology are to understand (1) the physiological and neurochemical mechanisms that are responsible for behavior as well as (2) how drugs interact with brain chemistry to modify that behavior. The tools and techniques of neuroscience allow us to combine results from studies using both humans and other animals. Lesioning selected brain areas using a stereotaxic device is the oldest of the methods, but modifications to this method that use neurotoxins to destroy cell bodies without damaging axons passing through the area have distinct advantages. Neurotoxins that are selective for a particular neurotransmitter provide the chance to lesion cells based on neurochemical identity. By implanting cannulas to deliver minute amounts of drugs, either agonists or antagonists, to functioning animals, we can test our knowledge of the role of specific receptors in behavior. Electrical stimulation and recording of the brain likewise provides a method to evaluate the role of particular cells in a behavioral response.

Emphasizing the role of receptors in pharmacology, the radioligand binding method has been developed to evaluate the number and affinity of specific receptor molecules. To locate these receptors more precisely in the brain, receptor

autoradiography, both in vitro and in vivo, is used. The ability to make antibodies to various proteins paves the way for more precise cellular localization of receptors or other protein components of cells like enzymes. Immunocytochemistry uses the antibodies to precisely locate cells containing a particular protein, while a complementary technique, in situ hybridization, can tell us which cells are manufacturing a given molecule by labeling cells with an appropriate mRNA probe. DNA microarrays provide a means to simultaneously evaluate the expression of thousands of genes to identify those involved in complex clinical diseases along with potential therapeutics to combat the disorders.

It is now possible to visualize cognitive functioning in the human brain and use animals to examine the cellular details of that functioning. Computerized tomography and MRI provide detailed representations of the human brain. PET, SPECT, and fMRI each provide a slightly different window into the working activity of the human brain using advanced computer technology to evaluate changes in cell function. Based on the premise that active brain cells use more glucose and oxygen and receive increased cerebral blood flow, the computerized methods are analogous to autoradiography but can be accomplished in an awake and functioning subject.

Clearly the use of genetic engineering to create transgenic or knockout mice provides the most sophisticated type of lesioning yet devised. By modifying a single piece of genetic material, the expression of a specific protein can be modified or eliminated to identify the biochemical and/or behavioral function of that protein.

Bear in mind that under normal circumstances several of these techniques are used in tandem to approach a problem in neuroscience from several directions (see Box 4.1). The power of these experimental tools is that when they are used together a more reasonable picture emerges and conflicting results can be incorporated into the larger picture. Only in this way can we uncover the neurobiological substrates of cognitive function and dysfunction. In every case, interpretation of these sophisticated approaches is subject to the same scrutiny that the earliest lesion experiments required. Remember, healthy skepticism is central to the scientific method.

Techniques in Behavioral Pharmacology

Evaluating Animal Behavior

The techniques of behavioral pharmacology allow scientists to evaluate the relationship between an experimental manipulation such as a lesion or drug administration and changes in behavior. In a well-designed experiment, it is necessary to compare the behavior of the experimental treatment group with that of placebo control subjects. The neurobiological

The Cutting Edge

Using the Techniques of Neuropsychopharmacology

The techniques of neuropharmacology and behavioral pharmacology are most often combined to test hypotheses of how drugs act on CNS neurons to alter behavior. Approaching a problem from several different directions reinforces the underlying model if results are consistent. Any discrepancies will cause the conceptual model to be changed and provide an avenue for future research. In one recent study, Picciotto and colleagues (1998) created knockout (KO) mice that lacked one specific subunit of the acetylcholine receptor. Such a mutation did not produce animals lacking all acetylcholine receptors, but only those containing the β_2-subunit. What they discovered was that although the KO animals looked just like their littermate controls, receptor binding studies showed that they lacked the ability to bind nicotine in the brain.

Several different methods were used to show the animals' lack of sensitivity to nicotine. Using in vivo microdialysis in combination with HPLC, they found that in contrast to control animals, intraperitoneal nicotine administration failed to cause dopamine to be released in the striatum of the KO mice (Figure A). Evaluating the electrophysiological discharge rate of dopaminergic neurons also showed no response to nicotine in brain slices from the KO mice, while controls responded with a moderate increase in frequency (Figure B).

The ability of nicotine to increase motor activity and produce reinforcing effects is believed to be due to nicotine-induced increase in dopamine function. The previous experiments showed that the KO animals failed to respond to nicotine with an increase in dopamine. Hence the researchers predicted that the mutant mice might show differences in locomotion and also fail to self-administer nicotine. Surprisingly, behavioral measures showed no differences between the two groups in spontaneous exploration in a novel environment (Figure C). However, when they were in a familiar environment, locomotor activity was reduced by 50% in the KO animals compared to controls. These results suggest that endogenous (normally occurring) acetylcholine might act through this subtype of acetylcholine receptor to regulate locomotion but not

exploratory behavior in a novel environment. The differences measured in these two tests of motor activity show why even simple behavioral measures must be evaluated cautiously.

To see whether nicotine is reinforcing for the KO mice, a self-administration experiment was devised. The animals were trained to work for intravenous cocaine injection. Once a stable baseline of responding for cocaine was achieved, the cocaine was replaced with nicotine or saline. Control mice maintained a significant amount of responding for nicotine over a 5-day period, but the response of mutant mice was significantly different (Figure D). The KO mice showed a decrease in response over the 5 days, suggesting that the available nicotine injections were not reinforcing. The response for nicotine in KO mice resembled the low response rate produced by a replacement with saline in normal mice. It would seem that altering the acetylcholine receptor prevents the stimulation of dopamine neurons and also prevents the self-administration of nicotine. From these data and other evidence (Stolerman et al., 1995), the authors

(A) Dopamine release

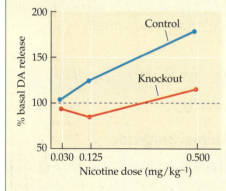

(B) Discharge rate of dopaminergic neurons

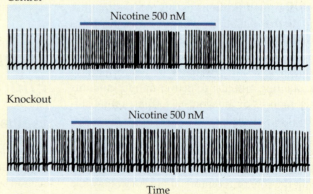

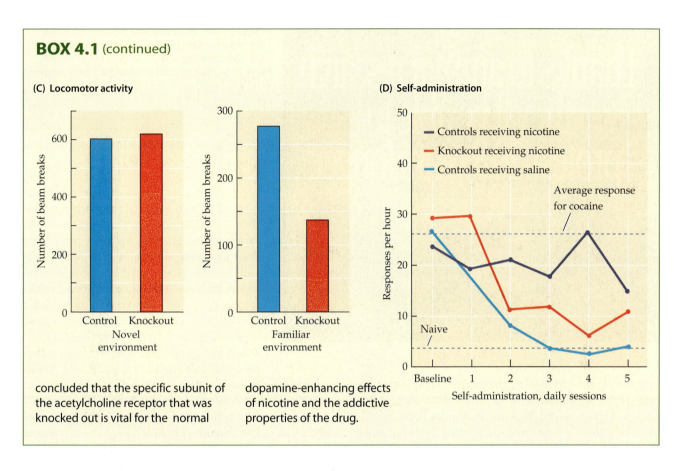

BOX 4.1 (continued)

(C) Locomotor activity

Number of beam breaks (axis: 0, 200, 400, 600)

Control   Knockout
Novel
environment

Number of beam breaks (axis: 0, 100, 200, 300)

Control   Knockout
Familiar
environment

(D) Self-administration

Responses per hour (axis: 0, 10, 20, 30, 40, 50)

— Controls receiving nicotine
— Knockout receiving nicotine
— Controls receiving saline

Average response
for cocaine

Naive

Baseline   1   2   3   4   5
Self-administration, daily sessions

concluded that the specific subunit of the acetylcholine receptor that was knocked out is vital for the normal dopamine-enhancing effects of nicotine and the addictive properties of the drug.

---

techniques (such as selective lesioning and intracerebral drug administration) described earlier tell us very little unless we have an objective measure of the behavioral consequences. Behavioral measures are crucial for (1) understanding the neurochemical basis of behavior as well as drug-induced changes in that behavior; (2) developing animal models of psychiatric disorders; and (3) screening the large number of newly designed and synthesized drug molecules in preclinical pharmaceutical settings.

Animal testing needs to be valid and reliable to produce useful information

Animal studies clearly have several advantages over studies using human subjects. The most obvious advantage is the use of rigorous controls. The living conditions (e.g., diet, exercise, room temperature, exposure to stress, day–night cycle) of animal subjects can be regulated far more precisely than those of humans. In addition, the histories of animal subjects are well known and the genetic backgrounds of a group of animals are very similar and well characterized. Finally, animals are the most appropriate subjects for the study of mechanisms of drug action because an understanding of the electophysiological and neurochemical bases of drug effects often requires invasive techniques that are obviously unethical with human

subjects. Consider, for example, the valuable information gained from transgenically manipulated animals. In addition, drugs can be administered to animal subjects in ways not generally appropriate for humans, for example, over long periods of time to determine toxic effects or the potential for addiction. Finally, the brains and behavior of nonhuman mammals and humans are similar enough to allow generalization across species. For example, lesions of the central nucleus of the amygdala of rats produce profound changes in the animals' conditioned emotional response. Likewise, tumors, strokes, or surgical procedures that damage the human amygdaloid complex produce profound changes in fearfulness, anxiety, and emotional memory.

The impact of animal testing in biomedical research on the quality of human life (Figure 4.17) and its alternatives is discussed in a thought-provoking manner by Hollinger (1997). The need for animal experimentation is best seen under conditions when research is impossible using human subjects, as when testing the effects of alcohol on fetal development. Ethical constraints prohibit researchers from administering varying doses of alcohol to groups of pregnant women to evaluate the effects on their newborns. Instead, data collected on alcohol consumption during pregnancy and the occurrence of fetal alcohol syndrome (FAS) suggests a relationship that tells us that the more alcohol a

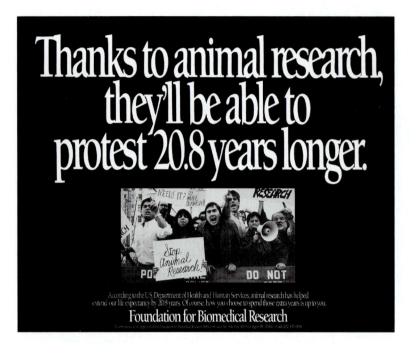

Figure 4.17 A poster used to counter the claims of animal rights activists increases public awareness about the benefits of animal research. (Courtesy of the Foundation for Biomedical Research.)

pregnant female consumes, the more likely it is that her infant will show signs of FAS. Although we know that infants of mothers who consume alcohol are more likely to show fetal abnormalities, the type of study described shows only a **correlational relationship;** we cannot assume alcohol *causes* FAS since other factors may be responsible for both. For example, poverty, poor diet, or other drug use may both lead to increased alcohol consumption *and* cause developmental defects in the fetus. Therefore, to learn more about how alcohol affects fetal development, we need to perform animal studies. Since animal testing remains an important part of new drug development and evaluation, strict animal care guidelines have been developed to ensure proper treatment of subjects. The animal-testing stage provides an important step between basic science and the treatment of human conditions.

The Health Extension Act of 1985 provides strict guidelines for the care of animals used in biomedical and behavioral research. The goal of the legislation is humane animal maintenance and experimentation that limits both the use of animals and animal distress. Each research institution must have an animal care committee that reviews each scientific protocol with three considerations in mind: (1) the research should be relevant to human or animal health, advancement of knowledge, or the good of society; (2) alternative methods such as computer simulations that do not require animal subjects must be considered; and (3) procedures must avoid or minimize discomfort, distress, and pain. Periodic inspections of living conditions assure that they are appropriate for their species and contribute to health and comfort: size, temperature, lighting, cleanliness, access to food and water, sanitation, and medical care are ensured. Animal care and use committees have the ability to veto any studies that they feel do not meet all the predetermined criteria.

Some animal tests used to evaluate drug effects on physiological measures such as blood pressure or body temperature closely resemble the test used for humans. These tests have high **face validity.** However, for many psychiatric disorders the symptoms are described in typically human terms, such as a certain facial expression, altered mood, or disordered thinking. In these cases a correlated, quantifiable measure in an animal is substituted for a more cognitive human behavior for testing purposes. When the correlation is strong, a drug that modifies rat behavior in a specific way can be expected to predictably alter a particular human behavior, even though the two behaviors seem unrelated. For instance, if a new drug were to reduce apomorphine-induced hyperactivity in rats, tests on humans might show it to be effective in treating schizophrenia (see Chapter 17). Tests such as these have low face validity. However, if the drug effects in the laboratory test closely parallel or predict the clinical effect, the tests may be said to demonstrate **construct validity,** or **empirical validity.** To be optimal, an animal behavioral test should also:

1. Be *specific* for the class of drug being screened. If antidepressants, for example, produce a consistent response in a behavioral test, we would probably not want to see analgesic drugs producing the same effect.
2. Be *sensitive* so that the doses used are in a normal therapeutic range and show a dose–response relationship.
3. Demonstrate the same *rank order of potency* (i.e., ranking drugs according to the dose that is effective) as the drugs' order of potency in therapeutic action.

In addition, good behavioral measures have high **reliability,** meaning that the same results will be recorded each time the test is used (Treit, 1985). Valid and reliable animal tests are an important component of the preclinical trials for new drug development (Box 4.2).

A wide variety of behaviors are evaluated by psychopharmacologists

There are many behavioral tests used by psychopharmacologists and they vary considerably in complexity, time needed to be carried out, and cost, as well as validity and reliability. In this next section we will describe just a few of the

Clinical Applications

Drug Development and Testing

All new drugs produced and sold by pharmaceutical companies must be approved by the Food and Drug Administration (FDA). For approval they must be demonstrated to be both effective and safe. Design and testing of new drugs is a long, complex, and expensive procedure involving extensive evaluation in both laboratory and clinical settings. The process utilizes many of the methods we have discussed so far in addition to extensive testing in humans (Zivin, 2000).

The figure shows a timeline of typical drug development beginning with preclinical trials, which include in vitro neuropharmacological methods, such as receptor binding, autoradiography, and so forth. In vivo animal studies provide important information about pharmacokinetics (absorption, distribution, and metabolism), the effective dose range, and the toxic and lethal doses. In addition, animal behavioral models and animal models of neurological and psychiatric disorders pro-

vide a means to screen and evaluate potentially useful drugs. Following preclinical testing, a drug considered safe is tested with humans in three distinct phases. In Phase 1, the drug is evaluated for toxicity and pharmacokinetic data in a small group of healthy human volunteers. In Phase 2, limited clinical testing is conducted to evaluate the drug's effectiveness in treating a particular disease. Finally, the drug is tested again in large clinical trials (Phase 3) involving thousands of patients and multiple testing sites around the country. After the third phase is completed, the FDA can evaluate the data collected on both effectiveness and safety. Finally, if the drug receives FDA approval, it can be marketed and sold. Once in general use, the drug may still be evaluated periodically and new warnings issued to maximize safety by monitoring adverse reactions, dangerous drug interactions, and product defects. Although arguments that new drugs are excessively expensive to the consumer are valid, it is important to understand that as few as 20% of new drugs tested reach final approval. That means that the remaining 80% are eliminated only after testing that is

both time-consuming and expensive. The clinical phases, for example, cost approximately $10 million (Phase 1), $20 million (Phase 2), and $45 million (Phase 3).

To protect its investment, a pharmaceutical company is encouraged to patent its drug so that no other company can sell it for a period of 20 years. The company develops a trade name (also called a proprietary name) and has exclusive rights to market that product. After 20 years the drug becomes "generic," and other companies can manufacture and sell their own formulations of the drug after proving to the FDA that they are equivalent to the original, with similar bioavailability. Once the patent has expired, the drug may acquire a variety of trade names, each developed by the individual manufacturer. For example, the newly patented drug buspirone is called BuSpar by its manufacturer. In contrast, since the patent on chlordiazepoxide has expired, the original manufacturer is still marketing Librium, but other pharmaceutical companies now produce chlordiazepoxide under the trade names Reposans, Sereen, and Mitran.

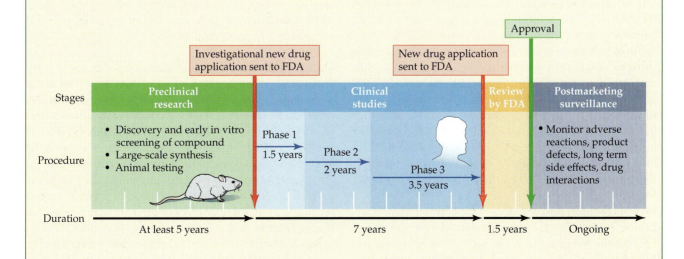

available procedures, many of which will be referred to in subsequent chapters.

Simple behavioral observation   Many simple observations of untrained behaviors require little or no instrumentation. Among the observations made are measures of tremors, ptosis (drooping eyelids), salivation, defecation, catalepsy, reflexes, response to tail pinch, and changes in eating or drinking. Animals demonstrating **catalepsy** are still and immobile and will sometimes remain in an unusual posture if positioned by the experimenter. The time it takes for the animal to return to normal posture gives an indication of the extent of catalepsy. The use of catalepsy as a test to identify antipsychotic drugs that produce motor side effects demonstrates the usefulness of screening tests that are not clearly related to human behavior (see Chapter 17).

Measures of motor activity   These measures identify drugs that produce sleep, sedation, or loss of coordination or, in contrast, drugs that stimulate activity. Spontaneous activity can be measured in a variety of ways. One popular method counts the number of times infrared light beams (invisible to rodents) directed across a designated space are broken. Automated video tracking with computerized analysis is a second method. A third, less automated technique (**open field test**) involves placing the animal in a prescribed area that is divided into squares so the investigator can record the number of squares traversed in a unit of time. It is also possible to count the number of fecal droppings and to observe the amount of time an animal spends along the walls of the chamber rather than venturing toward the open space. High fecal counts and low activity that is primarily at the perimeter of the cage are common indicators of anxiety.

Measures of analgesia   Analgesia is the reduction of perceived pain without loss of consciousness. Analgesia testing with human subjects is difficult because the response to experimentally induced pain is quite different than that to chronic or pathological pain, in which anxiety and the anticipation of more pain influence the individual's response. Of course, we cannot know whether an animal "feels pain" in the same way that a human does, but we can measure the animal's avoidance of a noxious stimulus. One simple test is the **tail-flick test,** in which heat produced by a beam of light (the intensity of which is controlled by a rheostat) is focused on a portion of a rat's tail (Figure 4.18). The latency between onset of the stimulus and the animal's removal of its tail from the beam of light is assumed to be correlated with pain intensity.

Tests of learning and memory   Objective measures of learning and memory, accompanied by careful interpretation of the results, are important whether you are using animal or human subjects. Keep in mind that these tests very often do not determine whether altered responses are due to drug-induced changes in attention or motivation, consolidation or

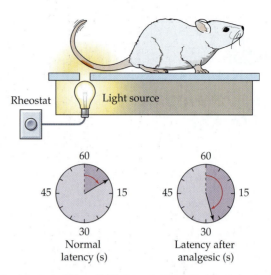

Figure 4.18 The tail-flick test of analgesia measures the response of the animal to a thermal stimulus. The quantitative measure made is the time between the onset of the light beam, which provides heat, and the movement of the tail. The clocks show that the response to the noxious stimulus is delayed following treatment with an analgesic that is known to reduce pain in humans. (After Hamilton and Timmons, 1990.)

retrieval of the memory, or other factors contributing to overall performance. Unless these other factors are considered, tests of learning are open to misinterpretation. Despite the challenges posed, finding new ways to manipulate the neurotransmitters involved in these functions will be central to developing drugs that are useful in treating memory deficits due to normal aging or neurological injuries or diseases such as Alzheimer's and other dementias. There are a wide variety of tests available that depend on the presentation of information (training stage) followed by a delay and then the opportunity for performance (test stage). Higher cognitive processes can be evaluated by creating situations in which reorganization of the information presented is necessary before the appropriate response can be made.

Mazes   Although the size and complexity of mazes can vary dramatically, what they have in common is a start box at the beginning of an alley with one (**T-maze**) or more (**multiple T-maze**) choice points that lead to the final goal box, which contains a small piece of food or other reward. A hungry rat is initially given an opportunity to explore the maze and find the food goal. On subsequent trials, learning is evaluated based on the number of errors at choice points and/or the time taken to reach the goal box. Careful evaluation of results is needed because drug-induced changes in behavior may be due to a change in either learning or motivation (e.g., does the drug make the animal more or less hungry? sedated? disoriented?).

Spatial learning tasks help us investigate the role of specific brain areas and neurotransmitters, such as acetylcholine, in forming memories for the relative locations of objects in

Figure 4.19 The radial arm maze has a central start box (S) and a number of arms or alleys radiating from the center. Goal areas (G) containing food are at the end of each arm.

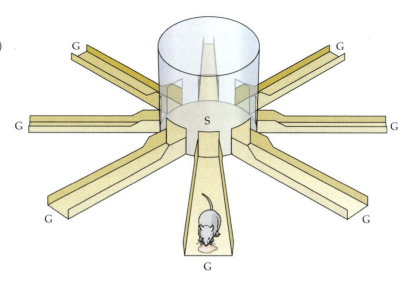

the environment. One special type of maze, the **radial arm maze,** is made up of multiple arms radiating away from a central choice point (Figure 4.19) with a small piece of food at the end of each arm. With very little experience, normal rats learn to forage efficiently by visiting each arm only once on a given day, indicating effective spatial memory for that particular episode. The task can be made more complex by blocking some arms on the initial trial before the animal is returned to the central choice point. The animal is expected to remember which arms have already been entered and move down only those that still contain food. For a normal rat the task is not complex, since it mimics the foraging behavior of animals in the wild, where they must remember where food has been found. But animals with selective lesions in the hippocampus (and other areas) as well as those injected with a cholinergic-blocking drug show significant impairment. Low doses of alcohol also interfere with spatial memory. Because the arms are identical, the animals must use cues in the environment to orient themselves in the maze, hence the need for spatial memory. The task is similar to our daily activity of driving home from work. Not only do we need to recognize each of the landmarks along our route, but we must learn the relative locations of the objects with respect to each other. As we move along our route, our perceptions of the objects and their relative locations to us tell us where we are and where we should be going. Failure in this complex cognitive process is characteristic of Alzheimer's patients who wander away and fail to find their way home.

A second test of spatial learning, the **Morris water maze,** uses a large circular pool of water that has been made opaque by the addition of milk or a dye. Animals placed in the pool must swim until they find the escape platform that is hidden from view just below the surface of the water (Figure 4.20). The subject demonstrates that it has learned the spatial location of the submerged platform by navigating from different starting positions to the platform. Since there are no local cues to direct the escape behavior, successful escape requires the learning of the spatial position of the platform relative to landmarks outside the pool. When curtains surrounding the pool are drawn to block external visual cues, performance falls to chance lev-

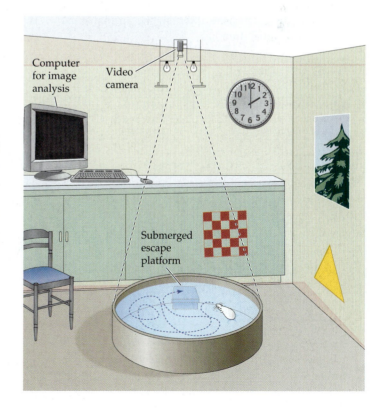

Figure 4.20 The Morris water maze is a circular pool filled with opaque water. The escape platform is approximately 1 cm below the water level. The rat's task is to locate the submerged, hidden platform by using visuospatial cues available in the room. A video camera is mounted above the pool and is connected to the video recorder and computer link to trace the individual swim path. (After Kolb and Whishaw, 1989.)

els, demonstrating the importance of visuospatial cues. As a laboratory technique, the water maze has several advantages. No extensive pretraining is required, and testing can be carried out over short periods of time. Escape from water motivates without the use of food or water deprivation or electric shock; this makes interpretation of drug studies easier, since drug-induced changes in motivation are less likely. One disadvantage, however, is that water immersion may cause endocrine or other stress effects that can interact with the drugs administered.

Delayed-response test   This design assesses the type of memory often impaired by damage to the prefrontal cortex in humans. It is similar to tasks included in the Wechsler Memory Scale, which is used to evaluate working memory deficits in humans. In this task (Figure 4.21), an animal watches the experimenter put a piece of food in one of the food boxes in front of it. The boxes are then closed, and a sliding screen is placed between the monkey and the boxes for a few seconds or minutes (the delay). At the end of the delay, the screen is removed and the animal has the opportunity to recall under which of the covers food is available.

Visual short-term memory can be tested by slightly modifying the procedure. At the beginning of the trial, an object or other stimulus is presented as the sample. After a short delay, during which the sample stimulus is removed, the animal is given a choice between two or more visual stimuli, one of which is the same as the sample. If the animal chooses the pattern that matches the sample, it is given a food reward; an incorrect response yields no reward (see the section on operant conditioning techniques later in the chapter). To make the correct choice after the interval, the animal must "remember" the initial stimulus.

Measures of anxiety   There are many biobehavioral measures available to identify novel antianxiety compounds and evaluate the neurochemical basis of anxiety. Most use induced fear as an analogy to human anxiety. Some use unconditioned animal reactions such as a tendency to avoid brightly lit places or heights, while others depend on traditional learning designs (see the conflict test described in the section on operant conditioning later in the chapter). The **light–dark crossing task** involves a two-compartment box with one side brightly lit (normally avoided by rodents) and the other side dark. Measures include the number of crossings between the bright and dark sections and the amount of time spent on each side, as well as total motor activity. Anxiety-reducing drugs produce a dose-dependent increase in the number of crossings and in overall activity while also increasing the amount of time spent in the light. The **elevated plus-maze** is a cross-shaped maze raised 50 cm off the floor that has two open arms (normally avoided due to aversion to heights) and two arms with enclosed sides. This quick and simple test shows a selective increase in open-arm exploration following treatment with antianxiety drugs and a reduction following treatment with caffeine and amphetamine, drugs considered to increase anxiety.

Measures of fear   In contrast to the spontaneous-behavior models described so far, tests based on learned behaviors require a certain amount of training and hence are generally more costly and time-consuming. The **conditioned emotional response** depends on presentation of a signal (a light or tone) followed by an unavoidable electric shock to form a classically conditioned association. When the warning signal is presented during ongoing behavior, the behavior is suppressed (i.e., "freezing" occurs). Although this method has

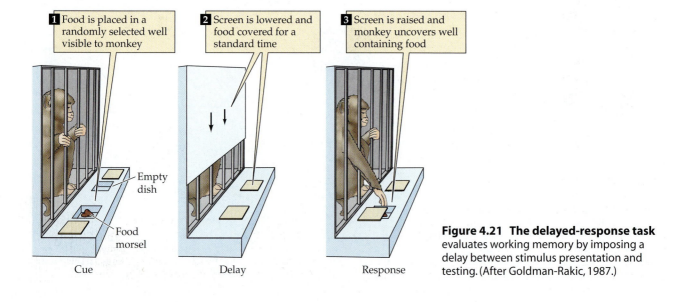

1 Food is placed in a randomly selected well visible to monkey

2 Screen is lowered and food covered for a standard time

3 Screen is raised and monkey uncovers well containing food

Empty dish

Food morsel

Cue

Delay

Response

Figure 4.21 The delayed-response task evaluates working memory by imposing a delay between stimulus presentation and testing. (After Goldman-Rakic, 1987.)

not always produced consistent results when used to screen antianxiety drugs, it has become an important tool in understanding the role of the amygdala and its neurochemistry in the conditioned fear response.

A second method is **fear-potentiated startle,** which refers to the enhancement of the basic startle response when the stimulus is preceded by the presentation of a conditioned fear stimulus. For example, if a light has been previously paired with a foot shock, the presentation of that light normally increases the magnitude of the startle response to a novel stimulus, such as a loud clap.

Measures of reward   Although several popular measures to evaluate the rewarding and reinforcing effects of drugs are operant techniques (described in the next section), a method called **conditioned place preference** relies on a classically conditioned association between drug effect and environment (Figure 4.22) During conditioning trials over several days, the animal is injected with either drug or saline and consistently placed in one compartment or the other so that it associates the environment with the drug state. The rewarding or aversive effect of the drug is determined in a test session in which the animal has access to both compartments and the amount of time spent in each is monitored. If the drug is rewarding, the animal spends much more time in the compartment associated with the drug. If the drug is aversive, the animal prefers the compartment associated with saline injection. Additionally, researchers may study the biological basis for the rewarding effects by pretreating animals with selected receptor antagonists or neurotoxins to modify the place preference. Stolerman (1992) reviews sev-

eral behavioral principles and methods related to drug reward and reinforcement.

Operant conditioning techniques provide a sensitive measure of drug effects

Operant conditioning has also made contributions to the study of drug effects on behavior. The underlying principle of operant conditioning is that consequences control behavior. An animal performs because it is reinforced for doing so. Animals learn to respond to obtain rewards and avoid punishment.

Although it is possible to train many types of operant responses, depending on the species of animal used, experiments are typically carried out in an operant chamber (Skinner box). An operant chamber is a soundproof box with a grid floor that can be electrified for shock delivery, a food or water dispenser for rewards, lights or loudspeaker for stimulus cue presentation, and levers that the animal can press (Figure 4.23). Computerized stimulus presentation and data collection provide the opportunity to measure the total number of responses per unit time. In addition, the technique records response rates and interresponse times, which provide a stable and sensitive measure of continuous behavior.

In a brief training session, the animal learns to press the lever to receive a food reinforcer. Once the behavior is established, the requirements for reinforcement can be altered according to a predetermined schedule (**schedule of reinforcement**). The rate and pattern of the animal's behavior is controlled by the schedule, and it allows us to examine the effect of a drug on the pattern of behavior. For instance, on a fixed-ratio (FR) schedule, reinforcement is delivered after a

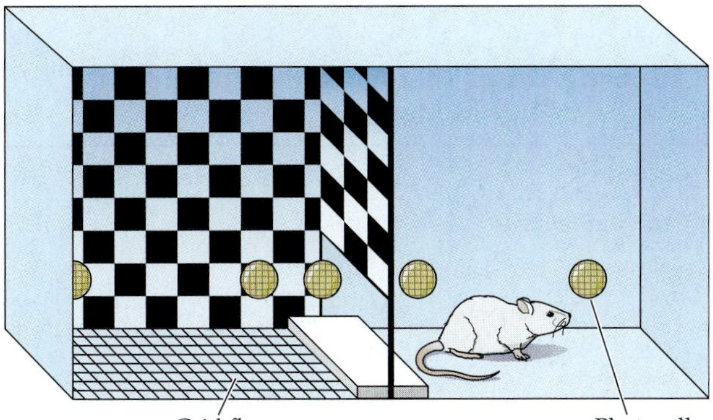

Figure 4.22 Place-conditioning apparatus The apparatus consists of two distinctly different compartments varying in the pattern and texture of floor and walls. Photocells monitor the animal's movement. Each compartment is repeatedly paired with either drug or saline injection. On the test day the animal is allowed free access to both compartments and the amount of time spent in each tells us whether the drug effect was rewarding or aversive. (After Stolerman, 1992.)

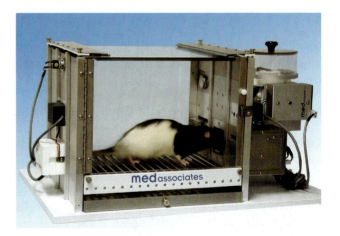

Figure 4.23 Rat in an operant chamber The rat can be trained to press the lever (response) to activate a food delivery mechanism (reinforcement). An animal can also learn to press the lever to terminate or postpone shocks that can be delivered through the grid floor. (Courtesy of Med Associates, Inc.)

fixed number of responses. Thus, an FR-3 schedule means that the animal must press the lever 3 times to receive 1 food pellet. Changing the fixed ratio from 3 to 20 or 45 will tell us how hard the animal is willing to work for the reinforcement. Interval schedules also are commonly used and are characterized by the availability of reinforcement after a certain amount of time has elapsed (rather than the number of bar presses). Thus, on an FI-2 schedule (fixed interval of 2 minutes), reinforcement follows the first response an animal makes after 2 minutes have passed since the last reinforcement. Responses made during the 2-minute interval are "wasted," that is, they elicit no reinforcement. This schedule produces a pattern of responding that includes a pause after each reinforcement and a gradual increase in the rate of responding as the interval ends. For a description of other variations in schedules and their use in drug testing see Carlton (1983).

Measuring anxiety   One classic method used to evaluate anxiety in animals is the **conflict test**, originally designed by Geller and Seifter. The animals are first trained to press a lever in the operant chamber for a standard (food or water) reinforcer. Once the behavior is established, the test sessions involve two stages. In the first, the animals press the lever for the reinforcer. After 10 or 15 minutes, a tone signals a change in the procedure: at this point lever pressing produces a reinforcer (approach) that is accompanied by a foot shock (avoidance), producing an approach–avoidance "conflict" for the subject. This situation is considered analogous to human anxiety experienced in approach–avoidance situations. As you would expect, lever pressing is steady during the reinforced situation but is reduced and variable during the conflict procedure. Antianxiety drugs have no effect on the reinforced schedule but increase the lever pressing during the conflict procedure, indicating that punishing situations are less inhibiting than normal. Naturally, one must be sure that the drugs being tested are not analgesics, which might also be expected to increase responding during the conflict session.

Methods of assessing drug reward and reinforcement

The simple FR schedule has been used very effectively in identifying drugs that have abuse potential—that is, drugs that are capable of inducing dependence. We assume that if an animal will press a lever in order to receive an injection of drug into the blood or into the brain, the drug must have reinforcing properties. The drug **self-administration method** (Figure 4.24) used with rodents is a very accurate indicator of abuse potential in humans. For instance, animals will readily self-administer morphine, cocaine, and amphetamine, drugs that we know are readily abused by humans. In contrast, drugs like aspirin, antidepressants, and antipsychotic drugs are neither self-administered by animals nor

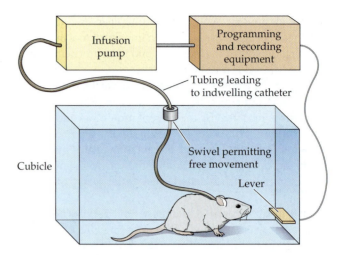

Figure 4.24 The drug self-administration method predicts abuse liability of psychoactive drugs. Pressing the lever according to a predetermined schedule of reinforcement triggers drug delivery into a vein or into discrete brain areas.

abused by humans. Table 4.2 lists some of the drugs that are reinforcing in rhesus monkeys. Compare this list with what you know about substances abused by humans.

Furthermore, we can ask the animal which of several drugs it prefers by placing two levers in the operant chamber and training the animal to press lever A for one drug and lever B for the alternative. Given free access to the levers, the animal's choice will be readily apparent. An additional question we can pose regards how much the animal really "likes" a particular drug. By varying the schedule of reinforcement from FR-10 to FR-40 or -65, we can tell how reinforcing the drug is by

TABLE 4.2 Drugs That Act as Reinforcers in the Rhesus Monkey

Category	Specific drug
Central stimulants	Cocaine
	Amphetamine
	Methylphenidate (Ritalin)
	Nicotine
	Caffeine
Opiates	Morphine
	Methadone
	Codeine
CNS depressants	Pentobarbital
	Amobarbital
	Chlordiazepoxide (Librium)
	Ethyl alcohol

how hard the animal works for the injection. The point at which the effort required exceeds the reinforcing value is called the **breaking point.** The higher the breaking point, the greater the reinforcement of the drug and presumably the greater the abuse potential in humans. Drugs like cocaine sustain incredibly high rates of responding: animals will lever-press for drug reinforcement until exhaustion.

A modification of the method allows the animal to self-administer a weak electric current to discrete brain areas via an indwelling electrode (**electrical self-stimulation).** The underlying assumption is that certain brain areas constitute "reward" pathways. It is assumed that when the animal works to stimulate a particular cluster of neurons, the electrical activation causes the release of neurotransmitters from the nerve terminals in the region, which in turn mediate a rewarding effect. The fact that pretreatment with certain drugs, such as morphine or heroin, increases the responding for even low levels of electrical stimulation indicates that the drugs enhance the brain reward mechanism (Esposito et al. 1989). In combination with mapping techniques, this method provides an excellent understanding of the neural mechanisms of reward and the effects of psychoactive drugs on those pathways.

Drugs as discriminative stimuli   A discriminative stimulus is any stimulus that signals reinforcement for a subject in an operant task. For example, "light on" in the chamber may signal that reinforcement is available following lever pressing, while "light out" signals that no reinforcement is available regardless of the animal's response. An animal that learns to press a lever in the presence of "light on" but not during the "light-out" period can discriminate between the two conditions. Although discriminative stimuli are usually changes in the physical environment, internal cues can also be discriminated. Thus an animal can learn to press the lever for reinforcement when it experiences the internal cues associated with a particular drug state (like the "light on") and to withhold responding in a nondrugged or different drug state (like the "light off"). The animal's response depends on its discriminating among internal cues produced by the drug. For example, if an animal has been trained to lever-press after receiving morphine, other opiates can be substituted for the internal cue and signal to the animal that reinforcement is present. Heroin or methadone are experienced like morphine. In contrast, drugs like amphetamine or marijuana, which apparently produce subjective effects very different from those of morphine, are treated by the animals as a nonreinforced cue. In this way novel drugs can be characterized according to how similar their internal cues are to those of the known drug. The same technique can be used to identify the neurochemical basis for a given drug cue. The drug cue can be challenged with increasing doses of a suspected antagonist until the cue has lost its effect. Likewise, neurotransmitter agonists can be substituted to find which more closely resembles the trained drug cue. Goudie and Leathley (1993) provide an excellent description of the basic methodology of drug discrimination as well as an assessment of potential pitfalls.

Negative reinforcement   A variation on the FR schedule utilizes negative reinforcement, which increases the probability of a response that terminates an averse condition. This technique can be easily applied to **operant analgesia testing.** First, the animal is trained to turn off an unpleasant foot shock by pressing the lever. In the test phase, the researcher administers increasing amounts of foot shock up to the point at which the animal responds by pressing the lever. The lowest shock intensity at which the animal first presses is considered the aversive threshold. Analgesic drugs would be expected to raise the threshold of electric shock. The method is very sensitive even to mild analgesics such as aspirin. However, an independent measure of sedation is necessary to distinguish between failure to respond due to analgesia and failure to respond due to behavioral depression.

Although clinical depression is typically a human condition, an animal model utilizing negative reinforcement called **learned helplessness** provides some fascinating insights. In this design, the subjects in each of two groups are exposed to aversive events (e.g., repetitive foot shocks). The difference between the two groups is that the control group has the opportunity to make a response (e.g., press a lever) that turns the shock off for both groups, while the experimental group has no control over the shock. Hence, although the experimental group cannot modify the shock, it receives the same amount of shock as the control group. The question to be asked is how the experimental group will behave in a new situation that provides them with the opportunity to help themselves. When the animals are placed in a situation in which they can run from an electrified shock chamber to a non-electrified chamber, the control group learns to escape very quickly (Figure 4.25), while the experimental group shows signs of anxiety but makes no appropriate response. Apparently, faced with their earlier experience in which their behavior had no effect on their environment, they have learned to be helpless and to make no attempt to cope. Human depression often follows a personal catastrophe over which the individual has had no control, such as death of a loved one, physical disability, disease, or rejection, and these individuals express feelings of hopelessness and the belief that nothing they do has an effect. This sense that they are passive victims of circumstance provides the theoretical framework for learned helplessness as a model for depression. The effectiveness of traditional antidepressant drugs in reversing the helpless behavior in the animals further validates the model. Chapter 15 discusses the neurochemical correlates of the experimental model and clinical depression and further examines drug effects upon the behavior.

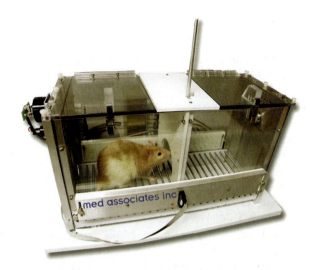

Figure 4.25 Measuring learned helplessness A shuttle box is a two-chambered box with a grid floor through which animals receive a foot shock after a warning tone. Since the shock is applied to only one side of the box, the animal can either avoid or escape the electric shock by moving to the other side. Animals that have experienced lack of control in an earlier aversive situation fail to learn the appropriate response despite showing signs of anxiety. Their "learned helplessness" is used as an animal model of depression. (Courtesy of Med Associates, Inc.)

Section Summary

Techniques in behavioral pharmacology provide a means to quantify animal behavior for drug testing, developing models for psychiatric disorders, and evaluating the neurochemical basis of behavior. The advantages of animal testing include having a subject population with similar genetic background and history, maintaining highly controlled living environments, and being able to use invasive neurobiological techniques.

Animal testing includes a wide range of measures varying not only in validity and reliability but also in complexity, time needed for completion, and cost. Some measures use simple quantitative observation of behaviors such as motor activity and response to noxious stimuli. Other methods assess more complex behaviors such as learning and memory using a variety of techniques such as the classic T-maze as well as mazes modified to target spatial learning: the radial arm maze and Morris water maze. Animal models of anxiety, depression, addiction, and response to pain provide the means to assess human conditions and examine the drugs that modify those responses. Operant conditioning has a special place in pharmacology and is the basis for many tests of addiction potential, anxiety, and analgesia. Each method has benefits and limitations and must be rigorously evaluated to provide data that produce nonbiased and valid conclusions.

Recommended Readings

Geyer, M. A., and Markou, A. (1995). Animal models of psychiatric disorders. In *Psychopharmacology: The Fourth Generation of Progress* (F. E. Bloom and D. J. Kupfer, eds.), pp. 787–798. Raven Press, New York.

Raichle, Marcus E. (1994). Visualizing the mind. *Sci. Am.*, 270, 58–65.

5 *Catecholamines*

*B*arry Kidston was a student and recreational drug user living in Bethesda, Maryland, in 1976. Kidston had studied some chemistry and used a home laboratory to synthesize drugs for his own use. On one occasion, he took some shortcuts in the course of making one of his favorite "designer" drugs, a compound abbreviated MPPP (this drug is chemically similar to the analgesic meperidine, or Demerol). When he injected himself with the resulting product, it produced a powerful burning sensation that had not occurred previously. More importantly, within 3 days Kidston suffered such great motor impairment that he was unable to speak or move. He was initially diagnosed as a catatonic schizophrenic and treated with antipsychotic drugs. When this treatment failed to improve his condition, Kidston was seen by a neurologist who recognized his condition as being indicative of Parkinson's disease.* This was a striking (although correct) diagnosis, since Parkinson's disease is almost always a disorder of aging. What contaminant found its way into Kidston's "home brew" that could cause such rapid and devastating effects? Can it tell us anything about the more typical, spontaneously occurring cases of Parkinson's disease in elderly people?

---

*Readers interested in learning more about this story and a group of related cases are referred to *The Case of the Frozen Addicts*, by Langston and Palfreman (1995).

Hand tremors are one of the cardinal symptoms of Parkinson's disease, a neurological disorder caused by degeneration of midbrain dopamine neurons.

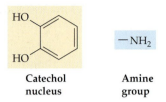

Figure 5.1 Structural features of catecholamines A catechol nucleus and amine group are found in all catecholamines.

We will learn more about Parkinson's disease later in this chapter. The point of mentioning it here concerns the fact that this disorder intimately involves a neurotransmitter called **dopamine (DA).** Dopamine and the related substances **norepinephrine (NE)** and **epinephrine (EPI)** comprise a small but important group of neurotransmitters and hormones called **catecholamines.** The term *catecholamine* comes from the fact that the members of this group all share two chemical similarities: a core structure of catechol and a nitrogen-containing group called an amine (Figure 5.1). The catecholamines, in turn, belong to a wider group of transmitters called either **monoamines** (transmitters that possess one amine group) or **biogenic amines** ("biogenic" refers to compounds made by living organisms). EPI and NE are sometimes called adrenaline and noradrenaline, respectively. It is important to note that the adjective forms for these substances are **adrenergic** and **noradrenergic,** although the term *adrenergic* is sometimes used broadly to refer to NE- as well as EPI-related features. The adjective form for DA is **dopaminergic.** Varying amounts of these substances are found within the central nervous system, the peripheral nervous system, and the inner part of the adrenal glands (adrenal medulla). The adrenal medulla secretes EPI and NE into the bloodstream, where they act as hormones. You will recall from Chapter 3 that the stimulation of catecholamine secretion from the adrenal glands is a vital part of the physiological response to stress.

The main emphasis in this chapter will be on DA and NE, as the neurotransmitter function of EPI is relatively minor. We will begin by considering the basic neurochemistry of the catecholamines, including their synthesis, release, and inactivation. This will be followed by a discussion of the neural systems for DA and NE, including the anatomy of these systems, the receptors for DA and NE, and some of the drugs that act on these receptors.

Catecholamine Synthesis, Release, and Inactivation

Tyrosine hydroxylase catalyzes the rate-limiting step in catecholamine synthesis

Classical transmitters (see Chapter 3) like the catecholamines are manufactured in one or more biochemical steps. These synthetic pathways offer neurons a mechanism for regulating the amount of transmitter available for release. At the same time, they offer us the opportunity to intervene with drugs that alter transmitter synthesis in specific ways. For example, we may administer a precursor that will be converted biochemically into a particular neurotransmitter. One application of this approach is in neurological disorders in which the neurons that make a certain transmitter have been damaged. Precursor therapy represents an attempt to boost transmitter synthesis and release in the remaining undamaged cells. Alternatively, we may give the subjects a drug that blocks a step in the biochemical pathway, thereby causing a depletion of the transmitter synthesized by that pathway. Neurotransmitter depletion is not as widely used clinically, but it can nevertheless be valuable in certain experimental settings.

The synthesis of catecholamine neurotransmitters occurs in several steps, as shown in Figure 5.2. The biochemical pathway begins with the amino acid **tyrosine.** Like other amino acids, tyrosine is obtained from dietary protein and is transported from the blood into the brain. Each of the steps in catecholamine formation depends on a specific enzyme that acts as a catalyst (an agent that increases the rate of a chemical reaction) for that step. Neurons that use DA as their transmitter contain only the first two enzymes, **tyrosine hydroxylase (TH)** and **aromatic amino acid decarboxylase (AADC),** and thus the biochemical pathway stops at DA. In contrast, neurons that need to synthesize NE also possess the third enzyme, which is called **dopamine β-hydroxylase (DBH).***

The conversion of tyrosine to DOPA by TH occurs at a slower rate than the subsequent reactions in the biochemical pathway. Consequently, TH is the **rate-limiting enzyme** in the pathway, because it determines the overall rate of DA or NE formation. The activity of TH is regulated by a variety of factors, including how much DA or NE is present within the nerve terminal. High catecholamine levels tend to inhibit TH, thus serving as a negative feedback mechanism. Another important factor is the rate of cell firing, since neuronal activity has a stimulatory effect on TH. These elegant mechanisms enable dopaminergic and noradrenergic neurons to carefully control their rate of neurotransmitter formation. When the levels are too high, TH is inhibited and catecholamine synthesis is slowed. But when the neurons are activated and firing at a high rate, such as during stress, TH is stimulated and catecholamine synthesis accelerates to keep up with the increased demand.

---

*It is worth noting some of the basics of how enzymes are named. Hydroxylases like TH and DBH add a hydroxyl group (—OH) to the molecule they're acting on. A decarboxylase like AADC removes a carboxyl group (—COOH) from the molecule. These reactions can be seen by following the biochemical pathway shown in Figure 5.2.

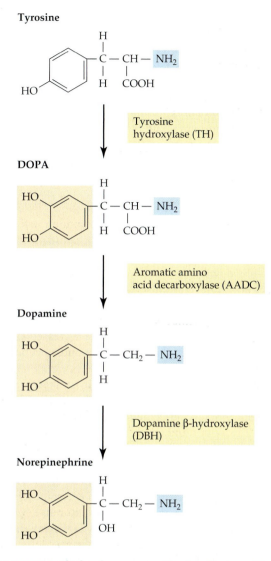

Figure 5.2 Catecholamines are synthesized in a multi-step pathway from the precursor amino acid tyrosine. Tyrosine hydroxylase and aromatic amino acid decarboxylase are found in all catecholaminergic neurons, whereas dopamine β-hydroxylase is present only in cells that use NE as their neurotransmitter.

As would be expected from our earlier discussion, catecholamine formation can be increased by the administration of a biochemical precursor such as L-**DOPA**. Indeed, for many years this compound has been the primary therapeutic agent used in the treatment of Parkinson's disease. Drugs that reduce catecholamine synthesis by inhibiting one of the synthetic enzymes are not as clinically important, but they have had widespread use in both animal and human research. The best example is a drug known as **α-methyl-*para*-tyrosine (AMPT)**. This compound blocks TH, thereby preventing overall catecholamine synthesis and causing a general depletion of these neurotransmitters. In one notable

series of psychiatric studies, AMPT treatment caused a return of depressive symptoms in patients who had previously recovered following treatment with antidepressant drugs that act selectively on the noradrenergic system (Heninger et al., 1996). This suggests that the patients' recovery was dependent on the maintenance of adequate catecholamine levels in the brain.

The enzymes needed to synthesize a classical neurotransmitter like DA, NE, acetylcholine, or serotonin are located to some extent throughout the neurons using that transmitter. Nevertheless, the rate of synthesis is greatest at the nerve endings, near the sites of transmitter release. As mentioned in Chapter 3, this is important for the refilling of recycling vesicles.

Catecholamines are stored in and released from synaptic vesicles

Once catecholamines have been synthesized, they are transported into synaptic vesicles for later release (Figure 5.3).

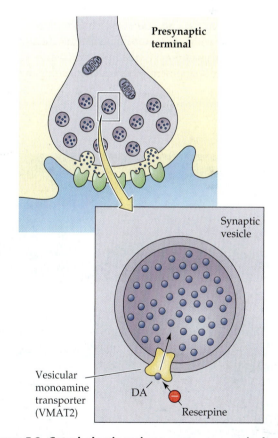

Figure 5.3 Catecholaminergic neurons use a vesicular monoamine transporter protein (VMAT2) to transport neurotransmitter molecules from the cytoplasm of the cell to the interior of the synaptic vesicles. This transport system is blocked by reserpine, which causes a marked depletion of catecholamine levels due to a lack of protection of the transmitter from metabolizing enzymes located outside of the vesicles.

Vesicular packaging is important not only because it provides a means for releasing a predetermined amount of neurotransmitter (usually several thousand molecules per vesicle) but also because it protects the neurotransmitter from degradation by enzymes within the nerve terminal (see the next section). A specific protein in the vesicle membrane is responsible for vesicular catecholamine uptake. This protein recognizes several different monoamine transmitters and is therefore called the **vesicular monoamine transporter (VMAT).** There are actually two related VMATs: VMAT1 is found in the adrenal medulla whereas VMAT2 is present in the brain. Both of these vesicular transporters are blocked by an interesting drug called **reserpine,** which comes from the roots of the plant *Rauwolfia serpentina* (snake root). Blocking the vesicular transporter means that DA and NE are no longer protected from breakdown within the nerve terminal. As a result, both transmitters temporarily drop to very low levels in the brain. The behavioral consequence of this neurochemical effect is sedation in animals and depressive symptoms in humans. Many years ago, a study by the eminent Swedish pharmacologist Arvid Carlsson and his colleagues (Carlsson et al., 1957) showed that reserpine's sedative effects could be reversed by restoration of catecholamines with DOPA, the immediate biochemical precursor of DA (Figure 5.4). Carlsson's work, which played a key role in the development of the catecholamine theory of depression (see Chapter 16), resulted in his being a co-recipient of the 2000 Nobel Prize in Physiology or Medicine.

Release of catecholamines normally occurs when a nerve impulse enters the terminal and triggers one or more vesicles to release their contents into the synaptic cleft by the process of exocytosis (see Chapter 3). Certain drugs, however, can cause a release of catecholamines independently of nerve cell firing. The most important of these compounds are the psychostimulants **amphetamine** and **methamphetamine.** In contrast to the behavioral sedation associated with reserpine-induced catecholamine depletion, catecholamine release leads to behavioral activation. In laboratory animals such as rats and mice, this activation may be shown by increased locomotor activity. At high doses, locomotor activation is replaced by **stereotyped behaviors** consisting of intense sniffing, repetitive head and limb movements, and licking and biting. Researchers believe that locomotion and stereotyped behaviors represent a continuum of behavioral activation that stems from increasing stimulation of DA receptors in the nucleus accumbens and striatum. In humans, amphetamine and methamphetamine cause increased alertness, heightened energy, euphoria, insomnia, and other behavioral effects (see Chapter 11).

Catecholamine release is inhibited by autoreceptors located on the cell bodies, terminals, and dendrites of dopaminergic and noradrenergic neurons. Terminal autoreceptors and other features of a typical dopaminergic neuron are illustrated in Figure 5.5. These autoreceptors inhibit catecholamine release by reducing the amount of calcium (Ca^{2+}) that enters the terminal in response to a nerve impulse (we saw in Chapter 3 that this Ca^{2+} entry is the triggering event for synaptic vesicle fusion with the presynaptic membrane). Thus, if a dopaminergic cell fires several action potentials in a row, we can imagine that DA released by the first few impulses stimulates the terminal autoreceptors and reduces the amount of DA released by the later action potentials. On the other hand, the somatodendritic autoreceptors function in a different way. As mentioned in

(A)

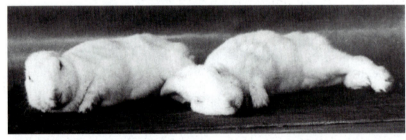

(B)

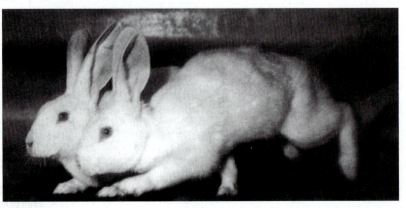

Figure 5.4 Role of catecholamine depletion in the behavioral depressant effects of reserpine (A) Rabbits injected with reserpine (5 mg/kg intravenously) showed extreme behavioral sedation that was reversed by subsequent treatment with DOPA (200 mg/kg intravenously) (B). (From Carlsson, 2001; photographs courtesy of Arvid Carlsson.)

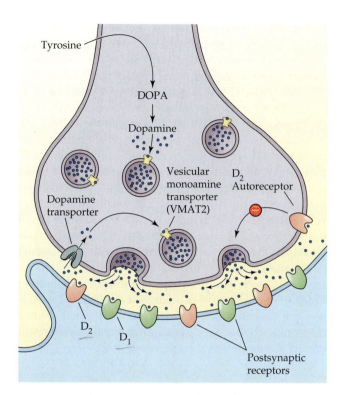

Figure 5.5 A typical dopaminergic neuron possesses autoreceptors on the membrane of its terminals. When these receptors are stimulated, they inhibit subsequent DA release by the cell.

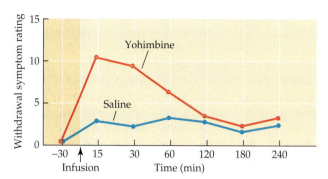

Figure 5.6 Noradrenergic activity contributes to the symptoms of opioid withdrawal When opioid-dependent patients were infused intravenously either with the α_2-receptor antagonist yohimbine (0.4 mg/kg) or a saline control solution, yohimbine but not saline caused a rapid increase in experimenter-rated withdrawal symptoms over the next 60 minutes. (After Stine et al., 2002.)

Chapter 3, these autoreceptors inhibit release indirectly by reducing the rate of firing of the cell.

As discussed below, the DA and NE systems possess a number of different subtypes of receptors. Here we will just mention that the DA autoreceptor is of the D_2 receptor subtype and the NE autoreceptor is of the α_2 subtype. Drugs that stimulate autoreceptors inhibit catecholamine release, just like the neurotransmitter itself. In contrast, autoreceptor antagonists tend to enhance the rate of release by preventing the normal inhibitory effect of the autoreceptors. We can see these effects illustrated dramatically in the case of the noradrenergic α_2-autoreceptor system. Withdrawal from opioid drugs such as heroin and morphine activates the noradrenergic system, which is one of the factors leading to withdrawal symptoms such as increased heart rate, elevated blood pressure, and diarrhea. For this reason, α_2-agonists such as **clonidine** are often used to treat the symptoms of opioid withdrawal due to their ability to stimulate the autoreceptors and inhibit noradrenergic cell firing. In contrast, experimental administration of the α_2-antagonist **yohimbine,** which blocks the autoreceptors and thus increases noradrenergic cell firing and NE release, was found to provoke withdrawal symptoms and drug craving in opioid-dependent patients (Stine et al., 2002) (Figure 5.6). Norepinephrine may also be

involved in producing feelings of anxiety, especially in patients suffering from a mental illness called panic disorder (see Chapter 17). Consequently, yohimbine induces anxiety in such patients and may even trigger a panic attack (Charney et al., 1998). Such an effect obviously has no therapeutic benefit, but it has provided useful research information concerning a possible role of NE in panic disorder and other anxiety-related disturbances.

Catecholamine inactivation occurs through a combination of reuptake and metabolism

The inactivation of catecholamines depends on the two different kinds of processes first mentioned in Chapter 3. The first process is reuptake. Much of the DA and NE that is released synaptically is taken up again into the nerve terminal by means of specific transporter proteins in the nerve cell membrane. That is, dopaminergic neurons contain a **DA transporter** (see Figure 5.5), whereas noradrenergic neurons contain a slightly different protein that is logically called the **NE transporter.** After the neurotransmitter molecules are returned to the terminal, some of them are repackaged into vesicles for re-release while the remainder are broken down and eliminated. It is important to keep in mind that neurotransmitter transporters differ in both their structure and function from the autoreceptors discussed earlier.

The importance of reuptake for catecholamine functioning can be seen when the DA or NE transporter is missing. For example, mutant mice lacking a functional gene for the DA transporter do not show the typical behavioral activation in response to psychostimulants like cocaine or amphetamine, whereas genetic deletion of the NE transporter gene causes increased sensitivity to these same drugs (F. Xu et al., 2000). A role for the NE transporter in cardiovascular function was demonstrated by a case study of identical twins carrying a mutation of the NE transporter gene (Shannon et al., 2000). The patients exhibited abnormally high NE levels in the bloodstream, along with heart rate and blood pressure abnormalities. These findings are consistent with animal studies showing that transporter-mediated uptake plays a vital role in the normal regulation of catecholamine activity.

Since the transporters are necessary for the rapid removal of catecholamines from the synaptic cleft, transporter-blocking drugs enhance the synaptic transmission of DA or NE by increasing the amount of neurotransmitter in the synaptic cleft. This is an important mechanism of action of several kinds of psychoactive drugs, including the **tricyclic antidepressants,** which inhibit the reuptake of both NE and the non-catecholamine transmitter serotonin (5-HT) (see Chapter 16). **Reboxetine** is a relatively new antidepressant that selectively inhibits NE reuptake by blocking only the NE transporter. Yet another important transporter-blocking drug is **cocaine,** which inhibits the reuptake of DA, NE, and 5-HT (see Chapter 11).

Although reuptake can quickly terminate the synaptic actions of catecholamines, there must also be processes of metabolic breakdown to prevent excessive neurotransmitter accumulation. The breakdown of catecholamines primarily involves two enzymes, **catechol-O-methyltransferase (COMT)** and **monoamine oxidase (MAO).** There are two types of MAO: MAO-A and MAO-B. The relative importance of each one depends on the species, brain area, and which neurotransmitter is being metabolized. The action of COMT and MAO, either individually or together, gives rise to several catecholamine **metabolites** (breakdown products). We will only mention the most important ones here. In humans, DA has only one major metabolite, which is called **homovanillic acid (HVA).** In contrast, NE breakdown gives rise to several important compounds, including **3-methoxy-4-hydroxy-phenylglycol (MHPG)** and **vanillylmandelic acid (VMA).** Metabolism of NE within the brain primarily leads to MHPG, whereas VMA is the more common metabolite in the peripheral nervous system. The brain metabolites HVA and MHPG make their way into the cerebrospinal fluid for subsequent clearance from the brain into the bloodstream and, along with VMA, are eventually excreted in the urine. The levels of these substances in the various fluid compartments (that is, blood and urine for all three metabolites and cerebrospinal fluid for HVA and MHPG) provide a rough indication of catecholaminergic activity in the nervous system. Such measurements have played an important role in determining the possible involvement of these neurotransmitters in mental disorders such as schizophrenia and depression (see Chapters 16 and 18).

Not surprisingly, drugs that inhibit catecholamine-metabolizing enzymes lead to an accumulation of these transmitters. Historically, this has been most important in the case of **MAO inhibitors** such as **phenelzine** or **tranylcypromine,** which have long been used in the treatment of clinical depression. More recently, COMT inhibitors such as **entacapone** (**Comtan**) and **tolcapone (Tasmar)** are being used as supplemental therapies to enhance the effectiveness of L-DOPA in treating Parkinson's disease. This is not so much to prevent the metabolism of DA but rather to block the metabolism of L-DOPA by COMT before the precursor reaches the brain.

Before we end this introductory section on catecholamines, it should be noted that at least some dopaminergic and noradrenergic nerve terminals do not seem to form traditional synaptic arrangements. As a result, the neurotransmitter molecules released from these terminals might reach multiple target cells after diffusing a short distance through the extracellular space. This phenomenon, called **volume transmission,** is somewhat like broadcasting a message to a group of people over a loudspeaker instead of talking only to the person next to you in the room, which would be the analogy for standard point-to-point synaptic transmission. Catecholamine systems are not the only ones in which volume transmission occurs (for example, the gaseous messenger nitric oxide operates exclusively through volume transmission), but they were among the first systems in which this phenomenon was demonstrated.

Section Summary

The major catecholamine transmitters in the brain are DA and NE. These substances are synthesized in several steps from the amino acid tyrosine. The first, and also rate-limiting, step in this biochemical pathway is catalyzed by the enzyme TH. Once they have been synthesized, catecholamines are stored in synaptic vesicles for subsequent release. The process of release is controlled by inhibitory autoreceptors located on the cell body, dendrites, and terminals of catecholamine neurons. DA autoreceptors are of the D_2 subtype, whereas NE autoreceptors are of the α_2 subtype. Catecholamines are inactivated by reuptake from the synaptic cleft and also by enzymatic degradation. MAO and COMT are two enzymes important in catecholamine metabolism. The major catecholamine metabolites are HVA for DA, and MHPG and VMA for NE. Certain drugs can modify catecholaminergic function by acting on the processes of synthesis, release, reuptake, or metabolism. Some of these compounds are used either clinically to treat various disorders or experimentally to study the DA or NE systems.

Organization and Function of the Dopaminergic System

Two important dopaminergic cell groups are found in the midbrain

In the early 1960s, Swedish researchers first began to map the location of DA- and NE-containing nerve cells and fibers in the brain (Dahlström and Fuxe, 1964). They developed a classification system in which the catecholamine cell groups (clusters of neurons that stained for either DA or NE) were designated with the letter "A" plus a number from 1 to 16. According to this system, cell groups A1 to A7 are noradrenergic, whereas groups A8 to A16 are dopaminergic. In this book, we will focus only a few catecholaminergic cell groups that are of particular interest to psychopharmacologists. To identify the various systems arising from these cells, we will use both the Swedish classification system and standard anatomical names.

Several dense clusters of dopaminergic neuronal cell bodies are located near the base of the mesencephalon (midbrain). Particularly important is the A9 cell group, which is associated with a structure called the **substantia nigra,** and the A10 group, which is found in a nearby area called the **ventral tegmental area (VTA).** Axons of dopaminergic neurons in the substantia nigra ascend to a forebrain structure known as the caudate-putamen or striatum. Nerve tracts in the central nervous system are often named by combining the site of origin of the fibers with their termination site. Hence, the pathway from the substantia nigra to the striatum is called the **nigrostriatal tract** (Figure 5.7A). This tract is severely damaged in Parkinson's disease (Box 5.1). Because the most prominent symptoms of Parkinson's disease reflect deficits in motor function (for example, tremors, postural disturbances, and difficulty in initiating voluntary movements), it is clear that the nigrostriatal DA tract plays a crucial role in the control of movement.

Two other important ascending dopaminergic systems arise from cells of the VTA. Some of the axons from these neurons travel to various structures of the limbic system, including the nucleus accumbens, septum, amygdala, and hippocampus. These diverse projections constitute the **mesolimbic dopamine pathway** ("meso" represents mesencephalon, which is the site of origin of the fibers; "limbic" stands for the termination of fibers in structures of the limbic system) (Figure 5.7B). Other DA-containing fibers from the VTA go to the cerebral cortex, particularly the prefrontal area. This group of fibers is termed the **mesocortical dopamine pathway** (Figure 5.7C). Together, the mesolimbic and mesocortical pathways are very important to psychopharmacologists because they have been implicated in the neural mechanisms underlying drug abuse (see Chapter 8) and also schizophrenia (see Chapter 18).

A few other sites of dopaminergic neurons can be mentioned briefly. For example, there is a small group of cells in the hypothalamus that gives rise to the **tuberohypophyseal dopamine pathway.** This pathway is important in controlling the secretion of the hormone prolactin by the pituitary gland. There are also DA-containing neurons within sensory structures such as the olfactory bulbs and the retina.

To examine the role of catecholamines in behavior, researchers sometimes damage these systems in ani-

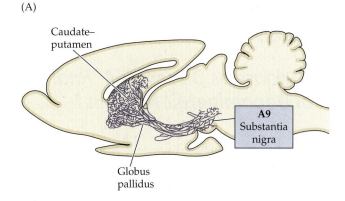

(A)

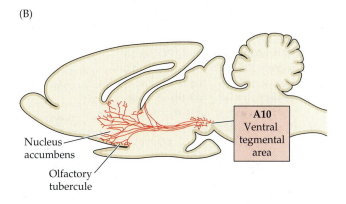

(B)

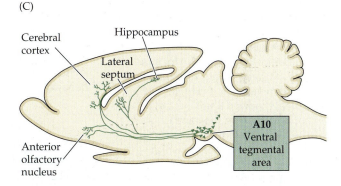

(C)

Figure 5.7 The ascending DA system can be divided into three pathways. The nigrostriatal pathway (A) originates in the substantia nigra (A9 cell cluster) and innervates the caudate–putamen (striatum). The mesolimbic pathway (B and C) originates in the ventral tegmental area (VTA) (A10 cell cluster) and innervates various limbic system structures such as the nucleus accumbens, hippocampus, lateral septum, and amygdala (not shown here). The mesocortical pathway (C) also originates in the VTA and innervates the cerebral cortex.

mals and then evaluate the resulting functional changes. Catecholamine pathways, particularly those using DA, can be lesioned using the substance **6-hydroxydopamine (6-OHDA).** This substance is a **neurotoxin,** which means that it causes injury or death to nerve cells. To lesion the cen-

BOX 5.1 Clinical Applications

Parkinson's Disease—A "Radical" Death of Dopaminergic Neurons?

Some diseases of the brain cause a progressive loss of neurons and their synaptic connections. Of these so-called neurodegenerative diseases, one of the best known is **Parkinson's disease (PD).** This disorder currently afflicts approximately 1.5 million Americans, most of whom are over 60 years old. The major symptoms of PD involve movement. They include tremors, rigidity, bradykinesia (poverty or slowing of movement), and postural disturbances. But PD is not just a motor disorder. Many patients exhibit varying degrees of cognitive dysfunction, sometimes so extreme as to constitute dementia (severe impairment of memory, abstract thinking, and language).

The London physician James Parkinson published the first clinical account of the "shaking palsy" (Parkinson's term for the disorder) in 1817. However, the neurological basis of PD remained unknown for more than 100 years, until a histopathological examination of the brains of PD patients showed a striking loss of nerve cells in the substantia nigra. The term substantia nigra actually means "black substance," which derives from the fact that the cells within this structure appear dark even when unstained because of their content of a neuronal pigment called neuromelanin. Indeed, these pigmented cells are exactly the ones that are lost in PD (Figure A).

More importantly, this collection of cells use DA as their main neurotransmitter. Thus, when one stains for TH immunohistochemically (as a marker for DA neurons) instead of relying on the cells' pigmentation, the same neuronal loss can be seen in the substantia nigra of PD patients. This cellular degeneration is accompanied by a severe decline (>80%) in DA content of the corpus striatum (caudate nucleus and putamen), the major termination point of the nigral axons.

There is no doubt that progressive damage to the ascending dopaminergic system, particularly the nigrostriatal pathway, is largely responsible for the motor disturbances of PD. This assertion is based on four types of findings.

1. Parkinsonian symptoms begin to appear once striatal DA levels decline by 70 to 80% from normal.

2. Beyond this threshold for symptom appearance, there is a correlation between the degree of damage to the dopaminergic system and symptom severity (Figure B).

3. Destruction of the nigrostriatal DA pathway or blockade of striatal DA receptors in either experimental animals or humans causes motor deficits resembling those seen in PD.

4. Pharmacotherapies aimed at increasing DA availability or stimulating DA receptors reduce the behavioral symptoms.

How does a loss of striatal DA result in such profound behavioral disturbances? The answer to this question revolves around the motor functions of the striatum and the interplay between DA and other transmitters within this structure and its related circuitry. The striatum, substantia nigra, and several other structures comprise a subcortical system known as the basal ganglia, which forms a loop with the cerebral cortex. One of the key functions of the basal ganglia is to "gate" movement commands originating in the motor cortex. In a sense, activity of the DA projection to the striatum helps keep the gate "open," whereas loss of this activity impairs gate opening, making it more difficult for the individual to initiate voluntary movements.

Although certain types of surgical procedures are reportedly helpful in reducing extreme tremors in some PD patients, this disease is almost always treated pharmacologically. As mentioned earlier in this chapter, the primary pharmacotherapy for PD involves administering the DA precursor L-DOPA. Unlike many of the classi-

Parkinson's disease   Normal

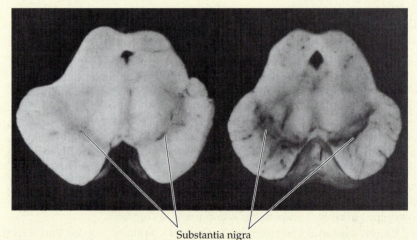

Substantia nigra

(A) Histopathology of Parkinson's disease Unstained sections through the brain stem of a normal individual and a Parkinson's disease patient illustrate the loss of pigmented neurons in the substantia nigra. (From Romanul, 1970.)

BOX 5.1 (continued)

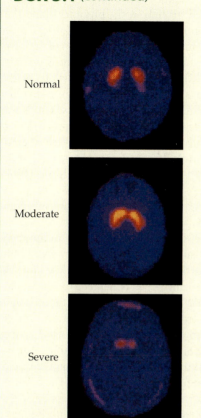

(B) Loss of dopaminergic innervation of the striatum correlates with symptom severity in PD. Subjects were imaged using [^{123}I]altropane , a drug that binds selectively to the DA transporter and is concentrated in the striatum due to the high density of dopaminergic nerve terminals there. The images are color-coded such that red represents the highest level of drug binding, yellow is less, and purple is the least. Striatal altropane binding is reduced in the patient with moderate PD and almost completely lost in the patient with an advanced case of PD. (Based on data from Fischman et al., 1998; images courtesy of Alan Fischman and Bertha Madras.)

cal drug treatments for psychiatric disorders that were discovered serendipitously (by chance), L-DOPA treatment was conceived as a "rational therapy" for PD because its aim is to replace the DA lost due to degeneration of the nigrostriatal tract. Unfortunately, there are many limitations of L-DOPA therapy, including a reduction in effectiveness over time, the development of dyskinesias (abnormal involuntary movements), and, in advanced cases, the possible occurrence of dopaminergic psychoses. These problems have led to a growing interest in DA receptor agonists as an alternative to L-DOPA, particularly in the early stages of PD.

A great deal has been learned about the histopathology of PD, yet the cause of this disorder remains enigmatic. PD is not inherited, and in contrast with Alzheimer's disease (see Chapter 6), genetics does not appear to play a major role except in rare forms of the disorder. The best current theory is that DA neurons are damaged and eventually killed due to oxyradical-induced oxidative stress. Oxyradicals are small, oxygen-containing free radicals (molecules containing an unpaired electron). They are highly reactive chemically, and if allowed to build up, they can cause severe damage to a cell's DNA, proteins, and membrane lipids. There is evidence that DA neurons in the substantia nigra are under increased oxidative stress in PD (Beal, 2003), although it is not yet conclusive that this difference is directly responsible for the accelerated loss of these cells.

Even if researchers confirm that oxidative stress is the immediate cause of PD, what is the source of this stress? Some have speculated that environmental toxins (industrial pollutants perhaps) could be the culprits. There is no direct evidence yet in support of this hypothesis, but we do know of certain toxic substances that can destroy DA neurons. Besides 6-OHDA, which is described in this section, another important DA neurotoxin is the drug 1-methyl-4-phenyl-1,2,3,6-tetrahydropyridine (MPTP). This compound was the accidental contaminant responsible for Barry Kidston's sudden onset of parkinsonian symptoms described at the beginning of this chapter. Later studies showed that monkeys treated with MPTP developed a behavioral syndrome very similar to PD that responded appropriately to L-DOPA (Burns et al., 1983). Biochemical and histological examination of the brains of these animals confirmed that their symptoms were due to a loss of DA neurons in the substantia nigra and a depletion of DA in the striatum.

No one is claiming that PD patients have been exposed specifically to MPTP, and in fact, oxidative stress is probably not the major mechanism by which this substance produces its neurotoxic effects. But studies on MPTP may nevertheless be useful in helping unravel the mechanisms underlying PD and developing methods for preventing this devastating disorder.

tral dopaminergic system, one must administer 6-OHDA directly into the brain, since the drug doesn't readily cross the blood–brain barrier. The toxin is taken up mainly by the catecholaminergic neurons (thus sparing neurons that use other neurotransmitters) due to its close structural similarity to DA. Once the toxin is inside, the nerve terminals are severely damaged and sometimes the entire cell dies. Animals with bilateral 6-OHDA lesions of the ascending dopaminer-

gic pathways show severe behavioral dysfunction. They exhibit sensory neglect (that is, they pay little attention to stimuli in the environment), motivational deficits (they show little interest in eating food or drinking water), and motor impairment (like patients with Parkinson's disease, they have difficulty initiating voluntary movements). It is also possible to damage the nigrostriatal DA pathway on only one side of the brain, as illustrated in Figure 5.8. In this case, the lesioned

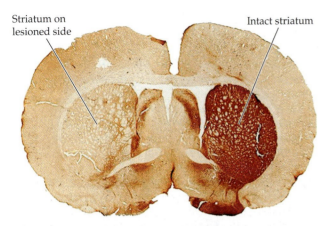

Striatum on lesioned side

Intact striatum

Figure 5.8 Damage to the nigrostriatal pathway on one side of the brain causes degeneration of dopaminergic fibers in the striatum on that side. This is shown in the photomicrograph of a tissue section through the brain of a rat that had received a unilateral 6-OHDA lesion of the medial forebrain bundle, which contains the axons of the nigrostriatal pathway. The section, which was stained using an antibody against tyrosine hydroxylase, depicts the loss of dopaminergic fibers and terminals in the striatum on the side of the lesion. (Photomicrograph courtesy of Michael Zigmond and Annie Cohen.)

animals display a postural asymmetry characterized by leaning and turning toward the damaged side of the brain due to the dominance of the untreated side. The profound abnormalities seen following either bilateral or unilateral lesions of the DA system indicate how important this neurotransmitter is for normal behavioral functioning.

There are five main subtypes of dopamine receptors organized into D₁- and D₂-like families

In the previous chapter, we discussed the concept of receptor subtypes. The neurotransmitter DA uses five main subtypes, designated D_1 to D_5, all of which are metabotropic receptors. That is, they interact with G proteins and they function, in part, through second messengers. Various studies have shown that the D_1 and D_5 receptors are very similar to each other, whereas the D_2, D_3, and D_4 receptors represent a separate family. The D_1 and D_2 receptors were discovered first, and they are also the most common subtypes in the brain. Both types of receptors are found in large numbers in the striatum and the nucleus accumbens, which are major termination sites of the nigrostriatal and mesolimbic DA pathways, respectively. Thus, D_2 receptors not only function as autoreceptors,

as mentioned earlier, but they also serve an important role as normal postsynaptic receptors. Interestingly, these receptors are additionally found on cells in the pituitary gland that make the hormone prolactin. Activation of D_2 receptors by DA from the hypothalamus leads to an inhibition of prolactin secretion, whereas the blockade of these receptors stimulates prolactin release. We will see in Chapter 18 that all current antischizophrenic drugs are D_2 receptor antagonists. In older studies, the receptor-blocking activity of these drugs was assessed by monitoring changes in circulating prolactin levels. Now, however, more direct information on receptor occupancy can be obtained by means of modern imaging techniques such as positron emission tomographic (PET) scanning.

In the early stages of research on DA receptors, investigators discovered that D_1 and D_2 have opposite effects on the second-messenger substance cyclic adenosine monophosphate (cAMP) (Kebabian and Calne, 1979). More specifically, D_1 receptors stimulate the enzyme adenylyl cyclase, which is responsible for synthesizing cAMP (Chapter 3). Consequently, the rate of cAMP formation is increased by stimulation of D_1 receptors. In contrast, D_2 receptor activation inhibits adenylyl cyclase, thereby decreasing the rate of cAMP synthesis (Figure 5.9). These opposing effects can occur because the receptors activate two different G proteins, G_s in the case of D_1 receptors and G_i in the case of D_2 receptors. The resulting changes in the level of cAMP within the postsynaptic cell alter the cell's excitability (that is, how readily it will fire nerve impulses) in complex ways that are beyond the scope of this discussion. A second important mechanism of D_2 receptor function involves the regulation of membrane ion channels for potassium (K^+). In some cells, D_2 receptor stimulation

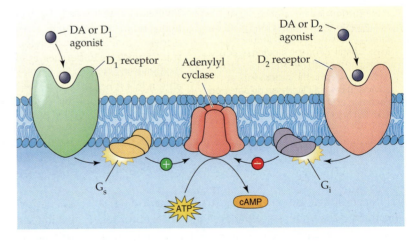

Figure 5.9 Signaling mechanisms of D₁ and D₂ receptors Activation of D_1 receptors stimulates the enzyme adenylyl cyclase and enhances DA synthesis, whereas activation of D_2 receptors inhibits adenylyl cyclase and decreases DA synthesis. These effects are produced by the activation of different G proteins in the postsynaptic cell membrane, namely G_s for the D_1 receptor and G_i for the D_2 receptor.

activates a G protein that subsequently enhances K⁺ channel opening. As we saw in Chapter 3, opening of such channels causes a hyperpolarization of the cell membrane, thus decreasing the cell's excitability and rate of firing.

Dopamine receptor agonists and antagonists affect locomotor activity and other behavioral functions

Many studies of DA pharmacology have used compounds that directly stimulate or block DA receptors. **Apomorphine** is a widely used agonist that stimulates both D_1 and D_2 receptors. At appropriate doses, apomorphine treatment causes behavioral activation similar to that seen with classical stimulants like amphetamine and cocaine. There is also a new use for apomorphine in treating erectile dysfunction in men (marketed under the trade name Uprima). At present, the best-known remedy for this disorder is, of course, Viagra. You will recall that the mechanism of action of Viagra, which involves inhibiting the breakdown of cyclic guanosine monophosphate (cGMP) in the penis, was discussed in Chapter 3. In contrast, apomorphine seems to increase penile blood flow (which is necessary for an erection) by acting through DA receptors in the brain. This effect of apomorphine has actually been known for some time, but clinical application for this purpose was previously thwarted by undesirable side effects (particularly nausea) and poor drug availability when taken orally. These problems have been overcome to some extent through the development of a lozenge that is taken sublingually (under the tongue), thereby bypassing the digestive system and delivering the drug directly into the bloodstream.

Psychopharmacologists also make use of drugs that are more selective for members of the D_1 or D_2 receptor family. Receptor-selective agonists and antagonists are extremely important in helping us understand which behaviors are under the control of a particular receptor subtype. The most commonly used agonist for D_1 receptors is a compound known as **SKF 38393.*** Administration of this compound to rats or mice elicits self-grooming behavior. **Quinpirole** is a drug that activates D_2 and D_3 receptors, and its effect is to increase locomotion and sniffing behavior. These responses are reminiscent of the effects of amphetamine or apomorphine, although quinpirole is not as powerful a stimulant as the former compounds.

The typical effect of administering a DA receptor antagonist is to suppress spontaneous exploratory and locomotor behavior. At higher doses, such drugs elicit a state known as

---

*Many drugs used in research never receive common names like *cocaine* or *reserpine*. In such instances, the drug is designated with an abbreviation for the pharmaceutical company at which it was developed, along with an identifying number. In the present instance, SKF stands for the Smith Kline & French company, which is now part of GlaxoSmithKline.

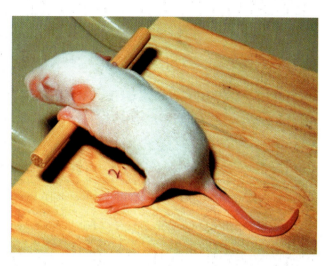

Figure 5.10 Catalepsy can be produced by DA receptor antagonists, particularly drugs that block D_2 receptors. Shown here is a 10-day-old rat pup that had received a subcutaneous injection of the D_2 antagonist haloperidol (1 mg/kg) 1 hour earlier. Pups treated in this manner often spent an entire 3-minute testing period immobile with their forepaws resting on the elevated bar, whereas control pups not given haloperidol got off the bar within a few seconds. (Photograph by Jerrold Meyer.)

catalepsy. Catalepsy refers to a lack of spontaneous movement, which is usually demonstrated experimentally by showing that the subject does not change position when placed in an awkward, presumably uncomfortable posture (Figure 5.10). Nevertheless, the subject is neither paralyzed nor asleep, and in fact it can be aroused to move by strong sensory stimuli such as being picked up by the experimenter. Catalepsy is usually associated with D_2 receptor blockers such as **haloperidol,** but it can also be elicited by giving a D_1 blocker such as **SCH 23390.** Given the important role of the nigrostriatal DA pathway in movement, it is not surprising that catalepsy is particularly related to the inhibition of DA receptors in the striatum. We mentioned earlier that D_2 receptor antagonists are used in the treatment of schizophrenia. The therapeutic benefit of these drugs is thought to derive from their blocking of DA receptors in the limbic system or the cortex. It should be clear from the present discussion, however, that the same drugs are also likely to produce inhibition of movement and other troublesome motor side effects because of the simultaneous interference with dopaminergic transmission in the striatum.

The various effects of DA receptor agonists and antagonists have given researchers a lot of useful information about the behavioral functions of DA. A newer approach is to manipulate the genes for individual components of the dopaminergic system and determine the behavioral consequences of such manipulations. The results from this approach are discussed in Box 5.2.

BOX 5.2 — The Cutting Edge

Using "Gene Knockout" Animals to Study the Dopaminergic System

In recent years, many researchers have begun to use techniques from molecular biology to investigate how neurotransmitter systems function and how they control various behaviors. One of the most exciting and powerful tools in this new field of molecular pharmacology is the production of gene knockout mice. As we saw in Chapter 4, these are strains of mice in which a particular gene of interest has been "knocked out" (that is, rendered inactive) by special genetic procedures. Application of this technology has yielded new clues as to how the dopaminergic system regulates various behavioral functions.

One interesting approach taken by Richard Palmiter and his colleagues at the University of Washington was to knock out the gene for tyrosine hydroxylase (TH) selectively in dopaminergic neurons. Although this required very skillful genetic manipulations, the investigators succeeded in creating mice that were virtually devoid of DA in the dopaminergic system but still possessed relatively normal amounts of NE. There is some similarity between these DA-deficient mice and genetically normal animals that have been given DA lesions with 6-OHDA, although one important difference is that the dopaminergic neurons themselves are undamaged in the genetic mutants. DA-deficient mice appear to behave and grow normally from birth until about 2 weeks of age, at which time they begin to show slower weight gain than wild-type (genetically normal) mice (Zhou and Palmiter, 1995). If untreated, they all die by 4 weeks of age. The DA-deficient mice can be saved by daily injections of L-DOPA, which bypasses the TH step (see Figure 5.2) in the bio-chemical pathway and therefore allows the neurons to make DA. But if the L-DOPA treatment is suspended, the mice show a tremendous reduction in movement and seem to have no interest in eating food or drinking, despite the fact that they can physically grasp food and swallow liquids that are placed directly into their mouths. The decreased movement in these animals is reminiscent of Parkinson's disease and supports a critical role for DA in spontaneous locomotor activity. Dopamine also seems to be involved in the neural systems governing food and water intake, although the exact nature of this involvement is still not clear.

Other strains of mutant mice have been generated that lack either the DA transporter or one of the DA receptors. It turns out that each gene knockout produces a unique behavioral phenotype (which means the behavior of the mutant strain compared to that of normal animals). The most obvious characteristic of DA transporter knockout mice is that they are extremely hyperactive (Giros et al., 1996) (Figure A). This effect is understandable in light of the fact that without a transporter on their terminals, the dopaminergic neurons cannot remove DA from the synaptic cleft. Consequently, the postsynaptic DA receptors are exposed to excessive amounts of transmitter, which has an activating effect on the animal's behavior.

The first DA receptor to be knocked out was the D_1 receptor (Drago et al., 1994). Like the DA-deficient mice, animals lacking this receptor subtype initially appear normal. By weaning age, though, they begin to show reduced growth. They may even die if their normally dry food isn't moistened to make it more palatable. Nevertheless, in the absence of drug treatment (see below), the locomotor activity of D_1 receptor knockouts is similar to that of wild-type mice.

Contrasting results have been obtained from knocking out the other DA receptors. Disrupting the gene for the D_2 receptor produces impairment in spontaneous movement and in coordination (Baik et al., 1995; Kelly et al., 1998). However, the degree of impairment seems to depend strongly on which genetic strain of mouse is used to create the mutation. This is partly because different strains already vary a lot in their behavior

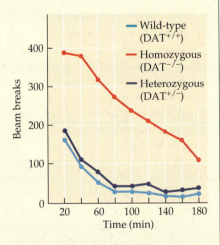

(A) Mutant mice lacking the dopamine transporter (DAT) (homozygous $DAT^{-/-}$) show increased locomotor activity compared to genetically normal wild-type mice ($DAT^{+/+}$) or heterozygous mice ($DAT^{+/-}$) that carry one copy of the DAT gene. Mice were tested in a photocell apparatus and the number of photobeam breaks was recorded every 20 minutes for a total of 3 hours. All groups showed a gradual habituation to the apparatus as indicated by decreasing beam breaks, but the activity of the DAT knockout mice ($DAT^{-/-}$) was consistently higher than that of the other two groups. (After Giros et al., 1996.)

BOX 5.2 (continued)

before any genes are knocked out. D_3 and D_4 receptor knockout mice have mainly been studied using tests thought to measure exploratory behavior and anxiety in rodents. D_3 receptor knockouts show signs of reduced anxiety in such tests (Steiner et al.,1998), whereas absence of the D_4 receptor has little apparent effect on anxiety but does produce reduced exploration of novel environmental stimuli (Dulawa et al.,1999). Finally, recent studies on D_5 receptor knockout mice found that the animals develop hypertension (high blood pressure) in adulthood, apparently due to increased sympathetic nervous system activity (Hollon et al., 2002). It will be interesting to see whether any cases of hypertension in humans are due to a defect in D_5 receptor expression or functioning.

Pharmacologists have naturally begun to study how these mutations of the DA system affect the reactions to different psychoactive drugs. Several studies have looked at behavioral responses to psychostimulant drugs such as cocaine, amphetamine, and methamphetamine, since DA is already known to play an important role in the effects of these compounds. Both DA transporter knockout mice and D_1 receptor knockouts show little or no increase in locomotion following psychostimulant treatment (Giros et al., 1996; M. Xu et al., 2000) (Figure B). Therefore, the DA transporter on the presynaptic side and the D_1 receptor on the postsynaptic side both play pivotal roles in the behavior-stimulating effects of cocaine and amphetamine (see Chapter 11). In contrast, mutant mice lacking the D_4 receptor are actually hypersensitive to the stimulating effects of

cocaine and methamphetamine (Rubinstein et al., 1997).

Another approach has been to test the effects of the DA receptor antagonist haloperidol in DA receptor knockout mice. Mice lacking D_1 or D_3 receptors still show catalepsy following haloperidol treatment (Boulay et al., 2000; Moratalla et al., 1996), whereas D_2 receptor knockouts are insensitive to the locomotor-inhibiting and cataleptic effects of this compound (Boulay et al., 2000; Kelly et al., 1998). These findings clearly show that D_2 receptors mediate the inhibitory effects of haloperidol on locomotor activity.

A few studies have also looked at behavioral responses to ethanol (alcohol). Ethanol can produce either locomotor stimulation or inhibition, depending on the dose and other factors. Mice lacking D_2 receptors are less sensitive to the locomotor-impairing effects of ethanol, and they also voluntarily drink less ethanol than control mice (Phillips et al., 1998). In contrast, D_4 receptor knockouts are hypersensitive to the locomotor-stimulating effects of ethanol, which coincides with their enhanced responsiveness to psychostimulant drugs as well (Rubinstein et al., 1997).

These results show us that by acting through different receptor subtypes, a single transmitter such as DA may influence many different behaviors and play a complicated role in the responses to psychoactive drugs. In some cases, genetically engineered mice have largely confirmed theories that researchers had previously formulated using more traditional pharmacological approaches. In other cases, however, the use of such animals has provided new and exciting

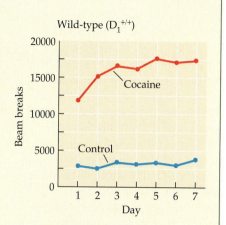

Wild-type ($D_1^{+/+}$)

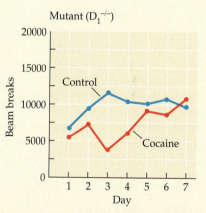

Mutant ($D_1^{-/-}$)

(B) Mutant mice lacking D_1 receptors are insensitive to the locomotor-stimulating effects of cocaine. Wild-type ($D_1^{+/+}$) and homozygous mutant mice ($D_1^{-/-}$) were injected twice daily for 7 consecutive days with either cocaine (20 mg/kg intraperitoneally) or a saline control solution. The animals were tested in a photocell apparatus for 30 minutes after each injection to record their locomotor activity. Cocaine greatly increased locomotor activity in the wild-type but not the mutant mice on all test days. (After M. Xu et al., 2000.)

insights into the interactions between neurotransmitters, drugs, and behavior.

We will conclude this section by considering the consequences of administering a D_2 receptor antagonist repeatedly rather than just once or twice. When haloperidol is given chronically to rats, the animals develop a syndrome called **behavioral supersensitivity.** This means that if the haloperidol treatment is stopped (to unblock the D_2 receptors) and the subjects are then given a DA agonist like apomorphine, they respond more strongly than control subjects not pretreated with haloperidol. Since the experimental and control animals both received the same dose of apomorphine, this finding suggests that somehow the DA receptors in the experimental group are more sensitive to the same pharmacological stimulation. A similar effect occurs following DA depletion by 6-OHDA. The similarity between haloperidol and 6-OHDA administration is that both treatments persistently reduce the amount of DA stimulation of D_2 receptors. Haloperidol accomplishes this by blocking the receptors, whereas 6-OHDA accomplishes the same result by causing a long-lasting depletion of DA. Various studies suggest that the supersensitivity associated with haloperidol or 6-OHDA treatment is related at least partly to an increase in the density of D_2 receptors on the postsynaptic cells in the striatum. This phenomenon, which is called **receptor up-regulation,** is considered to be an adaptive response whereby the lack of normal neurotransmitter (in this case DA) input causes the neurons to increase their sensitivity by making more receptors.

TABLE 5.1 Drugs That Affect the Dopaminergic System

Drug	Action
DOPA	Converted to DA in the brain
Phenelzine	Increases catecholamine levels by inhibiting MAO
α-Methyl-*para*-tyrosine (AMPT)	Depletes catecholamines by inhibiting tyrosine hydroxylase
Reserpine	Depletes catecholamines by inhibiting vesicular uptake
6-Hydroxydopamine (6-OHDA)	Damages or destroys catecholaminergic neurons
Amphetamine	Releases catecholamines
Cocaine and methylphenidate	Inhibit catecholamine reuptake
Apomorphine	Stimulates DA receptors generally (agonist)
SKF 38393	Stimulates D_1 receptors (agonist)
Quinpirole	Stimulates D_2 and D_3 receptors (agonist)
SCH 23390	Blocks D_1 receptors (antagonist)
Haloperidol	Blocks D_2 receptors (antagonist)

Section Summary

The dopaminergic neurons of greatest interest to neuropsychopharmacologists are found near the base of the midbrain in the substantia nigra (A9 cell group) and the VTA (A10 cell group). The neurons in the substantia nigra send their axons to the striatum, thus forming the nigrostriatal tract. This pathway plays an important role in the control of movement. It is severely damaged in the neurological disorder known as Parkinson's disease. The dopaminergic neurons in the VTA form two major dopaminergic systems. One is the mesolimbic system, which has terminations in several limbic system structures, including the nucleus accumbens, septum, amygdala, and hippocampus. The other is the mesocortical system, which terminates in the cerebral cortex, particularly the prefrontal cortex. The mesolimbic and mesocortical DA systems have been implicated in mechanisms of drug abuse as well as in schizophrenia.

Researchers have identified five main DA receptor subtypes, designated D_1 to D_5, all of which are metabotropic receptors. These subtypes fall into two families, the first consisting of D_1 and D_5 and the second consisting of D_2, D_3, and D_4. The most common subtypes are D_1 and D_2, both of which are found in large numbers in the striatum and the nucleus accumbens. These subtypes can be differentiated partly on the basis that D_1 receptors stimulate adenylyl cyclase, thus increasing the rate of cAMP synthesis, whereas D_2 receptors decrease the rate of cAMP synthesis by inhibiting adenylyl cyclase. Activation of D_2 receptors can also enhance the opening of K^+ channels in the cell membrane, which hyperpolarizes the membrane and therefore reduces the excitability of the cell.

Some of the drugs that affect the dopaminergic system, including DA receptor agonists and antagonists, are presented in Table 5.1. In general, enhancement of dopaminergic function has an activating effect on behavior, whereas interference with DA causes a suppression of normal behaviors ranging from temporary sedation and catalepsy to the profound deficits observed following 6-OHDA treatment. When D_2 receptor transmission is persistently impaired either by chronic antagonist administration or by denervation (e.g., 6-OHDA lesions), animals become supersensitive to treatment with a D_2 agonist. This response is mediated at least partially by an up-regulation of D_2 receptors by postsynaptic neurons in areas such as the striatum.

Organization and Function of the Noradrenergic System

The ascending noradrenergic system originates in the locus coeruleus

The NE-containing neurons within the brain are located in the parts of the brain stem called the pons and medulla. Of particular interest is a structure known as the **locus**

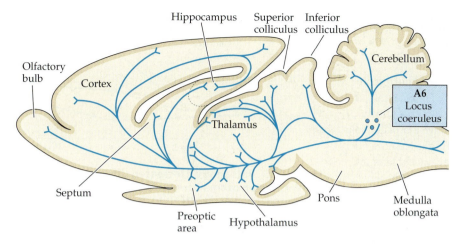

Figure 5.11 The locus coeruleus (LC) contains a dense cluster of noradenergic neurons designated the A6 cell group. These cells send their fibers to almost all regions of the forebrain as well as the cerebellum and spinal cord.

coeruleus (**LC**), a small area of the pons that contains a dense collection of noradrenergic neurons corresponding roughly to the A6 cell group (using the numbering system described previously). At first glance, the LC might not seem to be a very impressive structure, as the rat LC only contains a little more than 3000 nerve cells out of the millions of neurons present in the entire rat brain. Nevertheless, these cells send fibers into almost all areas of the forebrain, thereby providing nearly all of the NE in the cortex, limbic system, thalamus, and hypothalamus (Figure 5.11). The LC also provides noradrenergic input to the cerebellum and the spinal cord.

Norepinephrine also plays an important role in the peripheral nervous system. Many neurons that have their cell bodies in the ganglia of the sympathetic branch of the autonomic nervous system (see Chapter 2) use NE as their transmitter. These cells, which send out their fibers to various target organs throughout the body, are responsible for the autonomic actions of NE that are described later. We also mentioned earlier in the chapter that NE (as well as EPI) functions as a hormone secreted by the adrenal glands directly into the bloodstream. In this way, there are actually two routes by which NE can reach an organ such as the heart: it can be released from sympathetic noradrenergic neurons at synapse-like contacts with cardiac cells, and it can be released from the adrenal glands and travel to the heart through the circulatory system. On the other hand, blood-borne NE does

not reach the brain, because it is effectively excluded by the blood–brain barrier.

Modern techniques of neurophysiology make it possible to record the electrical firing of nerve cells in unanesthetized, freely moving animals. Aston-Jones and Bloom (1981a, 1981b) used this approach to determine how the activity of noradrenergic neurons in the LC of rats changed in relation to the behavior of the animals. The cells showed a low rate of firing (and sometimes even stopped altogether) when the rats were asleep. In contrast, presentation of novel sensory stimuli to the animals led to a short burst of LC cell firing. These and many other findings have led to the idea that the noradrenergic neurons of the LC play an important role in **vigilance** (that is, being alert to important stimuli in the environment) (Figure 5.12).

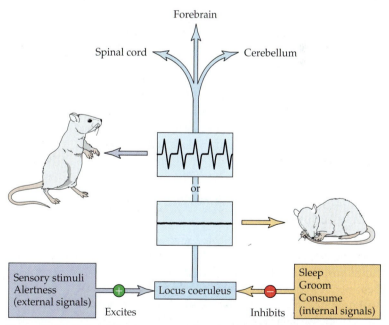

Figure 5.12 Role of the locus coeruleus in vigilance The firing of LC neurons is activated by arousing sensory stimuli and inhibited during the performance of maintenance behaviors such as sleeping, grooming, and consuming food. From these and other findings, Aston-Jones has hypothesized that NE plays an important role in vigilance, that is, attentiveness to important external stimuli. (After Aston-Jones, 1985.)

The cellular effects of norepinephrine and epinephrine are mediated by α- and β-adrenergic receptors

The receptors for NE and EPI are called adrenergic receptors (an alternate term is **adrenoceptors**). Like DA receptors, the adrenergic receptors all belong to the general family of metabotropic receptors. However, they serve a broader role by having to mediate both neurotransmitter (mainly NE) and hormonal (mainly EPI) actions of the catecholamines.

Early studies by Ahlquist (1948, 1979) and other investigators suggested the existence of two adrenoceptor subtypes, which were designated alpha (α) and beta (β). Since Ahlquist's pioneering research, many experiments have shown that the α- and β-adrenoceptors actually represent two families, each composed of several receptor subtypes. For present purposes, we will distinguish between α_1- and α_2-receptors, and also between β_1 and β_2. Postsynaptic adrenoceptors are found at high densities in many brain areas, including the cerebral cortex, thalamus, hypothalamus, cerebellum, and various limbic system structures such as the hippocampus and amygdala. In addition, α_2-autoreceptors are located on noradrenergic nerve terminals and on the cell bodies of noradrenergic neurons in the LC and elsewhere. These autoreceptors cause an inhibition of noradrenergic cell firing and a reduction in NE release from the terminals.

Like DA D_1 receptors, the β_1- and β_2-adrenoceptors both stimulate adenylyl cyclase and enhance the formation of cAMP. In contrast, α_2-receptors operate in a similar manner as D_2 receptors. That is, α_2-receptors reduce the rate of cAMP synthesis by inhibiting adenylyl cyclase, and they can also cause a hyperpolarization of the cell membrane by increasing K^+ channel opening. Yet another kind of mechanism is used by receptors of the α_1 subtype. These receptors operate through the phosphoinositide second-messenger system, which, as we saw in Chapter 3, leads to an increased concentration of free calcium (Ca^{2+}) ions within the postsynaptic cell.

Adrenergic agonists can stimulate arousal and eating behavior

Neurochemical and pharmacological studies in experimental animals indicate that NE is involved in many behavioral functions, including hunger and eating behavior, sexual behavior, fear and anxiety, pain, and sleep and arousal. We will provide a few pharmacological examples relevant to some of these functions.

We saw earlier that the firing of noradrenergic neurons of the LC is correlated with arousal and vigilance. The behavioral-activating functions of NE have also been investigated using pharmacological approaches. For example, Craig

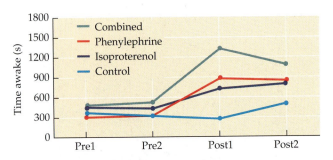

Figure 5.13 Rats showed increased time awake after administration of small amounts of either an α_1- or a β-adrenergic agonist directly into the medial septum. The α_1-agonist was phenylephrine (10×10^{-9} mol injected) and the β-agonist was isoproterenol (4×10^{-9} mol injected). Control injections were of the vehicle used to dissolve the active drugs. Behavioral state (asleep versus awake) was determined for two 30-minute intervals prior to drug administration (Pre1 and Pre2) as well as two 30-minute postdrug intervals (Post1 and Post2), the first of which began 15 minutes after the treatment. Note that the greatest effect was obtained with the combined injection of both drugs. (After Berridge et al., 2003.)

Berridge and his colleagues performed microinjections of the α_1-receptor agonist **phenylephrine** and/or the general β-receptor agonist **isoproterenol** into the rat medial septum, one of the brain areas believed to be important for NE's arousing effects (Berridge et al., 2003). The animals were then monitored to determine the amount of time they spent awake or asleep. As illustrated in Figure 5.13, each drug individually increased the amount of time spent awake, and at the low doses used in the study, the combination of the treatments produced the strongest effect. These results show that both α_1- and β-receptors are involved in NE-mediated arousal.

In both humans and animals, systemically administered α_2-receptor agonists have several behavioral effects related to activation of both autoreceptors and postsynaptic α_2-receptors. This can be seen in the properties of **dexmedetomidine (Precedex),** a recently introduced α_2-agonist with combined sedative, anxiolytic (antianxiety), and analgesic (pain-reducing) effects that is particularly useful for surgical patients in the intensive care unit. The sedative and anxiolytic effects of dexmedetomidine are believed to be mediated by α_2-autoreceptors in the LC, whereas the analgesic effect probably occurs at the level of the spinal cord.

Another behavioral function of NE concerns the regulation of hunger and eating behavior. The neural mechanisms underlying eating behavior are centered largely in the hypothalamus. One of the key areas within the hypothalamus is the paraventricular nucleus (PVN), a small paired structure that lies on either side of the third cerebral ventricle. The PVN receives noradrenergic input from the LC, and when

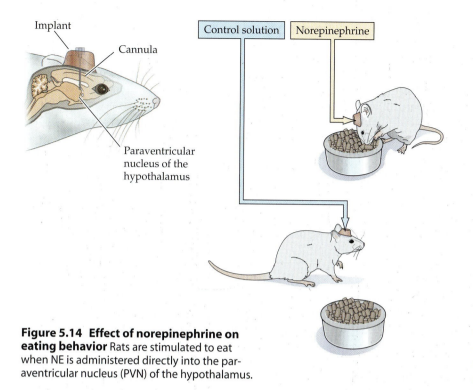

Figure 5.14 Effect of norepinephrine on eating behavior Rats are stimulated to eat when NE is administered directly into the paraventricular nucleus (PVN) of the hypothalamus.

NE is injected in small quantities directly into the PVN of awake rats, it elicits a robust eating response even if the animals were not previously food-deprived (Figure 5.14). This response to NE appears to be due to activation of α_2-receptors located within the PVN, because the response is blocked by administration of an α_2-antagonist and is mimicked when the α_2-agonist clonidine, instead of NE, is injected into the PVN (Wellman et al., 1993). Although we previously discussed the α_2 subtype as an autoreceptor, the PVN α_2-receptors responsible for triggering eating behavior are thought to lie on postsynaptic neurons that receive noradrenergic synapses.

A number of medications work by stimulating or inhibiting peripheral adrenergic receptors

Adrenergic agonists or antagonists are frequently used in the treatment of nonpsychiatric medical conditions. This is because of the widespread distribution and important functional role of adrenergic receptors in various peripheral organs (Table 5.2). For example, general adrenergic agonists that activate both α- and β-receptors have sometimes been used in the treatment of bronchial asthma. Stimulating the α-receptors causes constriction of the blood vessels in the bronchial lining, thus reducing congestion and edema (tissue swelling) by restricting blood flow to the tissue. On the other hand, β-receptor stimulation leads to relaxation of the bronchial muscles, thereby providing a wider airway. Although general adrenergic agonists can be effective antiasthma medications, they also cause a number of adverse side effects. For this reason, asthma is more commonly treated with a selective β-adrenoceptor agonist such as **albuterol.** Such drugs are packaged in an inhaler that delivers the compound directly to the respiratory system. The β-receptors found in the airways are of the β_2 subtype, in contrast to the heart, which contains mainly β_1-receptors. Consequently, albuterol is effective in alleviating the bronchial congestion of asthmatics without producing undesirable cardiovascular side effects.

Even over-the-counter cold medications are based on the properties of peripheral adrenergic receptors. Thus, the α_1-receptor agonist phenylephrine is the key ingredient in Neosynephrine. This drug is used as a nasal spray to constrict the blood vessels and reduce inflamed and swollen nasal

TABLE 5.2 Location and Physiological Actions of Peripheral α- and β-Adrenergic Receptors

Location	Action	Receptor subtype
Heart	Increased rate and force of contraction	β
Blood vessels	Constriction	α
	Dilation	β
Smooth muscle of the trachea and bronchi	Relaxation	β
Uterine smooth muscle	Contraction	α
Bladder	Contraction	α
	Relaxation	β
Spleen	Contraction	α
	Relaxation	β
Iris	Pupil dilation	α
Adipose (fat) tissue	Increased fat breakdown and release	β

membranes resulting from colds and allergies. In the form of eye drops, it is also used to stimulate α-receptors of the iris to dilate the pupil during eye examinations or before surgery of the eyes.

Alpha$_2$-receptor agonists such as clonidine are commonly used in the treatment of hypertension (high blood pressure). The therapeutic benefit of these drugs is due to their ability to inhibit activity of the sympathetic nervous system while stimulating the parasympathetic system. The combined effect of these actions is to reduce the patient's heart rate and blood pressure. As would be expected from our previous discussion of α$_2$-agonists, the typical side effects of clonidine treatment are sedation and feelings of sleepiness.

Adrenergic receptor antagonists likewise have varied clinical uses. For example, the α$_2$-antagonist yohimbine helps in the treatment of certain types of male sexual impotence. This compound increases parasympathetic and decreases sympathetic activity, which is thought to stimulate penile blood inflow and/or inhibit blood outflow.

The α$_1$-antagonist **prazosin** and the general β-adrenoceptor antagonist **propranolol** are both used clinically in the treatment of hypertension. Prazosin causes a dilation of blood vessels by blocking the α$_1$-receptors responsible for constricting these vessels. In contrast, the main function of propranolol is to block the β-receptors in the heart, thereby reducing the heart's contractile force. The discovery that β$_1$ is the major adrenoceptor subtype in the heart has led to the introduction of β$_1$-selective antagonists such as **metoprolol**. These compounds exhibit fewer side effects than the more general β-antagonist propranolol. Beta-receptor antagonists like propranolol and metoprolol are also useful in the treatment of cardiac arrhythmia (irregular heartbeat) and angina pectoris (feelings of pain and constriction around the heart caused by deficient blood flow and oxygen delivery to the heart).

Finally, it should be mentioned that propranolol and other β-antagonists have also been applied to the treatment of generalized anxiety disorder, which is one of the most common types of anxiety disorder (see Chapter 17). Many patients with generalized anxiety disorder suffer from physical symptoms such as palpitations, flushing, and tachycardia (racing heart). Beta-blockers do not alleviate anxiety per se, but instead they may help the patient feel better by reducing some of these distressing physical symptoms of the disorder.

Section Summary

The most important cluster of noradrenergic neurons is the A6 cell group, which is located in a region known as the locus coeruleus. These neurons innervate almost all areas of the forebrain and mediate many of the important behavioral functions of NE. Activity of LC cells depends on the behavioral state of the organism. The cells are relatively inactive during sleep, but they fire at a rapid rate in response to novel sensory stimuli. The noradrenergic system is thus thought to be important in the maintenance of vigilance.

NE and EPI activate a group of metabotropic receptors called adrenoceptors. They are divided into two broad families, α and β, which are further subdivided into α$_1$, α$_2$, β$_1$, and β$_2$. Both β-receptor subtypes enhance the synthesis of cAMP, whereas α$_2$-receptors inhibit cAMP formation. Another mechanism of action of α$_2$-receptors involves hyperpolarization of the cell membrane by stimulating K$^+$ channel opening. In contrast, α$_1$-receptors increase the intracellular concentration of Ca^{2+} ions by means of the phosphoinositide second-messenger system.

Some of the drugs that affect the noradrenergic system, including adrenergic receptor agonists and antagonists, are presented in Table 5.3. Adrenergic agonists are used therapeutically for various physiological and psychological disor-

TABLE 5.3 Drugs That Affect the Noradrenergic System

Drug	Action
Phenelzine	Increases catecholamine levels by inhibiting MAO
α-Methyl-*para*-tyrosine (AMPT)	Depletes catecholamines by inhibiting tyrosine hydroxylase
Reserpine	Depletes catecholamines by inhibiting vesicular uptake
6-Hydroxydopamine (6-OHDA)	Damages or destroys catecholaminergic neurons
Amphetamine	Releases catecholamines
Cocaine and methylphenidate	Inhibit catecholamine reuptake
Desipramine	Selectively inhibits NE reuptake
Phenylephrine	Stimulates α$_1$-receptors (agonist)
Clonidine	Stimulates α$_2$-receptors (agonist)
Albuterol	Stimulates β-receptors (partially selective for β$_2$)
Prazosin	Blocks α$_1$-receptors (antagonist)
Yohimbine	Blocks α$_2$-receptors (antagonist)
Propranolol	Blocks β-receptors generally (antagonist)
Metoprolol	Blocks β$_1$-receptors (antagonist)

ders. These include the α_1-agonist phenylephrine, which helps relieve nasal congestion; the α_2-agonist clonidine, which is used in the treatment of hypertension and drug withdrawal symptoms; and β_2-agonists such as albuterol, which is an important medication for relieving bronchial congestion in people suffering from asthma. Adrenergic receptor antagonists also have several clinical uses. The α_2-antagonist yohimbine is sometimes prescribed for male impotence. The α_1-antagonist prazosin, the general β-receptor antagonist propranolol, and several selective β_1-antagonists such as metoprolol are used in the treatment of hypertension. Beta-blockers also have a role in the treatment of generalized anxiety disorders, because these drugs reduce some of the somatic symptoms associated with strong anxiety. In general, the clinical application of adrenoceptor agonists and antagonists can be understood from the receptor subtypes in specific tissues or organs that they target and the resulting physiological effect of stimulating or blocking those receptors.

Recommended Readings

Berridge, C. W., and Waterhouse, B. D. (2003). The locus coeruleus-noradrenergic system: Modulation of behavioral state and state-dependent cognitive processes. *Brain Res. Rev.*, 42, 33–84.

Federoff, H. J., Burke, R. E., Fahn, S., and Fiskum, G. (eds.). (2003). *Parkinson's Disease: The Life Cycle of the Dopamine Neuron. Ann. N. Y. Acad. Sci.*, Vol. 991.

Neve, K. A., and Neve, R. L. (eds.). (1997). *The Dopamine Receptors.* Humana Press, Totowa, New Jersey.

Tan, S., Hermann, B., and Borrelli, E. (2003). Dopaminergic mouse mutants: Investigating the roles of the different dopamine receptor subtypes and the dopamine transporter. *Int. Rev. Neurobiol.*, 54, 145–197.

6

Acetylcholine and Serotonin

*I*magine that you are a United States soldier fighting in some future war. The conflict is not going well for your adversary, and recent military intelligence indicates that the enemy may be preparing to use chemical weapons (that is, nerve gas). Out on the battlefield, a missile explodes nearby, and you are suddenly enveloped in a fine mist emanating from the warhead. You experience a few moments of terror but then begin to relax when you realize that the antidote you took earlier in the day is doing its job. If you hadn't taken your pills as directed, you would now be sweating and salivating profusely, vomiting uncontrollably, gasping for breath, convulsing, and rapidly heading toward a gruesome death.

How does a nerve gas produce these horrible effects, and how would an antidote work? As we shall see in this chapter, nerve gases and their antidotes all revolve around a neurotransmitter called **acetylcholine** (**ACh;** adjective form **cholinergic**). ACh is a particularly fascinating transmitter—a molecule that is life-sustaining in its function but that is also the target of some of the most deadly known toxins, both naturally occurring and man-made. In the second part of this chapter, we will discuss another transmitter, serotonin, that also plays a central role in many behavioral and physiological functions.

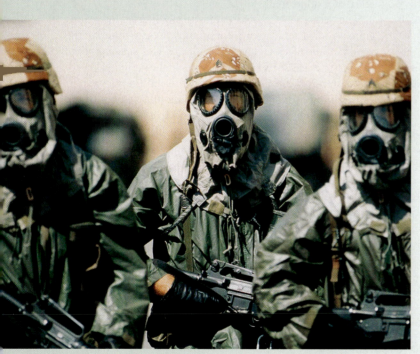

Gear such as this may be worn by soldiers to protect against nerve gases, which are agents that work through the cholinergic system.

Acetylcholine

Acetylcholine Synthesis, Release, and Inactivation

Acetylcholine synthesis is catalyzed by the enzyme choline acetyltransferase

In contrast to the multiple steps required to synthesize the catecholamine transmitters, ACh is formed in a single step from two precursors: **choline** and **acetyl coenzyme A (acetyl CoA)** (Figure 6.1). The choline comes mainly from fat in our diet (choline-containing lipids), although it is also produced in the liver. Acetyl CoA is generated within all cells by the metabolism of sugars and fats. The synthesis of ACh is catalyzed by the enzyme **choline acetyltransferase (ChAT)**, which does just what its name implies: it transfers the acetyl group (—COCH$_3$) from acetyl CoA to choline to form ACh. Choline acetyltransferase is present in the cytoplasm of the cell, and this enzyme is found only in neurons that use ACh as their transmitter. This specificity allows us to identify cholinergic neurons by staining for ChAT.

The rate of ACh synthesis is controlled by several factors, including the availability of its precursors inside the cell as well as the rate of cell firing. Thus cholinergic neurons make more ACh when more choline and/or acetyl CoA is available, and also when the neurons are stimulated to fire at a higher rate. Although knowledge of these regulatory processes has helped researchers understand how the ACh system functions, it has not yet led to the development of useful pharmacological agents. For example, it has been difficult to find highly selective inhibitors of ChAT, and even if such drugs are eventually isolated, it is not clear that inhibiting ACh synthesis has any obvious clinical usefulness. At one time, it was thought that boosting brain ACh levels by administering large doses of choline might be beneficial to patients suffering from Alzheimer's disease, since damage to the cholinergic system is one of the factors contributing to the cognitive deficits seen in that disorder. However, not only did choline treatment fail to produce symptom improvement, peripheral metabolism of this compound unfortunately caused the patients to give off a strong fishy odor!

Many different drugs and toxins can alter acetylcholine storage and release

The axon terminals of cholinergic neurons contain many small synaptic vesicles that store ACh for release when the nerve cell is active. It is estimated that a few thousand molecules of transmitter are present in each vesicle. Vesicles are loaded with ACh by a transport protein in the vesicle membrane called, appropriately, the **vesicular ACh transporter** (Figure 6.2). This protein can be blocked by a drug called **vesamicol.** What effect would you expect vesamicol to have on cholinergic neurons? Would you predict any drug-induced change in the distribution of ACh between the cytoplasm and the synaptic vesicles within the cholinergic nerve terminals? Furthermore, if there was a redistribution of ACh, what effect would this have on ACh release by the cells? If you predicted that vesamicol treatment would decrease vesicular ACh but increase the level of ACh in the cytoplasm, you were correct. This is because vesamicol doesn't affect the rate of ACh synthesis; therefore, ACh molecules that would normally have been transported into the vesicles remain in the cytoplasm of the terminal. Moreover, as ACh is only released from the vesicles when the cholinergic neurons fire, ACh release is reduced in the presence of vesamicol. We can imagine that the cholinergic vesicles are still present and are continuing to undergo exocytosis when the neurons are activated, but the amount of ACh available within the vesicles to be released is abnormally low.

The release of ACh is also dramatically affected by various animal and bacterial toxins. For example, a toxin found in the venom of the black widow spider, *Latrodectus mactans,* leads to a massive release of ACh at synapses in the peripheral nervous system (PNS). Overactivity of the cholinergic system causes numerous symptoms, including muscle pain in the abdomen or chest, tremors, nausea and vomiting, salivation, and copious sweating. Ounce for ounce, black widow spider venom is 15 times more toxic than prairie rattlesnake venom, but a single spider bite is rarely fatal in healthy young adults because of the small amount of venom injected into the victim. In contrast to the effects of black widow spider venom, the toxins that cause botulism poisoning potently inhibit ACh release. As described in Box 6.1, this inhibition of cholinergic activity can be deadly due to muscular paralysis.

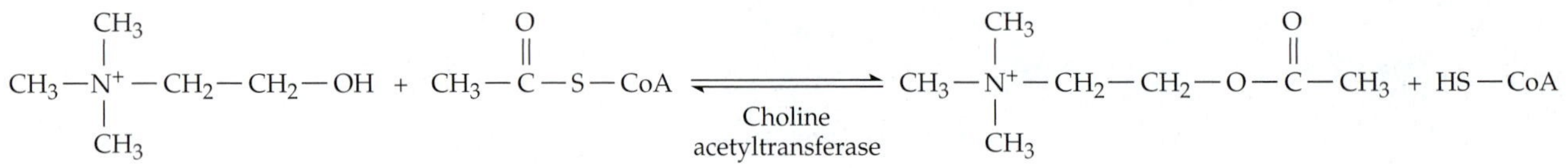

Figure 6.1 Synthesis of acetylcholine (ACh) by choline acetyltransferase

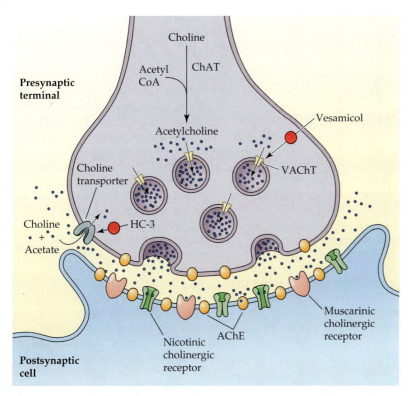

Figure 6.2 A cholinergic synapse illustrating the processes of ACh synthesis and metabolism, presynaptic choline uptake, and vesicular ACh uptake and release. Postsynaptic nicotinic and muscarinic ACh receptors are also shown.

Acetylcholinesterase is responsible for acetylcholine breakdown

Levels of ACh are carefully controlled by an enzyme called **acetylcholinesterase (AChE),** which breaks down the transmitter into choline and acetic acid (Figure 6.3). Within the cell, AChE is located in several strategic locations. One form of the enzyme is found inside the presynaptic cell, where it can metabolize excess ACh that may have been synthesized. Another form of AChE is present on the membrane of the postsynaptic cell to break down molecules of ACh after their release into the synaptic cleft. Finally, a unique type of AChE is found at neuromuscular junctions, which are specialized synapses between neurons and muscle cells where ACh is released by motor neurons to stimulate muscular contraction.

The muscle cells actually secrete AChE into the space between themselves and the cholinergic nerve endings, and the enzyme molecules become immobilized there by attaching to other proteins within the neuromuscular junction. This unique location helps the transmission process function very precisely at neuromuscular junctions. Immediately after a squirt of ACh causes a particular muscle to contract, the transmitter is metabolized extremely rapidly so that the muscle can relax until the next command arrives to squirt out some more ACh and contract that muscle once again.

Once ACh has been broken down within the synaptic cleft, a significant portion of the liberated choline is then taken back up into the cholinergic nerve terminal by a **choline transporter** in the membrane of the terminal (see Figure 6.2). If the choline transporter is blocked by means of the drug **hemicholinium-3 (HC-3),** the rate of ACh production declines. This tells us that reutilization of recycled choline plays an important role in maintaining ongoing ACh synthesis. HC-3 cannot cross the blood–brain barrier, but if central ACh is depleted by administration of HC-3 directly into the brain, rats show impaired performance on a task requiring visual attention (Muir et al., 1992). This finding is consistent with other evidence, to be presented later in this chapter, suggesting that ACh plays a role in various cognitive functions, including attention.

Drugs that block AChE prevent the inactivation of ACh, thereby increasing the transmitter's postsynaptic effects. One such drug is **physostigmine (Eserine),** a compound isolated from Calabar beans (the seeds of a woody plant found in the Calabar region of Nigeria). Physostigmine crosses the blood–brain barrier and thus exerts effects on the central nervous system (CNS). Accidental poisoning leads to slurred speech, mental confusion, hallucinations, loss of reflexes, convulsions, and even coma and death. Nineteenth-century missionaries to West Africa discovered societies that used extracts of the Calabar bean to determine the guilt of accused

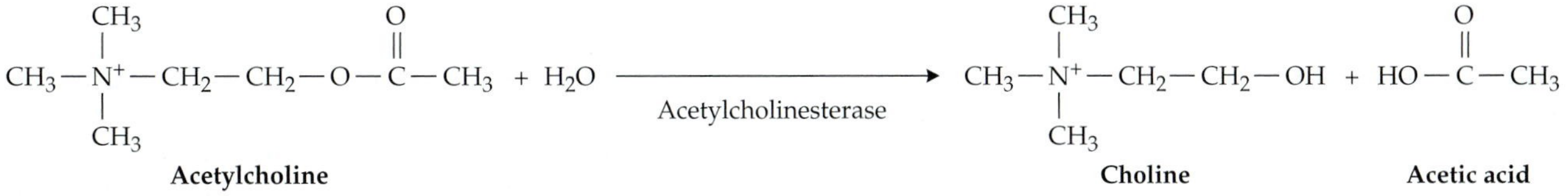

Figure 6.3 Breakdown of ACh by acetylcholinesterase

BOX 6.1 Pharmacology in Action

Botulinum Toxin—Deadly Poison, Therapeutic Remedy, and Cosmetic Aid

The bacterium *Clostridium botulinum*, which is responsible for botulism poisoning, produces what is perhaps the most potent toxin known to pharmacologists. The estimated lethal dose of botulinum toxin in humans is 0.3 µg; in other words, 1 gram (equivalent to the weight of three aspirin tablets) is enough to kill over 3 million individuals. *Clostridium botulinum* does not grow in the presence of oxygen; however, it can thrive in an anaerobic (oxygen-free) environment such as a sealed food can that has not been properly heated to kill the bacteria.

Botulinum toxin actually consists of a mixture of seven related proteins known as botulinum toxins A through G. These proteins are taken up selectively by the cholinergic neurons that innervate our skeletal muscles. The toxin molecules interfere with the process of ACh release at neuromuscular junctions, thereby causing muscle weakness and even paralysis (see figure). The symptoms of botulism poisoning include blurred vision, difficulty speaking and swallowing, muscle weakness, and gastrointestinal distress. Most victims recover, although a small percentage die due to severe muscle paralysis and eventual asphyxiation.

Once the mechanism of action of botulinum toxin became known,

researchers began to consider that this substance, if used carefully and at very low doses, might be helpful in treating clinical disorders characterized by involuntary muscle contractions. After appropriate testing, in 1989 the United States Food and Drug Administration approved the use of purified botulinum toxin A for the treatment of strabismus (crossed eyes), blepharospasm (spasm of the

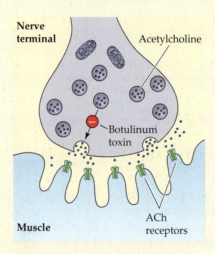

Mechanism of action of botulinum
Botulinum toxin blocks ACh release at the neuromuscular junction by preventing fusion of synaptic vesicles with the nerve terminal membrane.

eyelid), and hemifacial spasm (muscle spasms on just one side of the face). Since that time, this substance has also been administered for a variety of other disorders, including spastic cerebral palsy, dystonias (prolonged muscle contractions, sometimes seen as repeated jerking movements), and achalasia (failure of sphincter muscles to relax when appropriate).

Most remarkably, dermatologists have begun to use botulinum toxin (trade name Botox) for cosmetic purposes in patients with excessive frown lines, worry lines, or crow's-feet around the eyes. Such "dynamic wrinkles," as they are called, result from chronic contraction of specific facial muscles. When injected locally into a particular muscle or surrounding area, Botox causes a paralysis of that muscle due to a blockade of ACh release from the incoming motor nerve fibers. This leads to a reduction in the offending lines or wrinkles, although each treatment remains effective for only a few months, after which it must be repeated.

According to recent surveys, increasing numbers of people are turning to Botox treatments for purely cosmetic purposes. Depending on one's perspective, this trend might be considered either horrifying or liberating. Nevertheless, until true antiaging techniques are developed, it is safe to say that some folks will use whatever methods are available to appear younger than they really are.

---

prisoners (David, 1985). The defendant was considered innocent if he was fortunate enough to regurgitate the poison or, alternatively, if he could manage to walk 10 feet under the influence of the toxin (in which case vomiting was induced). Needless to say, however, most prisoners did neither, and were consequently judged guilty and permitted to die a horrible death.

Neostigmine (Prostigmin) and **pyridostigmine (Mestinon)** are synthetic analogs of physostigmine that do not cross the blood–brain barrier. These drugs are beneficial in the treatment of a serious neuromuscular disorder called **myas-**

thenia gravis. Because ACh is released at neuromuscular junctions, the muscle cells obviously possess cholinergic receptors so that they can respond to the neurotransmitter. For reasons that are not yet clear, patients with myasthenia gravis develop antibodies against their own muscle cholinergic receptors. Thus, myasthenia gravis is an example of an **autoimmune disorder,** a condition in which a part of the body is attacked by one's own immune system. In this case, the antibodies block the muscle acetylcholine receptors and eventually cause the receptors to be broken down by the muscle cells (Figure 6.4). The loss of receptor function causes the

Normal neuromuscular
junction

Neuromuscular junction in
myasthenia gravis

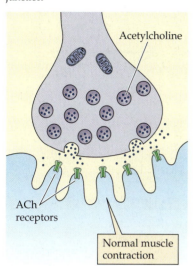
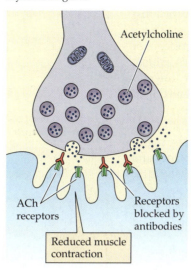

Figure 6.4 Myasthenia gravis, an autoimmune disorder In myasthenia gravis, antibodies interfere with cholinergic transmission at the neuromuscular junction by binding to and blocking the muscle ACh receptors.

dostigmine bromide (PB) were widely distributed to Allied troops for use as a nerve gas antidote. How can a reversible AChE inhibitor be an antidote against Sarin or Soman? It appears that the temporary interaction of PB with the enzyme protects AChE from permanent inactivation by the nerve gas. This protective effect, however, requires that the antidote be administered ahead of time, before exposure to the toxic agent. Therefore, soldiers were instructed to take three PB pills daily at times when they were thought to be at risk for nerve gas attack.* Previous animal studies had suggested that the PB itself would not cause any adverse effects because of low penetration across the blood–brain barrier. However, it appears that the blood–brain barrier can be "opened up" under stress, and indeed, a subsequent study showed that much more PB entered the brains of stressed mice than mice that hadn't undergone stress (Figure 6.5) (Fried-

patient's muscles to be less sensitive to ACh, which in turn leads to severe weakness and fatigue. By inhibiting AChE, neostigmine and pyridostigmine prolong the action of ACh at the neuromuscular junction, which causes increased stimulation of the remaining undamaged cholinergic receptors.

Physostigmine, neostigmine, and pyridostigmine are reversible AChE inhibitors, which means that ACh breakdown is restored after the drug dissociates from the enzyme. Certain other compounds, however, produce a nearly irreversible inhibition of AChE activity. Weaker versions of these chemicals are widely used as insecticides, since preventing ACh breakdown is just as harmful to ants and wasps as it is to humans. More-toxic varieties of irreversible AChE inhibitors have unfortunately been developed as "nerve gases" for use in chemical warfare. These agents go by names such as **Sarin** and **Soman.** They are designed to be dispersed as a vapor cloud or spray, which allows their entry into the body through skin contact or by inhalation. In either case, the drug quickly penetrates into the bloodstream and is distributed to all organs, including the brain. The symptoms of nerve gas poisoning, which were described in the opening passage of this chapter, are due to rapid ACh accumulation and overstimulation of cholinergic synapses throughout both the CNS and PNS. Death occurs through asphyxiation due to paralysis of the muscles of the diaphragm.

Sarin gas was used by terrorists in the infamous Tokyo subway attack in 1995. During the Persian Gulf War of 1990–1991 as well as the more recent conquest of Iraq, Allied forces were also very concerned about the possible use of this agent by the Iraqi army. Consequently, tablets of pyri-

*Although PB was only to be taken under presumed threat of a gas attack, one physician at a Veterans Administration Medical Center has stated that some military units participating in the Gulf War took the drug "every day they were in the Gulf" (Gavaghan, 1994).

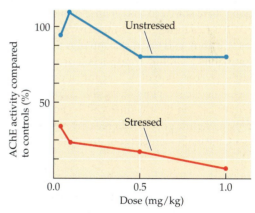

Figure 6.5 Stress increases pyridostigmine entry into the brain. Mice were stressed by a forced swim test, followed 10 minutes later by intraperitoneal injection of various doses of pyridostigmine. Other mice were unstressed prior to pyridostigmine administration. Brain tissues were subsequently analyzed for AChE to determine the amount of enzyme activity compared to unstressed control animals that had not received any drug. Unstressed mice showed relatively little AChE inhibition at any dose, indicating a lack of penetration of pyridostigmine into the brain under normal conditions. In contrast, the stressed mice showed a high degree of AChE inhibition even at low doses, showing that more pyridostigmine crossed the blood–brain barrier in these animals. (After Friedman et al., 1996.)

man et al., 1996). This raises the possibility of increased exposure of the brain to PB in Allied soldiers, who were not only engaged in combat but were additionally worried that they might be exposed to a deadly toxin. You may have heard of the so-called Gulf War syndrome, the existence of which has still not been resolved at the time of this writing. Some researchers claim to have identified three different syndromes, each with a distinct set of symptoms and caused by a different chemical exposure (Haley et al., 1997). The syndrome reportedly associated with the taking of PB has been termed confusion–ataxia and is manifested by cognitive impairment, dizziness, and problems of balance and coordination. However, it is still unclear whether the three proposed syndromes can be substantiated, and researchers have yet to convincingly demonstrate a causal relationship between PB exposure and any symptoms manifested by Gulf War veterans.

Section Summary

Acetylcholine is synthesized from choline and acetyl CoA in a single reaction catalyzed by the enzyme choline acetyltransferase. The rate of ACh synthesis is controlled by precursor availability and is also increased by cholinergic cell firing. The neurotransmitter is loaded into synaptic vesicles by a specific vesicular ACh transporter. A variety of animal and bacterial toxins influence the cholinergic system either by stimulating or inhibiting ACh release.

Following its release into the synapse or neuromuscular junction, ACh is rapidly degraded by the enzyme AChE. Much of the liberated choline is taken back up into the cholinergic nerve terminal by a choline transporter. Drugs that block AChE cause a prolongation of ACh action at postsynaptic or muscular cholinergic receptors. Reversible AChE antagonists are sometimes used in the treatment of the neuromuscular disorder myasthenia gravis, whereas irreversible AChE inhibitors are the main ingredients of dreaded nerve gases.

Organization and Function of the Cholinergic System

Cholinergic neurons play a key role in the functioning of both the peripheral and central nervous systems

Acetylcholine was first identified as a neurotransmitter in the PNS. We have already noted that ACh is the transmitter released at neuromuscular junctions throughout the body. This substance additionally plays a crucial role in both the sympathetic and parasympathetic branches of the autonomic nervous system. To briefly review the relevant features of

Parasympathetic branch

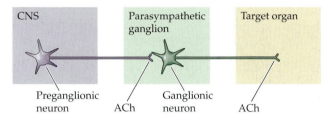

Sympathetic branch

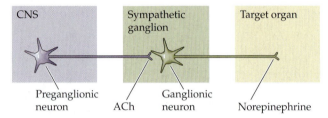

Figure 6.6 Cholinergic synapses in the parasympathetic and sympathetic branches of the autonomic nervous system

these branches of the autonomic nervous system, each consists of preganglionic neurons, which are cells located within the CNS that send their axons to the autonomic ganglia, as well as ganglionic neurons located within the ganglia that innervate various target organs throughout the body. The preganglionic neurons of both branches are cholinergic, as are the ganglionic neurons of the parasympathetic system (we saw in the previous chapter that norepinephrine is the transmitter of the sympathetic ganglionic neurons). Figure 6.6 illustrates the chemical coding of these cells and the synapses they make. The widespread involvement of ACh in both the neuromuscular and autonomic systems explains why drugs interfering with this transmitter exert such powerful physiological effects and are sometimes highly toxic.

Within the brain, the cell bodies of cholinergic neurons are clustered within just a few areas (Figure 6.7). Some of these nerve cells are interneurons, such as the ones found within the striatum. In the previous chapter, we saw that the dopaminergic input to the striatum plays a critical role in the regulation of movement. This regulation depends partly on the balance between ACh and dopamine (DA); that is, when DA is low, as in Parkinson's disease, the resulting neurotransmitter imbalance contributes to the motor symptoms of the disorder. Consequently, anticholinergic drugs such as **orphenadrine (Norflex), benztropine mesylate (Cogentin),** and **trihexyphenidyl (Artane)** are sometimes prescribed instead of L-DOPA in the early stages of Parkinson's disease.

Other cholinergic neurons send their axons longer distances to innervate many different brain areas. For example, there is a diffuse collection of cholinergic nerve cells called

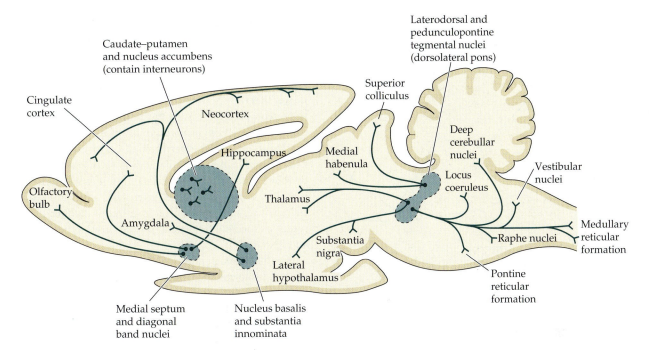

Figure 6.7 Anatomy of cholinergic pathways in the brain The cell bodies of cholinergic neurons are located primarily in the striatum, nucleus basalis, medial septum, diagonal band nuclei, substantia innominata, pedunculopontine tegmental nucleus, and dorsolateral tegmental nucleus. Note that the basal forebrain cholinergic cell groups send fibers to all areas of the cortex as well as to limbic system structures such as the hippocampus and amygdala. The cell groups of the pedunculopontine tegmental and dorsolateral tegmental nuclei primarily innervate subcortical structures that do not receive input from the basal forebrain system, caudate–putamen, and nucleus accumbens.

the **basal forebrain cholinergic system (BFCS)** that comprises neurons interspersed among several anatomical areas, including the nucleus basalis, substantia innominata, medial septal nucleus, and the diagonal band nuclei. The BFCS is the origin of a dense cholinergic innervation of the cerebral cortex as well as the hippocampus and other limbic system structures.

Research over many years has led to the view that ACh, and more specifically the BFCS, plays an important role in cognitive functioning. Early studies on rats and mice found that anticholinergic drugs such as atropine and scopolamine interfered with the acquisition and maintenance of many different kinds of learning tasks (Spencer and Lal, 1983). Both atropine and scopolamine block one subtype of ACh receptor, the muscarinic receptor, suggesting that this receptor subtype is necessary for the cognition-enhancing effects of ACh. However, this research could not tell us *where* the key cholinergic synapses are located, since peripherally administered atropine and scopolamine reach all parts of the brain and therefore block all central muscarinic receptors.

More-direct information concerning the role of the BFCS in cognitive functioning has been obtained from studies involving lesions of this system. An important innovation in this research area occurred with the introduction of a cholin-

ergic neurotoxin called **192 IgG–saporin.** This odd-sounding substance contains a monoclonal antibody, 192 IgG, that binds specifically to a cell surface protein carried by the basal forebrain cholinergic neurons. The other part of the molecule, saporin, is a cellular toxin obtained from the soapwort plant, *Saponaria officinalis*. When 192 IgG–saporin is injected into the brain's ventricular system, the basal forebrain cholinergic neurons take up the toxin due to binding of the antibody part of the molecule. As a result, those neurons are destroyed while neighboring noncholinergic cells are spared. Rats treated with 192 IgG–saporin exhibit disruptions in several different cognitive functions, including learning, memory, and attention (Wrenn and Wiley, 1998). One example is shown in Figure 6.8. Interestingly, some learning tasks require very large reductions (≥75 to 85%) in ACh levels before lesion-induced deficits are observed. It may be that only a relatively small amount of cholinergic input from the BFCS is required for most cognitive functions.

More than 20 years ago, Raymond Bartus and his colleagues proposed that the cognitive decline that often occurs with aging is due, at least in part, to a dysfunction of the BFCS (Bartus et al., 1982). This spurred tremendous interest in the BFCS, not only with respect to normal aging but also regarding a possible role in the age-related disorder,

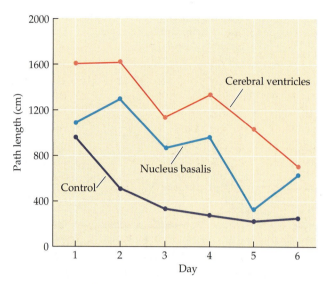

Figure 6.8 Cholinergic lesions produced by central infusions of 192 IgG–saporin impair spatial navigation learning in the Morris water maze. Rats were infused with 192 IgG–saporin either into the cerebral ventricles or into the nucleus basalis. Controls received saline injections at the same locations (data from all controls are pooled). The animals were later given 6 days of training in the water maze and their path lengths (swimming distance from the start position to finding the hidden platform; see Chapter 4) were recorded. Treatment with 192 IgG–saporin resulted in poorer maze learning in both groups, with the greatest deficits observed in the animals given the neurotoxin intraventricularly. (After Berger-Sweeney et al., 1994.)

Alzheimer's disease. As discussed in Box 6.2, while Alzheimer's disease does involve severe injury to the BFCS, other damaged neural systems undoubtedly contribute to the devastating psychological and behavioral effects of this disorder.

There are two acetylcholine receptor subtypes, nicotinic and muscarinic

Like dopamine (DA) and norepinephrine (NE), ACh has many different kinds of receptors. The story can be simplified a little by recognizing that the various cholinergic receptors belong to one of two families: **nicotinic receptors** and **muscarinic receptors.** Nicotinic receptors were named because they respond selectively to the agonist **nicotine,** an **alkaloid** found in the leaves of the tobacco plant.* The pharmacology of nicotine is discussed in Chapter 12. Muscarinic receptors are selectively stimulated by **muscarine,** another alkaloid, which was first isolated in 1869 from the fly agaric mushroom, *Amanita muscaria.*

---

*Alkaloids are nitrogen-containing compounds, usually bitter-tasting, that are often found in plants.

Nicotinic receptors   Nicotinic receptors are highly concentrated on muscle cells at neuromuscular junctions, on ganglionic neurons of both the sympathetic and parasympathetic system, and on certain neurons in the brain. They are ionotropic receptors, which, you will recall from Chapter 3, means that they possess an ion channel as an integral part of the receptor complex. When ACh binds to a nicotinic receptor, the channel opens very rapidly and sodium (Na^+) and calcium (Ca^{2+}) ions enter the neuron or muscle cell. This flow of ions causes a depolarization of the cell membrane, thereby increasing the cell's excitability. If the responding cell is a neuron, its likelihood of firing is increased. If it is a muscle cell, it responds by contracting. In this manner, nicotinic receptors mediate fast excitatory responses in both the CNS and PNS.

Another important function of nicotinic receptors within the brain is to enhance the release of neurotransmitters from nerve terminals. In this case, the nicotinic receptors are located presynaptically, right on the terminals. Thus, activation of nicotinic receptors by ACh can stimulate cell firing if the receptors are located postsynaptically on dendrites or cell bodies, or the receptors can stimulate neurotransmitter release without affecting the cell's firing rate if they are located presynaptically on nerve endings.

The structure of the nicotinic receptor has been known for many years. As members of the family of ionotropic receptors discussed in Chapter 3, nicotinic receptors comprise five proteins (subunits) that come together in the cell membrane, forming the ion channel in the center. As you can see in Figure 6.9, the subunits are labeled with Greek letters. There are two α-subunits, each of which helps form an ACh binding site on the receptor. Interestingly, both binding sites must be occupied by ACh molecules to open the nicotinic receptor channel.

Even though the nicotinic receptors of neurons and muscles possess five subunits (including two αs), the exact proteins making up neuronal and muscle receptors are different. This structural difference leads to significant pharmacological differences between the two types of receptors. For example, muscle nicotinic receptors are not as sensitive to nicotine as are the nicotinic receptors found in the brain and autonomic nervous system. This difference is very important to smokers, because it allows them to obtain the psychological effects of nicotine, which are dependent on activation of brain nicotinic receptors, without experiencing muscle contractions or spasms.

In a living organism, receptors are typically exposed to neurotransmitters in a somewhat sporadic manner. That is, at some moments, there are many transmitter molecules in the vicinity of a particular receptor, whereas at other moments, few transmitter molecules are nearby, because the releasing neuron has slowed its firing or perhaps become completely silent for a brief period of time. We can perform

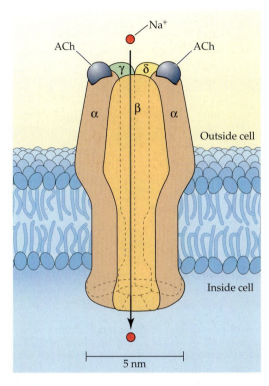

Figure 6.9 Structure of the nicotinic ACh receptor
The receptor comprises five protein subunits, two of which
(the α-subunits) are identical. Within the center of the receptor
is a channel that allows Na⁺ ions to flow into the cell when the
receptor is activated.

membrane is lost and the cell cannot be excited until the
agonist is removed and the membrane repolarized. A chemical relative of ACh called **succinylcholine** is a powerful muscle relaxant that is useful in certain surgical procedures where
anesthesia alone may not provide sufficient relaxation.
Unlike ACh, succinylcholine is resistant to breakdown by
AChE, and thus it continuously stimulates the nicotinic
receptors and induces a depolarization block of the muscle
cells. It is important to note that one of the paralyzed muscles is the diaphragm (the large muscle responsible for inflat-
ing and deflating the lungs), so the patient must be maintained on a ventilator until the succinylcholine is finally
eliminated and the effect wears off.

A well-known nicotinic receptor antagonist is D-**tubocu-
rarine.** This substance is the main active ingredient of
curare, a poison obtained from the tropical plant *Chondro-
dendron tomentosum.* Long before it came to the attention of
pharmacologists, curare was being used by South American
Indians as an arrow poison for hunting. D-Tubocurarine has
a high affinity for muscle nicotinic receptors, thus blocking
cholinergic transmission at neuromuscular junctions. Respiratory paralysis is the cause of death in curare poisoning, but
this effect can be overcome by treating the victim with an
anti-AChE drug such as neostigmine.

Muscarinic receptors   As mentioned earlier, muscarinic
receptors represent the other family of ACh receptors. Like

pharmacological experiments, however, in
which receptors are continuously exposed to
high concentrations of an agonist drug for
seconds or even longer intervals of minutes
or hours. When nicotinic receptors are subjected to continuous agonist exposure, they
become **desensitized** (Figure 6.10). Desensitization represents an altered state of the
receptor in which the channel remains
closed regardless of whether molecules of an
agonist such as ACh or nicotine are bound
to the receptor. After a short while, desensitized receptors spontaneously **resensitize**
and are then capable of responding again to
a nicotinic agonist.

Even if cells are continuously exposed to
nicotinic stimulation, the receptors are not
all desensitized. Those that remain active
produce a persistent depolarization of the
cell membrane. If this continues for very
long, a process called **depolarization block**
occurs, in which the resting potential of the

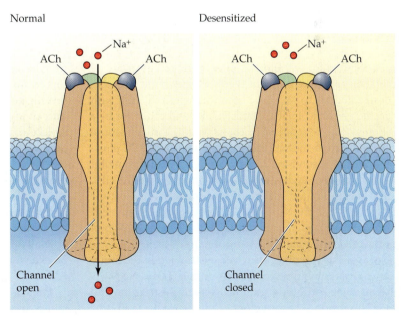

Figure 6.10 Nicotinic receptor desensitization When nicotinic receptors
are in a desensitized state, the channel does not open even in the presence of
ACh.

BOX 6.2   Clinical Applications

Alzheimer's Disease—A Tale of Two Proteins

As medical science continues to extend the human life span, we have become more prone to diseases of aging. None of these ailments strikes as much fear in the elderly as Alzheimer's disease (AD). In 1907, a German neurologist named Alois Alzheimer described a set of previously unidentified histological abnormalities in the brain of a 51-year-old woman who had been demented at the time of her death. Dementia refers to a major impairment of cognitive functions, including memory, language, and abstract thinking, and AD is the leading cause of dementia in the elderly.

The brain becomes severely damaged in the course of AD. Due to a loss of brain tissue, the cortical gyri (folds) become shrunken and the cerebral ventricles are enlarged. What

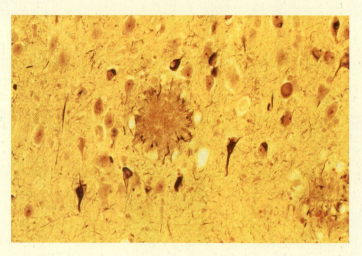

Photomicrograph of neuritic plaques and neurofibrillary tangles from the brain of a 69-year-old man suffering from severe Alzheimer's disease at the time of his death. Two plaques are visible: a large one near the center of the photomicrograph and part of a smaller plaque in the lower right-hand corner. Neurofibrillary tangles appear as darkly stained material that seems to fill the cytoplasm within some neurons in the center and left-hand parts of the photomicrograph. (Courtesy of Dennis Selkoe.)

Alzheimer noticed, however, was the presence of several pathological characteristics that are only visible under the microscope. Foremost among these are neuritic plaques and neurofibrillary tangles. The plaques are extracellular entities consisting of abnormal clusters of degenerating

---

the receptors for DA and NE, muscarinic receptors are all metabotropic. Five different types of muscarinic receptors (designated M_1 to M_5) have been characterized, each with specific pharmacological characteristics and coded for by a different gene. Muscarinic receptors operate through several different second-messenger systems. Some activate the phosphoinositide second-messenger system, while others inhibit the formation of cyclic adenosine monophosphate (cAMP). Another important mechanism of muscarinic receptor action is the stimulation of K^+ channel opening. As mentioned in previous chapters, this leads to a hyperpolarization of the cell membrane and a reduction in cell firing.

Muscarinic receptors are widely distributed in the brain. Some areas containing high levels of muscarinic receptors are the neocortex, hippocampus, thalamus, striatum, and basal forebrain. The receptors in the neocortex and hippocampus play an important role in the cognitive effects of ACh described earlier, whereas those in the striatum are involved in motor function. There is also recent evidence

from Basile and colleagues (2002) that M_5 muscarinic receptors are involved in morphine reward and dependence. These investigators compared genetically normal mice to mutant mice in which the M_5 receptor gene had been inactivated. In a place-conditioning paradigm, morphine doses that produced a robust place preference in the normal animals had no effect on the mutants (Figure 6.11). Loss of M_5 receptor function also reduced withdrawal symptoms in mice that were made dependent on morphine, but it had no effect on morphine-induced analgesia. These findings suggest that M_5 muscarinic receptors selectively influence the addictive properties of opiate drugs, and they raise the possibility that drugs targeted to these receptors could be useful in treating opiate addicts.

Outside of the brain, muscarinic receptors are found at high densities in the cardiac muscle of the heart and in the smooth muscle associated with many organs, such as the bronchioles, stomach, intestines, bladder, and urogenital organs. These peripheral muscarinic receptors are activated

BOX 6.2 (continued)

axons and dendrites surrounding a central core containing a small protein called β-amyloid protein (βAP) (see figure). In contrast, the tangles are intracellular masses of abnormal fibers containing a different protein, tau, which has been hyperphosphorylated. That is, an unusually large number of phosphate groups has been added to the tau protein, thus disturbing its function and somehow causing it to aggregate into these masses.

Microscopic examination of brains stricken with AD also reveals cell death and loss of synapses in the cortex and hippocampus, structures that play a critical role in various cognitive functions. Damage to these structures, therefore, helps explain the severe dementia characteristic of AD patients. The question is, what process causes this cellular damage? Although we don't yet completely know the answer to this question, most of the evidence indicates that βAP is the key element in the development of AD (Hardy and Selkoe, 2002). Of particular importance is the

mechanism by which βAP is generated in the brain. This small protein is derived from a larger precursor known as amyloid precursor protein (APP), which is normally found in the brain as well as in other organs. It appears that in healthy neurons, relatively little of the dangerous βAP is released from the precursor protein. In AD, however, larger amounts of βAP are created, which somehow eventually leads to plaque formation. Somewhere along the way, tau-containing tangles are also formed, and eventually the buildup of these toxic materials causes synaptic damage and nerve cell death.

So that is the tale of how two proteins, βAP and tau, are involved in the development of AD. But why is this disorder covered here in the chapter on ACh? In addition to the cortical and hippocampal cell loss mentioned in the previous paragraph, there is also severe damage to the basal forebrain cholinergic system that projects to the cortex and hippocampus. Consequently, researchers have long believed that

deficits in cholinergic activity play a major role in Alzheimer's dementia. This hypothesis resulted in the development of the first specific medications to treat AD, namely tacrine (Cognex), donepezil (Aricept), and rivastigmine (Exelon). These compounds are all AChE inhibitors and are thus thought to potentiate the activity of ACh released by the remaining cholinergic nerve terminals. Unfortunately, clinical trials have shown that anticholinesterase treatments generally produce only modest symptom improvement and only in patients with mild to moderate AD. Other cholinergic drugs are currently being tested for use in AD, including agonists at either nicotinic or muscarinic receptors. Although it is possible that some of these compounds will prove superior to the anticholinesterases, future treatment strategies will almost certainly be targeted at inhibiting βAP production or tau protein hyperphosphorylation and aggregation into neurofibrillary tangles.

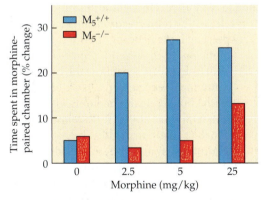

Figure 6.11 Genetic deletion of the M$_5$ muscarinic receptor reduces the rewarding effects of morphine. Genetically normal mice (also known as wild-type mice; shown as M$_5^{+/+}$) were compared to mutant mice lacking M$_5$ muscarinic receptors (also known as knockout mice; shown as M$_5^{-/-}$) in a place-conditioning test with morphine. Morphine reward in the wild-type animals was shown by increased time spent in the drug-paired chamber compared to controls given saline injections (0 mg/kg dose group). In the knockout animals, there was no rewarding effect of morphine except for a partial effect at the highest drug dose. (After Basile et al., 2002.)

by ACh released from postganglionic fibers of the parasympathetic nervous system. Stimulation of the parasympathetic system has two effects on the heart: a slowing of heart rate and a decrease in the strength of contraction, both of which are mediated by the muscarinic receptors in cardiac muscle. In contrast, smooth muscle cells are typically excited by muscarinic receptor activation, thus causing contraction of the muscle. Muscarinic receptors also mediate various secretory responses of the parasympathetic system, including salivation, sweating, and lacrimation (tearing). Unfortunately, many of the drugs used to treat depression, schizophrenia, and other major psychiatric disorders produce serious side effects due to their blockade of peripheral muscarinic receptors. Patients particularly complain about the so-called **dry-mouth effect** (technically referred to as xerostomia), which reflects the reduced production of saliva resulting from muscarinic antagonism. For some, the dry-mouth effect is severe enough to cause the patient to stop taking his or her medication. If the medication is continued, the chronic lack of salivation can lead to mouth sores, increased tooth decay, and difficulty in chewing and swallowing food. Later in the book, we will see that pharmaceutical companies have worked to develop newer medications that react less with muscarinic receptors and therefore do not produce the dry-mouth effect.

Several muscarinic receptor agonists occur in nature, including muscarine, from *Amanita muscaria;* **pilocarpine,** from the leaves of the South American shrub *Pilocarpus jaborandi;* and **arecoline,** which is found in the seeds of the betel nut palm *Areca catechu.* These substances are sometimes referred to as **parasympathomimetic agents,** because their ingestion mimics many of the effects of parasympathetic activation. Thus, poisoning due to accidental ingestion of *Amanita* or any of the other plants leads to exaggerated parasympathetic responses, including lacrimation, salivation, sweating, pinpoint pupils related to constriction of the iris, severe abdominal pain, strong contractions of the smooth muscles of the viscera, and painful diarrhea. High doses can even cause cardiovascular collapse, convulsions, coma, and death.

Given the autonomic effects of muscarinic agonists, it is understandable that antagonists of these receptors would inhibit the actions of the parasympathetic system. Such compounds, therefore, are called **parasympatholytic agents.** The major naturally occurring muscarinic antagonists are **atropine** (also sometimes called hyoscamine) and the closely related drug **scopolamine** (hyoscine). These alkaloids are found in a group of plants that includes the deadly nightshade *(Atropa belladonna)* and henbane *(Hyoscyamus niger)* (Figure 6.12). Extracts of these plants are toxic when taken systemically, a fact that was exploited during the Middle Ages, when the deadly nightshade was used as a lethal agent to settle many political and family intrigues. On the other hand, a cosmetic use of the plant also evolved, in which women instilled the juice of the berries into their eyes to cause pupillary dilation (by blocking the muscarinic receptors on the constrictor muscles of the iris). The effect was considered to make the user more attractive to men. Indeed, the name *Atropa belladonna* reflects these two facets of the plant, since *bella donna* means "beautiful woman" in Latin, whereas Atropos was a character in Greek mythology whose duty it was to cut the thread of life at the appropriate time.

Muscarinic antagonists have several current medical applications. Modern ophthalmologists use atropine just as did women of the Middle Ages, except in this case they are dilating the patient's pupils to obtain a better view of the interior of the eye. Another use is in human or veterinary surgery, where the drug reduces secretions that could clog the patient's airways. Atropine is also occasionally needed to counteract the effects of poisoning with a cholinergic agonist. Scopolamine in therapeutic doses produces drowsiness, euphoria, amnesia, fatigue, and dreamless sleep. It has sometimes been used along with narcotics as a preanesthetic medication before surgery or alone prior to childbirth to produce "twilight sleep," a condition characterized by drowsiness and amnesia for events occurring during the duration of drug use.

Despite their therapeutic uses, muscarinic antagonists can themselves be toxic when taken systemically at high doses. The CNS effects of atropine poisoning include restlessness, irritability, disorientation, hallucinations, and delirium. Even higher doses can lead to CNS depression, coma, and eventually death by respiratory paralysis. As in the case of nicotinic drugs, these toxic effects point to the delicate balance of cholinergic activity in both the CNS and PNS that is necessary for normal physiological functioning.

Section Summary

Acetylcholine is an important neurotransmitter in the PNS, where it is released by motor neurons innervating skeletal muscles, by preganglionic neurons of both the parasympathetic and sympathetic branches of the autonomic nervous system, and by ganglionic parasympathetic neurons. In the brain, there are many cholinergic interneurons within the striatum as well as a diffuse system of projection neurons that constitutes the basal forebrain cholinergic system. There is evidence that the BFCS plays an important role in cognitive functioning, and damage to this system may contribute to the dementia observed in Alzheimer's disease.

Cholinergic receptors are divided into two major families: nicotinic and muscarinic receptors. The nicotinic receptors are ionotropic receptors comprising five subunits. When the receptor channel opens, it produces a fast excitatory response due to an influx of Na^+ and Ca^{2+} ions across the cell membrane. Nicotinic receptors in neurons and muscles possess somewhat different subunits, which leads to significant

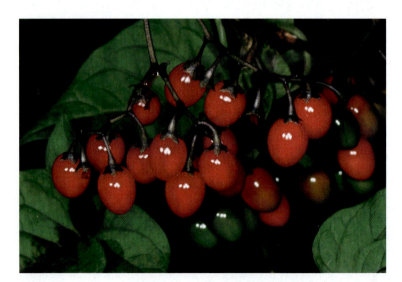

Figure 6.12 The deadly nightshade (*Atropa belladonna*), a natural source of the muscarinic antagonist atropine.

TABLE 6.1 Drugs and Toxins That Affect the Cholinergic System

Drug	Action
Vesamicol	Depletes ACh by inhibiting vesicular uptake
Black widow spider venom	Stimulates ACh release
Botulinum toxin	Inhibits ACh release
Hemicholinium-3	Depletes ACh by inhibiting choline uptake by the nerve terminal
Physostigmine, neostigmine, and pyridostigmine	Increase ACh levels by inhibiting acetylcholinesterase reversibly
Sarin and Soman	Inhibit acetylcholinesterase irreversibly
Nicotine	Stimulates nicotinic receptors (agonist)
Succinylcholine	Nicotinic receptor agonist that causes depolarization block
D-Tubocurarine	Blocks nicotinic receptors (antagonist)
Muscarine, pilocarpine, and arecoline	Stimulate muscarinic receptors (agonists)
Atropine and scopolamine	Block muscarinic receptors (antagonists)

pharmacological differences between the two types of receptors. With continuous stimulation by an agonist, nicotinic receptors are subject to a phenomenon called desensitization, in which the channel will not open despite the presence of the agonist. These receptors can also lead to a process of depolarization block involving temporary loss of the cell's resting potential and an inability of the cell to generate action potentials.

There are five kinds of muscarinic receptors, designated M_1 to M_5, all of which are metabotropic receptors. Muscarinic receptors function through several different signaling mechanisms, including activation of the phosphoinositide second-messenger system, inhibition of cAMP synthesis, and stimulation of K^+ channel opening. Muscarinic receptors are widely distributed in the brain, with particularly high densities in various forebrain structures. They are also found in the target organs of the parasympathetic system. Consequently, muscarinic agonists are called parasympathomimetic agents, whereas antagonists are considered parasympatholytic in their actions. Blockade of muscarinic receptors in the salivary glands leads to the dry-mouth effect, which is a serious side effect of many drugs used to treat various psychiatric disorders. Table 6.1 presents some of the drugs that affect the cholinergic system, including nicotinic and muscarinic receptor agonists and antagonists.

Serotonin

The National Institutes of Health declared the 1990s to be the "Decade of the Brain," to highlight the stunning advances in neuroscience being made at that time. If the 1990s was the decade of the brain for neuroscientists generally, then just as surely it was the "Decade of Serotonin" for psychopharmacologists. **Serotonin,** or, more technically speaking, **5-hydroxytryptamine (5-HT),** has been featured in the popular culture as the culprit in just about every human malady or vice, including depression, anxiety, obesity, impulsive aggression and violence, and even drug addiction. Can a single neurotransmitter really have such far-reaching behavioral consequences? The answer is not a simple one—5-HT probably does influence many different behavioral and physiological systems, yet the ability of this chemical to either destroy us (if imbalanced) or to cure all that ails us (if brought back into equilibrium) has unfortunately been oversold by a sensationalist media aided and abetted by a few publicity-seeking scientists. In this second part of Chapter 6, we learn about the neurochemistry, pharmacology, and functional characteristics of this fascinating neurotransmitter.

Serotonin Synthesis, Release, and Inactivation

Serotonin synthesis is regulated by the activity of tryptophan hydroxylase and the availability of the serotonin precursor tryptophan

Serotonin is synthesized from the amino acid **tryptophan,** which comes from protein in our diet. As shown in Figure 6.13, there are two steps in the biochemical pathway. The first step is catalyzed by the enzyme **tryptophan hydroxylase,** which converts tryptophan to **5-hydroxytryptophan (5-HTP).** 5-HTP is then acted upon by **aromatic amino acid decarboxylase (AADC)** to form 5-HT.

Many features of this pathway are similar to the pathway described in the previous chapter involving the formation of dopamine from the amino acid tyrosine. Just as the initial step in the synthesis of DA (that is, tyrosine to DOPA) is the rate-limiting step, the conversion of tryptophan to 5-HTP is rate-limiting in the 5-HT pathway. Furthermore, just as tyro-

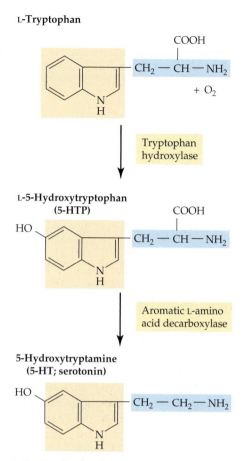

L-Tryptophan

L-5-Hydroxytryptophan
(5-HTP)

Tryptophan
hydroxylase

Aromatic L-amino
acid decarboxylase

5-Hydroxytryptamine
(5-HT; serotonin)

Figure 6.13 Synthesis of serotonin Serotonin (5-HT) is synthesized from the amino acid tryptophan in two steps catalyzed by the enzymes tryptophan hydroxylase and aromatic amino acid decarboxylase.

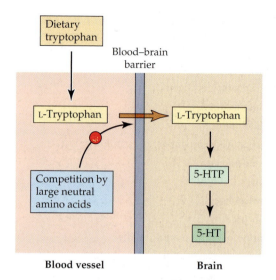

Figure 6.14 Tryptophan entry into the brain and 5-HT synthesis are regulated by the relative availability of tryptophan versus large neutral amino acids that compete with it for transport across the blood–brain barrier. In rats, a high-protein, low-carbohydrate meal does not increase brain tryptophan levels or 5-HT synthesis rate, due to this competitive process. However, the ratio of circulating tryptophan to large neutral amino acids is elevated following a high-carbohydrate, low-protein meal, thereby enhancing tryptophan entry into the brain and stimulating 5-HT synthesis.

sine hydroxylase is only found in neurons that synthesize catecholamines, tryptophan hydroxylase similarly is a specific marker for neurons that make 5-HT (these are called **serotonergic** neurons). Another important point is that the second enzyme in the pathway, AADC, is the same for both catecholamines and 5-HT.

Serotonin synthesis in the brain can be stimulated by giving animals a large dose of tryptophan, but 5-HTP administration is even more effective because it is converted so rapidly and efficiently to 5-HT. There is also an interesting link between food intake and 5-HT synthesis that was first discovered many years ago by John Fernstrom and Richard Wurtman (1972). Imagine a group of rats that has been fasted overnight and then fed a protein-rich meal. The level of tryptophan in their blood goes up, and thus you would probably expect brain 5-HT to rise as well, since an injection of pure tryptophan produces such an effect. Surprisingly, however, Fernstrom and Wurtman found that consumption of a protein-rich meal did not cause increases in either trypto-

phan or 5-HT in the brain, even though tryptophan levels in the bloodstream were elevated. The researchers explained this result by showing that tryptophan competes with a group of other amino acids (called large neutral amino acids) for transport from the blood to the brain across the blood–brain barrier (Figure 6.14). Consequently, it's the *ratio* between the amount of tryptophan in the blood and the overall amount of its competitors that counts. Most proteins contain larger amounts of these competitor amino acids than tryptophan, and thus when these proteins are consumed, the critical ratio either stays the same or even goes down.

Even more surprising was an additional finding of Fernstrom and Wurtman. When the researchers fed previously fasted rats a diet low in protein but high in carbohydrates, that experimental treatment led to increases in brain tryptophan and 5-HT levels. How could this be the case? You might already know that eating carbohydrates (starches and sugars) triggers a release of the hormone **insulin** from the pancreas. One important function of this insulin response is to stimulate the uptake of glucose from the bloodstream into various tissues, where it can be metabolized for energy. But glucose is not the only substance acted on by insulin. The hormone also stimulates the uptake of most amino acids from the bloodstream; tryptophan, however, is relatively unaffected. Because of this difference, we can see that a low-protein, high-carbohydrate meal will increase the ratio of tryptophan to competing amino acids, allowing more tryptophan to cross the blood–brain barrier and more 5-HT to be made in the brain.

Do the dietary effects observed in rats also occur in humans eating typical meals? Wurtman and colleagues (2003) recently addressed this issue by measuring the plasma ratio of tryptophan to large neutral amino acids in subjects eating either a high-carbohydrate, low-protein breakfast (consisting of waffles, maple syrup, orange juice, and coffee with sugar) or a high-protein, low-carbohydrate breakfast (consisting of turkey ham, Egg Beaters, cheese, grapefruit, and butter). As predicted, the high-carbohydrate, low-protein meal did increase the ratio of tryptophan to large neutral amino acids, whereas this ratio was decreased by the high-protein, low-carbohydrate meal. However, the average increase following the high-carbohydrate, low-protein meal was only about 14%, which may not have much effect on brain 5-HT levels.

Pharmacological depletion of 5-HT has been widely used to assess the role of this neurotransmitter in various behavioral functions. One method often used in rodent studies is to administer the drug *para*-**chlorophenylalanine (PCPA)**, which selectively blocks 5-HT synthesis by irreversibly inhibiting tryptophan hydroxylase. One or two high doses of PCPA can reduce brain 5-HT levels in rats 80 to 90% for as long as 2 weeks, until the serotonergic neurons make new molecules of tryptophan hydroxylase that haven't been exposed to the inhibitor. Because PCPA can cause adverse side effects in humans, researchers have developed an alternative approach that has been particularly valuable for studying the role of 5-HT in mood and mood disorders. Based in part on the rat studies of Fernstrom and Wurtman, this method involves the administration of an amino acid "cocktail" containing a large quantity of amino acids except for tryptophan. This cocktail leads to a temporary depletion of brain 5-HT for two reasons: (1) the surge of amino acids in the bloodstream stimulates protein synthesis by the liver, which reduces the level of plasma tryptophan below its starting point; and (2) the large neutral amino acids in the cocktail inhibit entry of the remaining tryptophan into the brain. The 5-HT depletion produced by this method is not nearly as great nor as long-lasting as that produced by PCPA. However, several studies have shown that giving the amino acid cocktail to previously depressed patients often causes a reappearance of depressive symptoms. In one case, 15 women who had suffered from repeated episodes of major depression but who were recovered at the time of the study were given either a tryptophan-free or tryptophan-containing amino acid mixture under double-blind conditions (Smith et al., 1997). Whereas the tryptophan-containing mixture had no effect on mood or depressive symptoms, the tryptophan-free mixture led to significant increases in

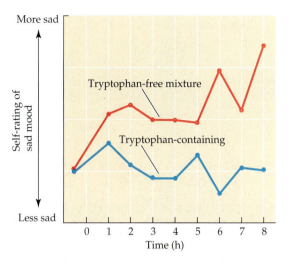

Figure 6.15 Rapid tryptophan depletion leads to symptom relapse in recovered depressed patients. The subjects were women who had a past history of recurrent depressive episodes, were currently in remission, and were not currently taking any antidepresssant medications. On separate occasions, each subject was given a mixture of amino acids either with or without tryptophan. The tryptophan-containing mixture had no effect on mood, whereas the tryptophan-free mixture elicited an increase in self-rated sadness. In two-thirds of the subjects, tryptophan depletion further caused clinically significant depressive symptoms, as determined by the Hamilton Depression Rating Scale (not shown). (After Smith et al., 1997.)

depression ratings for 10 of the subjects as well as an overall increase in self-reported feelings of sadness (Figure 6.15). Such findings implicate 5-HT in mood regulation and further suggest that in patients successfully treated with antidepressant medications, symptom improvement may depend on continued activity of the serotonergic system (see also Chapter 16).

The processes that regulate storage, release, and inactivation are similar for serotonin and the catecholamines

Serotonin is transported into synaptic vesicles using the same vesicular transporter, VMAT2 (vesicular monoamine transporter), found in dopaminergic and noradrenergic neurons. As with the catecholamines, storage of 5-HT in vesicles plays a critical role in protecting the transmitter from enzymatic breakdown in the nerve terminal. Consequently, the VMAT blocker reserpine depletes serotonergic neurons of 5-HT, just as it depletes catecholamines in dopaminergic and noradrenergic cells.

Serotonergic autoreceptors control 5-HT release in the same way as the DA and NE autoreceptors discussed in the previous chapter. Terminal autoreceptors directly inhibit 5-

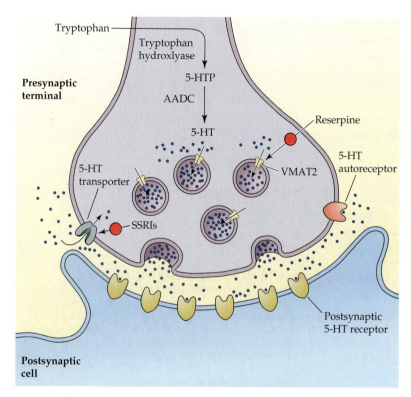

Figure 6.16 Features of a serotonergic neuron Serotonergic neurons express the vesicular monoamine transporter VMAT2, the 5-HT transporter, and 5-HT$_{1B}$ or 5-HT$_{1D}$ autoreceptors in their terminals.

on the nerve terminal known as the **5-HT transporter** (see Figure 6.16). This protein turns out to be a key target of drug action. For example, the introduction of **fluoxetine** (better known as **Prozac**) in late 1987 spawned a whole new class of antidepressant drugs based on the idea of inhibiting 5-HT reuptake. These compounds are, therefore, called **selective serotonin reuptake inhibitors (SSRIs)** (see Chapter 16). Certain abused drugs such as cocaine and MDMA likewise interact with the 5-HT transporter, but they are not selective in their effects because they also influence the DA transporter.

You will recall that DA and NE are metabolized by two different enzymes, monoamine oxidase (MAO) and catechol-O-methyltransferase (COMT). Since 5-HT is not a catecholamine, it is not affected by COMT. However, its breakdown is catalyzed by MAO to yield the metabolite **5-hydroxyindoleacetic acid (5-HIAA).** The level of 5-HIAA in the brains of animals or in the cerebrospinal fluid of humans or animals is often used as a measure of the activity of serotonergic neurons. This is based on research showing that when these neurons fire more rapidly, they make more 5-HT and there is a corresponding increase in the formation of 5-HIAA.

HT release, whereas other autoreceptors on the cell body and dendrites of the serotonergic neurons (somatodendritic autoreceptors) indirectly inhibit release by slowing the rate of firing of the neurons (Figure 6.16). Somatodendritic autoreceptors are of the 5-HT$_{1A}$ subtype, whereas the terminal autoreceptors are either of the 5-HT$_{1B}$ or 5-HT$_{1D}$ subtype, depending on the species (see later discussion of 5-HT receptors).

Release of 5-HT can be directly stimulated by a family of drugs based on the structure of amphetamine. These compounds include *para*-**chloroamphetamine,** which is mainly used experimentally; **fenfluramine,** which at one time was prescribed for appetite suppression in obese patients (Box 6.3); and **3,4-methylenedioxymethamphetamine (MDMA),** which is a recreational and abused drug. Besides their acute behavioral effects, these drugs (particularly *para*-chloroamphetamine and MDMA) can also exert toxic effects on the serotonergic system (see Chapter 11).

When we examine the processes responsible for inactivation of 5-HT after its release, there are again many similarities to the catecholamine systems. After 5-HT is released, it is rapidly removed from the synaptic cleft by a reuptake process. Analogously to DA and NE, this mechanism involves a protein

Section Summary

The neurotransmitter 5-HT is synthesized from the amino acid tryptophan in two biochemical reactions. The first and rate-limiting reaction is catalyzed by the enzyme tryptophan hydroxylase. Under appropriate conditions, the synthesis of brain 5-HT in rats can be enhanced by the consumption of a high-carbohydrate, low-protein meal. Administration of an amino acid mixture lacking tryptophan has been used to temporarily deplete 5-HT in human studies. Like the other transmitters previously discussed, 5-HT is stored in synaptic vesicles for subsequent release. Serotonin release is inhibited by autoreceptors located on the cell body, dendrites, and terminals of serotonergic neurons. The terminal autoreceptors are of either the 5-HT$_{1B}$ or 5-HT$_{1D}$ subtype, depending on the species, whereas the somatodendritic autoreceptors are of the 5-HT$_{1A}$ subtype. Serotonergic transmission is terminated by reuptake of 5-HT from the synaptic cleft. This process is mediated by the 5-HT transporter, which is an important target of several antidepressant drugs. Serotonin is ultimately metabolized by MAO to form the major breakdown product 5-HIAA.

Organization and Function of the Serotonergic System

The serotonergic system originates from cell bodies in the brain stem and projects to all forebrain areas

The Swedish researchers who first mapped the catecholamine systems in the 1960s (see Chapter 5) used the same experimental techniques to study the distribution of neurons and pathways using 5-HT. But in this case, they designated the 5-HT-containing cell groups with the letter "B" instead of "A," which they had used for the dopaminergic and noradrenergic cell groups. It turns out that almost all of the serotonergic neurons in the CNS are found along the midline of the brainstem (medulla, pons, and midbrain), loosely associated with a network of cell clusters called the **raphe nuclei.*** Of greatest interest to neuropharmacologists are the **dorsal raphe nucleus** and the **median raphe nucleus,** located in the area of the caudal midbrain and rostral pons. Together, these nuclei give rise to most of the serotonergic fibers in the forebrain. Virtually all forebrain regions receive a serotonergic innervation, including the neocortex, striatum and nucleus accumbens, thalamus and hypothalamus, and limbic system structures such as the hippocampus, amygdala, and septal area (Figure 6.17).

---

*The term *raphe* is Greek for "seam" or "suture." In biology, the term is applied to structures that look as if they are joined together in a line. This is applicable to the raphe nuclei, which are aligned with each other along the rostral–caudal axis of the brain stem.

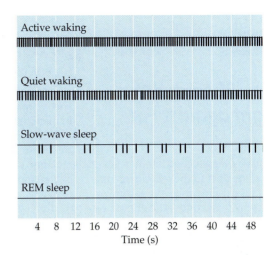

Figure 6.18 The firing rate of serotonergic neurons in the cat dorsal raphe is related to the animal's behavioral state. During quiet waking, the cells fire at a steady rate of approximately 2 action potentials per second. The firing rate is slightly increased during behavioral activity, but greatly diminishes during slow-wave sleep. Dorsal raphe cell firing is essentially abolished during REM sleep. (After Jacobs and Fornal, 1993.)

Barry Jacobs and his colleagues at Princeton University have discovered some interesting properties of serotonergic neurons in the dorsal raphe nucleus. The investigators recorded the firing of these cells in unanesthetized, freely moving cats under many different behavioral states. When a cat is awake, each cell fires at a relatively slow but very regular rate, almost like a ticking clock (Figure 6.18). When the cat

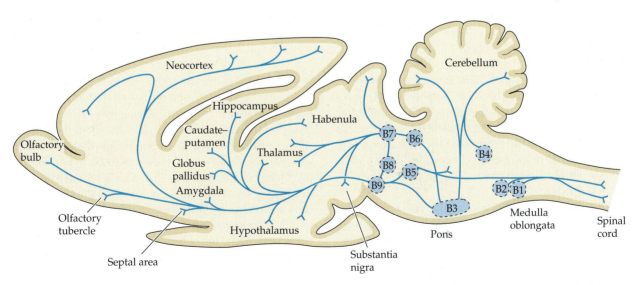

Figure 6.17 Anatomy of the serotonergic system The B7 cell group corresponds to the dorsal raphe and the B8 cell group corresponds to the median raphe.

BOX 6.3   Pharmacology in Action

Fen–Phen and the Fight against Fat

If you've ever watched infomercials on television or read the tabloid newspapers sold in supermarkets, you've probably seen ads or articles promoting the latest over-the-counter drug or herbal supplement "guaranteed" to help you lose weight. Indeed, obesity is a major health problem in the United States, and many pharmaceutical companies are working hard to develop effective antiobesity medications. In the mid-1990s, a diet pill combination called "Fen–Phen" was being touted as the new miracle treatment for obesity, but one of the drugs was later withdrawn from the marketplace. What were these compounds, how did they work, and what prompted withdrawal of one of the drugs?

The "Fen" part of the combo is fenfluramine, which we have already indicated releases 5-HT from serotonergic nerve terminals. Many studies in animals have shown that increasing serotonergic activity, such as by stimulating 5-HT release, leads to decreased food intake. Clinical studies also demonstrated reduced eating and weight loss in overweight humans, which led to the introduction of fenfluramine back in 1973 for the treatment of obesity. The initial formulation was a mixture of two closely related forms of the drug, dexfenfluramine and levofenfluramine. This mixture was marketed under the trade name Pondimin. Unfortunately, many patients regained their lost weight after ending the treatment, and therefore its long-term effectiveness was limited.

In 1992, Michael Weintraub and his colleagues at the University of Rochester published a study testing the extended use of two diet medications given together: fenfluramine and phentermine (the "Phen" in Fen–Phen). Phentermine had been in use even longer than fenfluramine (it was approved as an appetite suppressant in 1959), but it was thought to function through the catecholamine systems instead of 5-HT. Weintraub's group therefore reasoned that a combination of two drugs acting by different mechanisms might be more effective than either drug alone. Another possible benefit of the Fen–Phen mixture was related to the fact that fenfluramine tends to produce drowsiness as a side effect. In contrast, phentermine is a stimulant and was therefore expected to counteract the sedative effect of the fenfluramine.

The figure shows that in a clinical trial of the Fen–Phen combination used in conjunction with behavior modification therapy, dietary counseling, and exercise, subjects lost significant amounts of weight over a 34-week period (Weintraub et al., 1992). Word of these results spread, and many physicians began prescribing Fen–Phen for extended periods of time to overweight patients. It should be noted that the U.S. Food and Drug Administration (FDA) had licensed these medications only for short-term use (a few weeks), and it had never tested or approved the combined use of fenfluramine with phentermine. Such use of drugs, which is called "off-label use," is not illegal, but it should always been done with great caution. In 1996, pure dexfenfluramine, which is more pharmacologically active than the levo form of the drug, was approved for the treatment of obesity under the trade name Redux. Many patients then began taking Redux, either by itself or

enters slow-wave sleep, which is the stage of sleep in which large-amplitude, slow electroencephalographic (EEG) waves can be recorded in the cortex, the serotonergic neurons slow down and become more irregular. Most intriguingly, the cells are almost completely shut down when the cat is in rapid eye movement (REM) sleep, a stage of deep sleep characterized by side-to-side eye movements and low-amplitude, fast EEG waves in the cortex.

What do these changes in serotonergic activity mean for the animal? The key to understanding this strange pattern comes from other results obtained by Jacobs' lab. Some of the dorsal raphe neurons fired more rapidly during repetitive movements such as chewing, self-licking, or walking on a cat-sized treadmill. In contrast, cell firing was inhibited when the cat was exposed to a sudden sensory stimulus (such as opening the door to the room) that caught the animal's attention. It appears, therefore, that serotonergic neurons in the dorsal raphe are activated during movement (especially repetitive movement) but are quiescent when the animal is still because it is attending to a stimulus in the environment. You may also recall from a previous course in physiological psychology or neurobiology that muscle tone is lost during REM sleep, which is another state in which dorsal raphe neurons are silenced. From these results, Jacobs and Fornal (1993) hypothesized that one important function of brain 5-HT is to facilitate the output of motor systems in the brain (hence the activation of serotonergic neurons during waking in general and particularly during repetitive movement), while simultaneously suppressing sensory processing. When sensory information does need to be processed (as when a

BOX 6.3 (continued)

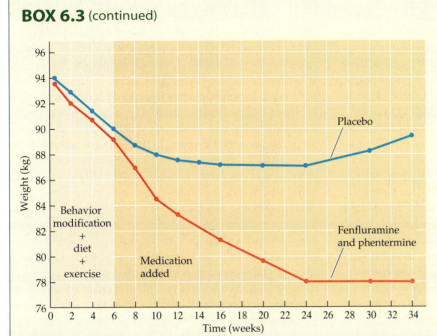

Combined fenfluramine and phentermine treatment reduces body weight in obese patients. Obese men and women were entered into a program of behavior modification, dietary counseling, and exercise. After 6 weeks, subjects were started on daily treatment with either fenfluramine and phentermine or placebo in a double-blind procedure. Greater weight loss occurred with drug treatment than placebo. (After Weintraub et al., 1992.)

as a replacement for Pondimin in the Fen–Phen combination.

We wish we could say that this story had a happy ending, and that millions of obese people were on their way to achieving a healthier body weight. Sadly, this was not to be the case. In 1996 and 1997, several studies were published suggesting an association of fenfluramine or dexfenfluramine use (with or without phentermine) with an increased risk for two different medical disorders: heart valve abnormalities and primary pulmonary hypertension (elevated blood pressure in the arteries between the heart and lungs). Both of these are serious problems, and primary pulmonary hypertension is often fatal. Consequently, upon the request of the FDA, Pondimin and Redux were both withdrawn from clinical use in September 1997. Phentermine is still being prescribed, as there is no evidence for its involvement in either medical disorder when taken alone.

It may be that the Fen–Phen story represents the final chapter in the use of serotonergic drugs to treat obesity. The new antiobesity compounds under development by the pharmaceutical industry do not act on the serotonergic system, instead targeting neuropeptides in the brain that regulate hunger or other chemicals that signal energy usage or energy storage (fat) by the body. The hope is that such approaches will lead to more-effective medications with better safety profiles. Since so many Americans seem unwilling or unable to make the lifestyle changes necessary to control their weight without using drugs, the health of a large percentage of our population hangs in the balance. Stay tuned!

new stimulus is presented to the animal), the serotonergic system has to be temporarily inhibited.

Correlating neuronal firing rate with behavioral state is only one way to assess the possible behavioral functions of 5-HT. Another approach is to damage the serotonergic neurons and then determine the behavioral changes produced by such lesions. Earlier we mentioned two drugs, *para*-chloroamphetamine and MDMA, that have neurotoxic effects on the serotonergic system. Another compound called **5,7-dihydroxytryptamine (5,7-DHT)** has also been widely used to produce serotonergic lesions in experimental animals, although one limitation of using 5,7-DHT is that it must be given directly into the brain since it doesn't cross the blood–brain barrier. All three neurotoxins cause extensive damage to serotonergic axons and nerve terminals in the forebrain, yet the cell bodies in the raphe nuclei are usually spared. Due to space limitations, we cannot review all of the behavioral effects produced by lesioning the serotonergic system; however, various studies have reported changes in food intake, reproductive behavior, pain sensitivity, anxiety, and learning and memory. These findings, along with the results of other experiments using serotonergic receptor agonists and antagonists (see the next section), indicate that 5-HT is involved in many functions besides the facilitation of motor output.

There is a large family of serotonin receptors, most of which are metabotropic

One of the remarkable properties of 5-HT is the number of receptors that have evolved for this transmitter. At the present time, pharmacologists have identified at least 15 5-HT receptor subtypes. Among these is a large family of 5-HT$_1$ receptors (that is, 5-HT$_{1A}$, 5-HT$_{1B}$, and so forth), a smaller family of 5-HT$_2$ receptors, and additional receptors designated 5-HT$_3$, 5-HT$_4$, 5-HT$_5$, 5-HT$_6$, and 5-HT$_7$. All of these receptors are metabotropic, except for the 5-HT$_3$ receptor, which is an excitatory ionotropic receptor. Here we will focus on the 5-HT$_{1A}$ and 5-HT$_{2A}$ receptors, which are the best-known serotonergic receptors in terms of their cellular and behavioral effects.

5-HT$_{1A}$ receptors   5-HT$_{1A}$ receptors are found in many brain areas, but they are particularly concentrated in the hippocampus, the septum, parts of the amygdala, and the dorsal raphe nucleus. In the forebrain, these receptors are located postsynaptically to 5-HT-containing nerve terminals. As mentioned earlier, 5-HT$_{1A}$ receptors additionally function as somatodendritic autoreceptors in the dorsal and median raphe nuclei.

5-HT$_{1A}$ receptors work through two major mechanisms. First, the receptors reduce the synthesis of cAMP by inhibiting adenylyl cyclase (Figure 6.19A). The second mechanism involves increased opening of K$^+$ channels and membrane hyperpolarization, which we have seen is a property shared by some cholinergic muscarinic receptors as well as by D$_2$ dopamine receptors and α$_2$-adrenergic receptors. You will recall that this hyperpolarization leads to a decrease in firing of either the postsynaptic cell (in the case of 5-HT$_{1A}$ receptors located postsynaptically) or the serotonergic neuron itself (in the case of the 5-HT$_{1A}$ autoreceptors).

A number of drugs act as 5-HT$_{1A}$ receptor agonists, including **buspirone, ipsapirone,** and **8-hydroxy-2-(di-n-**

propylamino)tetralin (8-OH-DPAT). The most widely used 5-HT$_{1A}$ receptor antagonist is the experimental drug **WAY 100635,** which was originally developed by the Wyeth-Ayerst pharmaceutical company (hence the WAY designation). Administration of a 5-HT$_{1A}$ receptor agonist produces several behavioral and physiological effects in animals. One consequence is **hyperphagia** (overeating). This effect is thought to be due to stimulation of the 5-HT$_{1A}$ autoreceptors, thereby inhibiting the activity of serotonergic neurons and reducing 5-HT release in the forebrain. In Box 6.3, we discussed the 5-HT-releasing drug fenfluramine, which is an appetite suppressant that was formerly prescribed for weight loss before being withdrawn from the market due to dangerous side effects. Serotonin generally tends to reduce appetite and food intake in both animals and humans (Leibowitz and Alexander, 1998), which explains why stimulation of serotonergic autoreceptors by a 5-HT$_{1A}$ agonist would lead to increased appetite and overeating. A second effect of 5-HT$_{1A}$ receptor stimulation is reduced anxiety, both in humans and in animal models of anxiety (see Chapter 17). Thus the 5-HT$_{1A}$ agonist buspirone (trade name **Buspar**) is prescribed as an antianxiety medication, whereas genetic knockout mice lacking 5-HT$_{1A}$ receptors exhibit increased anxiety in behavioral tests such as the elevated zero-maze (similar to the elevated plus-maze discussed in Chapter 4) (Figure 6.20; Heisler et al., 1998). Yet another potential use of 5-HT$_{1A}$ receptor agonists is in the area of substance abuse. There are genetic strains of rats that voluntarily consume significant amounts of alcohol. Administration of a 5-HT$_{1A}$ agonist inhibits this alcohol consumption, which raises the possibility that such compounds might provide some therapeutic benefit in the treatment of

(A)

(B)

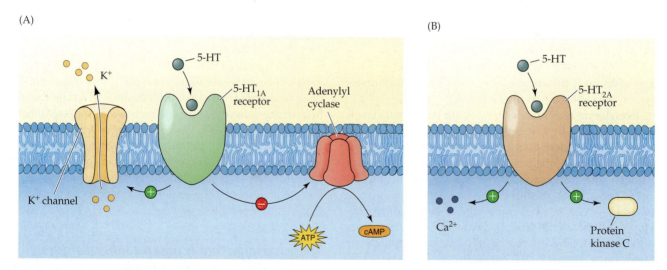

Figure 6.19 5-HT$_{1A}$ and 5-HT$_{2A}$ receptors operate through different signaling mechanisms. 5-HT$_{1A}$ receptors inhibit cAMP production and activate K$^+$ channel opening (A), whereas 5-HT$_{2A}$ receptors increase intracellular Ca^{2+} levels and stimulate protein kinase C via the phosphoinositide second-messenger system (B). For purposes of simplification, the G proteins required for coupling the receptors to their signaling pathways are not shown.

(A)   (B)

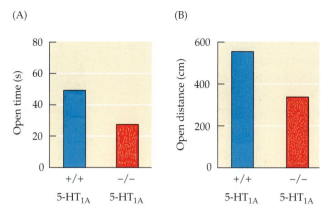

Figure 6.20 Genetic deletion of the 5-HT$_{1A}$ receptor increases anxiety-like behavior in the elevated zero-maze. Wild-type (5-HT$_{1A}$$^{+/+}$) and 5-HT$_{1A}$ knockout (5-HT$_{1A}$$^{-/-}$) mice were tested in the elevated zero-maze, which is a circular apparatus with open and closed areas like the elevated plus-maze. Compared to wild-type mice, the knockout animals showed increased anxiety, as indicated by less time spent (A) and less distance traveled (B) in the open areas of the maze. (After Heisler et al., 1998.)

alcoholism. Finally, 5-HT$_{1A}$ receptor agonists cause a modest amount of **hypothermia,** which is a lowering of body temperature. Together, these findings indicate that 5-HT, acting in some cases through the 5-HT$_{1A}$ receptor subtype, is involved in the regulation of eating behavior, anxiety, temperature regulation, and the motivation to consume alcohol.

5-HT$_{2A}$ receptors   Large numbers of 5-HT$_{2A}$ receptors are present in the cerebral cortex. This receptor subtype is also found in the striatum, nucleus accumbens, and a variety of other brain areas. Similar to some types of muscarinic receptors as well as to α_1-adrenergic receptors, 5-HT$_{2A}$ receptors function mainly by activating the phosphoinositide second-messenger system (Figure 6.19B). You will recall that this system increases Ca^{2+} levels within the postsynaptic cell and also activates protein kinase C (PKC). Thus our discussion of different neurotransmitters and their receptor subtypes has shown common mechanisms of transmitter action occurring over and over again. These mechanisms may involve a second messenger like cAMP or Ca^{2+}, or some type of ion channel such as K$^+$ channels, which are opened by a wide variety of receptors.

The best-known 5-HT$_{2A}$ receptor agonist is **1-(2,5-dimethoxy-4-iodophenyl)-2-aminopropane (DOI),** whereas **ketanserin** and **ritanserin** are widely used 5-HT$_{2A}$ antagonists. Giving rats or mice DOI or another 5-HT$_{2A}$ agonist leads to a characteristic "head-twitch" response (periodic, brief twitches of the head) that is a useful measure of 5-HT$_{2A}$ receptor stimulation in these species. More interesting is the fact that DOI and related drugs are **hallucinogenic** (hallucination-producing) in humans. Indeed, the hallucinogenic effects of **lysergic acid diethylamide (LSD)** are also believed to stem from its ability to stimulate 5-HT$_{2A}$ receptors. LSD and other hallucinogens are discussed in greater detail in Chapter 14.

In the past several years, blockade of 5-HT$_{2A}$ receptors has become a major topic of discussion and research with respect to the treatment of schizophrenia. As mentioned in the previous chapter, traditional antischizophrenic drugs that work by blocking D$_2$ dopamine receptors often produce serious movement-related side effects, some of which can even resemble Parkinson's disease. Such side effects are much less severe, however, with newer drugs such as **clozapine (Clozaril)** and **risperidone (Risperdal).** Clozapine and risperidone both block 5-HT$_{2A}$ receptors in addition to their effects on the dopamine system. This has led to the hypothesis that a combination of D$_2$ and 5-HT$_{2A}$ receptor antagonism is desirable for symptom improvement in schizophrenic patients while minimizing the side effects associated with previous antischizophrenic drugs that don't affect the 5-HT$_{2A}$ receptor (see Chapter 18).

Section Summary

Most of the serotonergic neurons in the CNS are associated with the raphe nuclei of the brain stem. Together, the dorsal and median raphe send 5-HT-containing fibers to virtually all forebrain areas. Studies on cats by Jacobs and his colleagues showed that serotonergic neurons in the dorsal raphe fire most rapidly when the animal is awake and active, particularly when it is engaged in some kind of rhythmic behavior. These cells are silent either when the cat is in REM sleep or when it is paying attention to a sensory stimulus. These findings led to the hypothesis that one function of 5-HT is to facilitate the output of motor systems while simultaneously inhibiting sensory processing.

At least 15 different 5-HT receptor subtypes have been identified. Some of these fall within groups, such as the 5-HT$_1$ and 5-HT$_2$ receptor families. All of the 5-HT receptors are metabotropic, except for the 5-HT$_3$ receptor, which is an excitatory ionotropic receptor.

Two of the best-characterized 5-HT receptor subtypes are the 5-HT$_{1A}$ and 5-HT$_{2A}$ receptors. High levels of 5-HT$_{1A}$ receptors have been found in the hippocampus, the septum, parts of the amygdala, and the dorsal raphe nucleus. In the raphe nuclei, including the dorsal raphe, these receptors are mainly somatodendritic autoreceptors on the serotonergic neurons themselves. In other brain areas, 5-HT$_{1A}$ receptors are found on postsynaptic neurons that receive a serotonergic input. 5-HT$_{1A}$ receptors function by inhibiting cAMP formation and by enhancing the opening of K$^+$ channels in the cell membrane. Administering a 5-HT$_{1A}$ agonist drug causes a number of behavioral and physiological effects,

TABLE 6.2 Drugs That Affect the Serotonergic System

Drug	Action
para-Chlorophenylalanine	Depletes 5-HT by inhibiting tryptophan hydroxylase
Reserpine	Depletes 5-HT by inhibiting vesicular uptake
para-Chloroamphetamine, fenfluramine, and MDMA	Release 5-HT from nerve terminals (MDMA and *para*-chloroamphetamine also have neurotoxic effects)
Fluoxetine	Inhibits 5-HT reuptake
5,7-Dihydroxytryptamine	5-HT neurotoxin
Buspirone, ipsapirone, and 8-OH-DPAT	Stimulate 5-HT$_{1A}$ receptors (agonists)
WAY 100635	Blocks 5-HT$_{1A}$ receptors (antagonist)
DOI	Stimulates 5-HT$_{2A}$ receptors (agonist)
Ketanserin and ritanserin	Block 5-HT$_{2A}$ receptors (antagonists)

including hyperphagia, reduced anxiety, decreased alcohol consumption in rats, and hypothermia.

5-HT$_{2A}$ receptors are present in the neocortex, striatum, nucleus accumbens, and other brain regions. This receptor subtype activates the phosphoinositide second-messenger system, which increases the amount of free Ca^{2+} within the cell. When given to rodents, 5-HT$_{2A}$ receptor agonists trigger a head-twitch response. In humans, such drugs (which include LSD) produce hallucinations. Certain drugs used in the treatment of schizophrenia can block 5-HT$_{2A}$ receptors, and some researchers hypothesize that such blockade may reduce certain harmful side effects usually associated with antischizophrenic medications. Table 6.2 lists some of the major drugs that influence serotonergic transmission, including 5-HT$_{1A}$ and 5-HT$_{2A}$ receptor agonists and antagonists.

Recommended Readings

Bell, C., Abrams, J., and Nutt, D. (2001). Tryptophan depletion and its implications for psychiatry. *Br. J. Psychiatry*, 178, 399–405.

Gingrich, J. A., and Hen, R. (2001). Dissecting the role of the serotonin system in neuropsychiatric disorders using knockout mice. *Psychopharmacology*, 155, 1–10.

Wess, J. (2003). Novel insights into muscarinic acetylcholine receptor function using gene targeting technology. *Trends Pharmacol. Sci.*, 24, 414–420.

7 *Glutamate and GABA*

*I*n 1966, Daniel Keyes published a science fiction novel entitled *Flowers for Algernon,* in which an experimental brain operation turns a mentally retarded young man into a genius. The book spawned an Oscar-winning movie adaptation called *Charly,* starring Cliff Robertson as the protagonist. Tragically, Charly's intellectual ascent was only temporary, and in any case, most people probably wouldn't want to endure brain surgery to increase their IQ. On the other hand, the possibility of a "smart pill" would be appealing to many. An informal survey conducted by Marilyn vos Savant (author of the "Ask Marilyn" column in the popular Sunday newspaper magazine *Parade*) found that if given a choice, a large majority of respondents would prefer raising their intelligence to improving their physical appearance. Likewise, most students would probably appreciate an easy way to improve their learning skills, perhaps enabling them to "ace" all their courses without too much difficulty.

Although no genius pills are yet in sight, researchers actually have been hard at work to find drugs that improve cognitive function. Some cognitive-enhancing compounds, which are called nootropics,* act on the cholinergic system (see Chapter 6). Others influence the amino acid neurotransmitter glutamate, which is the subject of the first part of the present chapter. The effects of nootropic drugs have thus far been relatively modest. However, a group of investigators headed by Joe Tsien at Princeton University made a big splash in September 1999, when they published an exciting paper showing that a genetic modification involving one of the receptors for glutamate could

The *Doogie* mouse, a genetically engineered strain that exhibits enhanced learning and memory.

enhance learning and long-term memory in mice (Tang et al., 1999). Tsien and his colleagues called their genetically engineered mouse the *Doogie* mouse, after the former TV show *Doogie Howser, M.D.,* which featured a boy genius who became a doctor at a young age. We will learn more about the *Doogie* mouse and the role of glutamate in learning and memory later in this chapter. The second part of the chapter covers γ-aminobutyric acid (GABA), another important amino acid neurotransmitter.

Glutamate

Glutamate is the term we use for the ionized (i.e., electrically charged) form of the amino acid glutamic acid. Since most of the glutamic acid in our bodies is in this ionized state, we will refer to it as glutamate throughout the text. Like other common amino acids, glutamate is used by all of our cells to help make new proteins. But glutamate also has numerous other biochemical functions (for example, in energy metabolism), which is reflected in the fact that it is the most abundant amino acid in the brain. Glutamate and **aspartate** (the name for the ionized form of aspartic acid) are the two principal members of a small family of **excitatory amino acid neurotransmitters.** These transmitters are so named because they cause a powerful excitatory response when applied to most neurons in the brain or spinal cord. We will focus on glutamate, which seems to be the more widely used excitatory amino acid transmitter and which has been more intensively studied than aspartate.

Glutamate Synthesis, Release, and Inactivation

Neurons generate glutamate from the precursor glutamine

When a nerve cell synthesizes a molecule of norepinephrine (NE), acetylcholine (ACh), or serotonin (5-HT), it is almost always for the purpose of neurotransmission. Moreover, in the brain these substances are localized specifically within the cells using them as transmitters. However, we must recognize that the situation is different for glutamate due to its roles in protein synthesis and general cellular metabolism. First, all neurons and glial cells contain significant amounts of glutamate, although neurons that use glutamate as a transmitter (called **glutamatergic neurons**) possess even greater concentrations than other cells in the brain. Second, glutamatergic neurons are thought to segregate the pool of glutamate they use for transmission from the pool of glutamate used

---

*The term *nootropic* comes from two Greek words: *noos,* which means "mind," and *tropein,* which means "toward."

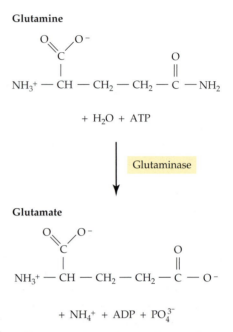

Figure 7.1 Glutamate is synthesized from glutamine by the enzyme glutaminase. This reaction requires energy provided by the breakdown of adenosine triphosphate (ATP) into adenosine diphosphate (ADP) and phosphate (PO_4^{3-}).

for other cellular functions. These facts complicate both our ability to determine which nerve cells actually are glutamatergic and our understanding of how these cells synthesize and dispose of the transmitter-related glutamate. Nevertheless, researchers have accumulated considerable information, which we summarize in this section.

Glutamate can be synthesized by several different chemical reactions. Most molecules of glutamate are derived ultimately from the normal metabolic breakdown of the sugar glucose. The more immediate precursor for much of the transmitter-related glutamate is a related substance known as **glutamine.** Neurons can transform glutamine into glutamate using an enzyme called **glutaminase** (Figure 7.1). We will see in the next section that the role of glutamine in glutamate synthesis involves a fascinating metabolic partnership between glutamatergic neurons and neighboring glial cells, specifically astrocytes.

Glutamate is released from vesicles and removed from the synaptic cleft by both neuronal and glial transport systems

For a long time, no one knew how glutamate got into synaptic vesicles for the purpose of storage and release. Then between the years 2000 and 2002, researchers discovered *three* distinct proteins that package glutamate into vesicles: **VGLUT1, VGLUT2,** and **VGLUT3** (**VGLUT** standing for vesicular glutamate transporter). These proteins provide good markers for glutamatergic neurons, because unlike glutamate itself, they are found only in cells that use glutamate as a neurotransmitter. Glutamatergic neurons generally possess either VGLUT1 or VGLUT2 (but not both), with VGLUT3 being less abundant than the other two transporters. As illustrated in Figure 7.2A and B, mRNAs for the *VGLUT1* and *VGLUT2* genes show very little overlap across different brain regions, confirming that the glutamatergic neurons in most regions manufacture only one VGLUT. What difference does it make which vesicular glutamate transporter is expressed by a particular nerve cell? This question is being investigated, but we don't yet have a clear answer.

After glutamate molecules are released into the synaptic cleft, they are rapidly removed by other glutamate transporters located on cell membranes. Always keep in mind that the plasma membrane transporters that remove neurotransmitters from the synaptic cleft are distinct from the transporters on the vesicle membranes that are responsible for loading the vesicles in preparation for transmitter release. In the case of glutamate, five different plasma membrane transporters have already been identified. Because these transporters take up aspartate as well as glutamate, they are called **EAAT1–EAAT5** (**EAAT** standing for **excitatory amino acid transporter**). Two of these transporters, EAAT1 and EAAT2, are located mainly on astrocytes instead of neurons. Of the neuronal transporters, EAAT3 is the most widely distributed in the brain. As we will see later, prolonged high levels of glutamate in the extracellular fluid are very dangerous, produc-

ing excessive neuronal excitation and even cell death. With this in mind, it is interesting to discover that uptake by astrocytes seems to be particularly important in controlling the amount of extracellular glutamate. For example, there is evidence that more than half of patients with **amyotrophic lateral sclerosis** (**ALS**; also known as Lou Gehrig's disease), a neurological disorder involving degeneration of motor neurons in the spinal cord and cortex, have abnormalities in EAAT2 in the affected areas of their nervous systems (Lin et al., 1998). In rats, inhibition of EAAT1 or EAAT2 synthesis led to large increases in extracellular glutamate levels in the striatum, indicating that these transporters are the most important ones for normal glutamate uptake in this brain area (Rothstein et al., 1996). Furthermore, there were signs of neural degeneration in the striatum in the treated animals, and all of the animals exhibited progressive motor deficits. In contrast, inhibition of the neuronal glutamate transporter EAAT3 was much less effective in producing either neural degeneration or behavioral symptoms.

Besides playing a key role in removing excess glutamate from the extracellular space, the astrocyte transporters are also intimately involved in the metabolic partnership between neurons and astrocytes. After astrocytes have taken up glutamate by means of EAAT1 or EAAT2, they convert a major portion of it to glutamine by means of an enzyme called **glutamine synthetase.** The glutamine is then transported out of the astrocytes and picked up by neurons, where it can be converted back into glutamate by glutaminase, as described earlier. This interplay between glutamatergic neu-

(A)   Inferior colliculus   Thalamus

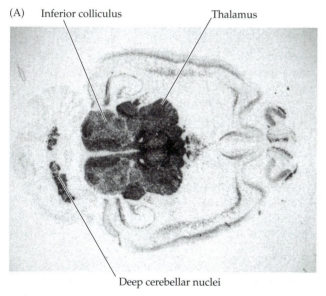

Deep cerebellar nuclei

(B)   Cerebellar cortex Hippocampus   Cortex

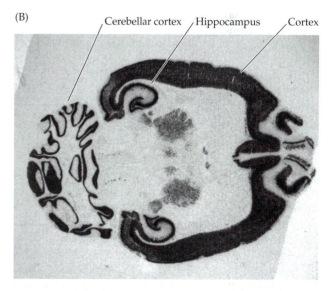

Figure 7.2 Distribution of VGLUTs in the brain Horizontal sections through rat brain showing the regional distribution of mRNAs for *VGLUT2* (A) and *VGLUT1* (B). Most brain regions express one of the transporters much more strongly than the other. (Images courtesy of Robert Edwards.)

Figure 7.3 Cycling of glutamate and glutamine between glutamatergic neurons and astrocytes After neurons release glutamate, it can be transported back into the nerve terminal by EAAT3 or transported into nearby astrocytes by EAAT1 or EAAT2. Inside the astrocyte, glutamate is converted into glutamine by the enzyme glutamine synthetase. The glutamine can be later released by the astrocytes, taken up by neurons, and converted back into glutamate by the enzyme glutaminase.

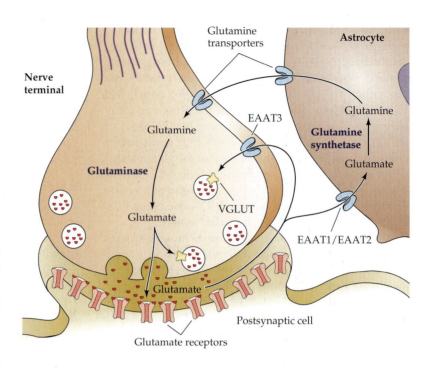

rons and neighboring astrocytes is illustrated in Figure 7.3. It is reasonable to wonder why such a complex system has evolved; why don't the neurons themselves have the primary responsibility for glutamate reuptake, as we have seen previously for the catecholamine neurotransmitters and for serotonin? Although we aren't certain about the answer to this question, it's worth noting that glutamine does not produce neuronal excitation and therefore is not potentially dangerous like glutamate. Hence, glial cell production of glutamine may be the brain's way of storing glutamate in a form that is "safe" but still available for use once the glutamine has been transferred to the neurons and reconverted to glutamate.

Section Summary

Glutamate and aspartate are amino acid neurotransmitters that have potent excitatory effects on neurons throughout the brain and spinal cord. Although glutamate is contained within all cells due to its multiple biochemical functions, glutamatergic neurons are thought to possess higher glutamate concentrations than other cells and to segregate their neurotransmitter pool of this amino acid. Many of the glutamate molecules that are released synaptically are synthesized from glutamine in a chemical reaction catalyzed by the enzyme glutaminase.

Glutamate is packaged into vesicles by the vesicular transporters VGLUT1, VGLUT2, and VGLUT3. After being released, glutamate molecules are removed from the extracellular space by several different excitatory amino acid transporters, designated EAAT1–EAAT5. EAAT1 and EAAT2 mediate glutamate uptake into astrocytes, after which some of the glutamate is converted into glutamine. This glutamine can subsequently be transported from the astrocytes to the glutamatergic neurons, where it is transformed back into glutamate and reutilized. This constitutes an important metabolic interplay between glutamatergic nerve cells and

their neighboring glial cells. The importance of EAAT2, in particular, is exemplified in recent findings that many patients suffering from the neurological disorder ALS seem to have abnormalities in this transporter.

Organization and Function of the Glutamatergic System

Glutamate is the neurotransmitter used in many excitatory pathways in the brain

Glutamate is considered to be the workhorse transmitter for fast excitatory signaling in the nervous system. Not only is it used in many excitatory neuronal pathways, but the most important receptors for glutamate are ionotropic receptors that produce fast postsynaptic responses (see the next section). We will not discuss a large number of glutamatergic pathways here, but simply mention a few that have been extensively studied. In the cerebral cortex, glutamate is the main neurotransmitter used by the pyramidal neurons. These cells, which are named on the basis of their pyramid-like shape, are the major output neurons of the cortex. Their axons project to numerous subcortical structures, including the striatum, the thalamus, various limbic system structures, and regions of the brain stem. Glutamate is also used in the numerous parallel fibers of the cerebellar cortex and in several excitatory pathways within the hippocampus.

Because glutamate is found throughout the brain, it is more difficult to assign specific functional roles to this neurotransmitter than it is for some of the other transmitters covered previously. Glutamate is undoubtedly involved in many different behavioral and physiological functions, but among the most important are synaptic plasticity (that is, changes in the strength of synaptic connections), learning, and memory. We discuss the role of glutamate in these processes in greater detail later.

Both ionotropic and metabotropic receptors mediate the synaptic effects of glutamate

Glutamate receptors are divided into two broad families: a group of ionotropic receptors for fast signaling and a group of slower metabotropic receptors that function by means of second-messenger systems. We will focus on the ionotropic receptors, since those are most important for understanding the mechanisms of glutamate action in the brain. Note that glutamate receptors are also used by aspartate and possibly by other excitatory amino acid transmitters that may exist. Hence, these receptors are sometimes called excitatory amino acid receptors rather than simply glutamate receptors.

Ionotropic glutamate receptors   There are three subtypes of ionotropic glutamate receptors. Each is named for a relatively selective agonist for that receptor subtype. First is the **AMPA receptor,** which is named for the selective agonist AMPA (α-amino-3-hydroxy-5-methyl-4-isoxazole proprionic acid), a synthetic (not naturally occurring) amino acid analog. Most fast excitatory responses to glutamate are mediated by stimulation of AMPA receptors. The second ionotropic receptor subtype is the **kainate receptor,** which is named for the selective agonist kainic acid. Even though kainic acid powerfully stimulates kainate receptors in the mammalian brain, this substance actually comes from a type of seaweed called *Digenea simplex*. The third ionotropic glutamate receptor is the **NMDA receptor,** the agonist of which is obviously NMDA (*N*-methyl-D-aspartate). Like AMPA, NMDA is a synthetic amino acid. Thus, we see that pharmacologists have had to take advantage of several unusual compounds (either man-made or plant-derived) to distinguish between the different ionotropic receptor subtypes, since glutamate itself obviously must activate all of these receptors.

Like the nicotinic receptors discussed in the previous chapter, ionotropic glutamate receptors depolarize the membrane of the postsynaptic cell, which leads to an excitatory response. For the AMPA and kainate receptors, this depolarizing effect is produced mainly by the flow of sodium (Na^+) ions into the cell through the receptor channel. In the case of NMDA receptors, the channel conducts not only Na^+ but also significant amounts of calcium (Ca^{2+}). Since Ca^{2+} can function as a second messenger in the postsynaptic cell (see Chapter 3), this is an interesting case where an ionotropic receptor (the NMDA receptor) directly activates a second-messenger system (Figure 7.4).

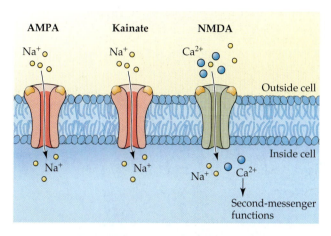

Figure 7.4   All ionotropic glutamate receptor channels conduct Na⁺ ions into the cell but NMDA receptor channels also conduct Ca^{2+} ions. Once inside the cell, Ca^{2+} can activate a number of important second-messenger functions.

Going back to the nicotinic receptor again, recall that the complete receptor contains five separate proteins (subunits) that come together in the membrane to form the receptor channel. Ionotropic glutamate receptors are also formed from multiple subunits, but the subunits are different for each receptor subtype (AMPA, kainate, and NMDA). Not surprisingly, this is why the three subtypes differ in their pharmacology. Not only does each subtype have its own selective agonist, but various receptor antagonists have also been developed that have helped us understand the behavioral and physiological functions of these receptors.

One widely used antagonist called **NBQX** (6-nitro-7-sulfamoyl-benzo(f)-quinoxaline-2,3-dione) can block both AMPA and kainate receptors, although it is somewhat more effective against the former subtype. The compound has no effect on NMDA receptors. Rats or mice treated with high doses of NBQX exhibit sedation, reduced locomotor activity and ataxia (impaired coordination in movement; an example in humans is staggering), poor performance in the rotarod task (another test of coordination), and protection against electrically or chemically induced seizures. These findings indicate a broad role for AMPA (and possibly also kainate) receptors in locomotor activity, coordination, and brain excitability (as shown by the seizure results).

NMDA receptors possess a number of characteristics not found in the other glutamate ionotropic receptors (Figure 7.5). First, we've already mentioned that unlike AMPA and kainate receptor channels, the channels for NMDA receptors allow Ca^{2+} ions to flow into the postsynaptic cell, thus triggering Ca^{2+}-dependent second-messenger activities. Second, NMDA receptors are very unusual in that there are actually two different neurotransmitters required to stimulate the

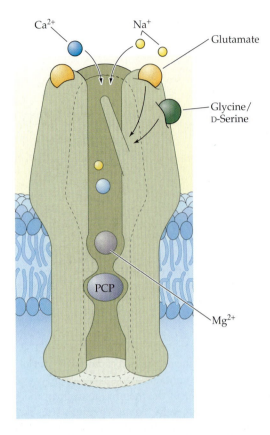

Figure 7.5 NMDA receptor properties The NMDA receptor is activated by simultaneous binding of glutamate and a co-agonist, either glycine or D-serine. The receptor channel can be blocked by Mg^{2+} ions under resting conditions and also by the presence of the abused drug phencyclidine (PCP).

receptor and open its ion channel. The first neurotransmitter, of course, is glutamate. But in addition to the binding site for glutamate on the NMDA receptor complex, there is also a binding site that recognizes the amino acid **glycine.** The importance of this is that if the glycine binding site isn't occupied at the same time as the glutamate binding site, the NMDA receptor channel remains closed. If that wasn't complicated enough, it appears that another amino acid, **D-serine,** may be more important than glycine for interacting with the second binding site. In any case, either glycine or D-serine is considered to be a **co-agonist** with glutamate at the NMDA receptor, since one or the other of these substances is just as necessary as glutamate for receptor activation. However, because the co-agonist binding site is thought to be occupied under most conditions, the presence or absence of glutamate is the more important factor in determining channel opening.

There are two additional binding sites on the NMDA receptor that affect its function. One is a site within the receptor channel that binds magnesium (Mg^{2+}) ions. When the cell membrane is at the resting potential (typically –60 or –70

mV), Mg^{2+} ions are bound to this site relatively tightly. This causes the receptor channel to be blocked, even if glutamate and glycine or D-serine are present to activate the receptor. However, if the membrane becomes depolarized, then the Mg^{2+} ions dissociate from the receptor and permit the channel to open if glutamate and glycine or D-serine are present. Consider the implications of this property of NMDA receptors. How does the membrane become depolarized? The answer, of course, is that some other source of excitation (other than through NMDA receptors) must have already activated the cell. This other source of excitation could have been either glutamate acting through AMPA (or potentially kainate) receptors, or a different transmitter such as acetylcholine acting through nicotinic receptors. The point is that an NMDA receptor is a kind of biological "coincidence detector." That is, the channel only opens when two events occur close together in time: (1) glutamate is released onto the NMDA receptor, and (2) the cell membrane is depolarized by stimulation of a different excitatory receptor (Figure 7.6).

The second site, which is also located within the receptor channel, recognizes the abused drugs **phencyclidine (PCP)**

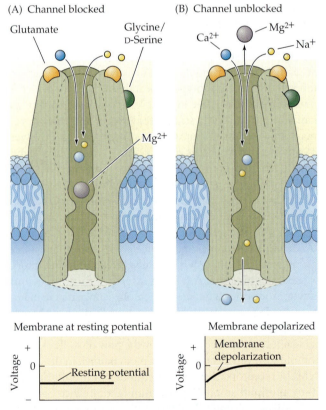

Figure 7.6 Role of the membrane potential in NMDA receptor activation Even in the presence of agonist binding, NMDA receptor channels cannot open unless the cell membrane is depolarized, thereby removing the Mg^{2+} block.

and **ketamine,** as well as **MK-801 (dizocilpine),** which is a compound more commonly used for research purposes. When any of these drugs binds to the PCP site, it blocks the channel and thus prevents ion flow. Because these compounds do not interfere with the ability of glutamate to bind to its site on the receptor, they are noncompetitive rather than competitive antagonists of the NMDA receptor. As will be discussed further in Chapter 14, most of the behavioral effects of PCP and ketamine are due to NMDA receptor antagonism.

Metabotropic glutamate receptors   Besides the three ionotropic receptors, there are also eight different metabotropic glutamate receptors. They are designated **mGluR1–mGluR8.** Through their coupling to G proteins, some of these receptors inhibit cyclic adenosine monophosphate (cAMP) formation, whereas others activate the phosphoinositide second-messenger system. Finally, certain metabotropic glutamate receptors are located on nerve terminals, where they act as presynaptic autoreceptors to inhibit glutamate release. The novel amino acid L-**AP4** (L-**2-amino-4-phosphonobutyrate)** is a selective agonist at these glutamate autoreceptors, thereby suppressing glutamatergic synaptic transmission.

We previously saw that functioning AMPA receptors are necessary for normal locomotor activity, motor coordination, and learning. The same is also true for at least some of the metabotropic glutamate receptors, such as mGluR1. Mutant mice in which the *mGluR1* receptor gene has been inactivated show reduced locomotion, an ataxic gait, poor coordination, and deficits in several kinds of learning tasks (Aiba et al., 1994a; Aiba et al., 1994b; Conquet et al., 1994). Moreover, one study found that restoration of the *mGluR1* gene *just* in the Purkinje cells of the cerebellum (these are the major output neurons of the cerebellar cortex) reinstated normal locomotion and motor coordination in the mice (learning was not tested in this study) (Ichise et al., 2000; Figure 7.7). From this intriguing result, the authors concluded that the mGluR1 receptor in Purkinje cells is required for the normal cerebellar regulation of motor function. Various metabotropic glutamate receptors also participate in many other behavioral and physiological functions, including pain perception, anxiety, and the regulation of brain excitability.

NMDA receptors play a key role in learning and memory

Earlier, we mentioned that NMDA receptors are thought to play an important role in learning and memory, and the coincidence detection feature of the NMDA receptor is one possible aspect of this role. Many forms of learning are associative, meaning that they involve the pairing of two events, such as two different stimuli or a stimulus and a response.

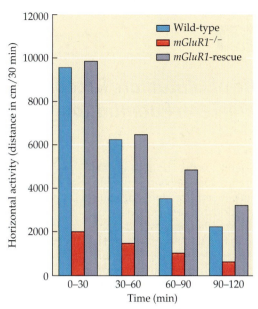

Figure 7.7 Role of *mGluR1* in locomotor activity Genetically normal (wild-type) mice, *mGluR1* knockout mice (*mGluR1⁻/⁻*), and mice in which the *mGluR1* gene was restored just in cerebellar Purkinje cells (*mGluR1*-rescue) were tested for horizontal activity over a 120-minute period in an open field. Activity in the wild-type mice was high during the first 30-minute time block and then gradually decreased as the animals habituated to the novel environment. The *mGluR1* knockout mice showed low levels of activity throughout the test session, whereas rescue of the *mGluR1* gene in cerebellar Purkinje cells completely restored the normal activity pattern. (From Ichise et al., 2000.)

One kind of simple associative learning is classical conditioning, as exemplified by Pavlov's original experiment with dogs. Like the opening of an NMDA receptor channel, classical conditioning is based on the close timing of two events: the pairing of a conditioned stimulus (the bell in Pavlov's experiment) with an unconditioned stimulus (the meat powder). You can see that the NMDA receptor represents a biochemical mechanism that could be involved not only in classical conditioning but in other forms of associative learning.

There are other, more direct lines of evidence linking NMDA receptors with learning. First, a number of studies have found that treatment with NMDA receptor antagonists leads to impaired acquisition of various tasks, especially those involving spatial learning. This makes sense in light of the fact that the hippocampus, a brain area that is necessary for spatial learning, contains a high density of NMDA receptors. Second, NMDA receptors are critically involved in an important type of synaptic plasticity known as **long-term potentiation (LTP)** (Box 7.1). Many investigators believe that LTP could underlie various kinds of learning, particularly those mediated by the hippocampus.

The Cutting Edge

Role of Glutamate Receptors in Long-Term Potentiation

Long-term potentiation (LTP) refers to a persistent (at least 1 hour) increase in synaptic strength produced by a burst of activity in the presynaptic neuron. This burst of firing is produced experimentally by a single brief train of electrical stimuli (for example, 100 stimuli over a period of 1 second) that is sometimes called a **tetanic stimulus** (or simply a **tetanus**). The synaptic enhancement produced by the tetanus is measured by changes in the excitatory postsynaptic potential (EPSP) recorded in the postsynaptic cell.

Although LTP occurs in many brain areas, it was first discovered in the hippocampus and has been studied most extensively in that structure. The hippocampus from a rat or mouse is cut into slices around 200 μm (0.2 mm) in thickness. These slices are then placed in a dish where the neurons can be maintained in a healthy state for many hours while the investigator stimulates them and records their electrophysiological responses. The important cellular anatomy of a hippocampal slice is illustrated in Figure A. Without going into great detail, it is sufficient to know that all of the pathways shown in the diagram use glutamate as their transmitter and that LTP occurs at all of the synaptic connections depicted. However, the majority of LTP studies have focused on the pyramidal neurons of the CA1 region of the hippocampus, which receive excitatory glutamatergic inputs from the CA3 neurons via the Schaffer collaterals.

Figure B depicts what happens to a typical synapse on a CA1 pyramidal neuron before, during, and after the tetanic stimulus. A test pulse (single electrical stimulation) of the presynaptic cell is used to assess the

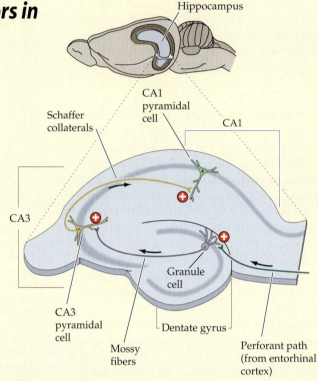

(A) Long-term potentiation of synaptic transmission can be studied in vitro using the hippocampal slice preparation.

strength of the synaptic connection. The test pulse elicits the release of a small amount of glutamate from the presynaptic nerve endings. As shown in the left panel, this glutamate binds to both AMPA and NMDA receptors in the postsynaptic membrane. There is a small EPSP that is produced mainly by the AMPA receptors. However, the NMDA receptor channels fail to open because the membrane is not depolarized sufficiently to release the Mg^{2+} block of those channels. As long as the test pulses are separated in time, you can give many of these pulses and not see any enhancement of the EPSP. But look at what happens in response to a tetanic stimulus (middle panel). Much more glutamate is released, which causes a prolonged activation of the AMPA receptors and

a greater postsynaptic depolarization. This permits Mg^{2+} ions to dissociate from the NMDA receptor channels and Ca^{2+} ions to enter the cell through these channels. Acting as a second messenger, these Ca^{2+} ions alter the functioning of the postsynaptic cell so that the same test pulse given before now produces an enhanced EPSP (right panel).

LTP can be divided into two phases: an **induction phase,** which takes place during and immediately after the tetanic stimulation, and an **expression phase,** which represents the enhanced synaptic strength measured at a later time. NMDA receptors play a critical role in the induction phase but not the expression phase. We know this because application of an NMDA receptor

BOX 7.1 (continued)

Single stimulus

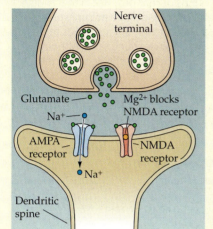

Tetanus

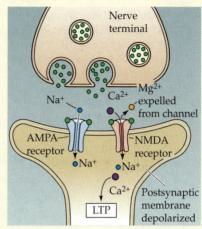

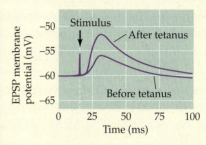

(B) Long-term potentiation is induced by a tetanic stimulation of the presynaptic input.

antagonist to the hippocampal slice during the tetanus blocks induction, but the same drug applied during the test pulse does not prevent the enhanced EPSP. In contrast, AMPA receptors are necessary for LTP expression, since it is an AMPA receptor–mediated EPSP that is facilitated in LTP.

The biochemical mechanisms thought to underlie LTP are illustrated in Figure C. The influx of Ca^{2+} ions through the NMDA receptor channels activates several protein kinases, including one type of calcium/calmodulin protein kinase called CaMKII (see Chapter 3). CaMKII and the other kinases phosphorylate the AMPA receptors, which has two consequences. First, the sensitivity of the receptors to glutamate is enhanced. Second, more AMPA receptors are inserted into the postsynaptic membrane. Both of these mechanisms enhance the strength of signaling at potentiated synapses. The tetanic stimulation that gives rise to LTP may

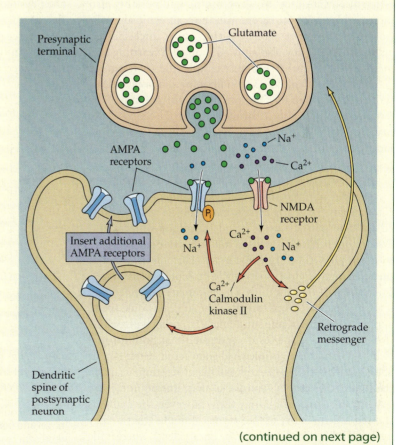

(C) The mechanism underlying LTP involves modification of AMPA receptors in the postsynaptic cell.

(continued on next page)

The third line of evidence brings us back to the *Doogie* mouse mentioned at the beginning of this chapter. Unlike the knockout mice that we have discussed in previous chapters, this strain of mouse was genetically engineered to *overexpress* one of the subunits of the NMDA receptor, namely the NR2B subunit (Tang et al., 1999). This resulted in more-efficient NMDA receptor functioning and possibly also increased levels of the receptor in the transgenic animals. Compared to normal controls, the *Doogie* mice showed enhanced LTP. They also showed improved learning and memory on several tasks. For example, the *Doogie* mice demonstrated enhanced fear conditioning and faster extinction of the learned fear response than normal mice. The transgenic animals also performed better in the Morris water maze, which is a spatial navigation task (see Chapter 4). Finally, the subjects were tested in a novel-object-recognition task in which they were initially allowed to explore two objects for a period of 5 minutes (see chapter opening photo for examples of objects used in this task). After an interval of 1 hour, 1 day, 3 days, or 1 week, a novel object was substituted for one of the two original (familiar) objects and exploratory behavior was again tested. Because subjects tend to spend more time exploring unfamiliar objects, recall of the remaining original object would be demonstrated by less exploration of that stimulus. The researchers expected that if the original object was forgotten, the subjects would spend approximately equal amounts of time exploring both objects in the recall test. The results indicated that both normal (wild-type) and *Doogie* mice had good recall at the 1-hour test, because both groups explored the novel stimulus much more than the original stimulus at that time point (Figure 7.8). At the 1-day and 3-day tests, however, the controls showed little memory of the original stimulus (that is, they explored both stimuli to about the same extent), whereas the transgenic mice continued to show a clear preference for the

novel object. At the 1-week recall interval, neither group of mice remembered the original stimulus. Thus enhancement of NMDA receptor function produced a significant improvement of long-term memory, although this improvement was gone by 1 week after the initial stimulus exposure.

Genetic manipulations often produce multiple behavioral and physiological effects, some of which may be undesirable. Indeed, that is what was later found for the *Doogie* mouse. NMDA receptors are involved in many functions besides learning and memory, one of which is pain perception. As a result, overexpression of the NR2B receptor subunit in the

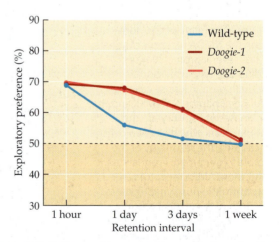

Figure 7.8 Enhanced memory shown by *Doogie* mice in the novel-object-recognition task The graph illustrates exploratory preference for the novel object measured as a percentage of the total exploration time that was spent exploring the novel object (a 50% score indicates equal exploration of the novel and familiar objects). Note that *Doogie-1* and *Doogie-2* represent two different strains of transgenic mice, which behaved similarly on this task. (From Tang et al., 1999.)

Doogie mouse caused the animals to have increased sensitivity to inflammation-related pain (Wei et al., 2001). Perhaps we should heed the tragic lesson of Charly in the book *Flowers for Algernon,* that altering the brain may carry risks in addition to the potential benefits.

High levels of glutamate can be toxic to nerve cells

Despite the vital role of glutamate in normal neural and behavioral functioning, there is also a dark side to this neurotransmitter system. More than 40 years ago, two researchers published a report showing retinal damage in mice following subcutaneous injection of the sodium salt of glutamic acid, monosodium glutamate (MSG) (Lucas and Newhouse, 1957). Furthermore, this toxic effect of glutamate was more severe in infant than in adult mice. Twelve years later, Olney (1969) presented the first evidence that MSG also produces brain damage in young mice. As shown in Figure 7.9A and B, one of the injured areas was a part of the hypothalamus known as the arcuate nucleus. The arcuate nucleus plays an important role in controlling the endocrine system. Consequently, MSG-induced damage to this structure produced devastating effects as the animals matured, including stunted skeletal growth, extreme obesity, and reproductive abnormalities, particularly in the female subjects.

Subsequent research showed that glutamate could lesion any brain area of adult animals when injected directly into that structure. This effect was shared by other excitatory amino acids, including kainate and NMDA, and the damage was shown to occur at postsynaptic sites but not at nerve terminals. These and other findings led to the **excitotoxicity hypothesis,** which proposed that the effects produced by

excessive exposure to glutamate and related excitatory amino acids are caused by a prolonged depolarization of receptive neurons that in some way leads to their eventual damage or death. Administration of an excitatory amino acid kills nerve cells but spares fibers of passage (that is, axons from distant cells that are merely passing through the lesioned area). Thus excitotoxic lesions are more selective than lesions produced by passing electric current through the targeted area (which are called electrolytic lesions), since the latter method damages both cells and fibers of passage. For this reason, excitotoxic lesions have replaced electrolytic lesions in many research applications.

The mechanisms underlying amino acid excitoxicity have been studied primarily using cultured nerve cells. In such tissue culture models, neuronal cell death is most readily triggered by strong activation of NMDA receptors. Nevertheless, non-NMDA receptors (AMPA and/or kainate receptors) may contribute to the excitotoxic effects of glutamate, and under certain conditions these receptors can even mediate cell death themselves without NMDA receptor involvement. When both NMDA and non-NMDA receptors are subjected to prolonged stimulation by a high concentration of glutamate, then a large percentage of the cells die within a few hours. The mode of cell death in this case is called **necrosis,** which is characterized by **lysis** (bursting) of the cell due to osmotic swelling and other injurious consequences of prolonged glutamate receptor activation. But a different pattern occurs if either the neurotransmitter concentration or time of exposure is significantly reduced. In that case, the osmotic swelling is temporary and the cells appear to return to a normal state. However, there may be a delayed response that emerges over the succeeding hours and that is characterized by a gradual disintegration of the cells and their eventual

(A)

(B)

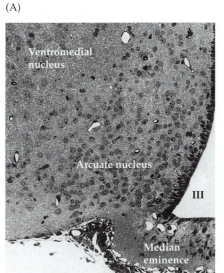
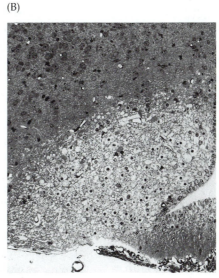

Figure 7.9 Damage to the arcuate nucleus following administration of MSG (A) The arcuate nucleus of the hypothalamus of an untreated 10-day-old mouse. (B) Damage to the arcuate nucleus is revealed by the loss of cell staining in a littermate subject injected 6 hours earlier with MSG. (From Olney et al., 1971; courtesy of John Olney.)

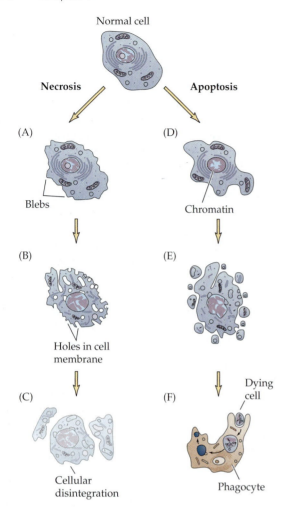

Normal cell

Necrosis — Apoptosis

(A)

Blebs

(B)

Holes in cell
membrane

(C)

Cellular
disintegration

(D)

Chromatin

(E)

(F)

Dying
cell

Phagocyte

Figure 7.10 Cell death by necrosis versus apoptosis
During the initial stages of necrosis (A), the cell swells and the
membrane forms protrusions called blebs. In the next stage (B),
the membrane begins to break up and release the contents of
the cell cytoplasm. Finally, the cell disintegrates completely (C).
In apoptotic cell death, the cell also blebs (D), but instead of
swelling, it shrinks. At the same time, the chromatin (genetic
material) condenses within the cell nucleus. The cell then breaks
up into smaller pieces (E) that are subsequently engulfed and
digested by phagocytes (F).

death. This delayed excitotoxic reaction is highly dependent
on NMDA receptor activation, since it can be elicited by the
selective application of NMDA or blocked by the presence of
an NMDA receptor antagonist such as MK-801.

In contrast to the necrotic reaction, which occurs relatively quickly, the later-appearing type of cell death is known
as **apoptosis** (sometimes also called **programmed cell
death**). Apoptosis involves a complex cascade of biochemical events that leads to disruption of the cell's nucleus, DNA
breakup, and ultimately cell death. One of the differences
between necrosis and apoptosis is that apoptotic cells do not
lyse and spill their contents into the extracellular space.
Instead, they are cleared away by other cells in a process
called phagocytosis (Figure 7.10). A significant amount of

apoptosis occurs normally during fetal brain development,
because the brain generates more cells than will be needed
later on. However, under the right conditions, it appears that
excitotoxic treatments can also activate the cell death program, thereby leading to inappropriate and excessive loss of
nerve cells.

Does excitotoxicity ever occur in humans? The answer
appears to be yes. The most well-established example of excitotoxic brain damage in humans is the damage produced by
ingesting large amounts of an excitatory amino acid called
domoic acid. This toxin is made by several species of marine
algae; taken up and concentrated by certain shellfish, crabs,
and fish; and passed on to humans who eat the tainted food.
Domoic acid poisoning first came to the attention of health
officials in 1987, when more than 100 people in Prince
Edward Island, Canada, were afflicted after consuming blue
mussels contaminated with domoic acid. The victims developed various neurological symptoms such as headache,
dizziness, muscle weakness, mental confusion, and in some
cases a permanent loss of short-term memory. Three people
died. Since then, unsafe levels of domoic acid in seafood have
periodically been found off the west coast of the United
States and Canada. Fortunately, government officials have
taken appropriate actions to minimize the danger to local
residents. But because it is impossible to prevent all wildlife
from being exposed to the toxin, many dolphins, sea lions,
and seabirds have become ill and died from ingesting domoic
acid. In fact, Alfred Hitchcock's film *The Birds* is reportedly
based on a 1961 incident in the town of Capitola, California,
in which domoic acid–poisoned seabirds began crashing into
pedestrians, automobiles, and buildings. In reality, the birds
were not attacking the town, but rather had become weak
and disoriented due to the effects of the toxin.

Excitotoxic brain damage is also believed to occur in people who experience brain **ischemia,** which is an interruption
of blood flow to the brain. Ischemia can result from either a
stroke (focal ischemia, where the interruption is localized to
the specific region of the stroke) or a heart attack (global
ischemia, where blood flow to the entire brain is interrupted). One consequence of ischemia is a massive release of glutamate in the affected area, thereby leading to prolonged
NMDA receptor activation. Many animal studies have found
that treatment with an NMDA receptor antagonist successfully reduces the amount of ischemic cell loss, particularly in
models of focal ischemia. Unfortunately, human clinical trials with the same drugs have thus far been largely disappointing. Compounds that appeared promising in preclinical
studies failed to show therapeutic benefit in patients and
sometimes led to severe side effects. Indeed, noncompetitive
NMDA receptor antagonists that bind to the PCP site within
the receptor channel can produce psychotic-like symptoms
in people (see Chapter 14). A more promising approach may
be to use drugs that block the glycine binding site on the
NMDA receptor, since there is reason to believe that antago-

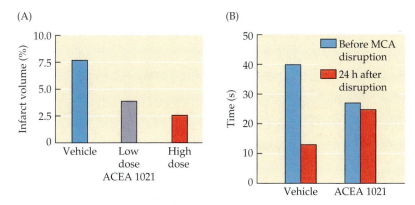

Figure 7.11 Neuroprotective effects of the NMDA receptor glycine-site antagonist ACEA 1021 in a rat model of ischemic stroke (A) Rats were subjected to permanent focal ischemia by disruption of blood flow through the middle cerebral artery (MCA). Animals given ACEA 1021 received either a low dose (a 5-mg/kg intravenous injection 15 minutes after ischemia onset followed by a 6-hour infusion at 3.5 mg/kg/h) or a high dose (a 10-mg/kg injection followed by a 7-mg/kg/h infusion) of the drug. Controls received only the injection vehicle. Rats were killed 24 hours after ischemia onset, their brains were removed, and the volume of infarcted (stroke-damaged) tissue was determined. Treatment with ACEA 1021 led to a dose-dependent reduction in infarct volume. (B) Functional consequences of ACEA 1021 administration were assessed using a test of grip strength. A 1-cm-diameter rope was suspended vertically and the rats were tested before and 24 hours after MCA disruption to determine how long they were able to cling to the rope using their forepaws. High-dose treatment with ACEA 1021 completely protected the animals from ischemia-induced deficits on this task. (After Petty et al., 2003.)

nists at this site may produce fewer side effects than compounds targeting other parts of the receptor. For example, one recent study showed that treatment with the glycine-site antagonist ACEA 1021 reduced both the observable brain damage and the resulting behavioral deficits in a rat model of ischemic stroke (Figure 7.11A and B; Petty et al., 2003). Future studies will hopefully show that such drugs produce a clinical benefit when given to stroke patients.

Section Summary

Glutamate is believed to be the workhorse for fast excitatory signaling in the nervous system. There are numerous glutamatergic pathways in the brain, including the projections of the pyramidal neurons of the cerebral cortex, the parallel fibers of the cerebellar cortex, and several excitatory pathways within the hippocampus.

AMPA, kainate, and NMDA receptors constitute the three subtypes of ionotropic glutamate receptors. Each is named for an agonist that is relatively selective for that subtype. All of these receptors permit Na^+ ions to cross the cell membrane, thereby producing membrane depolarization and an excitatory postsynaptic response. NMDA receptors also con-

duct Ca^{2+} ions and can trigger Ca^{2+}-dependent second-messenger actions within the postsynaptic cell.

AMPA and kainate receptors possess different protein subunits that give them somewhat different electrophysiological and pharmacological properties. Behavioral functions of AMPA receptors have been revealed through the use of the antagonist NBQX. Administration of high doses of this compound to rodents leads to sedation, ataxia, deficient rotarod performance, and protection against seizures, indicating an involvement of this receptor subtype in locomotor activity, coordination, and brain excitability.

NMDA receptors are distinct from the AMPA and kainate receptor subtypes in several ways in addition to the difference in ionic conductances. First, the opening of NMDA receptor channels requires a co-agonist in addition to glutamate. This co-agonist may be either glycine or D-serine. Second, NMDA receptors possess a binding site for Mg^{2+} ions within the receptor channel. When the cell membrane is at the resting potential, this site is occupied and the channel is blocked even if the receptor has been activated by agonists. However, depolarization of the membrane reduces the Mg^{2+} binding, thus allowing the channel to open. Consequently, for the NMDA receptor to function, some other synaptic input must excite the cell at the same time that glutamate and glycine or D-serine bind to the receptor. Third, NMDA receptors also possess a channel binding site that recognizes PCP, ketamine, and MK-801. These compounds act as noncompetitive antagonists of the NMDA receptor.

There are also eight different metabotropic receptors for glutamate, designated mGluR1–mGluR8. These G protein–coupled receptors typically either inhibit cAMP formation or stimulate the phosphoinositide second-messenger system. Some metabotropic receptors, those that are sensitive to the selective agonist L-AP4, function as presynaptic autoreceptors to inhibit glutamate release. Furthermore, mutant mice deficient in mGluR1 show reduced locomotion, ataxia, poor coordination, and learning deficits. The motor abnormalities are reversed by restoring the mGluR1 receptor to the Purkinje cells of the cerebellar cortex.

NMDA receptors are believed to play an important role in learning and memory. First, NMDA receptor antagonists impair the acquisition of various learning tasks. Second, activation of this receptor is necessary for the induction of hippocampal LTP. LTP is a process of synaptic strengthening that may underlie certain types of learning. Third, *Doogie* mice in which there is overexpression of one of the NMDA receptor subunits exhibit enhanced LTP and improved performance on a fear conditioning task, the Morris water maze spatial learning task, and a novel-object-recognition task.

Excessive exposure to glutamate and other excitatory amino acids can damage or even kill nerve cells through a process of depolarization-induced excitotoxicity. This process is usually mediated primarily by NMDA receptors, with some contribution from AMPA and/or kainate receptors. One type of excitotoxic cell death occurs via necrosis, which involves cellular swelling and eventual lysis. Alternatively, delayed cell death may occur via apoptosis, which involves disruption of the cell nucleus and breakdown of DNA. In humans, excitotoxic cell death can be caused by ingestion of food contaminated with the algal toxin domoic acid. Excitotoxicity is also thought to be a major contributory factor to the brain damage that occurs in focal ischemia (for example, stroke). NMDA receptor antagonists have proven beneficial in treating animal models of focal ischemia, but human trials with such compounds have thus far been mostly disappointing. An alternative approach that may prove more beneficial is to use an antagonist at the glycine binding site on the NMDA receptor.

GABA

Earlier in this chapter we saw that glutamate and, to a lesser extent, aspartate play a dominant role in fast excitatory transmission in the central nervous system (CNS). Inhibitory transmission is equally important in behavioral control mechanisms. The significance of neural inhibition is evident from the fact that blocking the action of either of the two major inhibitory amino acid transmitters leads to convulsions and even death. These two transmitters are **GABA (γ-aminobutyric acid)** and **glycine**. The remainder of this chapter focuses primarily on GABA, which is the more important of the two transmitters in the brain.*

GABA Synthesis, Release, and Inactivation

GABA is synthesized by the enzyme glutamic acid decarboxylase

Whereas the amino acids glutamate and aspartate participate widely in cellular metabolism, including protein synthesis, the only function of GABA is to serve as a neurotransmitter. Hence, it is only manufactured by GABAergic neurons. GABA is synthesized from glutamate in a single biochemical step, which is catalyzed by the enzyme **glutamic acid decarboxylase (GAD)** (Figure 7.12). It is interesting to note that the principal inhibitory neurotransmitter in the brain, namely GABA, is

*Although glycinergic neurons are present in the brain, their role has been studied more extensively in the spinal cord.

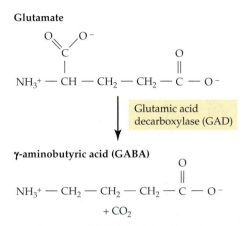

Figure 7.12 GABA is synthesized from glutamate by the enzyme glutamic acid decarboxylase (GAD).

made from the principal excitatory transmitter, glutamate. GAD is localized specifically to GABAergic neurons, and therefore researchers can identify such neurons by staining for GAD.

Several drugs are known to block GABA synthesis, including **allylglycine, thiosemicarbazide,** and **3-mercaptopropionic acid.** As noted earlier, a significant reduction in GABA synthesis leads to convulsions, which indicates the importance of this transmitter in regulating brain excitability. On the other hand, it also means that GAD inhibitors are normally used to study GABAergic transmission only in vitro, not in vivo.

Specific transporter proteins are used to transport GABA into synaptic vesicles and nerve terminals following release

Like the vesicular transporters that take up glutamate into synaptic vesicles, the **vesicular GABA transporter (VGAT)** was discovered fairly recently. Subsequent studies revealed an interesting and unexpected feature of this protein, namely that it is also found in neurons that use glycine as a transmitter. Thus the same transporter is used to load either GABA or glycine into synaptic vesicles. This situation is similar to the previously discussed example of VMAT, the vesicular monoamine transporter, which is responsible for vesicle filling of three different neurotransmitters: DA, NE, and 5-HT.

Following the synaptic release of GABA, it is removed from the cleft by three different transporters on the membranes of nerve cells and glia, designated **GAT-1, GAT-2,** and **GAT-3.** GAT-1 and GAT-2 seem to be expressed in both neurons and astrocytes, whereas GAT-3 is found in astrocytes only. GAT-1 has received particular attention for two reasons. First, this transporter has been found at the nerve terminals of GABAergic neurons, and therefore it is likely to be important for GABA reuptake by these cells. Second, in contrast to GAT-2 and GAT-3, there is a selective inhibitor of GAT-1 available for pharmacological study. Administration of this compound, **tiagabine,** elevates extracellular GABA levels and enhances

GABAergic transmission in several brain areas, including the cortex and hippocampus. Based on the fact that depleting GABA (for example, by blocking GAD activity) causes seizures, we might predict that tiagabine protects against seizure onset. Indeed, tiagabine was licensed in 1997 under the trade name **Gabitril** for use as an adjunctive therapy (an additional treatment given along with more-standard antiepileptic drugs) in treatment-resistant patients with partial seizures (seizures involving only part of the body). Tiagabine appears to be clinically beneficial in this role, and this compound is also being tested as a monotherapy (single treatment) for certain kinds of epilepsy.

Whereas the immediate inactivation of GABA in the synapse occurs through a combination of neuronal and astroglial uptake, there is also a cellular mechanism for metabolizing and recycling this neurotransmitter. GABA breakdown occurs through several steps, beginning with the enzyme **GABA aminotransferase (GABA-T)** and leading eventually to the final product, succinate. It is worth noting that a by-product of this metabolic pathway is the formation of one molecule of glutamate for every molecule of GABA that is broken down. GABA-T is found in both GABAergic neurons and astrocytes. Hence, in the GABAergic neurons, some of the glutamate regenerated by the action of GABA-T could be used to synthesize more GABA. Moreover, some of the glutamate produced by GABA-T in astrocytes could be converted to glutamine by astrocytic glutamine synthetase, and the glutamine could subsequently be transported to the GABAergic neurons to be converted back to glutamate by the enzyme glutaminase (Figure 7.13). This shows that the metabolic interplay between neurons and glial cells discussed earlier for glutamate is equally important for GABA.

Vigabatrin is an irreversible inhibitor of GABA-T. By preventing GABA metabolism, administration of this drug leads to a buildup of GABA levels in the brain. By now, you should be able to predict correctly that vigabatrin has anticonvulsant effects in animals and humans. Like tiagabine, vigabatrin (trade name **Sabril**) is being used clinically as either an adjunctive treatment or as the primary therapeutic agent for certain types of epilepsy, particularly infantile spasms (repeated generalized seizures in young infants). However, there are a number of recent reports that vigabatrin use can lead to constriction of the visual field in both adults and children. Since there are GABAergic interneurons in the retina, visual abnormalities could be related to drug effects on these cells. In light

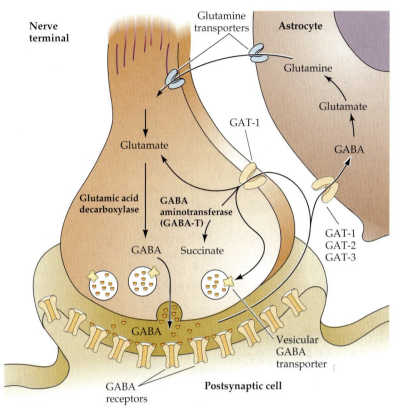

Figure 7.13 Cycling of GABA between glutamatergic neurons and astrocytes After neurons release GABA, it can be transported back into the nerve terminal by GAT-1 or transported into nearby astrocytes by GAT-2 or GAT-3. Inside the cell, GABA is metabolized to glutamate and succinate by GABA aminotransferase (GABA-T). In the case of astrocytes, the glutamate is converted into glutamine by the enzyme glutamine synthetase. The glutamine can later be released by the astrocytes, taken up by neurons, converted back into glutamate by the enzyme glutaminase, and finally used to resynthesize GABA.

of these findings, physicians must consider the risk-to-benefit ratio when considering vigabatrin treatment of epileptic patients.

Section Summary

GABA is the major inhibitory amino acid neurotransmitter in the brain. This transmitter is synthesized from glutamate in a single biochemical reaction catalyzed by GAD, an enzyme found only in GABAergic neurons. Because of GABA's widespread inhibitory effects on neuronal excitability, treatment with drugs that inhibit GABA synthesis by blocking GAD leads to seizures.

GABA is taken up into synaptic vesicles by the vesicular transporter VGAT. After release into the synaptic cleft, GABA is removed from the cleft by three different transporters designated GAT-1, GAT-2, and GAT-3. Astrocytes express all three of these transporters and therefore must play a significant role in GABA uptake. GAT-1 is also found in GABAergic neurons, and the GAT-1 inhibitor tiagabine (Gabitril) is used clinically in the treatment of some epileptic patients.

In addition to uptake, the other process that regulates GABAergic transmission is GABA metabolism. The key enzyme in GABA breakdown is GABA-T, which is present in both GABAergic neurons and astrocytes. A by-product of the reaction catalyzed by GABA-T is glutamate, which is the precursor of GABA. Hence, GABA breakdown either in neurons or glial cells may involve a recycling process that assists in the formation of new GABA molecules.

Vigabatrin (Sabril) is an irreversible inhibitor of GABA-T, thereby elevating GABA levels in the brain. Like tiagabine, vigabatrin has been licensed for treating certain types of epilepsy. However, there are reports that repeated vigabatrin use can lead to visual system abnormalities in adults and children, which means that caution should be exercised in the administration of this compound to patients.

Organization and Function of the GABAergic System

Some GABAergic neurons are interneurons, while others are projection neurons

Fonnum (1987) has estimated that as many as 10 to 40% of the nerve terminals in the cerebral cortex, hippocampus, and substantia nigra use GABA as their neurotransmitter. Even the lower range of this estimate indicates that a lot of GABAergic transmission takes place, when you consider the dozens of different neurotransmitters that may be present within a specific brain region. In addition to the three structures just mentioned, other brain areas rich in GABA are the cerebellum, striatum, globus pallidus, and olfactory bulbs.

In some structures, such as the cortex and hippocampus, GABA is found in large numbers of local interneurons. However, there are also GABAergic projection neurons that carry inhibitory information longer distances within the brain. For example, GABAergic neurons of the striatum project to the globus pallidus and the substantia nigra. When the DA input to the striatum is damaged in Parkinson's disease, the result is abnormal firing of the striatal GABAergic neurons, which causes the motor abnormalities seen in this neurological disorder (see Chapter 5). GABA is also the transmitter used by the Purkinje cells of the cerebellar cortex. These neurons, which project to the deep cerebellar nuclei and to the brain stem, have an important function in fine muscle control and coordination. This is illustrated in a rare disorder involving degeneration of the cerebellar Purkinje cells. Patients suffering from this disorder, which is known as Holmes cerebellar degeneration, show ataxia when walking, impaired fine hand movements, defective speech, and tremors.

The actions of GABA are mediated by ionotropic GABA$_A$ receptors and metabotropic GABA$_B$ receptors

Like glutamate, GABA makes use of both ionotropic and metabotropic receptors. However, there is only one type of each: the **GABA$_A$ receptor,** which is ionotropic, and the **GABA$_B$ receptor,** which is metabotropic. Our discussion will concentrate on the GABA$_A$ receptor because of its prominent role in GABAergic transmission and because it is a crucial target of many important psychoactive drugs.

Structure and function of the GABA$_A$ receptor   GABA$_A$ receptors are ion channels that permit Cl$^-$ ions to move across the cell membrane from the outside to the inside. This causes inhibition of the postsynaptic cell due to membrane hyperpolarization. More Cl$^-$ ions flow through open GABA$_A$ receptor channels when the membrane has previously been depolarized by excitatory synaptic inputs. In such cases, these receptors function to blunt the depolarization and prevent the cell from firing an action potential.

Structurally, each GABA$_A$ receptor contains five subunits. Three or four different *kinds* of subunits may be found within a particular GABA$_A$ receptor complex. These different kinds of subunits are designated with the Greek letters α, β, γ, and δ. Most GABA$_A$ receptors are thought to contain either (1) two α-subunits, two β-subunits, and one γ-subunit or (2) two α-subunits, one β-subunit, and two γ-subunits. A small number of receptors contain a δ-subunit instead of γ. With this information in mind, the likely structure of a typical GABA$_A$ receptor is illustrated in Figure 7.14.

The classic agonist for the GABA$_A$ receptor is a drug called **muscimol.** This compound is found in the mushroom *Amanita muscaria* (Figure 7.15), which was mentioned in the last chapter as the original source of the cholinergic agonist muscarine. In earlier times, the mushroom would apparently be chopped up and placed in a dish with milk to attract flies. Ingestion of muscimol and the related compound ibotenic acid would make the flies stuporous and easy to catch. The common name for *A. muscaria* is therefore "fly agaric" (*agaric* is an old term meaning "mushroom"). Rudgley (1999) discusses the custom of eating fly agaric, which various Siberian peoples have practiced for hundreds of years. The mushroom was prized for its stimulatory and hallucinogenic qualities, effects that can also be obtained by drinking urine from an intoxicated individual (not a very appealing idea to most Westerners!).* One of the interesting kinds of hallucinatory effects produced by the fly agaric is

---

*Fly agaric intoxication was apparently enjoyed not only by Siberians but by their reindeer as well. Animals were observed to eat the mushrooms of their own accord, and were also sometimes given urine to drink from a person who had previously partaken.

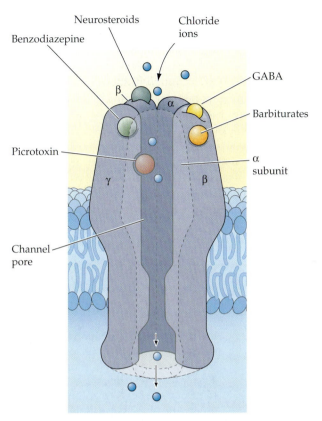

Figure 7.14 The GABA$_A$ receptor consists of five subunits that form a chloride-conducting channel. In addition to the GABA binding site on the receptor complex, there are additional modulatory sites for benzodiazepines, barbiturates, neurosteroids, and picrotoxin. Note that the locations of the various binding sites are depicted arbitrarily and are not meant to imply the actual locations of these sites on the receptor.

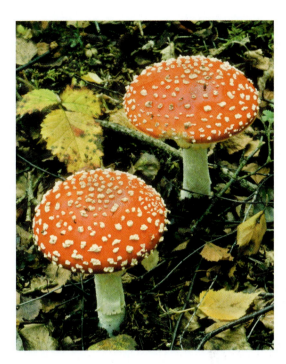

Figure 7.15 The fly agaric mushroom, *Amanita muscaria*

macroscopia, which refers to the perception of objects as being larger than they really are. When administered to humans at relatively high doses, pure muscimol causes an intoxication characterized by hyperthermia (elevated body temperature), pupil dilation, elevation of mood, difficulties in concentration, anorexia (loss of appetite), ataxia, catalepsy, and hallucinations. Many of these effects are similar to those associated with more-traditional hallucinogenic drugs such as LSD (see Chapter 14).

Bicuculline is the best-known competitive antagonist for the GABA$_A$ receptor. It blocks the binding of GABA to the GABA$_A$ receptor, and when taken systemically, it has a potent convulsant effect. **Pentylenetetrazol (Metrazol)** and **picrotoxin** are two other convulsant drugs that inhibit GABA$_A$ receptor function by acting at sites distinct from the binding site of GABA itself. Pentylenetetrazol is a synthetic compound that once was used as a convulsant therapy for major depression. Although it is no longer used for that purpose, it still has value for the induction of experimental seizures in

laboratory animals. Picrotoxin is obtained from the seeds of the East Indian shrub *Anirmirta cocculus*. Since neither pentylenetetrazol nor picrotoxin blocks GABA from interacting with the GABA$_A$ receptor, they are noncompetitive rather than competitive receptor antagonists.

For psychopharmacologists, the most remarkable property of the GABA$_A$ receptor is its sensitivity to certain CNS-depressant drugs that display an anxiolytic (antianxiety), sedative–hypnotic (sedating and sleep-inducing), and anticonvulsant profile. Among such drugs are the **benzodiazepines (BDZs)** and the **barbiturates.** There is overwhelming evidence that the principal mechanism of action of BDZs and barbiturates involves potentiating the effects of GABA on the GABA$_A$ receptor. **Ethanol** (drinking alcohol) is another CNS-depressant drug that has many of the same properties as BDZs and barbiturates. Although the actions of ethanol are complex, one of its major effects is likewise to enhance GABA$_A$ receptor activity.

How do BDZs, barbiturates, and ethanol exert their influence on the GABA$_A$ receptor? The first two classes of drugs interact with sites on the receptor complex that are distinct from the GABA binding site. This concept is illustrated in Figure 7.14, which also shows the presence of a modulatory site for picrotoxin and related convulsant drugs. Details of the interaction of ethanol with the GABA$_A$ receptor are still being worked out. The pharmacology of ethanol and of the BDZs and barbiturates are discussed in greater detail in Chapters 9 and 17. However, it is worth noting some of the key features of the interactions of BDZs with the GABA$_A$ receptor before concluding this section of the chapter.

The recognition site for BDZs on the GABA$_A$ receptor complex is considered a bona fide BDZ receptor, since these drugs bind directly to the site, and such binding is necessary for BDZs to exert their behavioral and physiological effects. When a BDZ such as **diazepam** (trade name **Valium**) binds to the BDZ receptor, it increases the potency of GABA to open the receptor channel. BDZs cannot activate the GABA$_A$ receptor by themselves; thus, they have no effect in the absence of GABA.

Diazepam and related BDZs are agonists at the BDZ receptor on the GABA$_A$ receptor complex. Researchers have also discovered certain compounds that modulate the

GABA$_A$ receptor in the opposite direction as a BDZ agonist. Such compounds have been termed **inverse agonists** at the BDZ receptor. If a BDZ agonist enhances the effectiveness of GABA on the receptor, then a BDZ inverse agonist reduces GABA's effectiveness, although it doesn't actually block GABA like a GABA receptor antagonist. Like a BDZ agonist, an inverse agonist has no effect in the absence of GABA. The behavioral profile of a BDZ inverse agonist is the opposite of that seen with BDZ agonists. Consequently, BDZ inverse agonists are anxiogenic (anxiety-producing), arousing, and proconvulsant (seizure-promoting) instead of anxiolytic, sedating, and anticonvulsant. Finally, let us think about what it means for the brain to have a receptor (that is, the BDZ

BOX 7.2 Pharmacology in Action

What Is the Endogenous Ligand for the Benzodiazepine Receptor?

Pharmacologists sometimes work in seemingly strange ways. Traditionally, you identify a new neurotransmitter and then search for the receptors for that transmitter. Sometimes, however, a receptor is discovered that is not responsive to any known neurotransmitter, hormone, or other signaling agent. Such a receptor is termed an **orphan receptor.** If you discover one of these, then you need to work "backwards," in that you must try to find the neurotransmitter that activates your orphan receptor.

What if you discover a new receptor by virtue of its sensitivity to either a plant-derived substance or a synthetic drug? As an example, the existence of opioid receptors was hypothesized and subsequently proven based on the behavioral and physiological effects of morphine, a substance found only in the opium poppy. The same reasoning led more recently to the discovery of cannabinoid receptors, which are activated by the psychoactive substances present in cannabis plants. In this chapter, we have seen that there are BDZ receptors in the brain that are activated by synthetic drugs. Is it possible that the

brain possesses receptors whose sole function is to respond to either plant-derived or synthetic compounds? Evolutionary theory argues against such a possibility. Consequently, these receptors must have arisen in the course of evolutionary history in order to serve signaling molecules that are made in our own brains as well as the brains of animals. We use the term **endogenous ligand** to designate the body's own signaling molecule(s) used to activate a receptor that was initially discovered because of its sensitivity to plant-derived or synthetic substances. *Endogenous* means "occurring within the body," and *lig-*

and refers to any compound that binds to a receptor (see Chapter 1).

As shown in the table, endogenous ligands have been discovered for some of these novel receptors but not others. The two success stories involve the discovery of endorphins and enkephalins as endogenous ligands for opioid receptors (see Chapter 10) and the later discovery of anandamide as an endogenous ligand for cannabinoid receptors (see Chapter 13). Receptors for which the endogenous ligand has still not been conclusively identified include the phencyclidine (PCP) receptor (as mentioned earlier, this is a site within the NMDA receptor channel) and the BDZ receptor.

Although there is still uncertainty regarding the endogenous ligand for BDZ receptors, several candidates have been proposed. One of the

Drugs, Receptors, and Endogenous Ligands in the Brain

Drug	Source	Receptor(s)	Endogenous ligand(s)
Morphine	Opium poppy	Opioid receptors	Endorphins and enkephalins
Cannabinoids	Cannabis plant	Cannabinoid receptors	Anandamide
Phencyclidine	Synthetic	PCP receptor	?
BDZs	Synthetic	BDZ receptor	?

receptor) that responds to a class of synthetic drugs* rather than one of the brain's own neurotransmitters. This last point is the subject of Box 7.2.

The GABA$_A$ receptor is additionally modulated by a family of substances known as **neurosteroids.** These substances are made from cholesterol and possess a steroid structure like that of the glucocorticoids and gonadal steroids (see Chapter 3). However, they are synthesized in the brain (hence the term *neuro*steroid) and they are thought to act as local signaling molecules rather than as hormones. Allopregnanolone, tetrahydrodeoxycorticosterone, and dehydroepiandrosterone (DHEA) are among the most extensively studied neurosteroids. Like BDZ agonists, most neurosteroids enhance GABA$_A$ receptor function and produce sedative–hypnotic and anxiolytic effects behaviorally. As depicted in Figure 7.14, though, neurosteroids seem to interact with the receptor at a site other than the BDZ binding site.

Structure and function of the GABA$_B$ receptor
As mentioned earlier, the other GABA receptor subtype is a metabotropic receptor termed GABA$_B$. GABA$_B$ receptors

---

*BDZs were developed by pharmaceutical companies and do not occur naturally in the brain except perhaps in small quantities (and even the evidence for that is inconclusive).

BOX 7.2 (continued)

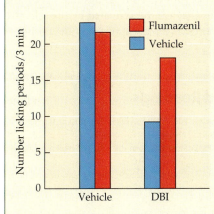

Diazepam binding inhibitor has a proconflict effect in rats Drinking behavior by water-deprived rats was measured under conditions in which a 0.25-mA shock was delivered through the drinking tube. Intracerebroventricular administration of 100 µg of DBI reduced the amount of punished drinking, an effect that was largely blocked by the benzodiazepine receptor antagonist flumazenil (1 mg/kg intravenously). (After Guidotti et al., 1983.)

major contenders is a large peptide called **diazepam binding inhibitor (DBI),** along with two smaller peptides (abbreviated ODN and TTN) derived from DBI. DBI was isolated from rat brain more than 20 years ago based on its ability to inhibit diazepam binding to the BDZ site on the GABA$_A$ receptor (Guidotti et al., 1983). Subsequent studies showed that DBI is present in both neurons and glial cells in the brains of many species, including humans (Costa and Guidotti, 1991; Ferrero et al., 1986a). It is also found in numerous peripheral tissues including the liver, kidney, and certain endocrine glands.

The behavioral effects of DBI and ODN were assessed in the Vogel conflict test. This test involves training thirsty rats to drink water by licking a metal sipper tube and then giving them a mild shock through the tube. The degree of lick suppression is taken as a measure of the conflict (anxiety) produced by the electric shock. BDZs produce an anticonflict effect that is seen as an increased amount of postshock licking, presumably due to their enhancement of GABA$_A$ receptor function. In contrast, because BDZ inverse agonists reduce GABA$_A$ receptor activity, they produce a proconflict effect, manifested by decreased licking compared to control animals. Interestingly, when either DBI or ODN was administered directly into the brains of rats, a proconflict effect was observed (Guidotti et al., 1983; Ferrero et al., 1986b) (see figure). Moreover, in both cases this effect was blocked by treatment with flumazenil, a BDZ receptor antagonist. These findings indicate that DBI and ODN act as inverse agonists at the BDZ receptor. There is also a report that ODN is localized together with GABA in cultured nerve cells and that the two substances are released together upon stimulation (Ferrarese et al., 1987). However, these findings have not yet been replicated by other researchers. Thus, while the DBI story raises intriguing possibilities, the physiological role of this family of peptides has not yet been established conclusively.

Yet another line of research has led to the hypothesis that the brain contains small nonpeptide molecules that have BDZ-like activity on GABA$_A$ receptors (Rothstein et al., 1992) and that can be mapped using antibodies against BDZs (Sánchez et al., 1991). These substances have been termed **endozepines** (endogenous benzodiazepines), although their exact chemical identity remains uncertain. It is possible that our level of anxiety is controlled in a complex way by the competing effects of BDZ inverse agonists (DBI and ODN), which increase feelings of anxiety, and agonist compounds (endozepines), which reduce such feelings. But such a scenario is highly speculative at the present time and must await the results of many more studies identifying and characterizing the endogenous ligands of the BDZ receptor.

function by several mechanisms, including inhibition of cAMP formation and stimulation of K$^+$ channel opening. Drugs that function as agonists or antagonists at GABA$_A$ receptors have no effect on the GABA$_B$ receptor. However, GABA$_B$ receptors can be activated by a selective agonist called **baclofen (Lioresal),** which has been used for a number of years as a muscle relaxant and antispastic agent.

Section Summary

Many brain areas are rich in GABA, including the cerebral cortex, hippocampus, substantia nigra, cerebellum, striatum, globus pallidus, and olfactory bulbs. GABAergic neurons may function as interneurons, as in the cortex and hippocampus, or they may function as projection neurons, as in pathways originating in the striatum and in the cerebellar Purkinje cells.

There are two general GABA receptor subtypes: ionotropic GABA$_A$ receptors and metabotropic GABA$_B$ receptors. GABA$_A$ receptors conduct Cl$^-$ ions into the postsynaptic cell, causing a membrane hyperpolarization and an inhibitory effect on cell excitability. Each receptor is composed of five subunits, usually including two α-subunits, two βs, and one γ or two αs, one β, and two γs. Muscimol is a GABA$_A$ receptor agonist derived from the mushroom *Amanita muscaria* (fly agaric). Ingestion of this mushroom or of pure muscimol causes hallucinations (including macroscopia) and other behavioral and physiological effects similar to those associated with LSD. GABA$_A$ receptor antagonists include the competitive antagonist bicuculline and the noncompetitive inhibitors pentylenetetrazol (Metrazol) and picrotoxin, all of which are seizure-inducing.

The effects of GABA on the GABA$_A$ receptor are enhanced by several kinds of CNS-depressant drugs, such as BDZs, barbiturates, and ethanol. With respect to their effects on behavior, these compounds display anxiolytic, sedative–hypnotic, and anticonvulsant properties. BDZs bind to a specific site on the GABA$_A$ receptor complex that is considered to be a BDZ receptor. Although BDZs amplify the effect of GABA, they have no effect on GABA$_A$ receptor function in the absence of the neurotransmitter. Inverse agonists at the BDZ receptor also require the presence of GABA, but such compounds reduce instead of enhance GABA's effectiveness in activating the GABA$_A$ receptor. BDZ inverse agonists produce the opposite behavioral effects as BDZ agonists, namely anxiety, arousal, and increased susceptibility to seizures. Researchers continue to search for an endogenous ligand for the BDZ receptor.

The metabotropic GABA$_B$ receptors function by inhibiting cAMP formation and stimulating K$^+$ channel opening. These receptors are not influenced by drugs that act on the GABA$_A$ receptor, but they can be activated by the selective agonist baclofen (Lioresal), a muscle relaxant and antispastic agent.

Recommended Readings

Ashton, H., and Young, A. H. (2003). GABA-Ergic drugs: Exit stage left, enter stage right. *J. Psychopharmacol.,* 17, 174–178.

Moghaddam, B. (ed.) (2003). Glutamate and disorders of cognition and motivation. *Ann. N. Y. Acad. Sci.,* Vol. 1003.

Sattler, R., and Tymianski, M. (2001). Molecular mechanisms of glutamate receptor-mediated excitotoxic neuronal cell death. *Mol. Neurobiol.,* 24, 107–129.

Squire, L. R., and Kandel, E. R. (1999). *Memory: From Mind to Molecules.* Scientific American Library, New York.

8 Drug Abuse, Dependence, and Addiction

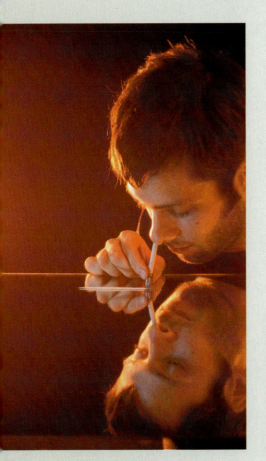

The problem of drug abuse and addiction is exemplified by a user snorting a line of cocaine.

ob had begun drinking at the age of 12, sneaking beers from his family's refrigerator. Thirty years later, when he and his wife Kathy sought counseling for their marital problems, alcohol had come to dominate much of Bob's life. According to his conversations with the counselor, his drinking had gotten "really bad" after his marriage and the birth of his children.

Around that time, he began to feel trapped in an undesirable job because of the needed income. In addition, the demands of child care caused his wife to pay less attention to him than before, and their sexual relations became much less frequent.

Bob's response to these problems was to increase his drinking. Upon returning home from work, he would have "a cocktail or two" before dinner. After a while, one or two cocktails became three, four, or even more. Furthermore, Bob didn't want to be bothered with the family's problems until he was "relaxed," meaning intoxicated. Unfortunately, the combination of his intoxication and feelings of guilt made him impatient and irritable when he was approached by family members. Eventually, Kathy and the children began to avoid him much of the time, leading their own lives and dealing with their problems without Bob's input.

Bob's situation at work was also deteriorating. At lunchtime, he frequently went out to a nearby bar for a sandwich and cocktails instead of joining his coworkers at the company cafeteria. He got away with this for a while, but finally his boss smelled liquor on his breath. Although he wasn't fired, his performance evaluations began to suffer and he received a stern warning that another incident of drinking during working hours would lead to disciplinary action.

By the time Bob and Kathy went to the counselor after 20 years of marriage, Bob's life was a mess. Despite attempts to control his habit, he was continuing to drink daily and had developed a powerful tolerance to alcohol. His marriage was in crisis. His job was in jeopardy. He was two years behind on his income tax returns and was in debt to the government for several thousand dollars. According to Kathy, their house was in danger of falling apart due to numerous repair projects that Bob had promised to carry out but had never done. Their son, who was a freshman in college, was failing half his courses. Their younger daughter "hated" Bob, and her main interactions with him were either to fight or to ridicule him.

The above is an actual case study presented by Joseph Nowinski (1996) in a discussion of 12-step recovery from drug addiction. It dramatically illustrates what we might call the "paradox" of addiction. That is, how can a person develop and maintain a pattern of behavior (in this case, repeated, heavy alcohol consumption) that is so obviously destructive to the individual's life? No one has a complete explanation of this paradox, but a variety of model theories have been proposed. The aim of this chapter is to introduce you to several facets of this intriguing problem. We first consider the discovery and use of psychoactive drugs in early times, the history of drug laws in the United States, and the definition and characteristics of addiction. Later parts of the chapter survey and critique several classical and contemporary models of addiction. Treatment approaches for addiction are presented in subsequent chapters covering specific drugs of abuse.

Introduction to Drug Abuse and Addiction

Drugs of abuse are widely consumed in our society

Each year, the Substance Abuse and Mental Health Services Administration conducts a National Survey on Drug Use and Health, which estimates the prevalence and incidence of drug use among civilians 12 years of age and older. According to the 2002 survey, approximately 19.5 million Americans (8.3% of the population) were current users of at least one illicit drug at that time. As shown in Figure 8.1A, more than 50% of these illicit drug users confined their use to marijuana. Figure 8.1B illustrates that the incidence of illicit drug use peaks between the ages of 16 and 25 years and declines slowly thereafter. Not surprisingly, legal drugs such as tobacco and alcohol are consumed even more widely than illicit substances. The 2002 survey estimated that more than 71 million Americans were current tobacco users (mostly cigarette smokers), 120 million drank alcohol, and of the latter, almost 16 million were heavy drinkers (defined as consuming 5 or more drinks at one time

on 5 or more days within a single month). How did we reach a state where psychoactive drug use and abuse are so prevalent?

Drug use in our society has increased and become more heavily regulated over time

Historical trends   Psychoactive drugs have been a part of human culture since antiquity. Many psychoactive substances such as nicotine, caffeine, morphine, cocaine, and tetrahydrocannabinol are made by plants and were available to ancient peoples in their native forms. Likewise, alcohol is a naturally occurring product of sugar fermentation by yeast. In his 1989 book *Intoxication: Life in Pursuit of Artificial Paradise*, Ronald Siegel presents many anecdotal accounts of wild animals becoming intoxicated after eating drug-containing plants. He goes on to suggest that early societies may have come to identify the pharmacological properties of such plants after first observing the behaviors of these intoxicated animals. More historical information on individual abused drugs is covered in later chapters. Here, we will focus on the history of drug use and cultural attitudes in the United States over the past 200 years.

(A)

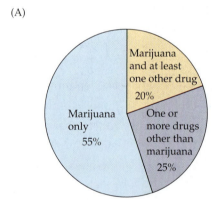

(B)

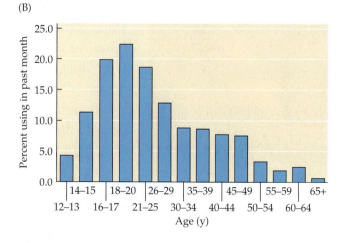

Figure 8.1 Data on illicit drug use in the United States from the 2002 National Survey on Drug Use and Health. (A) shows the percentage of drug users who were taking marijuana alone, marijuana and at least one other illicit substance, or only illicit substances other than marijuana at the time of the survey. (B) depicts the age distribution of illicit drug users.

Compared to the wide variety of psychoactive drugs available (legally or illegally) to twenty-first-century Americans, the situation was quite different 200 years ago. Alcohol and caffeine were widely used, and although the modern cigarette had not yet been invented, tobacco chewing was becoming increasingly popular within a large segment of the male population. Opium, either alone or in the form of laudanum (opium extract in alcohol), was available for the purpose of pain relief. On the other hand, there was no cocaine, heroin, marijuana, MDMA ("Ecstasy"), methamphetamine, barbiturates, LSD, or PCP. There were also few drug control laws, and especially none at the federal level.

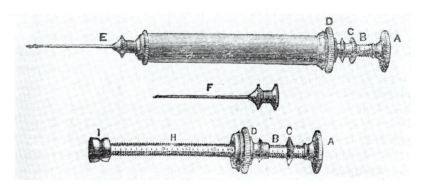

Figure 8.2   An early hypodermic syringe and needle used in the 1870s (From Morgan, 1981; original photograph from H. H. Kane, *The Hypodermic Injection of Morphia,* 1880, p. 21.)

As time went on, however, a number of events and cultural trends occurred that set us on the path to where we are today. First, the alcohol temperance movement started gaining strength. The founding of this movement, which promoted abstention from hard liquor in favor of moderate beer or wine consumption, is generally credited to a highly regarded Philadelphia physician named Benjamin Rush. Rush not only identified a number of adverse physiological consequences of excessive drinking, he also argued that such consumption impaired the drinker's moral faculty, leading to irresponsible and even criminal acts. Although the temperance movement reached its height in the failed twentieth-century attempt at complete alcohol prohibition (except for "medicinal" use), its aftermath still colors the attitudes of many people toward the problem of alcohol and drug abuse. In particular, the equating of drug use with criminal behavior can be seen in the "War on Drugs" that has pervaded our society for so many years.

Second, advances in chemistry during the nineteenth century made it possible to purify the primary active ingredient of opium, namely morphine, and then later the active ingredient of coca, which of course is cocaine. This allowed the drugs to be taken in much more concentrated form, increasing their addictive potential. But since the route of administration is also important, an equally significant event was the development of the hypodermic syringe in 1858 (Figure 8.2), which permitted the purified substances to be injected directly into the bloodstream. One consequence of this marriage of purified drug and improved delivery vehicle was the widespread use of morphine to treat wounded and ill soldiers during the Civil War. Many developed an opiate addiction, which was called "soldier's disease" in the common parlance.

Third, the increasing availability of purified drugs combined with the lack of drug control laws led to a growing use of these substances in many different forms. Cocaine was the major ingredient in a variety of tonics and patent medicines

sold over-the-counter. The most notorious of these was *Vin Mariani,* which was made by the French chemist Angelo Mariani by soaking coca leaves in wine along with spices and other flavorings. Heroin was synthesized by the Bayer Laboratories in 1874 and first marketed 14 years later as a nonaddicting (!) substitute for codeine. If you've ever had a severe cough, the doctor probably prescribed a codeine-containing cough syrup. At the turn of the twentieth century, you could purchase heroin-containing cough syrup at any neighborhood pharmacy without a prescription (Figure 8.3). It does not surprise us

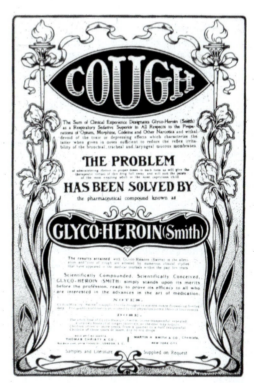

Figure 8.3   An early ad for heroin-containing cough syrup

now that the ready availability of these substances led many people to become dependent on them.

The last factor that we wish to mention here is the medicalization of drug addiction that occurred primarily in the second half of the twentieth century. The medicalization of addiction had two components: that addiction was now thought of as a disease and that drug addicts should be treated by the medical establishment. We can trace the origin of these views to the American Association for the Cure of Inebriates, an organization founded in 1870 that stated that inebriety (excessive drinking) was a disease and proposed that inebriates (alcoholics) be admitted to hospitals and sanitaria for help. However, this medical approach to alcoholism and drug abuse later faded and was not seriously revived until the early 1950s, when alcoholism was declared a disease first by the World Health Organization and subsequently by the American Medical Association. Alcoholics Anonymous (AA), which embraces many aspects of the disease model of alcoholism, was also gaining prominence during this period. The disease model of drug addiction continues to be strongly promoted by the treatment community, by self-help groups such as AA and Narcotics Anonymous, and by much of the research establishment (including the National Institute on Drug Abuse, an agency of the National Institutes of Health). It is also the view most widely accepted by the lay public. On the other hand, this model has also been the subject of some criticism, as we shall see later in the chapter.

Drugs and the law   Since 1980, the United States has witnessed the introduction of "crack" cocaine, the increased potency of heroin and marijuana sold on the street, an upsurge in methamphetamine use, and the rise of so-called club drugs such as MDMA and GHB. Although these developments led to the establishment and continuation of our government's "War on Drugs," illicit drug use continues on a massive scale despite the best efforts of the drug warriors. At the federal level, the current political climate is strongly against any consideration of legalization or even decriminalization of any currently illegal drugs, including marijuana. Indeed, when Dr. Joycelyn Elders, President Bill Clinton's first Surgeon General, innocently mentioned in December 1993 that perhaps the issue of drug legalization should at least be openly discussed, it led to a tremendous public outcry and an immediate retraction by the Clinton administration. A year later, Dr. Elders was fired. Although she had made other controversial remarks before her dismissal, no one doubted that her first misstep was to bring up the notion of drug legalization.

TABLE 8.1 History of Federal Drug Legislation in the United States

Name of law	Year enacted	Purpose
Pure Food and Drug Act	1906	Regulated labeling of patent medicines and created the FDA
Harrison Act	1914	Regulated dispensing and use of opioid drugs and cocaine
Eighteenth Constitutional Amendment (Prohibition)	1920	Banned alcohol sales except for medicinal use (repealed in 1933)
Marijuana Tax Act	1937	Banned nonmedical use of cannabis (overturned by U.S. Supreme Court in 1969)
Controlled Substances Act	1970	Established the schedule of controlled substances and created the DEA

Given the recent history of drug politics in the United States, it is easy to forget that things were not always this way. As discussed earlier, by the beginning of the twentieth century, there was widespread use of cocaine, opium, and heroin in over-the-counter or patent medicines. In the absence of any federal regulations governing the marketing, distribution, or purchase of these preparations, sales increased from $3.5 million in 1859 to $74 million in 1904 (Hollinger, 1995). Over time, however, the federal government became increasingly involved in controlling the commercialization of drugs (Table 8.1). This involvement began with an initial concern about the quality and purity of both medications and food, which led to the passage in 1906 of the Pure Food and Drug Act. The new law mandated the accurate labeling of patent medicines so that the consumer would be aware of the presence of alcohol, cocaine, opiates, or marijuana in such products. It also created the Food and Drug Administration (FDA), which is charged with assessing the potential hazards and benefits of new medications and with licensing their use. The Pure Food and Drug Act was clearly an educational approach to the drug problem, since the law did not make any of the above-mentioned substances illegal to sell or use.

Around the same time that drug labeling and purity were under discussion, there was a growing concern over the burgeoning problem of drug abuse and dependency. For example, importation of opium grew rapidly between 1870 and 1900. Rightly or wrongly, opium smoking had become associated with Chinese laborers who had immigrated to the United States following the Civil War to work on the railroads. Meanwhile, China itself began a vigorous campaign against opium, viewing it as symbol of Western imperialism.* These events

---

*In the eighteenth and nineteenth centuries, England profited enormously from Chinese purchase of opium obtained through the British colony in India. The Opium Wars of the mid-1800s at least partially revolved around the desire of Western powers to maintain this lucrative drug trade against China's wishes. Although the United States was not a participant in the wars, it benefited from favorable trade agreements negotiated after the conclusion of hostilities.

culminated in the convening of the first International Opium Conference in 1911, where participating countries each agreed to enact their own legislation restricting narcotic drug use except for legitimate medical purposes.

It took the United States several more years for its antinarcotic law to pass, the Harrison Act of 1914. A major reason for the delay was lobbying by drug and patent medicine manufacturers who objected to the initial wording of the bill. The Act was designed to regulate the dispensing and use of opiates (opium and its derivatives such as morphine) and cocaine by means of the following provisions:

1. Use of these substances for nonmedical purposes was prohibited.
2. Pharmacists and physicians were required to register with the Treasury Department and to keep records of their inventory of narcotics.
3. Retail sellers of narcotics and practicing physicians had to pay a yearly $1 tax to the federal government.
4. Patent medicines containing small amounts of opium, morphine, heroin, or cocaine remained legal and could continue to be sold by mail order or in retail establishments.

Because of the third and fourth provisions, we can see that the principal aims of the Harrison Act were to control rather than abolish the use of opiates and cocaine and to link narcotic use with government revenue through taxation (it's worth noting that during the Prohibition era, the federal government finally managed to convict the notorious gangster Al Capone not on alcohol trafficking per se, but rather on tax evasion!).

Many physicians had previously been providing maintenance doses of opiates or cocaine to patients who were addicted to these substances. However, because addiction was not considered a disease by government authorities at that time, one immediate effect of the Harrison Act was to cut addicts off from this source of drugs. The consequences are easily predicted. Addicts were forced to turn to street dealers and the prices skyrocketed. According to Hollinger (1995), the cost of heroin increased from $6.50 per ounce to roughly $100 (a huge sum in the early 1900s). People who could not afford to pay these prices were forced into abstinence and withdrawal. One result of these events was the establishment of many municipal clinics to treat drug addicts. The clinic in New York City registered approximately 7700 patients between April 1919 and March 1920 (Morgan, 1981). Unfortunately, these clinics failed to solve the problem, since most addicts went back to using street drugs soon after their treatment, and illegal drug sales continued to flourish.

The Harrison Act did not regulate the use of alcohol, which had nevertheless been a major social problem in the United States for many years. As a consequence of increasing support for the alcohol temperance movement mentioned previously, the Eighteenth Amendment to the Constitution went into effect in 1920. The new Prohibition law banned the dispensing of any beverage with an alcohol content greater than 0.5 % (1/10 the typical alcohol content of regular beer) except by physicians for medicinal purposes. Once again, the consequences were disastrous. Speakeasies (establishments where alcohol was sold illegally) sprang up everywhere, and the organized crime movement really took off during this period. The experiment in Prohibition finally ended in 1933.

Cannabis was another substance disregarded by the Harrison Act. The practice of marijuana smoking was initially associated with Mexican immigrants who entered the United States in the early 1900s. After World War I, public opposition to marijuana grew, and eventually numerous state laws were passed against its possession or sale. The federal government subsequently entered the picture with the passage of the Marijuana Tax Act of 1937. This law was similar to the Harrison Act in banning nonmedical use of cannabis and levying a tax on importers, sellers, and dispensers of marijuana.

The Marijuana Tax Act was declared unconstitutional and overturned by the United States Supreme Court in 1969. But in the very next year, the federal government passed a much broader law meant to apply to all potentially addictive substances. This was the Comprehensive Drug Abuse Prevention and Control Act (sometimes called the Controlled Substances Act [CSA]) of 1970. The CSA replaced or updated virtually all previous federal legislation concerning narcotic drugs and other substances thought to have abuse or addiction potential. Among other provisions, the CSA established five schedules of controlled substances, which are discussed later in this chapter. It also created the Drug Enforcement Agency (DEA), which was charged with enforcement of the CSA. Although this law has been revised several times since its inception, it remains the cornerstone of federal drug control legislation. Moreover, many states have adopted the Uniform Controlled Substances Act, a model drug control law patterned after the CSA.

Several conclusions emerge from this brief survey of the history of federal drug laws. The first is that each time the federal government became more involved in drug regulation, the action resulted from increases in drug use and/or perceived societal dangers posed by such use. Those who wish to make drug laws more lenient must start by changing such antidrug perceptions. The second conclusion is that existing laws are not entirely consistent with available medical and scientific evidence. For example, we will see later that nicotine (obtained via tobacco) is more addictive than marijuana by all established criteria, yet tobacco smoking is legal whereas marijuana smoking is not. A final conclusion is that legal mechanisms have only limited effectiveness in preventing drug use. This is most obvious in the events that occurred during Prohibition, as well as the current widespread use of marijuana. We acknowledge that cocaine and heroin use would almost certainly be greater than it is now if those substances were legal. But millions of people have little trouble obtaining cocaine, heroin, or any other illicit drug they desire. Many would argue that a more important restraint on drug use is the individual's own concerns that a particular substance might harm her health, jeopardize other important goals or values, or put her at risk for becoming addicted to that substance.

Features of Drug Abuse and Dependence

Drug addiction is a chronic, relapsing behavioral disorder

Before proceeding further, try writing down your definition of drug addiction in one or two sentences. Were you easily able to come up with a satisfactory definition? If not, don't be concerned, because addiction is not a simple concept. This problem was highlighted by Burglass and Shaffer (1984) in the following (not entirely frivolous) description of addiction: "Certain individuals use certain substances in certain ways thought at certain times to be unacceptable by certain other individuals for reasons both certain and uncertain." The medical establishment has attempted to develop a broadly acceptable definition, yet experts continue to disagree about what it means to be addicted to a drug (Walters and Gilbert, 2000).

Early views of drug addiction emphasized the importance of physical dependence. As you learned in Chapter 1, this means that abstinence from the drug leads to highly unpleasant withdrawal symptoms that motivate the individual to reinstate his or her drug use. It is true that some drugs of abuse, such as alcohol and opiates, can create strong physical dependence and severe withdrawal symptoms in dependent individuals. Certain other substances, however, produce relatively minor physical dependence. It may surprise you to learn that cocaine is one such substance, and that there was a time when cocaine was not considered to be addictive because of this lack of an opiate-like withdrawal syndrome.

Recent conceptions of addiction have focused more on other features of this phenomenon. First, there is an emphasis on behavior, specifically the compulsive nature of drug seeking and drug use in the addict. The addict is often driven by a strong urge to take the drug, which is called drug **craving.** Second, addiction is thought of as a chronic, relapsing disorder. This means that individuals remain addicted for long periods of time, and that drug-free periods (**remissions**) are often followed by **relapses** in which drug use recurs. In recent years, the medical profession has classified obesity in much the same way, since obese people typically struggle to lose weight for many years (sometimes their whole lives), go on frequent diets during which they lose some weight (remissions), and almost always regain the weight after each diet (relapse). A third important feature is that drug use persists despite serious harmful consequences to the addict. This is the paradox of addiction mentioned earlier in the chapter. One widely cited definition of addiction that encompasses the first two of the three features just described is as follows: "a behavioral pattern of drug use, characterized by overwhelming involvement with the use of a drug (compulsive use), the securing of its supply, and a high tendency to relapse after withdrawal" (Goldstein, 1989).

The term *addiction* has strong negative emotional associations for most of us. Despite the fact that drug addicts live in all parts of the country and come from all walks of life, we usually think of them as urban and poor. Our mental images are those of an unwashed heroin user huddled in an alley "shooting up" with a dirty syringe, or an emaciated "crackhead" engulfed in a cloud of cocaine vapor in an inner-city crack house, or a wino staggering down the street begging for a little change to buy his next bottle. Although some drug addicts fit these images, many others do not. For this reason as well as the conflicting definitions of addiction, the American Psychiatric Association stopped using the terms *addiction* and *addict* in its professional writings. This can be seen in the association's *Diagnostic and Statistical Manual of Mental Disorders (DSM)* (American Psychiatric Association, 2000). The *DSM* represents an attempt to classify the entire range of psychiatric disorders, with objective criteria provided for the diagnosis of each disorder. Instead of using the term *drug addiction,* the *DSM* specifies a group of substance-related disorders, where *substance* refers to typical drugs of abuse as well as some psychoactive medications that have abuse potential. Within the category of substance-related disorders are two general disorders called **substance dependence** and **substance abuse.** Substance dependence, which is the more severe disorder, corresponds roughly to the notion of addiction. Substance abuse is a less severe disorder that may or may not lead subsequently to substance dependence. The diagnostic criteria for these disorders are shown in Table 8.2. You can see that there is no single criterion for either substance abuse or substance dependence. This reflects the fact that maladaptive drug use may result in many different adverse consequences, depending on which drug is being taken as well as the amount and pattern of drug taking. Of course, someone with a long-standing, severe case of substance dependence may meet virtually all of the listed criteria, not just three or four.

In addition to the general categories of substance dependence and substance abuse, the *DSM* also includes specific diagnostic criteria for the abuse of or dependence on alcohol, amphetamines, cannabis, cocaine, hallucinogens, inhalants, nicotine, opioid drugs such as heroin, phencyclidine (PCP), and sedative–hypnotic and anxiolytic (antianxiety) drugs. All of these compounds are covered in detail in subsequent chapters of the book. Finally, the *DSM* identifies a number of **substance-induced disorders** involving the acute intoxicating

TABLE 8.2 *DSM-IV* Criteria for Substance Dependence and Substance Abuse

The following are *DSM-IV* criteria for substance dependence:

A maladaptive pattern of substance use leading to clinically significant impairment of distress, as manifested by three (or more) of the following, occurring at any time in the same 12-month period:

1. Tolerance, as defined by either of the following:

    a. A need for markedly increased amounts of the substance to achieve intoxication or designed effect

    b. Markedly diminished effect with continued use of the same amount of the substance

2. Withdrawal, as manifested by either of the following:

    a. The characteristic withdrawal syndrome for the substance

    b. The same (or a closely related) substance is taken to relieve or avoid withdrawal symptoms

3. The substance is often taken in larger amounts or over a longer period than was intended

4. There is a persistent desire or unsuccessful efforts to cut down or control substance use

5. A great deal of time is spent in activities necessary to obtain the substance (e.g., visiting multiple doctors or driving long distances), use the substance (e.g., chain-smoking), or recover from its effects

6. Important social, occupational, or recreational activities are given up or reduced because of substance use

7. The substance use is continued despite knowledge of having a persistent or recurrent physical or psychological problem that is likely to have been caused or exacerbated by the substance (e.g., current cocaine use despite recognition of cocaine-induced depression, or continued drinking despite recognition that an ulcer was made worse by alcohol consumption).

The following are *DSM-IV* criteria for substance abuse:

A. A maladaptive pattern of substance use leading to clinically significant impairment or distress, as manifested by one (or more) of the following, occurring within a 12-month period:

    1. Recurrent substance use resulting in a failure to fulfill major role obligations at work, school, or home (e.g., repeated absences or poor work performance related to substance use; substance-related absences, suspensions or expulsions from school; neglect of children or household)

    2. Recurrent substance use in situations in which it is physically hazardous (e.g., driving an automobile or operating a machine when impaired by substance use)

    3. Recurrent substance-related legal problems (e.g., arrests for substance-related disorderly conduct)

    4. Continued substance use despite having persistent or recurrent social or interpersonal problems caused or exacerbated by the effects of the substance (e.g., arguments with spouse about consequences of intoxication, physical fights)

B. The symptoms have never met the criteria for Substance Dependence for this class of substance.

Source: From American Psychiatric Association, 2000.

effects of particular substances as well as withdrawal symptoms in cases where such symptoms have been well characterized.

It is important to note that mere use of any drug, whether alcohol, tobacco, marijuana, cocaine, or heroin, does not constitute substance abuse or dependence. As indicated in the *DSM*, the use must be maladaptive, which means that harm is occurring to the user. Someone who snorts cocaine occasionally may be doing something illegal and dangerous, in that there is a potential for harm and for the subsequent development of a pattern of abuse or dependence. But if the *DSM* criteria for substance abuse or dependence are not met, then we cannot claim that the person is an addict or even that she is abusing the drug.

There are two types of progressions in drug use

Drug use can involve two different kinds of progressions. In one type of progression characteristic of many young peo-ple, the individual starts out taking a legal substance such as alcohol or tobacco, later progresses to marijuana, and in a small percentage of cases moves on to cocaine, heroin, other illicit substances, or illegally obtained prescription drugs. One theory that attempts to account for this type of progression is discussed in Box 8.1.

The second kind of progression pertains to changes in the amount, pattern, and consequences of drug use as they affect the user's health and functioning. This progression can be portrayed as a **continuum of drug use** (Figure 8.4). Once an individual first experiments with an abused drug, he may or may not progress to regular, nonproblem use or beyond. Despite the popular view that drugs like cocaine and heroin are instantly and automatically addictive, that is not the case. Why, then, do some people who experiment with these (or other) substances become dependent, while others do not? This is one of the central questions that must be addressed by any good theory or model of drug addiction.

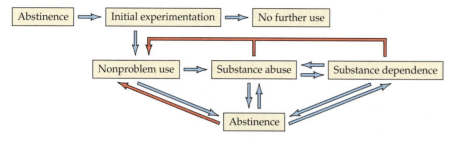

Figure 8.4 The continuum of drug use Over the course of their drug use history, individuals may move frequently from one stage to another along the continuum. The red lines represent possible movement to nonproblem drug use from a stage of substance abuse, substance dependence, or abstinence (in a previously abusing or dependent person). Whether or not individuals can successfully make such changes in their drug use is discussed later in the chapter.

Another important feature of drug use shown in Figure 8.4 is that people can move in both directions along the continuum. Regardless of whether they're using heroin, cocaine, or alcohol, long-term drug addicts often have a history of numerous shifts along the continuum involving changes in the frequency and amount of drug use as well as periodic intervals of abstinence that are often associated with participation in a treatment program or incarceration in prison. Figure 8.5 illustrates one example of this phenomenon taken from a longitudinal study of male opioid (heroin) addicts in

San Antonio, Texas (Maddux and Desmond, 1981). The figure presents drug status data over periods ranging from 7 to 20 years for 10 representative subjects out of a total of nearly 250. Particularly striking is the diversity of patterns among the subjects. For example, subject 111 exhibited periods of either occasional or daily use interspersed with long intervals of abstinence. In contrast, subject 162 used daily for most of the 20-year period except when he was institutionalized in a hospital or prison. When considered across all 10 subjects, the numerous instances of abstinence followed by renewed drug use supports the view mentioned earlier that addiction is a chronic, relapsing disorder.

For many people, the use of both alcohol and illicit drugs such as marijuana naturally declines once they reach adulthood and begin to take on the responsibilities associated with earning a living and having a family. This pattern is consistent with the data shown in Figure 8.1 as well as longitudinal studies documenting a reduction in drug use beyond the period of adolescence (Chen and Kandel, 1995). Some writers have called this process "maturing out" of a drug-using lifestyle. There are scattered reports that maturing out may even occur in some cases of substance dependence and not merely heavy use; however, recovery from substance dependence is a complex process that cannot be accounted for by any single factor (Waldorf, 1983).

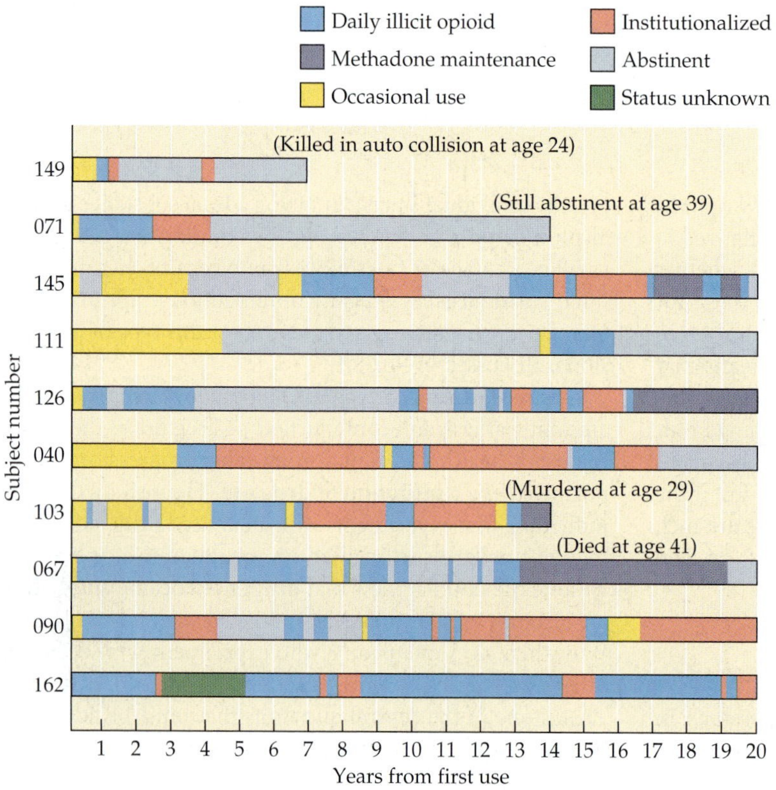

Which drugs are the most addictive?

Just as we all have mental images of drug addicts, we also have ideas about which drugs are the most addictive. Drugs thought to have a high addictive potential are sometimes called "hard drugs." There are two sets of standards by which we might classify drugs according to their addictive potential. The first are legal standards. As discussed earlier, the Controlled Substances Act of 1970 established a system by which most substances with abuse potential are classified into one of five different schedules. These schedules, along with representa-

Figure 8.5 Patterns of opioid drug use over a 20-year period in ten heroin addicts (After Maddux and Desmond, 1981.)

BOX 8.1

Drugs and Society

The "Gateway" Theory of Drug Use

Numerous studies of adolescent drug use have shown that there is a typical sequence of use, such that teenagers or preteens usually use alcohol and/or cigarettes before trying marijuana. Some of these studies further indicate that almost all adolescents who become involved with illicit drugs other than marijuana don't start with those drugs, but instead begin with alcohol or cigarettes and then marijuana. Results from one representative study are illustrated in the table. The data were obtained from a sample of 1108 twelfth-grade students (540 males and 568 females) attending public or private schools in New York State in 1988. It is readily apparent that within this subject population, alcohol and cigarettes tended to be used first, followed by marijuana, and then by cocaine. Initial use of crack cocaine occurred either after other forms of the drug (that is, powdered cocaine) or sometimes at the same time (Kandel and Yamaguchi, 1993).

Findings such as these have led to the "gateway" theory of adolescent drug progression. According to this theory, individuals who drink or smoke cigarettes are at increased risk for going on to marijuana use, and marijuana use in turn raises a person's risk of trying other, more dangerous substances such as cocaine. Thus, alcohol and cigarettes are "gateways" for marijuana, and marijuana is a gateway for other illicit drugs (Kandel et al., 1992).

Because of its apparently strong experimental support, the gateway theory has become widely accepted by many researchers, counselors, and drug policy makers. A massive effort has been made to reduce adolescent use of proposed gateway drugs (for example, the DARE Program), in the hope that this will diminish the num-ber of people who later become dependent on substances such as cocaine or heroin. However, objections to the gateway theory can be raised on at least two different grounds. First, the studies upon which the theory is based have been carried out mainly using school surveys. The majority of drug users in a typical high school are probably occasional rather than heavy or "hard-core" users, particularly if we focus on illicit drugs other than marijuana. This is not only because hard-core users represent a relatively small percentage of the adolescent population, but also because these individuals often drop out of school.

Since many of the destructive effects of drugs on our society arise from hard-core use, we need to ask whether a progression from alcohol and cigarettes to marijuana and then beyond is characteristic of heavy drug users. Two studies of serious drug abusers in New York City have addressed this question. In one study of 994 subjects, most of whom had used cocaine and other illicit substances, marijuana use reliably occurred before that of cocaine or other "hard" drugs. However, in contrast to the prediction of the gateway theory, marijuana was often the first substance used, even before alcohol (Golub and Johnson, 1994). Another study carried out on 233 regular cocaine and heroin users found that the standard progression of alcohol to marijuana to "hard" drugs was true for only 33% of the subjects (Mackesy-Amiti et al., 1997). The remainder showed several different patterns, sometimes starting with alcohol, then proceeding to illicit drugs other than marijuana and then marijuana (17%); or starting with marijuana before any other drugs (28%); or even starting off with other illicit drugs and then later taking up marijuana and alcohol (22%). These findings suggest that the standard gateway theory may not be a good predictor of the progression of drug use for many people who go on to become hard-core users.

Second, even if we stick to the adolescent population usually considered in the gateway theory, the causal rela-

(continued on next page)

Pairwise Comparison of the Order of Age of Initiation for Five Classes of Drugs among Twelfth Graders Who Used Both Classes of Drugs

		Proportion of Specified Ordering			
Drug A	Drug B	Drug A before B (%)	Same age (%)	Drug B before A (%)	Total (n)
Alcohol	Cigarettes	47.2	24.9	27.9	789
Alcohol	Marijuana	80.3	15.0	4.7	578
Alcohol	Crack	96.1	0.0	3.9	118
Cigarettes	Marijuana	70.8	20.7	8.5	534
Cigarettes	Any cocaine	89.7	9.1	1.1	143
Cigarettes	Crack	89.7	5.9	4.4	32
Marijuana	Any cocaine	88.0	11.2	0.8	150
Marijuana	Crack	82.6	7.0	10.4	36
Any cocaine	Crack	44.2	42.5	13.3	35

Source: From Kandel and Yamaguchi, 1993.

BOX 8.1 (continued)

tionships implied by the theory are difficult to prove. It may be the case, for example, that most adolescent cocaine users tried marijuana first. But merely demonstrating this fact is far from proving that the marijuana use somehow *caused* the individual to progress to cocaine, particularly since most adolescent marijuana users do *not* progress to more-addictive substances. Indeed, Morral and coworkers (2002) found that the relationship between marijuana use and progression to hard drugs could be accounted for by a common factor they called drug use propensity, which refers to the tendency to use both marijuana and other illicit drugs. Other researchers have proposed a more general alternative to the gateway theory termed either the common syndrome theory or the problem behavior theory. According to this idea, certain adolescents exhibit a

number of problem behaviors, such as delinquency, sexual promiscuity, misconduct, parental defiance, and substance use, all of which "reflect a single, underlying factor" (Donovan and Jessor, 1985). This proposed personality factor would increase an individual's likelihood of experimenting with more-addictive substances. Furthermore, the observed progression that is usually taken as support for the gateway theory might be due to differences in availability and perceived risk. Even though alcohol and cigarettes cannot be purchased legally by minors, they are nevertheless readily available and are often considered harmless by young people. Likewise, marijuana is more easily obtained than drugs like cocaine and heroin, and its use would be considered less risky. Finally, as individuals exhibiting problem behaviors move through their teenage years into late adoles-

cence and young adulthood, they may develop a belief that taking riskier substances is necessary to demonstrate their newfound maturity.

In summary, there is a well-described progression of substance use among adolescents, although this pattern may differ somewhat for those who eventually become serious drug abusers. The gateway theory proposes that initial use of alcohol and/or cigarettes increases an adolescent's risk of progressing to marijuana and that marijuana use is a risk factor for "hard" drugs such as cocaine and heroin. Yet it remains to be demonstrated that there is a causal connection involved in the progression of drug use. Moreover, there are alternative approaches such as the problem behavior theory that may be able to account for a progression of drug use without one substance serving as a gateway for another.

---

tive drugs, are shown in Table 8.3. Schedule I substances are considered to have no medicinal value and thus can be obtained only for research use by registered investigators.* Items listed under Schedules II to V are available for medicinal purposes with a prescription from a medical professional such

*For all controlled substances, but particularly for Schedule I and II items, there are strict federal requirements for investigator registration, ordering, and recordkeeping. The substances must be maintained securely, such as in a locked safe, with careful control over who has access to the drug supply.

TABLE 8.3 Schedule of Controlled Substances

Schedule	Description	Representative substances
I	Substances that have no accepted medical use in the U.S. and have a high abuse potential	Heroin, LSD, mescaline, marijuana, THC, MDMA
II	Substances that have a high abuse potential with severe psychic or physical dependence liability	Opium, morphine, codeine, meperidine (Demerol), cocaine, amphetamine, methylphenidate (Ritalin), pentobarbital, phencyclidine (PCP)
III	Substances that have an abuse potential less than those in Schedules I and II, including compounds containing limited quantities of certain narcotics and nonnarcotic drugs	Paregoric, barbiturates other than those listed in another schedule
IV	Substances that have an abuse potential less than those in Schedule III	Phenobarbital, chloral hydrate, diazepam (Valium), alprazolam (Xanax)
V	Substances that have an abuse potential less than those in Schedule IV, consisting of preparations containing limited amounts of certain narcotic drugs generally for antitussive (cough suppressant) and antidiarrheal purposes	

as a physician, dentist, or veterinarian. They can also be obtained for research use. Note that the **Schedule of Controlled Substances** specifically excludes alcohol and tobacco, thus permitting these substances to be purchased and used legally without registration or prescription.

The Schedule of Controlled Substances was formulated more than 30 years ago and was based not only on the scientific knowledge of that time but also partly on political considerations. Although it has been updated periodically since its inception, we may still ask whether this classification system accurately reflects our current understanding of various abused substances. For example, marijuana and its major active ingredient, Δ^9-tetrahydrocannabinol (THC), are in Schedule I, which means that they are considered to have no medicinal value as well as a high level of abuse potential. In Chapter 13, we discuss the possibility that marijuana or THC may be useful in some therapeutic situations. For now, let's consider the second point regarding marijuana's potential for producing abuse or dependence.

Several years ago, two leading addiction experts rated various substances for their abuse potential in five different categories: (1) presence and severity of *withdrawal* symptoms; (2) strength of the drug's *reinforcing* effects based on human and animal studies; (3) degree of *tolerance* produced by the drug; (4) degree of *dependence* produced by the drug based on difficulty quitting, relapse rates, and the percentage of users who become dependent; and (5) degree of *intoxication*

produced by the drug. The ratings were made by Dr. Jack Henningfield, formerly Chief of Clinical Pharmacology at the Addiction Research Center of the National Institute on Drug Abuse, and Dr. Neil Benowitz, a prominent addiction researcher at the University of California at San Francisco. Their ratings are shown in Table 8.4, with 1 representing the most serious and 6 being the least serious. We can see that the two sets of ratings are fairly consistent with each other in most cases. Furthermore, if we determine the combined mean ratings for each substance across categories, the results indicate that heroin was considered the most problematic substance (mean rating of 1.9), followed by alcohol (2.5) and cocaine (2.65), and then nicotine (3.35). The least problematic substances were caffeine (5.0) and marijuana (5.4). It is important to remember that the above rating system did not account for the long-term health consequences of using these substances, only their abuse potential based on the listed criteria. Not only is this obviously important for tobacco smoking and lung disease, but there is also evidence for potentially serious consequences of heavy marijuana use over long periods of time (see Chapter 13). Nevertheless, the disparity between current scientific opinion (at least as represented by these two experts) and the Schedule of Controlled Substances is striking. Two of the top four substances in terms of their abuse liability (alcohol and nicotine) are legal, whereas one of the two least problematic substances (marijuana) is classified in Schedule I. At some point in the future,

TABLE 8.4 Abuse Potential of Different Substances as Rated by Two Addiction Experts[a]

Substance	Category				
	Withdrawal	Reinforcement	Tolerance	Dependence	Intoxication
Henningfield ratings					
Nicotine	3	4	2	1	5
Heroin	2	2	1	2	2
Cocaine	4	1	4	3	3
Alcohol	1	3	3	4	1
Caffeine	5	6	5	5	6
Marijuana	6	5	6	6	4
Benowitz ratings					
Nicotine	3.5	4	4	1	6
Heroin	2	2	2	2	2
Cocaine	3.5	1	1	3	3
Alcohol	1	3	4	4	1
Caffeine	5	5	3	5	5
Marijuana	6	6	5	6	4

Source: From Hilts, 1994.

[a] In this rating system, 1 = most serious, 6 = least serious. Note that for the category of withdrawal, Benowitz gave equal ratings of 3 to nicotine and cocaine, and ratings of 4 and 5 to caffeine and marijuana, respectively. These ratings were altered as shown so that every category would add up to the same value.

the political climate in this country might be more receptive than it is now to bringing federal regulations in line with the weight of scientific evidence.

Section Summary

High levels of drug use continue in our society despite significant governmental attempts to control such use. Although early ideas about addiction emphasized the role of physical dependence, recent conceptions have focused on the compulsive features of drug seeking and use (despite the potentially harmful consequences) and the concept of drug addiction as a chronic, relapsing disorder characterized by repeated periods of remission followed by relapses. The *DSM* specifies a disorder called substance dependence, the characteristics of which correspond closely to those usually associated with addiction. Maladaptive drug use that does not meet the criteria for substance dependence is called substance abuse.

Young people often progress from legal substances like alcohol or tobacco to marijuana, and some even go on to try cocaine, heroin, or illegally obtained prescription drugs. The gateway theory attempts to account for this progression, although other explanations have also been offered to explain the same findings. A second kind of progression consists of movement along a continuum of drug use. Movement may occur in both directions along this continuum, and even in heavy users, there are often periods of abstinence interspersed among the intervals of regular drug consumption.

The Schedule of Controlled Substances classifies drugs with abuse potential into five categories, or schedules, based on their abuse potential and medicinal value. Alcohol and tobacco are not listed on the schedule, so they can be purchased for recreational use and without a prescription. Although the Schedule of Controlled Substances is a reasonable classification system in most cases, it is not entirely consistent with current scientific knowledge concerning the abuse liability and potential medicinal use of certain substances, particularly marijuana.

Models of Drug Abuse and Dependence

Over the years, many different explanations of drug abuse, dependence, and addiction have been proposed. Some of these explanations are meant to be mutually exclusive (that is, both explanations cannot be true at the same time). In other cases, however, two competing explanations might recognize many of the same factors as contributing to maladaptive drug-taking behavior but place a different emphasis on certain factors above others. For this reason, it is appropriate to talk about "models" rather than "theories" of addiction. In this section of the chapter, we discuss several of the most influential models of drug abuse, dependence, and addiction. Each model is summarized and then its strengths and weaknesses are evaluated with respect to our current understanding of addictive behaviors.

The physical dependence model emphasizes the withdrawal symptoms associated with drug abstinence

One important model of addiction is the **physical dependence model.** As mentioned earlier, certain drugs of abuse such as opiates (for example, heroin or morphine) and alcohol can lead to physical dependence when taken repeatedly. Some researchers have proposed that this process plays a key role in the establishment and maintenance of drug addiction. The simplest form of the physical dependence model is illustrated in Figure 8.6. According to this model, once an individual has become physically dependent due to repeated drug use, attempts at abstinence lead to highly unpleasant withdrawal symptoms (also called an **abstinence syndrome**). This motivates the user to take the drug again (relapse) to alleviate the symptoms. In the language of learning theory, relief of withdrawal symptoms promotes drug-taking behavior through a process of negative reinforcement, thus leading ultimately to a continuous behavioral loop consisting of repeated abstinence attempts followed by relapses.*

One of the most influential proponents of the physical dependence model was Abraham Wikler, who studied and

---

*Recall that negative reinforcement refers to the concept of reinforcement by removal of an undesirable stimulus (in this case, painful or distressing withdrawal symptoms).

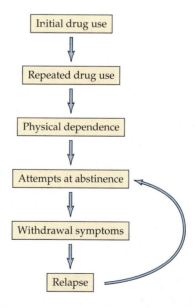

Figure 8.6 The physical dependence model of addiction

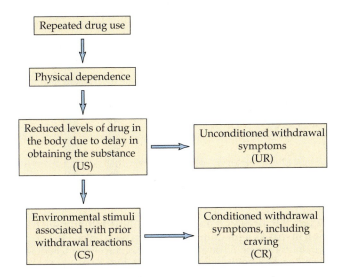

Figure 8.7 Development of conditioned drug withdrawal responses in dependent drug users US, unconditioned stimulus; UR, unconditioned response; CS, conditioned stimulus; CR, conditioned response.

treated heroin addicts over a period of several decades. Due to lack of money or other factors, addicts do not have constant access to heroin. Over time, therefore, they are likely to undergo many episodes of withdrawal. Wikler argued that if these withdrawal reactions repeatedly occur in specific environments, such as the places where the addict either "hustles" for or takes the drug, the responses will become classically conditioned to the stimuli associated with those environments (Wikler, 1980). Consequently, even if an addict has been drug free for some length of time and is therefore no longer experiencing an acute abstinence syndrome, withdrawal symptoms can be triggered by exposure to the conditioned stimuli (Figure 8.7).

As shown in the figure, drug craving is considered to be one of the crucial symptoms associated with conditioned withdrawal. Anna Rose Childress, Charles O'Brien, and their colleagues at the University of Pennsylvania School of Medicine have been studying conditioned craving as well as other behavioral and physiological responses to drug-associated cues. For example, cocaine-dependent but not control subjects experienced a significant craving for cocaine, the desire for a cocaine-induced "rush" (see Chapter 11), and even the feeling of a "cocaine high" when watching a video that simulated a person obtaining, preparing, and then smoking crack cocaine (Childress et al., 1999; Figure 8.8). Brain scans measuring regional cerebral blood flow during the video watching showed that these subjective responses were correlated with increased activation of the amygdala and the anterior cingulate cortex along with decreased activation of the basal ganglia. Thus stimuli associated with the procurement and use of cocaine evoked craving and other drug-related responses as

well as specific changes in brain activity. The conditioned nature of these responses is shown by the fact they occurred only in the cocaine-dependent subjects, not in control subjects who had not had any experience with this substance.

Critique of the physical dependence model For drugs that produce significant physical dependence, such dependence undoubtedly is an important contributor to the maintenance of addiction because unpleasant withdrawal symptoms provide motivation to obtain and take the drug again. Nevertheless, there are several problems with the physical dependence model as a comprehensive explanation of addiction. First, as we mentioned earlier, some major drugs of abuse including cocaine do not produce strong physical dependence. How, then, do we explain addiction to these drugs? Second, although this model may help us understand what happens *after* a person becomes dependent, it does not account for the earlier drug use that led to development of the physical dependence. Third, the physical dependence model has a problem with relapse of addicts after they have gone through **drug detoxification** (elimination of the drug from one's system and passage through the abstinence syndrome). After the withdrawal symptoms have gone away, what still motivates an addict to take heroin again, for example?

Wikler explained relapse as being motivated by conditioned withdrawal and drug craving that are triggered by environmental stimuli associated with prior instances of

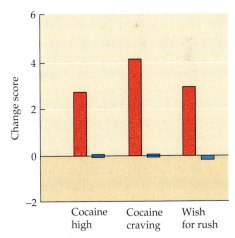

Figure 8.8 Subjective responses to a cocaine-related video were obtained from cocaine-dependent men and control subjects who had never taken cocaine. All subjects watched a 25-minute video depicting the acquisition and use of crack cocaine. Self-ratings of cocaine-related states were provided before and after the video, and change scores (after video minus before video) were determined. The cocaine-dependent group (red bars) showed significant increases in "cocaine high," "cocaine craving," and "wish for rush." For the control subjects, there was no change in "cocaine high" or "cocaine craving" and a small, statistically nonsignificant decrease in "wish for rush" (blue bars). (After Childress et al., 1999.)

withdrawal. Both human and animal studies have demonstrated that sensory stimuli can become conditioned to the effects of drug administration as well as drug withdrawal. But we do not yet have convincing evidence that such conditioning plays a role in the actual relapse of previously abstinent addicts. Whereas Wikler's subjects gave anecdotal accounts of sudden withdrawal symptoms when they encountered drug-associated stimuli on the street, subsequent studies have not consistently confirmed this finding. When questioned, addicts usually give other explanations for their relapse. Moreover, even if an addict experiences a sudden craving for the drug, cravings are more appropriately considered psychological rather than physiological responses and therefore do not support a strict physical dependence model. Thus, although physical dependence is one factor that can contribute to drug addiction, it does not provide a good overall addiction model, for the reasons stated above.

The positive reinforcement model is based on the rewarding and reinforcing effects of abused drugs

Whereas the physical dependence model emphasizes the role of negative reinforcement in drug addiction, the **positive reinforcement model** focuses on the ability of many abused drugs to serve as positively reinforcing stimuli. This means that consuming the drug strengthens whatever preceding behavior was performed by the organism. The rewarding and reinforcing properties of abused drugs have been demonstrated in numerous animal studies using several different experimental techniques. The most important of these procedures is drug self-administration, which was introduced in Chapter 4. As you will recall, an experimental animal such as a rat, mouse, or monkey is fitted with an intravenous catheter attached to a drug-filled syringe. When the animal performs an operant response such as pressing a lever, a pump is briefly activated that slightly depresses the plunger of the syringe and delivers a small dose of the drug directly into the subject's bloodstream. This is directly analogous to a drug addict giving himself an intravenous drug injection. The ability of animals to learn and maintain the lever-pressing response or for addicts to learn and maintain drug-seeking and drug-using behaviors means that the drug is acting as a reinforcer, just as food is a reinforcer for those who are hungry.

We can measure the relative strength of drug reinforcement using a **progressive-ratio** procedure. In this procedure, the animals are initially trained to lever-press on a continuous-reinforcement (CR) schedule, which means that each press is followed by drug delivery. In the second phase, the animals are switched to a low fixed-ratio (FR) schedule, such as an FR-5 (1 drug delivery for every 5 responses). Finally, the FR schedule is progressively increased until the animals stop responding, presumably because the dose being deliv-

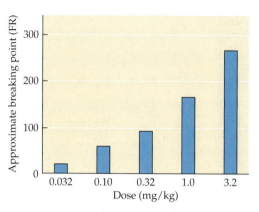

Figure 8.9 Breaking point for morphine self-administration in rats as a function of dose Rats were trained to self-administer morphine on a continuous-reinforcement schedule, then switched to a fixed-ratio (FR) schedule. The FR was increased daily (progressive-ratio schedule) until the breaking point was reached, as defined in this study by fewer than four drug injections in a day. The graph illustrates the estimated breaking points according to morphine dose per infusion. Within the dose range tested, it is clear that the drug's reinforcing properties rise dramatically as the dose is increased. (After Weeks and Collins, 1987.)

ered is not sufficiently reinforcing to support the amount of effort required. The response ratio at which responding ceases is called the **breaking point.** Breaking points vary across drugs and also across doses. What do you think is the relationship between dose and breaking point? If you guessed that breaking point generally increases with higher doses, then you were correct. This is illustrated in a study conducted by Weeks and Collins (1987) in which they compared the approximate breaking points for a range of morphine doses in rats. As the dose of morphine was increased, the breaking point also rose by a large amount (Figure 8.9). Keep in mind, however, that if the dose of the drug being tested becomes too high, determination of the breaking point may be compromised, either because the drug is exerting unpleasant side effects that reduce its reinforcing efficacy or because the drug is interfering with the lever-press response (for example, due to a sedating effect in the case of depressant drugs or to the elicitation of extreme hyperactivity or stereotyped behaviors in the case of psychostimulants).

Most drugs that are abused by humans are self-administered by animals, although some substances are more powerful reinforcers than others. Students sometimes wonder whether animals can become so addicted to drugs that they kill themselves. This actually can occur with cocaine and, to a lesser extent, with heroin if the subjects are given unlimited (around-the-clock) access to the drug by intravenous self-administration. Under such conditions, animals given cocaine will continue their self-administration even following full-blown seizures, and they become so disorganized in their other activities that they lose large amounts of body weight and stop grooming themselves before finally succumbing (Bozarth and Wise, 1985). For these reasons, researchers normally permit only a few hours per day of drug access when self-administration studies are being carried out.

Although no one would argue against the idea that abused drugs are reinforcing, a number of authors have pointed out that this doesn't explain *why* such reinforcement occurs. In other words, what does the drug do to a person or an animal that causes the organism to repeat the experience? At the neurobiological level, researchers have discovered that drugs of abuse engage (and in a sense "hijack") a system within the brain that's intimately involved in natural rewards (Box 8.2). This certainly helps us understand why such drugs can be so powerfully reinforcing. At the subjective level, drugs of abuse are often reported to cause **euphoria,** which means a feeling of well-being or elevated mood. We are, of course, referring to the "high" produced by many of these drugs. Human drug users can give us a verbal report of the drug-induced high, and we may speculate that animals experience something analogous to this feeling. Considering this additional factor, we can now present the positive reinforcement model in Figure 8.10. In this model, the euphoria produced by initial drug use serves as reinforcement for further use. When the user attempts to abstain from taking the drug, she suffers from a craving that can be conceptualized as an overwhelming desire to re-experience drug-induced euphoria. This craving then leads to relapse.

Critique of the positive reinforcement model

There are several strong points to the positive reinforcement model. The animal experiments we discussed support an important role for positive reinforcement in drug-taking behavior, and they also show how drugs of abuse interact with brain reward mechanisms. In addition, studies have shown that addicts greatly value the drug high and that a desire to get high is at least one important explanation (though not the only one) for relapse.

However, there are also some significant limitations of the positive reinforcement model of addiction. For example, users clearly display greater drug craving after many doses have been consumed than after the first few doses. Yet the magnitude of the drug high does not correlate with this increase in craving. Instead, there may be less of a high after many doses due to drug-induced tolerance. Moreover, controlled human studies have sometimes found dissociations between self-reported high and either the desire or willingness to work for the drug.

Even if drug use is acknowledged to be powerfully reinforcing, we may ask why the negative consequences of drug addiction (which may include such extreme effects as family breakup, loss of one's job and financial destitution, engaging in criminal activity to support drug purchases, damage to one's health, contracting needle-borne diseases such as AIDS or hepatitis, and even fatal overdose for some drugs) don't effectively counteract the positive reinforcement so that the individual stops using and remains abstinent. One possible answer concerns the temporal relationship between drug consumption and the positive or negative effects. Drug-induced euphoria occurs very quickly after consumption, particularly in the case of intravenous injection or inhalation (including smoking). In contrast, the negative consequences occur later in time and, in most cases, are linked to a long pattern of use rather than to a specific occasion of drug consumption. According to well-established principles of reinforcement, an event (euphoria) that occurs very soon after a response (drug consumption) exerts much greater control over that response than events (negative consequences) that occur later in time. Even for humans, who have the ability to plan and to foresee the consequences of their actions in ways that animals cannot, this property of reinforcers has considerable influence over many behaviors, not just drug use. On the other hand, many individuals who take drugs once or even a few times stop their drug use before they develop a compulsive pattern and become addicted. This is true even for highly reinforcing drugs like cocaine and heroin. Thus a significant problem with this model is its failure to account for why some individuals succumb to the reinforcing effects of drugs while others do not.

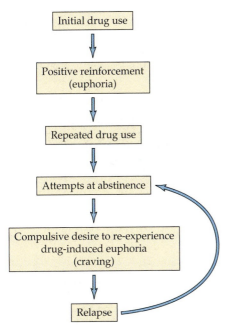

Figure 8.10 The positive reinforcement model of addiction

BOX 8.2

The Cutting Edge

Drugs of Abuse and the Neural Mechanisms of Reward

The positive reinforcement model proposes that addiction occurs due to the rewarding/euphoric effects of drugs. Is there a neural mechanism of reward that most or all drugs of abuse might be acting on to produce these effects? There does appear to be a neural "reward circuit," as indicated by the eagerness with which laboratory animals and even humans will electrically stimulate specific parts of their brain if given the opportunity. This phenomenon of intracranial self-stimulation (ICSS) was first demonstrated many years ago by James Olds and has been extensively studied since then. One important kind of evidence for an interaction between drugs of abuse and the reward circuit concerns drug-induced changes in the threshold for ICSS. Researchers can experimentally determine how much current must be delivered for the electrical stimulation to be reinforcing (that is, to promote an operant response such as lever pressing). The lower the threshold, the more sensitive is the reward circuit. As shown in the table, a variety of different abused drugs all reduce the threshold for ICSS when given acutely. Such results indicate that the underlying neural circuitry for drug reward overlaps with the circuitry for brain stimulation reward. On the other hand, withdrawal of animals from chronic treatment with these substances causes an increased ICSS threshold. A similar phenomenon occurring in a drug-dependent addict might contribute to the negative mood state and difficulty in experiencing pleasure that are often reported during withdrawal.

Another important link between abused drugs and reward mechanisms is provided by the neurotransmitter dopamine (DA). The mesolimbic DA pathway from the ventral tegmental area (VTA) to the nucleus accumbens is an important component of the reward circuit. Moreover, the same drugs that acutely reduce the threshold for ICSS also increase synaptic DA levels in the accumbens, either by enhancing the firing of VTA neurons (opiates, nicotine, ethanol, and THC) or by stimulating DA release and/or inhibiting DA reuptake from the nerve terminals (psychostimulants). Finally, just as withdrawal from these drugs leads to decreased brain reward (as indicated by elevated thresholds for ICSS), it can also produce subnormal DA levels in the nucleus accumbens.

These findings suggest that the mesolimbic DA pathway plays a significant role in the reinforcing effects of many (perhaps most) drugs of abuse. Further discussion on this topic can be found in later chapters covering specific drugs or drug classes. Here, however, we would like to dispel two widely held ideas about DA that are not correct: first, that enhanced DA transmission in the nucleus accumbens is always required for drug reinforcement, and second, that DA in the accumbens directly produces feelings of pleasure (or, in animals, whatever is analogous to human pleasure). Concerning the first point, there are several ways of experimentally testing whether the mesolimbic DA pathway from the VTA to the nucleus accumbens is essential for drug reinforcement. One of the most direct tests is to lesion the dopaminergic nerve terminals in the accumbens with the catecholamine neurotoxin 6-hydroxydopamine (6-OHDA) (see Chapter 5) and see whether this blocks drug self-administration. For the psychostimulants cocaine and amphetamine, self-administration *is* abolished by such lesions, lending strong support to the notion that accumbens DA is essential for the reinforcing effects of these compounds. In contrast, many other drugs including alcohol and heroin

Drug Effects on Thresholds for Rewarding Brain Stimulation

Drug class	Acute administration	Withdrawal from chronic treatment
Psychostimulants (cocaine, amphetamine)	↓	↑
Opiates (morphine, heroin)	↓	↑
Nicotine	↓	↑
Sedative–hypnotic drugs (ethanol)	↓	↑
THC	↓	↑

Manifest affective response — Underlying opponent processes — Stimulus event

Figure 8.
(After Solo

induced e
individu
drome is
More
have pre:
opponent
more spe
tive chan
ment of
Robinsor
hypothes
primary a
nic (pleas
sumption
process, v
is called **c**
be strengt
Corbit. A
model, h
set point
rienced by
ic user ex
mood sta
starting p

Figure 8.
process r
1977.)

BOX 8.2 (continued)

continue to be self-administered even after severe damage to the VTA–accumbens DA pathway. This does not rule out the possibility that DA release contributes to the reinforcing properties of these substances, but it does strongly argue that accumbens DA is not *required* for reinforcement by drugs other than cocaine and amphetamine.

The second idea of DA as the "pleasure neurotransmitter" has been even more pervasive, but it, too, is contradicted by various experimental findings. In one important set of studies carried out by Wolfram Schultz and his colleagues, the investigators recorded the firing of midbrain DA neurons (substantia nigra and VTA) in awake monkeys under different behavioral conditions (Schultz, 1998). As illustrated in the figure, these cells showed a burst of activity in response to a novel sensory stimulus or an unsignaled (unexpected) reward such as a food treat. Interestingly, if the reward was paired in a classical conditioning paradigm with a conditioned stimulus (CS) so that the CS reliably predicted the reward, DA cell firing came to be elicited by the CS rather than the reward itself. Finally, if the conditioned monkeys were presented with the CS and then no reward followed, there was actually a depression in DA cell firing. According to Schultz, therefore, one function of DA neuronal firing is to signal the difference between prediction and actual occurrence of rewards. An unpredicted reward leads to increased firing, a predicted reward causes no change, and the failure of a reward to occur after being predicted leads to a brief depression in cellular activity. Redgrave and coworkers (1999) offered an alternative hypothesis, namely that DA cell firing under these conditions is critically involved

in switching the animal's attention and behavior toward unexpected, behaviorally significant events that can include reward. In neither case is DA proposed to mediate "pleasure" per se.

An even more startling finding was obtained by a group of researchers headed by Mark Wightman (Garris et al., 1999). In this case, in vivo voltammetry was used to monitor DA release in the nucleus accumbens of rats during electrical stimulation of the VTA or substantia nigra. For most of the subjects, experimenter-controlled application of the electrical stimulus led to significant DA release in the accumbens. These animals learned to press a lever to obtain ICSS through the same electrode. Surprisingly, however, ICSS only evoked DA release during the beginning of a test session and not afterwards. Thus, as the sessions progressed, rats were repeatedly pressing the lever to obtain the rewarding brain stimulation without a measurable increase in DA transmission in the nucleus accumbens. These results are inconsistent with the idea that DA release in the accumbens mediates feelings of reward or pleasure.

We have seen that drugs of abuse interact with the neural circuit that mediates reward. Although the mesolimbic DA pathway from the VTA to the nucleus accumbens is part of this circuit and many drugs of abuse stimulate DA release in the accumbens, such release is required for drug reinforcement only in the case of cocaine, amphetamine, and closely related psychostimulants. DA seems to play some kind of role in the learning or anticipation of reward, or orienting toward salient stimuli, but it is clearly not a "pleasure transmitter" as is sometimes claimed.

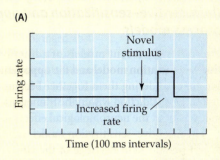
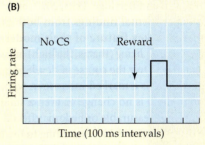
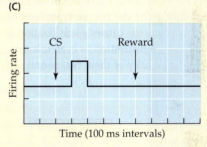
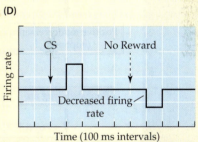

Dopamine cell firing under various behavioral conditions Under baseline conditions, midbrain DA cells in monkeys fire intermittently at a low rate, as depicted by the straight horizontal lines. Brief (about 100 ms long) bursts of firing occur in response to novel stimuli (A), presentation of an unexpected reward (B), and presentation of a CS associated with reward (C). If an expected reward is withheld, then DA cell firing is transiently suppressed (D).

Two relative
tive–sensitiz
We are consi
account for a
mation abou

The incen
Robinson an
(Robinson an
ous experim
research. A I
between drug
is, craving). C
argue, there i
though there
liking (the pl
the drug) (Fi;
ity occurs be
responsible f
repeated drug
tem but no se
tem. The ide

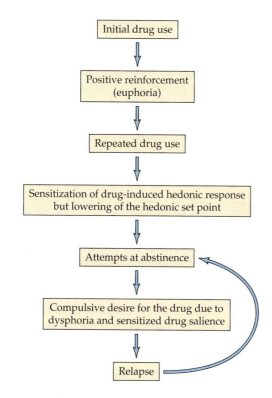

Figure 8.14   The opponent–process model of addiction

model is preferable to the physical dependence and positive reinforcement models. Comparing the two approaches, the incentive–sensitization model seems to provide a more satisfactory explanation of drug craving by addicts, whereas the opponent–process model is better at accounting for the dysphoria experienced by users during withdrawal and abstinence. Neither model, however, attempts to deal with the earliest stages of drug use when individuals first begin to experiment with these substances. In addition, these models incorporate only some of the many psychosocial factors that interact with neurobiological mechanisms in the development and maintenance of an addictive pattern of drug use.

The disease model treats addiction as a medical disorder

The most widely accepted model of addiction in our society is the **disease model.** Not only has this view been popularized in the mass media, but addicts themselves and their treatment providers usually ascribe to this model. The disease model of addiction arose from early work with alcoholics and remains most closely associated with alco-

holism. Benjamin Rush, the Philadelphia physician who founded the alcohol temperance movement, was also the first to consider alcoholism a disease. This view was later expanded and promoted by E. M. Jellinek in his influential book *The Disease Concept of Alcoholism* (Jellinek, 1960). For many years now, alcoholism has been formally considered a disease by medical organizations such as the World Health Organization and the American Medical Association. Indeed, the disease model is sometimes also called a **medical model.** Not surprisingly, it is the leading model used both in the professional treatment of alcoholics and other drug addicts (in 12-step programs, for example) and in self-help groups such as Alcoholics Anonymous (AA) and Narcotics Anonymous.

Despite the widespread popularity of the disease model, there remains some confusion about its exact nature. This is partly because there are two different types of disease models, which differ in their emphasis. Early disease models, such as the one proposed by Jellinek for alcoholism, can be called **susceptibility models.** As shown in Figure 8.15, this kind of model proposes that the disease of addiction stems primarily from an inherited susceptibility to uncontrolled drug use. In the case of Jellinek's alcoholism model, **loss of control** meant that once a vulnerable person took any amount of alcohol, he could not stop drinking until he became intoxicated. Likewise, if an individual with an inherited susceptibility to cocaine addiction began using cocaine, he would suffer a similar loss of control and become addicted to that substance. In a susceptibility model, therefore, "addicts are born, not made."

During the time when susceptibility models were first proposed, little was known about the genetic contributions to complex human traits. Geneticists now recognize that complex traits, including drug addiction, are controlled by many different genes working together and that these genetic influences interact in important ways with various social and environmental factors. Moreover, studies of long-term drug

Sens
salie

Cc
a :

Figure 8.11
addiction

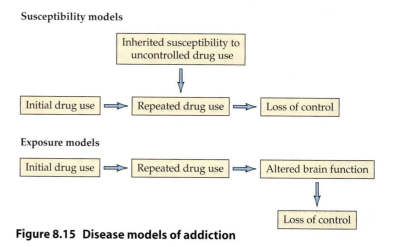

Figure 8.15   Disease models of addiction

effects on experimental animals along with the application of brain imaging techniques to drug-addicted subjects have shown that the structure and functioning of the brain can be altered dramatically by repeated exposure to substances of abuse. These findings have given rise to **exposure models** of addiction. According to this type of model, chronic drug use leads to significant alterations in the brain that are responsible for loss of control and the other key features of addictive behavior (Figure 8.15). Most current neuroscience-based disease models are variations on this theme. A general summary of such models was presented in an article entitled "Addiction Is a Brain Disease, and It Matters" by Alan Leshner, former Director of the National Institute on Drug Abuse. Leshner said, "That addiction is tied to changes in brain structure and function is what makes it, fundamentally, a brain disease. A metaphorical switch in the brain seems to be thrown as a result of prolonged drug use. Initially, drug use is a voluntary behavior, but when the switch is thrown, the individual moves into the state of addiction, characterized by compulsive drug seeking and use" (Leshner, 1997).

These two kinds of disease models are not mutually exclusive. Susceptibility models may include a role for drug-induced physiological (including neural) changes, and exposure models typically hypothesize that some individuals are more susceptible genetically to developing the neurobiological changes that lead to addiction. However, the difference in emphasis between these approaches has potential consequences for both research and clinical treatment. For example, one logical outcome of susceptibility models is that an addict must completely abstain from the substance, since loss of control is an inborn trait. As this kind of model underlies the teachings of AA as well as various 12-step treatment programs patterned after AA, such organizations and programs only permit complete abstinence as a treatment goal. In contrast, an exposure model might or might not require abstinence. It depends on whether the hypothesized neural changes are reversible or not. If it is possible for the addict's brain to return to a relatively normal state during a sufficient period of abstinence, then it might also be possible for the individual to begin using the substance again but in a controlled manner. There is some evidence, though controversial, that some people who are heavy alcohol users but not yet severely dependent can establish a pattern of controlled drinking (Rosenberg, 1993). However, substance abuse treatment providers rarely consider this option, based partly on their interpretation of the disease model and partly on their own clinical experience with failed attempts of clients to maintain controlled substance use. Consequently, clients are almost always advised to strive for total abstinence as the desired treatment outcome.

Critique of the disease model   The disease model has had a tremendously valuable impact on society's reaction toward drug abuse and addiction. For a long time, excessive drug use and addiction were seen primarily as signs of personal and moral weakness. Indeed, this earlier view has sometimes been termed a **moral model** of addiction. Initial development of the disease model sought to remove the social stigma of addiction (after all, no one *blames* you for coming down with a disease) and to involve the medical profession in helping addicts deal with their problem through treatment programs. It is important to note, though, that our society is still ambivalent about disease versus moral conceptions of drug use. Although you can get treatment for alcohol or tobacco abuse without fear of prosecution, because these substances are legal, abuse of heroin, cocaine, or marijuana often leads to a jail sentence instead of medical help.

A second key benefit of the disease model is reducing the sense of guilt experienced by the recovering addict. For example, there may be strong feelings of remorse for past problems caused by the person's drug use. If such problems are viewed as stemming from a disease, then the therapeutic process may benefit. As one alcoholic put it, "Calling it [alcoholism] a disease allows us to put the guilt aside so that we can do the work that we need to do" (Thombs, 1999, p. 71). In addition, even for a highly motivated individual in an intensive treatment program, there is a great likelihood that one or more lapses (brief instances of drug use) will occur before long-term abstinence is attained. The danger is that the resulting feelings of guilt and diminished self-worth will engender a sense of hopelessness that leads to a complete loss of control and full-blown relapse back into compulsive use. Belief that such lapses are the consequence of a disease process instead of a moral failing is thought to help the individual resist these destructive feelings, although it obviously does not guarantee a successful treatment outcome.

Despite its wide acceptance, however, the disease model of addiction has been criticized by some writers, both within and outside of the research community. To understand these criticisms, we must first consider what a disease is. According to one medical dictionary, a disease is "a pathological condition of the body that presents a group of clinical signs and symptoms and laboratory findings peculiar to it and that sets the condition apart as an abnormal entity differing from other normal or pathological body states" (Thomas, 1993). Let's see how this definition applies to a classical infectious disease such as bacterial pneumonia. The patient arrives at the doctor's office complaining of severe cough, shortness of breath, pain in the chest, chills, and a high fever. These are the clinical signs and symptoms that are the initial indicators of a possible diagnosis. The doctor suspects bacterial pneumonia and orders a chest X-ray and a sputum culture. The X-ray shows inflammation of the lungs and the culture comes back positive for *Pneumococcus,* one of the bacterial strains that cause pneumonia. These laboratory findings confirm a diagnosis of pneumococcal pneumonia and call for the patient to be placed on an appropriate antibiotic (which the doctor has probably already started based on her preliminary findings).

Do the same principles apply to addiction? Imagine a second patient arriving at the doctor's office with the following symptoms: he has had at least six or seven drinks of liquor almost every day for the past 8 years; he often has cravings for alcohol; he doesn't become drunk even after four or five drinks; if he doesn't drink any alcohol for a day or two, he becomes extremely irritable, anxious, and unable to sleep; he has tried to stop drinking numerous times without success; he recently lost his job due to repeated tardiness and absence from work; and he has been arrested twice for driving under the influence of alcohol. These are very clear signs and symptoms of alcohol dependence. Can the doctor now perform some laboratory tests to confirm the diagnosis? She might test his liver function and determine that he suffers from cirrhosis (a serious liver condition that occurs in some chronic alcoholics), but cirrhosis is a *consequence* of alcohol dependence, not a cause. In fact, there are no laboratory tests that can identify the etiology (cause) of an addictive process in the same way that a sputum culture can identify the source of someone's pneumonia or a tissue biopsy can identify the source of another person's cancer. Addiction or substance dependence can be diagnosed *only* through the clinical signs and symptoms.

One criticism of the disease model of addiction emphasizes this difference between addiction and most other recognized disease conditions (for example, see Schaler, 2000). However, a key counterargument is that *all* psychiatric disorders, not just addiction, must be diagnosed by means of the patient's mental and behavioral symptoms. Just as there are no blood tests or brain scans that can identify someone who is suffering from addiction (or, using *DSM* terminology, substance dependence), there are no laboratory tests that enable a psychiatrist to determine whether a patient has schizophrenia, major depression, or obsessive–compulsive disorder. Therefore, the lack of such a test for addiction cannot be used to disqualify it as a disease unless we are willing to similarly disqualify all other psychiatric disorders.

The fact that we presently have no anatomical, biochemical, or neurological tests to identify drug-addicted individuals does not conflict with the evidence mentioned earlier that chronic drug exposure can produce long-term alterations in brain structure and function. First of all, we do not yet know whether the same neural changes underlie all drug addictions. Researchers have long believed that what we call schizophrenia is actually a number of diseases that have been grouped together due to a core symptom cluster. The same could be true of addiction. Second, it is likely that complex *patterns* of neural abnormalities are responsible for psychiatric illnesses such as addiction. If so, then it will be difficult to find any one or two differences between drug-addicted and nonaddicted people that are sufficiently reliable to serve as diagnostic indicators.

A second criticism of the disease model stems from the observation that the levels of drug consumption and the behavioral symptoms of addiction lie on a continuum. There is no sharp dividing line between those we label addicts and nonaddicts either in the amount of drugs consumed or the behaviors used to characterize addiction. Consider Figure 8.16, which illustrates the distribution of alcohol purchases (including wine and distilled spirits such as whiskey, rum, gin, vodka, and liqueurs) within five areas of Ontario, Canada, during a single month in the early 1960s (de Lint and Schmidt, 1968). Clearly, nonproblem social drinkers lie toward the left-hand part of the distribution, whereas problem drinkers and alcoholics are in the right-hand part of the

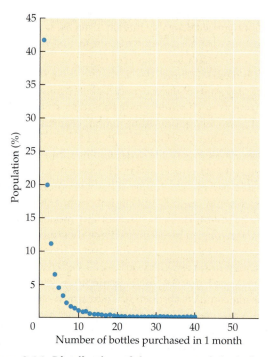

Figure 8.16 Distribution of the amount of alcohol purchased by 21,513 people over a 1-month period in Ontario, Canada. A survey of alcohol purchases (including wine and distilled spirits such as whiskey and other liquors, but not including beer) was conducted in the early 1960s within five areas of Ontario. The graph depicts the percentage of the population that purchased differing numbers of bottles of alcohol (from 1 to 40) over a 1-month period. Because of the lower alcohol content of wine compared to distilled spirits, each bottle of wine was only counted as a half bottle in the data analysis. It is apparent that during the sampling period, more than 40% of the surveyed people purchased one bottle or its equivalent, 20% purchased two bottles, about 11% purchased three bottles, and so forth. Note that data points from 20 to 40 that appear to be on the *x*-axis are not actually at zero, but represent percentages under 0.1% that cannot be discriminated on a graph this size. Furthermore, there are even a few individuals who purchased more than 40 bottles in 1 month who are not shown in the figure. (After de Lint and Schmidt, 1968.)

distribution. But there is nothing intrinsic to the graph that tells us where to draw the line. Even if we plotted the distribution of behavioral symptoms of alcohol dependence instead of alcohol purchases, there wouldn't be a clean break in the distribution telling us where to separate those who have the disease and those who do not.

Defenders of the disease model can point to other medical disorders that share this feature of addiction. Two such disorders are essential hypertension (high blood pressure that isn't a secondary consequence of a known disease process) and obesity. In both cases, there is a continuum of symptomatology (blood pressure and body weight, respectively) between healthy individuals and those suffering from the disease. Consequently, doctors have had to set arbitrary cutoff points to define the disease state. Moreover, most cases of hypertension and obesity are thought to result from a combination of interacting genetic, psychosocial, and behavioral factors, all of which must also be included in any comprehensive theory of addiction.

Finally, the disease model is criticized by theoreticians and practitioners who use behavioral approaches to understanding and treating substance abuse and addiction. While not excluding genetic and neurochemical factors, such approaches emphasize the role of learning and other cognitive processes in both the development and treatment of substance abuse problems (Rotgers, 1996). Accordingly, addiction is viewed not as a disease but as a behavior pattern that comes about due to an interaction between many factors, including the person's environment (for example, the availability of drugs and peer pressure to use them), behavioral modeling of drug use by others, the positive-reinforcing effects of abused drugs, the reinforcing consequences of avoiding or eliminating drug withdrawal, and conditioning to drug-related stimuli.

In summary, the disease model of addiction can be defended, but only with certain restrictions. First, we believe that classic susceptibility models like Jellinek's for alcoholism have too many problems to be given serious consideration. Exposure models emphasizing drug effects on brain function are more consistent with current research findings. Second, the idea that addicts possess distinctive qualities (whether genetic, neurochemical, psychological, or behavioral) that readily separate them from nonaddicts may not be correct. A better model may be one that places the signs and symptoms of addiction along a continuum, similar to what is done with essential hypertension or obesity. Third, it seems clear that a good model of addiction, whether a disease model or not, must incorporate multiple etiologic factors at all levels of analysis, from social to molecular. We offer some ideas along this line in the last section of the chapter. In the final analysis, it may not make much difference to researchers whether addiction is considered a disease or not, as long as the full range of contributory factors is acknowledged. As we mentioned earlier, however, the disease model continues to play a

central role in addiction treatment. As George Vaillant states in his landmark study of alcoholism, "In our attempts to *understand* and to *study* alcoholism, it behooves us to employ the models of the social scientist and of the learning theorist [we would also include the models of the neuroscientist]. But in order to *treat* alcoholics effectively, we need to invoke the model of the medical practitioner" (Vaillant, 1995, p. 22).

Toward a Comprehensive Model of Drug Abuse and Dependence

None of the models presented above attempts to provide a comprehensive account of drug abuse, dependence, or addiction. Indeed, no one has yet offered a complete model of this complex phenomenon. However, we hope in this final section to offer a glimpse of what a comprehensive addiction model might look like. This can be termed a **biopsychosocial model,** because it incorporates a range of biological, psychological, and sociological factors in explaining the phenomenon of addiction.

People who become addicted to drugs often began using these substances relatively early in life. Thus, it is important to understand the factors underlying initial experimentation with drugs of abuse, particularly because these factors may differ somewhat from those responsible for later development and maintenance of an addictive pattern of use. There are at least two reasons for postulating such a difference. First, whereas initial experimentation with drugs of abuse (typically alcohol and tobacco) almost always occurs during the teenage years or even younger, there is usually a significant time interval (ranging from a few years to several decades, as with some alcoholics) before the onset of substance dependence. The many psychosocial differences between teenagers and adults can have a profound influence on the motivation to use drugs. Second, the repeated drug consumption that leads to addiction alters the user's neural and behavioral functioning, as emphasized by some of the models described earlier. There are also significant changes to the person's social milieu that may involve disruption of relationships within his circle of family and friends, problems at work (if he's even still employed), and possibly criminal activities and incarceration. Thus drug use under these conditions is bound to be driven by many factors not present at the time of initial experimentation. Because of the need for a separate consideration of experimental substance use, we shall begin developing our model with that topic.

Three types of factors are involved in experimental substance use

Petraitis and colleagues (1995) reviewed many theories of experimental substance use in adolescents. They argue that

TABLE 8.5 Factors Influencing Experimental Substance Use in Adolescents

Level of influence	Type of influence		
	Social/interpersonal	Cultural/attitudinal	Intrapersonal
Proximal	Peer pressure to use substances and beliefs that such use is normal	Belief that the benefits of substance use outweigh the risks or costs	Belief that one has the ability to control one's substance use
Distal	Stronger attachments to peers than to family members along with positive peer attitudes toward drug use	Social alienation; rejection of conventional values; desire for short-term gratification; rebelliousness	Low self-esteem; poor social, academic, or coping skills; feelings of stress, anxiety, or depression
Ultimate	Lack of parental support, reinforcement, or supervision; negative evaluations from parents; familial stress, including parental divorce or separation	Local environmental factors such as ready availability of drugs, high crime rates, inadequate schools, and poor career opportunities	Genetic susceptibility to addiction; personality traits such as impulsivity, risk-taking, emotional instability, aggressiveness, and sociability

Source: Adapted from Petraitis et al., 1995.

there are three types of factors influencing experimental substance use and three levels of influence, thereby leading to the 3 × 3 matrix presented in Table 8.5. Social/interpersonal factors have been emphasized most in previous theories, but cultural/attitudinal and intrapersonal factors can also play important roles. The different levels relate to how closely or immediately specific factors govern experimental substance use. Thus proximal factors are those thought to have the most direct influence on this behavior and to be most highly predictive of its occurrence. At the other extreme, ultimate factors are not immediately involved in the decision to experiment with drugs, but they are hypothesized to increase the long-term risk for such experimentation to occur. Distal factors are intermediate between proximal and ultimate.

From Table 8.5, we see that some of the factors hypothesized to be most important in experimental substance use are positive beliefs concerning such use; strong peer attachments and peer pressure toward substance use; rejection of conventional social values; poor life skills; and feelings of stress, anxiety, or depression. At the ultimate level, certain personality traits, familial problems, and local environmental factors can also play a role. Personality traits commonly associated with experimental substance use, such as impulsivity, risk taking, and so forth, have a heritable component (meaning that individual differences in these traits are under genetic influence). This seems to be the principal way that biology may contribute to the early phase of drug-seeking behavior.

Different factors are involved in the development and maintenance of compulsive substance use

The major factors that contribute to the development and maintenance of compulsive drug seeking and drug use (that

is, addiction) are illustrated in Figure 8.17. The first four types of factors are related to various drug effects that together exert direct control over drug use. The remaining two categories include factors that don't directly influence drug use but indirectly either increase (risk factors) or decrease (protective factors) the likelihood of developing or maintaining a compulsive pattern of use.

Drug-related factors The first type of factor is the positive-reinforcing effects of drugs of abuse. This is the same

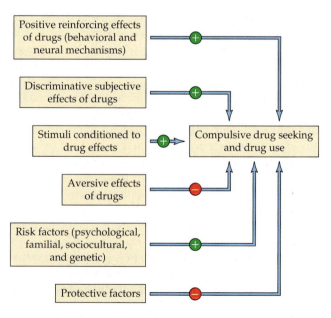

Figure 8.17 Factors involved in the development and maintenance of compulsive drug use (Adapted from Stolerman, 1992.)

influence discussed previously in the section on the positive reinforcement model of addiction, but here it is just one of several relevant kinds of drug effects. We can elaborate briefly on some of the behavioral and neural mechanisms that underlie this positive reinforcement. At a behavioral level, we may attribute the reinforcing effects of drugs of abuse to:

- Mood elevation/euphoria, as emphasized in the positive reinforcement model;
- Relief from unpleasant withdrawal symptoms,* as proposed by the physical dependence model of addiction;
- Relief from feelings of anxiety; or
- Functional enhancement, for example, increased alertness.

It is clear that different substances vary in the degree to which they fit these differing categories of reinforcement. Most drugs of abuse produce mood elevation or euphoria, but not all. As we saw earlier, relief from withdrawal symptoms may be important for substances that produce strong dependence but not for those that do not. Anxiety relief may play a role in the use of sedative–anxiolytic drugs (drugs that cause relaxation and anxiety reduction) like barbiturates, benzodiazepines (for example, Valium), or alcohol, but it is not involved in addiction to stimulants like cocaine or amphetamine that tend to heighten rather than diminish feelings of anxiety. Enhancement of alertness or other cognitive functions has been associated with nicotine and caffeine use, whereas sedative drugs have the opposite effect on cognitive performance.

At the neural level, we have already pointed out that the mesolimbic dopamine system seems to be a key part of the brain circuit responsible for the reinforcing effects of many drugs. However, we also noted that the importance of this system varies with different substances. Other neurotransmitter systems are undoubtedly also involved in drug reinforcement, depending on each particular drug of abuse. These include the GABA (γ-aminobutyric acid) system for the sedative–anxiolytic drugs mentioned in the previous paragraph, the opioid system for opiate drugs such as heroin and morphine, and the cannabinoid system for marijuana. Some of these systems were presented in previous chapters, while others are discussed in forthcoming chapters on specific classes of abused drugs.

Psychoactive drugs, including drugs of abuse, often produce powerful discriminative stimulus effects in animal studies. As summarized in Chapter 4, this means that the drugs produce internal states that can serve as cues controlling the animal's behavior in a learning task. Discriminative stimulus effects of drugs in animals are considered to be analogous to the subjective effects that people experience when they take the same substances. Experienced users come to expect these subjective effects, and such expectations are thought to contribute to the persistence of drug-seeking and drug-using behaviors.

It is a truism to say that every episode of drug use occurs in the presence of some set of environmental stimuli. The powerful role of environment was seen when U.S. soldiers were returning from the war in Vietnam in the 1970s. Although many soldiers were frequent heroin users in Vietnam, most had little difficulty "kicking the habit" once they returned home (Robins et al., 1975). While there are undoubtedly many factors involved in this situation, one important factor is thought to be removal from the environmental stimuli that had previously been associated with the drug. There are many ways that drug effects can be paired with specific stimuli. For example, the user might always meet her supplier at a particular street corner. A crack cocaine addict might always use a favorite crack pipe to smoke the drug. In such cases, this repeated association leads to conditioning of the stimulus or stimuli to the drug. What are the consequences of being exposed to drug-conditioned stimuli in the absence of the drug itself (for example, seeing the crack pipe with no cocaine on hand)? The answer is complex and depends on the exact circumstances of the conditioning. But in general, exposure to drug-conditioned stimuli will lead to either druglike effects or drug-opposite effects. Druglike effects (that is, responses similar to those produced by the drug itself) may serve as **primers,** promoting subsequent drug seeking and using by reminding the individual of how the drug feels when it's "on board." Interestingly, because drug-opposite effects are manifested as withdrawal symptoms, including drug craving, they also drive the user toward obtaining and taking the drug. Thus stimuli conditioned to drug effects can be potent motivators in the cycle of compulsive drug seeking and drug use.

Interestingly, drugs of abuse can sometimes be shown to exert aversive effects on animals or humans. For example, even though rats will self-administer nicotine under some conditions, they will also learn to press a lever to prevent experimenter-controlled infusions of the same drug. There is considerable evidence that a number of substances are reinforcing when under the animal's control but either not as reinforcing or even aversive when administered by the experimenter. For humans as well, drugs may produce aversive psychological or behavioral effects in addition to their reinforcing effects. One example is the ability of cocaine to bring about feelings of anxiety that follow soon after the initial period of drug-induced euphoria. However, even though such aversive effects presumably inhibit the tendency toward future drug seeking and drug use, they may not be sufficient to outweigh the many factors promoting these behaviors.

---

*Strictly speaking, taking a drug to alleviate withdrawal symptoms could be classified as negative rather than positive reinforcement; however, this distinction is not important for the present discussion.

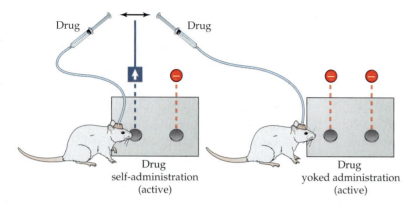

Drug

Drug

Drug
self-administration
(active)

Drug
yoked administration
(active)

Figure 8.18 The yoked-control drug administration procedure This is a procedure designed to investigate potential differences in the consequences of passive drug exposure versus active, controlled drug self-administration. The self-administration group learns to perform an operant response to trigger an intravenous infusion of the test drug. The required response may be a lever press or, as in the illustration, a nose poke into a hole in the wall of the experimental chamber (upward arrow). An inactive lever or hole (minus sign) is used for control purposes to demonstrate the specificity of the learned response (there should be little or no responding to the inactive device). The yoked animals are given the same two levers or holes as the self-administration group, but in this case both devices are inactive. Instead, each animal in the yoked group is paired with a counterpart in the self-administration group, and the yoked animal receives the exact same drug dose whenever its counterpart has earned an infusion due to its responding. Thus, we can see that the two animals receive identical drug exposure, but the self-administering animal has control over the amount and timing of this exposure that the yoked animal lacks.

In concluding this section on drug-related factors, it is worth noting that many kinds of drug effects in animals (and probably humans, as well) vary depending on whether drug administration is under the organism's control. This is tested experimentally by comparing two different treatment groups, one that is permitted to self-administer the drug and a second group that is yoked to the first. That is, each animal in the self-administration group has a counterpart in the yoked group, and each time the first animal gives itself a drug injection by performing the necessary operant response, its counterpart receives the same injection (Figure 8.18). Thus, the exact dose and patterning of drug treatments are the same in the self-administering and yoked groups, but they differ in that only the first group has control over the treatment. Using this paradigm, researchers have found many examples in which drug-induced neurotransmitter release and turnover, changes in receptor density, and alterations in gene expression vary as a function of whether the drug was self-administered or not (Jacobs et al., 2003). These findings emphasize that psychoactive drugs interact with the organism's state—the effects will differ depending on whether drug exposure is uncontrolled and unpredictable or whether the organism can optimize the pattern of administration and

can anticipate when the next dose will be delivered.

Risk factors   There are many modulating factors that can influence either the likelihood of someone becoming a drug addict or the probability that they will be able to achieve stable abstinence once addicted. One important environmental factor is the occurrence of stress and the ability of the person to cope with such stress. The life histories of drug addicts often show instances in which stressful events either promoted increased drug use or precipitated relapse from a previous period of abstinence. Numerous animal studies have confirmed that stress can increase the self-administration of abused drugs (Piazza and Le Moal, 1998) as well as trigger renewed drug-taking behavior in models of relapse (Stewart, 2000). For this reason, many treatment providers teach their clients new coping skills to deal with life stresses without relapsing.

At the psychological level, there is an abundance of research on the relationship between personality variables and alcoholism or other types of drug addiction (Sher et al., 1999). Moreover, there is significant **comorbidity** of drug abuse or addiction with various personality or mood disorders. This means that addicts or drug abusers are often diagnosed with one or more psychiatric disorders in addition to their drug problem. Interestingly, a recent review of this literature found that comorbidity of substance use problems with other psychiatric disorders is more common in women than in men (Zilberman et al., 2003). Furthermore, whereas substance abuse or addiction is typically the primary diagnosis in men (meaning that it came before the other psychiatric disorder), the comorbid diagnosis (for example, depression) is more commonly the primary one in women. This gender difference should be taken into account by treatment providers working with clients suffering from comorbid disorders involving substance abuse.

Verheul and van den Brink (2000) proposed three different personality-related pathways to addiction: (1) behavioral disinhibition; (2) stress reduction; and (3) reward sensitivity. The behavioral disinihibition pathway hypothesizes that deviant behaviors such as substance abuse are linked to a trait cluster of impulsivity, antisociality, unconventionality, and aggressiveness, combined with low levels of constraint and harm avoidance. This pathway may be particularly relevant for drug abusers suffering from antisocial or borderline personality disorder. According to the stress reduction pathway, high scores on traits such as stress reactivity, anxiety, and neuroticism are indicative of a heightened vulnerability to stressful life events. Such events, therefore, trigger anxiety and mood disorders (for example, depression), which in turn can lead to substance use in an attempt at self-medication. Indeed, this idea has sometimes been called the **self-medication hypothesis.** It predicts that individuals suffering from elevated anxiety should prefer alcohol and other sedative–anxiolytic drugs, whereas depressed individuals should seek out stimulant drugs such as cocaine or amphetamine. The third pathway, termed reward sensitivity, relates drug abuse to the personality traits of sensation seeking, reward seeking, extraversion, and gregariousness. It suggests that individuals scoring high on these traits seek out drugs for their positive-reinforcing qualities.

Familial and sociocultural influences can also influence the risk of developing a pattern of drug abuse or addiction. Familial factors have been studied most extensively in conjunction with the risk of alcoholism. For example, adult children of alcoholics are at increased risk for having alcohol or other substance abuse problems (Windle and Davies, 1999). In the case of alcohol itself, this may be related in part to modeling (imitation) of the parent's drinking behavior or to a heightened expectancy that drinking will lead to positive mood changes. Sociocultural studies have identified at least four different functions served by drug abuse (Thombs, 1999). The first involves social facilitation. Alcohol and other drugs are often consumed in a group setting where the substance may enhance social bonds between the participants. The second function is to remove the user from normal social roles and responsibilities, thereby allowing an escape from the burdens that may be associated with these responsibilities. Third, substance use may promote group solidarity within a particular ethnic group. A good example of this phenomenon is the association of Irish culture with heavy alcohol use and a high rate of alcoholism. Finally, substance abuse sometimes occurs within a "drug subculture" that embraces social rituals surrounding a particular subculture and rejects conventional social norms and lifestyles. Sociological studies have identified distinct subcultures for many different substances, including heroin, cocaine, alcohol, marijuana, methamphetamine, and PCP. This is not to say that all users of a particular substance participate in the rituals of a subculture, or that users necessarily limit themselves to just one substance. Nevertheless, one can find groups of individuals who share their common experiences with a specific drug of abuse and who have a similar disdain for the "straight" lifestyle.

Finally, genes play a modulatory but not a deterministic role in substance abuse, as mentioned earlier. Genetic differences may enter the picture in numerous ways, from altering the sensitivity of neurotransmitter receptors (and thus to the drugs that act via those same neurotransmitters) to influenc-

ing drug pharmacokinetics by changing the activity of key drug-metabolizing enzymes. Some examples of genetic modulation of drug use or abuse are presented in subsequent chapters.

Protective factors   There are two different ways that we can think about protective factors in drug addiction. First, an absence of the various risk factors described in the previous section should be relatively protective with respect to drug abuse or addiction. Put another way, individuals who do not suffer from a preexisting personality or mood disorder, who do not exhibit the trait clusters mentioned earlier, who come from a stable family without any substance abuse, who do not belong to an ethnic group that promotes substance use, and who do not become involved in the social rituals surrounding drug use are at reduced risk for becoming addicted.

The second way that protective factors can operate is to help maintain a stable abstinence in previously drug-abusing or addicted individuals. Drug addicts who seek treatment tend to be the most heavily dependent and seriously affected individuals. Some will be able to overcome their dependence, but current research indicates that the majority will struggle with their drug problems for much of their remaining life. However, there are also reports of heavy drug users achieving long-term abstinence with little or no treatment (Bischof et al., 2001; Klingemann, 1992; Sobell et al., 2000). This has been termed natural recovery or spontaneous recovery. These individuals are probably less dependent overall than those seen by the treatment community. Even though this difference may be significant in facilitating spontaneous recovery, very few recovered drug abusers report that they no longer have any desire for drugs. Therefore, it is important to know how the decision was made to stop drug use and what experiences or actions may help protect these individuals from relapsing.

Recovered (that is, stably abstinent) drug addicts or abusers recount many different tales of how they made and kept the decision to quit using drugs. It is often thought that the addict must hit "rock bottom" or go through an "existential crisis" before he'll be sufficiently motivated to stop using. Although this kind of experience is reported in some cases, many individuals find the means to abstain without reaching such a crisis situation. Spontaneous recovery from drug abuse or addiction may be triggered by a variety of major life changes. Some of these are positive changes such as marriage or having a spiritual/religious experience, whereas others are negative consequences of drug use such as health problems, financial problems, loss of one's job, social pressures, fear of imprisonment, or death of a drug-abusing friend. Once the decision is made, the risk of relapse is reduced by such actions as moving to a new area, developing new social relationships with nonusers, obtaining employment, and engaging in substitute activities like physical exercise or meditation. The relative importance of different factors also varies somewhat with different drugs of abuse. For example, health concerns are particularly important in motivating tobacco smokers to stop smoking, and much more than other drug users, they cite simple willpower as a critical factor in maintaining abstinence (Walters, 2000).

In conclusion, achievement of stable abstinence either spontaneously or with the aid of treatment is greatly facilitated by certain behavioral changes that help protect the drug addict from relapse. Some of these changes involve avoidance of drug-associated cues (for example, moving to a new location and shunning drug-using acquaintances), whereas other changes serve to provide substitutes for the former substance use, new sources of reinforcement, a new social support network, financial stability, and general structure to the individual's life.

Section Summary

Various models have been proposed to account for the development and maintenance of drug abuse or addiction. One of the earliest models proposes that addictive drug use is caused by the development of physical dependence and the resulting unpleasant withdrawal symptoms that result when an addict attempts to abstain from drug taking. Conditioned craving may also occur in response to drug-associated stimuli in the environment and may serve as an important factor in relapse even after detoxification. The second model discussed emphasizes that drugs of abuse are taken for their positive-reinforcing effects. This model is supported by human reports of drug-induced euphoria and by the ability of the same substances to support self-administration in animals. Two recent models of addiction are the incentive-sensitization model and the opponent-process model. The incentive-sensitization model of Robinson and Berridge is based on the idea that with repeated exposure, there is an increase in drug wanting (craving) due to sensitization of the underlying neural mechanisms, but there is no equivalent enhancement of drug liking. The opponent-process model put forward by Koob and Le Moal proposes that any affective stimulus triggers an opposing reaction that is experienced after the initial response has ended. Repeated drug use is thought to sensitize the primary affective response (drug-induced euphoria) but, at the same time, to lower the hedonic set point so that the addict experiences a dysphoric mood state in the absence of the drug.

The most influential model of addiction in our society is the disease or medical model. As these names imply, this model proposes that addiction should be considered a disease requiring medical treatment. There are actually two types of disease models, susceptibility and exposure models. In the first type, addiction is thought to stem primarily from

an inherited susceptibility to uncontrolled drug use. The other type of disease model involves the notion that chronic drug use leads to alterations in brain function that are responsible for loss of control and compulsive drug-seeking and drug-taking behaviors.

Disease models have played an important role in helping people deal with guilt associated with their addiction and also in promoting social acceptance of medical treatment for drug addicts. However, it is important to recognize that, like other psychiatric disorders, addiction must be diagnosed solely on the basis of the individual's mental and behavioral symptoms. The disease concept of addiction seems to work best when compared to certain other diseases like obesity or essential hypertension. Like addiction, these disorders are thought to result from a combination of interacting genetic, psychosocial, and behavioral factors and to involve a continuum of symptomatology between healthy individuals and those suffering from the disease.

In formulating a more comprehensive, biopsychosocial model of addiction, it is appropriate to begin with the factors involved in initial or experimental substance use. These can be categorized as proximal, distal, or ultimate, depending on how closely or immediately they govern experimental substance use. Among the factors thought to be most important are positive beliefs concerning substance use; strong peer attachments and peer pressure toward substance use; rejection of conventional social values; poor life skills; and feelings of stress, anxiety, or depression.

Several types of factors contribute to the development and maintenance of compulsive drug seeking and drug use. These include four categories of factors related directly to drug effects, as well as various risk or protective factors that modify the likelihood of developing or maintaining a compulsive pattern of use. Drugs can exert positive-reinforcing effects through mood elevation/euphoria, relief from unpleasant withdrawal symptoms, relief from anxiety, or functional enhancement. There are discriminative stimulus effects of drugs that can be demonstrated in animals and are thought to correspond to the subjective effects produced by these same compounds in human users. Through conditioning, environmental stimuli can either elicit druglike or drug-opposite effects, both of which can motivate subsequent drug seeking and drug taking. Drugs also sometimes produce aversive effects, although these may not be sufficiently strong to outweigh other factors that promote compulsive drug use.

Although there is no specific "addictive personality," certain personality traits are associated with increased risk for drug addiction. Three different personality-related pathways to addiction have been termed the behavioral disinhibition, stress reduction, and reward sensitivity pathways. There is also significant comorbidity of drug abuse or addiction with various personality or mood disorders, and the self-medication hypothesis proposes that some individuals take drugs in an attempt to treat these coexisting disorders. The risk of developing a pattern of drug abuse or addiction is also affected by familial and sociocultural influences. For example, drugs may promote social facilitation, remove the user from normal social roles and responsibilities, promote solidarity within a particular ethnic group, or lead to association with a specific drug subculture.

Finally, there are also various protective factors that can reduce the likelihood of an individual becoming addicted or help prevent relapse in drug users attempting to maintain stable abstinence. These factors encompass the person's personality structure, social (including family) life, and environment. It seems to be possible for some substance abusers to achieve abstinence without formal treatment, but heavily dependent individuals typically need the assistance of a structured treatment program.

Recommended Readings

Caan, W., and de Belleroche, J. (2002). *Drink, Drugs and Dependence: From Science to Clinical Practice.* Routledge, New York.

Goldstein, A. (2001). *Addiction: From Biology to Drug Policy.* Oxford University Press, New York.

Marlatt, G. A., and VandenBos, G. R. (eds.) (1997). *Addictive Behaviors. Readings on Etiology, Prevention, and Treatment.* American Psychological Association, Washington.

Rasmussen, S. (2000). *Addiction Treatment: Theory and Practice.* Sage Publications, Thousand Oaks, California.

9 *Alcohol*

*I*magine yourself at a Friday night rager just getting under way. Students are mingling and dancing to pop music while someone taps a keg behind the bar. When we look around an hour later, some changes have occurred. Guys from the soccer team are chanting the time as one of their number performs a keg stand. In the middle of the dance floor, an upperclassman grinds with a freshman girl, their hands all over each other. Many other students dance wildly, their glazed eyes indicating that the fun they are having will probably not be remembered in the morning. A group of Asians come in, and most grab beers, but unlike most students, several decline, knowing how sick the alcohol will make them within minutes. Nobody notices the girl passed out in the chair in the corner, with much more attention focused on the two guys yelling and shoving each other next to the Beirut table.

Alcohol, an amazing beverage, used by people all over the world for thousands of years, is responsible, we assume, for all the effects we see here: loss of coordination and judgment, enhanced sexuality, memory loss and stupor, increased hostility and aggression, and, for some, the potential for unpleasant side effects. Can such a simple molecule chemically produce all these diverse effects by acting on specific neurotransmitters, or might the setting, the mood of the participants, and their expectations be major contributors?

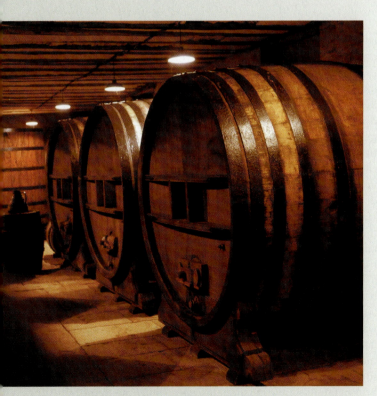

Wine making is an ancient tradition requiring the fermentation of the sugar in grapes with yeast to form alcohol.

Psychopharmacology of Alcohol

Alcohol, after caffeine, is the most commonly used psychoactive drug in America and is certainly the drug most abused. Despite the fact that alcohol has dramatic effects on mood, behavior, and thinking, and that its chronic use is damaging to the individual, his family, and society, the majority of people accept its use. In fact, many people do not consider alcohol to be a drug. How many people do you know who shun taking over-the-counter or prescription medicines because they don't want to take "drugs" but will have a beer at a party or a cocktail before dinner? How many parents of high school students have you heard say that they are relieved that their child was only caught drinking alcohol illegally and not using "real" drugs? How many books and magazine articles have been titled "Drugs and Alcohol," as though alcohol was not included in the drug category? The popularity of alcohol use means that almost everyone has an idea about its effects. Some of these ideas are based on fact, but frequently people's beliefs about alcohol are misconceptions and based on myth and "common" wisdom. Our job is to present the empirical evidence that describes not only the acute effects of the drug and its mechanism of action in the brain but also some of the long-term effects on other organ systems.

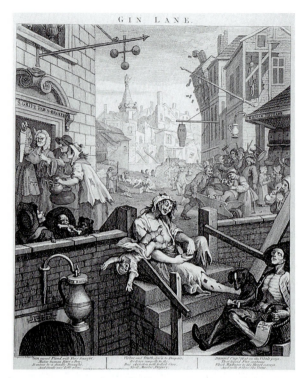

Figure 9.1 Engraving of "Gin Lane" by artist William Hogarth (1697–1764), depicting the popular opinion that the "lower classes" drank gin and got drunk.

Alcohol has a long history of use

Alcohol use in America began with the very first immigrants, but its history is really very much longer than that. Perhaps as early as 8000 B.C., mead was brewed from fermented honey, producing the first alcoholic beverage. Archeological evidence shows that around 3700 B.C., the Egyptians prepared the first very hearty beer, called *hek,* which might have been thick enough to stand up a spoon, and wine may have first come from Babylonia in 1700 B.C. Later still, the popularity of alcohol among the Romans may have contributed to the decline of the Empire. Certainly many historians believe that the civilization was doomed by the corruption of society, alcohol intemperance, and moral decay, but the mental instability of the Roman nobility is an additional factor. Those signs of confusion and dementia may have been due to lead poisoning caused by alcohol prepared with a flavor enhancer having a high lead content. Aqua vitae (meaning "the water of life" in Latin) represents the first distilled conversion of wine into brandy during the Middle Ages in Italy. Production of gin by the Dutch is frequently credited with beginning serious alcohol abuse in Europe. Not only was gin far more potent than wine and very inexpensive to buy, but it was introduced during a time of social upheaval. Gin turned out to be a common method of dealing with the poor living conditions and social instability caused by the newly created urban societies following the feudal period. Gin consumption became associated with the lower class, while the more respectable middle class drank beer (Figure 9.1).

Colonial Americans brought their habits of heavy drinking from Europe, and alcohol had a large part in their daily lives. The American tavern was not just a place for food and drink and overnight accommodation, it was also the focal point in each town for conducting business and local politics, and for mail delivery. The Continental Army supplied each soldier with a daily ration of rum, and employers and farmers supplied their workers with liquor on the job. Students, then as now, had reputations for hard drinking, and Harvard University operated its own brewery. At some point the celebrations at graduation ceremonies became so wild and unrestrained that the administration developed strict rules of behavior. American drinking of alcohol remained at a high level until the 1830s, when the temperance movement began a campaign to educate society about the dangers of long-term alcohol consumption. Although their initial goal was to reduce alcohol consumption rather than prevent it, later offshoots of the group used social and religious arguments to convince Americans that alcohol itself was the source of evil in the world and was directly responsible for broken families, poverty, social disorder, and crime. Some of the same arguments are currently being used to regulate other drugs in our society, such as marijuana, heroin, and cocaine.

In 1917, Congress passed a law that in 1920 became the Eighteenth Amendment to the American Constitution, prohibiting the "manufacture, sale, transportation, and importation" of liquor. Despite its intent, the period of Prohibition increased illegal manufacturing that often produced highly toxic forms of alcohol, increased consumption of distilled spirits rather than beer because it was easier to hide and store, and made drinking in illegal speakeasies a fad. Medicinal "tonics" containing up to 75% alcohol became increasingly popular. Worst of all, Prohibition increased the activity of organized crime mobs that were heavily involved in the sale and distribution of alcohol. By 1933, most Americans realized the experiment was a failure, and the Eighteenth Amendment was repealed by Congress during the presidency of Franklin D. Roosevelt. (For a brief history of alcohol use in America, see Goode, 1993.) Today, the use of alcohol is restricted by age and circumstance (prohibited when operating a motor vehicle) and regulated to some extent by an increased tax on the cost of consumption (the "sin tax").

What is an alcohol and where does it come from?

Alcohols come in many forms, and although they have similarities in structure, they have very different uses. Ethyl alcohol is the alcohol we are most familiar with because it is used as a beverage. Ethyl alcohol has only two carbon atoms, a complement of hydrogens, plus the —OH (hydroxyl group) characteristic of all alcohols (Figure 9.2). Methyl alcohol, or wood alcohol, has an even simpler chemical structure but is highly toxic if consumed, because the liver metabolites of methyl alcohol include formic acid and formaldehyde.

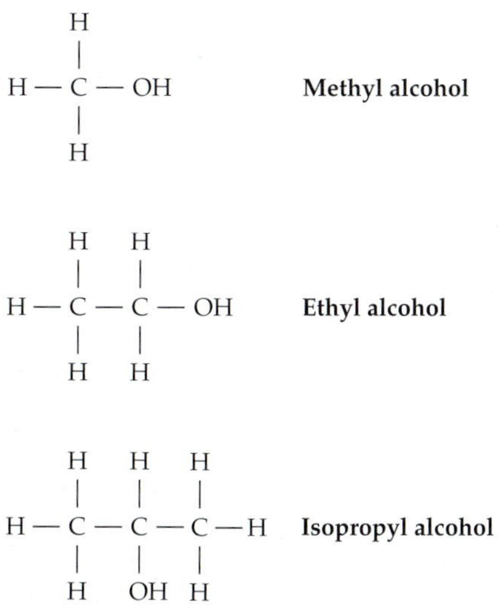

Figure 9.2 Chemical structures of three commonly used forms of alcohol

Drinking wood alcohol causes blindness, coma, and death. It is commonly used as a fuel, an antifreeze, and an industrial solvent. Isopropyl alcohol has a small molecular side chain that changes its characteristics and makes it most useful as rubbing alcohol or as a disinfectant. It is also dangerous to consume.

Ethyl alcohol (or ethanol) is the form we focus on in this chapter. It is produced by fermentation, a process that occurs naturally whenever microscopic yeast cells in the air fall on a product containing sugar, such as honey, fruit, sugar cane, or grains like rye, corn, and others. The material that provides the sugar determines the type of alcoholic beverage, for example, wine (grapes), sake (rice), or beer (grains). The yeast converts each sugar molecule into two molecules of alcohol and two molecules of carbon dioxide. This fermentation process is entirely natural and explains why alcohol has been discovered in cultures all over the world. The fermentation process continues until the concentration of alcohol is about 15%, at which point the yeast dies. Most wines have an alcohol content in that range. To achieve higher alcohol concentration, distillation is necessary. Distillation requires heating the fermented mixture to the point where the alcohol boils off in steam (since it has a lower boiling point than water), leaving some of the water behind. The alcohol vapor passes through a series of cooling tubes (called a still) and condenses to be collected as "hard liquor," or distilled spirits, such as whiskey, brandy, rum, tequila, and so forth. The alcohol concentration of these beverages varies from 40 to 50%. A second way to increase alcohol concentrations above 15% is to add additional alcohol, a procedure used to make fortified wines such as sherry. Flavoring and sugar may also be added to produce liqueurs such as crème de menthe (mint), amaretto (almond), or ouzo (anise). Regardless of the form, alcohol is high in calories, which means that it provides heat or energy when it is metabolized. However, there is no nutritional value with those calories because alcohol provides no proteins, vitamins, or minerals that are a necessary component of a normal diet. For this reason, individuals who chronically consume large quantities of alcohol in lieu of food frequently suffer from inadequate nutrition, leading to health problems and brain damage.

Although it would make the most sense to describe alcohol content as a percentage, if you look at a bottle of distilled spirits you are more likely to see alcohol content described according to "proof." This convention is based on an old British army custom of testing an alcoholic product by pouring it on gunpowder and attempting to light it. If the alcohol content is 50%, the gunpowder burns, but if the alcohol is less concentrated, the remaining water content prevents the burning. Hence, the burning of the sample was 100% "proof" that it was at least 50% alcohol. The proof number now corresponds to twice the percent of alcohol concentration.

The pharmacokinetics of alcohol determine its bioavailability

In order to evaluate the effects of alcohol in the central nervous system (CNS), we need to know how much alcohol is freely available to enter the brain from the blood (i.e., its bioavailability). Ethyl alcohol is a unique drug in several respects. Although alcohol is a small, simple molecule that cannot be ionized, it nevertheless readily mixes with water and is not high in lipid solubility. Despite these characteristics, it is easily absorbed from the gastrointestinal (GI) tract and diffuses throughout the body, readily entering most tissues, including the brain. The rates of absorption, distribution, and clearance of alcohol are modified by many factors, all of which contribute to the highly variable blood levels that occur following ingestion of a fixed amount of the drug. For this reason, behavioral effects are described based on **blood alcohol concentration (BAC)** rather than on the amount ingested. In general, it takes a BAC of 0.04% (i.e., 40 milliliters of alcohol per 100 milliliters of blood) to produce measurable behavioral effects. Keep in mind that one "drink" may take the form of one 12-ounce can of beer, one 5-ounce glass of wine, a cocktail with 1.25 ounces of spirits, or a 12-ounce wine cooler, but each will raise your blood level by the equivalent amount (Figure 9.3).

Absorption and distribution   Since oral administration is about the only way the drug is used recreationally, absorption will necessarily be from the GI tract: about 10% from the stomach and 90% from the small intestine. The small mole-

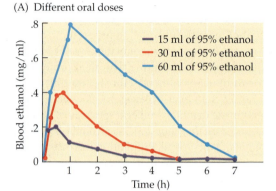

(A) Different oral doses

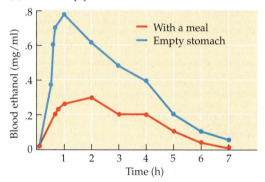

(B) Full or empty stomach

Figure 9.4 Blood levels of alcohol after oral administration (A) Larger oral doses of alcohol produce higher concentrations in the stomach, which causes faster absorption and higher peak blood levels. (B) The presence of food in the stomach slows absorption of alcohol and prevents the sharp peak in blood level.

cules move across the membrane barriers by passive diffusion from the higher concentration on one side (the GI tract) to the lower concentration on the other (blood). Of course, this means that the more alcohol you drink in a short period of time or the more alcohol you drink in an undiluted form (i.e., more concentrated), the more rapid the movement from stomach and intestine to blood, producing a higher blood level (Figure 9.4A). The presence of food in the stomach slows absorption because it delays the movement into the small intestine through the pyloric sphincter, a muscle that regulates the movement of material from stomach to intestine (Figure 9.4B). Milk seems to be particularly effective in delaying absorption. In contrast, carbonated alcoholic beverages such as champagne are absorbed more rapidly because the carbonation speeds the movement of materials from the stomach into the intestine.

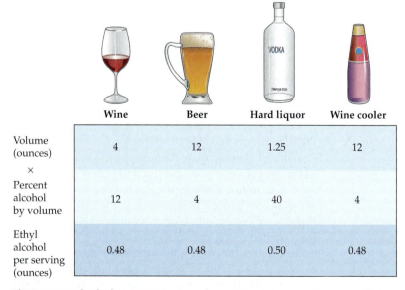

	Wine	Beer	Hard liquor	Wine cooler
Volume (ounces)	4	12	1.25	12
×				
Percent alcohol by volume	12	4	40	4
Ethyl alcohol per serving (ounces)	0.48	0.48	0.50	0.48

Figure 9.3 Alcohol content A comparison of alcohol content in various beverages shows an equivalent amount despite differences in volume. To calculate the amount of alcohol in a given beverage, multiply the number of ounces in the container by the percent alcohol content by volume. Note that the alcohol content of beer varies from 3% up to 6% for some microbrews.

Gender differences also exist in the absorption of alcohol from the stomach because certain enzymes (particularly alcohol dehydrogenase) that are present in gastric fluid are about 60% more active in men than in women, leaving a higher concentration of alcohol that will be absorbed more rapidly in women (Freeza et al., 1990). Further, taking aspirin generally inhibits gastric alcohol dehydrogenase, but to a greater extent in women than in men. Since women have lower levels of alcohol dehydrogenase to begin with, aspirin use before drinking may essentially eliminate any gastric metabolism of alcohol in women (Roine et al., 1990). Ulcer medications (such as Tagamet or Zantac) also impair gastric metabolism, increasing alcohol concentrations and hence increasing absorption.

Once alcohol is in the blood, it circulates throughout the body. It readily moves by passive diffusion from the higher concentration in the blood to all tissues and fluid compartments. Body size and gender differences also play a part in the distribution of alcohol and in the magnitude of its effect. The same amount of alcohol, say one beer, is much more concentrated in the average woman compared to a man because her fluid volume is much smaller due to her size and because women have a higher fat-to-water ratio. Furthermore, alcohol readily passes the placental barrier, so the alcohol that a pregnant female drinks is delivered almost immediately to her fetus as well, producing potentially damaging effects to the developing infant. Fetal alcohol syndrome is discussed in Box 9.1.

Metabolism   Of the alcohol that reaches the general circulation, approximately 95% is metabolized by the liver before being excreted as carbon dioxide and water in the urine. The remaining 5% is excreted by the lungs and can be measured in one's breath using a Breathalyzer, which provides law enforcement officials a means to calculate alcohol levels. Alcohol metabolism is different from that of most other drugs in that the rate of oxidation is constant over time and does not occur more quickly when the drug is more concentrated in the blood. The rate of metabolism is quite variable from one person to another, but the average rate is approximately 1 to 1.5 ounces or 12–18 ml of 80-proof alcohol per hour. Since the metabolic rate is constant for an individual, if the rate of consumption is faster than the rate of metabolism, alcohol accumulates in the body and the individual becomes intoxicated.

Several enzyme systems in the liver are capable of oxidizing alcohol. The most important is **alcohol dehydrogenase,** which we already know is also found in the stomach and reduces the amount of available alcohol for absorption. Alcohol dehydrogenase converts alcohol to acetaldehyde, a potentially toxic intermediate, which normally is rapidly modified further by **acetaldehyde dehydrogenase (ALDH)** to form acetic acid. Further oxidation yields carbon dioxide, water, and energy (Figure 9.5A). ALDH exists in several genetically determined forms with varying activities. About 10% of

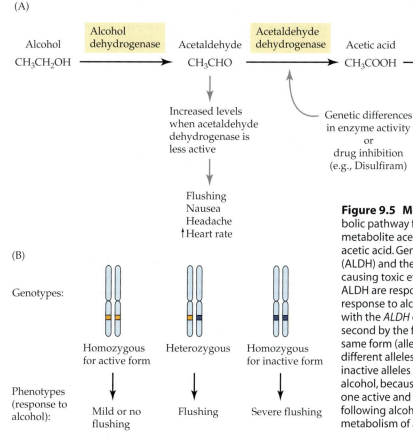

(A)

Alcohol   →[Alcohol dehydrogenase]→   Acetaldehyde   →[Acetaldehyde dehydrogenase]→   Acetic acid   →[Oxidation reaction]→   Carbon dioxide
CH_3CH_2OH ——————→ CH_3CHO ——————→ CH_3COOH ——————→ $CO_2 + H_2O + Energy$

Increased levels when acetaldehyde dehydrogenase is less active

Genetic differences in enzyme activity or drug inhibition (e.g., Disulfiram)

Flushing
Nausea
Headache
↑Heart rate

(B)

Genotypes:

Homozygous for active form   Heterozygous   Homozygous for inactive form

Phenotypes (response to alcohol):

Mild or no flushing   Flushing   Severe flushing

Figure 9.5 Metabolism of alcohol (A) The principal metabolic pathway for alcohol involves the formation of the toxic metabolite acetaldehyde, which must be further degraded to acetic acid. Genetic differences in acetaldehyde dehydrogenase (ALDH) and the use of certain drugs can inhibit enzyme activity, causing toxic effects. (B) Three possible genetic variations of ALDH are responsible for large individual differences in response to alcohol. Each person has a pair of chromosomes with the *ALDH* gene, one contributed by the mother and the second by the father. The two chromosomes can have either the same form (allele), making the individual homozygous, or two different alleles, making him heterozygous. Individuals with two inactive alleles experience a severe reaction if they consume alcohol, because acetaldehyde levels remain high. Those with one active and one inactive allele show some flushing response following alcohol ingestion. Two active alleles produce normal metabolism of acetaldehyde.

BOX 9.1

Clinical Applications

Fetal Alcohol Syndrome

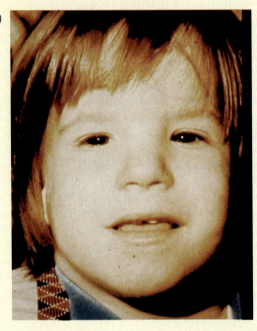

(A)

One of the greatest tragedies of fetal alcohol syndrome (FAS) is that it occurs at all. Fetal alcohol exposure is the most common cause of mental retardation in the United States and could be prevented. Although the damaging effects of alcohol on an adult generally take decades of heavy drinking, the developing embryo is far more susceptible. The major and minor birth defects that constitute FAS present a challenge to families, social services, and the educational system. The cost for serving those individuals with only the most severe symptoms is over $321 million a year in the United States, and billions more might be spent on special care for the less impaired (Williams et al., 1994).

The diagnostic signs and symptoms include:

1. *Mental retardation and other developmental delays.* The average IQ for an individual with FAS is 68. Such an individual generally attains an average reading level of a fourth-grader and the average math skills of second grade. The development of typical motor milestones is delayed, and evidence of poor coordination, slow response times, and language disabilities is common.

2. *Low birthweight* (below the 10th percentile). In addition, the infants fail to thrive, producing poor catch-up growth.

3. *Neurological problems.* Some infants are born with high alcohol levels and experience withdrawal from the drug, which includes tremors and seizures starting within 6 to 12 hours of birth and lasting as long as a week. Abnormal electroencephalogram recordings per-

sist, and the infant shows a high degree of irritability and hypersensitivity to sound. These infants show poor sucking reflexes, hyperactivity, attentional deficits, and poor sleep patterns.

4. *Distinctive craniofacial malformations.* These include a small head, small wide-set eyes with drooping eyelids, a short upturned nose, a thin upper lip, and flattening of the vertical groove between the nose and upper lip (Figure A). The infants may also show low-set and nonparallel ears, malformations of the ear that produce hearing deficits, cleft palate, and reduced growth of the lower jaw.

5. *Other physical abnormalities.* Cardiac defects such as a hole between the chambers or deformed blood vessels in the heart, failure of kidney development, undescended testes, and skeletal abnormalities in fingers and toes are common.

How sure are we that alcohol itself is **teratogenic** (i.e., causes birth defects)? After all, women using high

doses of alcohol often have poor nutrition, smoke cigarettes or use other drugs, have poor health overall, and get poor prenatal care. These issues have been well controlled in animal research that can regulate the amount of alcohol, the pattern of consumption, the timing of alcohol use during the pregnancy, and the diet of the mother. Early conclusions and subsequent research agree that prenatal alcohol does induce both physical defects and behavioral deficits in animals that closely resemble those in humans. Single large doses of alcohol given to pregnant mice produced abnormalities in the developing fetuses (Figure B), including eye damage, smaller brains, and facial deformities similar to those seen in human babies with FAS. The amount of alcohol responsible was equivalent to a woman drinking a quart of whiskey over 24 hours.

The blood alcohol level is important in estimating the risk and severity of teratogenic effects, but the pattern of alcohol use that contributes to the peak maternal blood alcohol level is

BOX 9.1 (continued)

(B) Normal

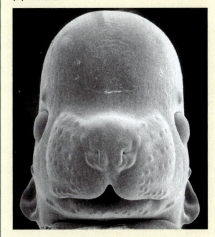

Exposed to alcohol

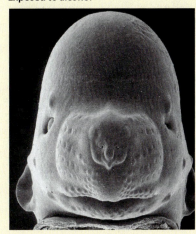

equally important. In one rodent study, 12 equally spaced doses of alcohol that produced maternal blood levels up to 0.12% did not affect fetal brain growth. In contrast, the same total amount of alcohol given in condensed fashion raised maternal blood levels to a range between 0.20 to 0.35% and caused a significant decrease in brain weight (Randall et al., 1990). Although that blood level is quite high, it is consistent with blood levels following binge drinking in humans.

In addition to the amount and pattern of alcohol ingestion, the develop-mental stage of the fetus when exposed to alcohol is critical in determining the specific effects. Organ systems are most vulnerable to damage during the period of most rapid development. Alcohol ingestion at the time of conception significantly increases the risk of teratogenic effects, and within the first 3 weeks the fetus may not survive. Alcohol use during the fourth to ninth weeks, a time when many women are unaware of their pregnancy, produces the most severe formative damage and severe mental retardation. Alcohol use later in the pregnancy causes slowed growth. Since the brain is one of the first organ systems to begin to develop but also is the last to be complete, alcohol use at any point in the pregnancy can have damaging effects on the CNS. Obviously, if drinking is constant throughout the fetal development, the effects will be much greater than if drinking is stopped mid-pregnancy.

Although the damaging effects of fetal alcohol exposure are clear, its precise mechanism is less certain. There are some suggestions that acetaldehyde may be the toxic agent, while other possible mechanisms include decreased blood flow in the uterine artery, reducing oxygen availability; or placental dysfunction, reducing the transport of vital amino acids, glucose, folate, or zinc. Hormone-like substances called prostaglandins are also suspected of mediating teratogenic effects, because inhibitors of prostaglandins, such as aspirin, reduce alcohol-induced birth defects in animals. Recent research also finds that ethanol acting on both glutamate and GABA neural transmission may trigger significant cell death (apoptosis) in the developing brain (Ikonomidou et al., 2000). (Figure A from Jones et al., 1973; Figure B from Sulik et al., 1981.)

Asian individuals (e.g., Japanese, Korean, Chinese) have genes that code only for an inactive form of the enzyme (Figure 9.5B). For these individuals, drinking even small amounts of alcohol produces very high levels of acetaldehyde, causing intense flushing, nausea and vomiting, tachycardia, headache, sweating, dizziness, and confusion. Because these individuals almost always totally abstain from using alcohol, they have no risk for alcoholism. Another 40% of the Asian population have genes that code for both the active and inactive enzyme. These heterozygous individuals have a more intense response to alcohol but not necessarily an unpleasant one. They are partially protected from alcohol dependence and have a lower vulnerability, making the *ALDH* gene a marker for low risk of alcoholism.

The second class of liver enzymes are those that belong to the **cytochrome P450** family, which metabolize many drugs in addition to alcohol. Because when alcohol is consumed along with these other drugs they must compete for the same enzyme molecules, alcohol consumption may lead to high and potentially dangerous levels of the other drugs. Be sure to look for warnings on both prescription and over-the-counter medications before consuming alcohol with any other drug. In contrast to the acute effect, when alcohol is consumed on a regular basis these liver enzymes *increase* in number, which increases the rate of metabolism of alcohol as well as any other drugs normally metabolized by these enzymes. The process is called **induction** of liver enzymes and is the basis for drug disposition tolerance, which is described in the next section. Finally, prolonged heavy use of alcohol causes liver damage that significantly impairs metabolism of alcohol and many other drugs.

Based on the pharmacokinetic factors just described, you know that the amount of alcohol in your blood depends on how much you have consumed and also on the rate of

TABLE 9.1 Estimated BAC and Impairment as a Function of Time for Men and Women According to Body Weight[a]

Drinks	Approximate Blood Alcohol Concentration[b] (Men) Body weight (pounds)							
	100	120	140	160	180	200	220	240
0	.00	.00	.00	.00	.00	.00	.00	.00
1	.04	.03	.03	.02	.02	.02	.02	.02
2	.08	.06	.05	.05	.04	.04	.03	.03
3	.11	.09	.08	.07	.06	.06	.05	.05
4	.15	.12	.11	.09	.08	.08	.07	.06
5	.19	.16	.13	.12	.11	.09	.09	.08
6	.23	.19	.16	.14	.13	.11	.10	.09
7	.26	.22	.19	.16	.15	.13	.12	.11
8	.30	.25	.21	.19	.17	.15	.14	.13
9	.34	.28	.24	.21	.19	.17	.15	.14
10	.38	.31	.27	.23	.21	.19	.17	.16

Drinks	Approximate Blood Alcohol Concentration (Women) Body weight (pounds)							
	90	100	120	140	160	180	200	220
0	.00	.00	.00	.00	.00	.00	.00	.00
1	.05	.05	.04	.03	.03	.03	.02	.02
2	.10	.09	.08	.07	.06	.05	.05	.04
3	.15	.14	.11	.10	.09	.08	.07	.06
4	.20	.18	.15	.13	.11	.10	.09	.08
5	.25	.23	.19	.16	.14	.13	.11	.10
6	.30	.27	.23	.19	.17	.15	.14	.12
7	.35	.32	.27	.23	.20	.18	.16	.14
8	.40	.36	.30	.26	.23	.20	.18	.17
9	.45	.41	.34	.29	.26	.23	.20	.19
10	.51	.45	.38	.32	.28	.25	.23	.21

Source: Pennsylvania Liquor Control Board, 1995.

[a]Note: Your body can get rid of one drink per hour.

[b]0.2–.04 = Impairment begins; .05–.07 = Impaired driving; .08 and greater = Legal intoxication

absorption and metabolism. Table 9.1 provides a rough estimate of BAC based on the number of drinks consumed in 1 hour and the body weight of the individual, assuming the metabolism of approximately 1 ounce per hour.

Chronic alcohol use leads to both tolerance and physical dependence

Tolerance The effects of alcohol are significantly reduced when the drug is administered repeatedly; hence, **tolerance** occurs. There is also **cross-tolerance** with a variety of other

drugs in the sedative–hypnotic class, including the barbiturates and the benzodiazepines. Each of the four mechanisms that we described in Chapter 1 contributes to alcohol tolerance.

1. **Acute tolerance** occurs within a single exposure to alcohol. Several of the subjective and behavioral drug effects are greater while the blood level of alcohol is increasing and are less while the blood level is falling (Figure 9.6A). LeBlanc and colleagues (1975) found that alcohol-induced incoordination in rats was 50% less while blood levels were falling as measured by the amount of time off a mini-treadmill during a single exposure to alcohol. Why acute tolerance occurs is not entirely clear, but some rapid adaptation of neuronal membranes is one possibility.

2. Chronic alcohol use increases both alcohol dehydrogenase and the P450 liver microsomal enzymes that metabolize the drug. More rapid metabolism means that blood levels of the drug will be reduced (Figure 9.6B), producing diminished effects (**drug disposition tolerance**).

3. Neurons also adapt to the continued presence of alcohol by making compensatory changes in cell function. The mechanism of this **pharmacodynamic tolerance** is described in later sections dealing with specific neurotransmitters.

4. Finally, there is also clear evidence of **behavioral tolerance.** Rats, like humans, seem to be able to learn to adjust their behaviors when allowed to practice while under the influence of alcohol (Wenger et al., 1981). Although initially unsuccessful, rats readily learned to run on a treadmill despite the administration of alcohol. Other rats given the same amount of drug each day *after* their treadmill session showed only minimal improvement when tested on the treadmill under the influence of alcohol. That small amount of improvement may have been due to drug disposition tolerance.

Classical conditioning may also contribute to behavioral tolerance. In animal experiments alcohol initially reduces body

(A) Acute tolerance

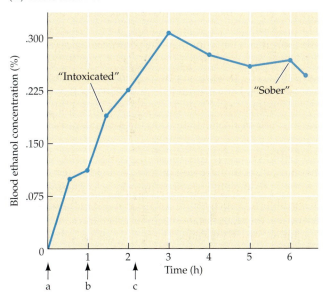

(B) Drug disposition tolerance

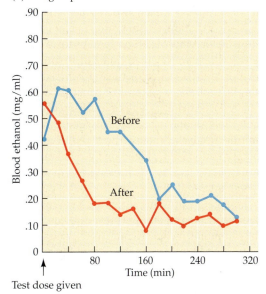

Test dose given

Figure 9.6 Tolerance to alcohol (A) After three doses of alcohol (a, b, c), signs of intoxication (such as incoordination in the balance beam test) appeared during the rising phase of blood alcohol levels at about 0.20%. However, as blood alcohol was declining, the human subject became sober at a higher concentration (about 0.265%), showing that acute tolerance had occurred. Note that the high blood levels for intoxication reflect the fact that the subject was a chronically heavy user of alcohol.

(B) Blood alcohol levels were calculated at 20-minute intervals after a test dose was given at time zero. The blue line represents blood levels before a 7-day period of drinking; the red line shows blood levels in the same person after 7 days of drinking (3.2 grams of ethanol per kilogram of body weight per day in individual doses). Tolerance following repeated alcohol consumption is shown by the more rapid decrease in blood alcohol. (A after Mirsky et al., 1941; B after Goldstein et al., 1974.)

temperature, but when the drug is administered repeatedly in the same environment, a compensatory increase in body temperature occurs, which reduces the initial hypothermia (low body temperature). If these animals are given saline instead of alcohol in this environment, they show *only* the compensatory mechanism and their body temperature rises (hyperthermia). The importance of environment is further demonstrated by evidence that in a novel environment the tolerance is significantly less because there is no conditioned hyperthermia (Le et al., 1979).

Physical dependence   We know that prolonged use of alcohol produces **physical dependence,** because a significant withdrawal syndrome occurs when drinking is terminated. As you already know, the intensity and duration of abstinence signs are dependent on the amount and duration of drug taking (Figure 9.7). In addition, alcohol shows **cross dependence** with other drugs in the sedative–hypnotic class, including barbiturates and benzodiazepines. A quick review of Chapter 1 will remind you that withdrawal signs can be eliminated by taking the drug again or by taking any drug in the same class that shows cross dependence.

Some investigators suggest that the **"hangover"** that occurs after even a single bout of heavy drinking may in fact also be evidence of withdrawal, although others consider it

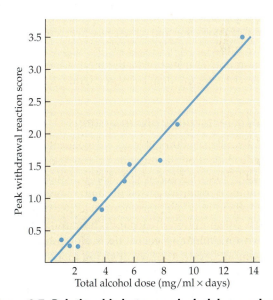

Figure 9.7 Relationship between alcohol dose and withdrawal severity A linear relationship exists between the total alcohol dose (amount of alcohol consumed multiplied by number of days of alcohol exposure) and the maximum withdrawal response at abstinence in mice. Withdrawal response was calculated based on standard physiological and behavioral measures. (After Goldstein, 1972.)

a sign of acute toxicity. Possible explanations for hangover symptoms include residual acetaldehyde in the body; alcohol-induced gastric irritation; rebound drop in blood sugar; excess fluid loss the previous night; or perhaps toxic effects from congeners, which are small amounts of by-products from fermentation and distillation that may accumulate after heavy drinking. The classic symptoms of hangover are recognized by many social drinkers who on occasion consume an excess of alcohol. Among the usual signs are nausea and perhaps vomiting, headache, intense thirst and dry mouth that feels a bit like cotton balls, fatigue, and general malaise.

Withdrawal from repeated heavy drinking over months or years produces an intense abstinence syndrome that develops within a few hours after drinking stops and may continue over 2 to 4 days, depending on the dose previously consumed. Generally, the symptoms include tremor (the "shakes") and intense anxiety, high blood pressure and rapid heart rate, excessive sweating, rapid breathing, and nausea and vomiting. A small percentage of alcoholics undergoing withdrawal demonstrate more-severe effects called **delirium tremens,** or DTs. Signs of DTs include irritability, headaches, agitation, and confusion. In addition, convulsions; vivid and frightening hallucinations that include snakes, rats, or insects crawling on their bodies; total disorientation; and delirium may occur. Some of the withdrawal signs, such as unstable blood pressure, depression and anxiety including panic attacks, and sleep disturbances, may last for several weeks. Since the most extreme symptoms are potentially life-threatening, detoxification of an alcoholic individual (see the section on alcoholism later in the chapter) should always be done under medical supervision. The syndrome is characteristically a "rebound" phenomenon and represents a hyperexcitable state of the nervous system following the prolonged depressant effects of alcohol. The neuroadaptive mechanisms responsible are described more completely later in this chapter.

Alcohol affects many organ systems

Alcohol, like all drugs, produces dose-dependent effects that are also dependent on the duration of drug taking. Since it is so readily absorbed and widely distributed, alcohol has effects on most organ systems of the body. As you read this section, keep in mind that there is no evidence that light to moderate consumption of alcohol is harmful, and it may even have some minor beneficial effects. However, the transition from moderate to heavy drinking that leads to the chronic intoxication associated with alcoholism is a part of the same dose–response curve, and the precise point at which alcohol becomes damaging is not clear for a particular individual.

A second thing to keep in mind is that the environment and expectation have a great influence on many of the behav-

ioral effects of alcohol. A host of well-controlled studies clearly show that a subject's *belief* that alcohol will produce relaxation, sexual desire, or aggression may have far more effect on the individual's behavior than the pharmacological effects of the drug, at least at low to moderate doses. Pronounced behavioral effects occur in placebo conditions if the individual believes he has ingested alcohol. Refer to Box 9.2 for a demonstration. As you might expect, the environment plays less of a role in alcohol's effects as the dose increases.

CNS effects   As is true for all the drugs in the sedative–hypnotic class, at the lowest doses an individual feels relaxed and less anxious. In a quiet setting she may feel somewhat sleepy, but in a social setting where sensory stimulation is increased, the relaxed state is demonstrated by reduced social inhibition, which may make the individual more gregarious, talkative, and friendly or inappropriately outspoken. Self-perception and judgment are somewhat impaired, and one may feel more confident than reality proves true. Reduced judgment and overconfidence may increase risk-taking behaviors and may make sexual encounters more likely. Of additional concern is the alcohol-induced loss of judgment on the initiation of unsafe sex practices that may lead to increased risk of AIDS and other sexually transmitted diseases. In a large representative sample of 12,069 young men and women, a significant relationship between alcohol use and sexual risk taking was found even after controlling for age, education, and family income (Parker et al., 1994). Since the relationship between alcohol use and unsafe sex is correlational, no clear cause-and-effect relationship can be assumed and other factors such as rebellion against societal expectations may be responsible for both.

Acute effects of alcohol on memory vary with dose and task difficulty (Jung, 2001). At low doses, memory deficits are based more on expectation than on the quantity of alcohol actually consumed. Further, under high-stress conditions, alcohol may enhance performance by minimizing the damaging effects of anxiety. However, high doses of alcohol rapidly consumed may produce total amnesia for the events that occur during intoxication, despite the fact that the individual is behaving quite normally. This amnesia is called a **blackout,** and it is a common occurrence for alcoholics but also occurs in about 25% of social drinkers (Campbell and Hodgins, 1993).

Reduced coordination leads to slurred speech, impaired fine-motor skills, and delayed reaction time. Reductions in reaction times for multiple stimuli along with reductions in attention, increased sedation and drowsiness, and impaired judgment and emotional control all contribute to the increased probability of being involved in automobile accidents. Alcohol is involved in about half of all highway deaths, and there is a distinct temporal pattern of high-risk alcohol-

BOX 9.2   Pharmacology in Action

The Role of Expectation in Alcohol-Enhanced Human Sexual Response

One problem in evaluating the effects of alcohol on behavior is that individuals have expectations about how alcohol will affect them. It is frequently believed (in our culture) that alcohol will increase sociability, reduce anxiety and tension, increase aggression, and enhance sexual responses. However, many of the effects of alcohol, especially at low doses, are due to the individual's expectation of effect more than the drug's pharmacological effect (Marlatt and Rohsenow, 1980).

As you probably recall, experiments measuring drug effects have at least two groups of subjects: a drug treatment group and a placebo (non-drug) group who generally assume they are also receiving the drug. Since both groups expect to receive the drug, any difference in their scores reflects the effect of the drug alone. However, since both groups believe they are getting the drug, there is no direct measure of the extent of **expectancy.** A further elaboration of the research design that more specifically tests the role that expectation plays is a four-block or 2×2 design (see figure). In this design, half the subjects are *told* that they will get alcohol and half are *told* that they will get placebo. Half of each of the two groups will actually get alcohol. Thus, there are two groups who get what they are expecting and two groups who are deceived and receive the opposite treatment.

In order to be effective, these experiments must completely deceive the subjects, which includes providing the alcohol in a way that it cannot be detected, such as combining vodka and tonic and at relatively low doses. In addition, subjects must also be deceived about the purpose of the experiment, for instance, by being told they are involved in a taste test of either different vodkas or different tonic waters.

Results from experiments using the 2×2 design support the hypothesis that when subjects think they have received alcohol, their behavior reflects their *expectations* of the drug effect. For example, in one study, college students watched erotic videos showing heterosexual and homosexual activity. The low dose of alcohol administered (0.04%) did not have an effect on physiological arousal, as measured by penile tumescence, but an expectancy effect occurred. The group *expecting* to receive alcohol showed more physical and subjective arousal than the group that did not expect to receive alcohol, regardless of whether they actually received alcohol or not (Wilson and Lawson, 1976b). This seems to be a case when a drinker's beliefs about the effects of a drug become a self-fulfilling prophecy and their actions match their expectations.

An additional way to isolate pharmacological effects from expectation is to look at cross-cultural studies. Those of us who drink alcohol or observe others drinking may believe that alcohol induces our amorous nature, makes us more sexually appealing, and enhances our basic sexuality. But does it really? The observations of the anthropologists MacAndrew and Edgerton (1969) say something quite different. They found, for example, that the Camba of Bolivia are a people with strong, almost puritanical taboos regarding sexual activities. When intoxicated, they become extremely gregarious and outgoing, maintaining festivities long into the night. However, regardless of the revelry, they never fail to maintain strict sexual limits. The Tarhumara of Mexico also strictly limit sexual encounters under normal conditions. However, when they are drunk, mate swapping becomes the norm and is not considered inappropriate. For the Lepcha of Sikkim, sex is the primary recreation beginning at age 10 or 11 and continuing through old age. Adultery is expected and generates no ill will. Sex is an open topic for conversation and humor. During harvest festival time, large amounts of homemade liquor are consumed and the Lepchas' casual sexual customs become wildly promiscuous in order to enhance the harvest. With adult encouragement, even 4- and 5-year-olds imitate copulation with each other. Nevertheless, their very strict guidelines regarding incest taboos are never broken even when the Lepcha are quite drunk.

How can we explain experiences so different from our own? Does alcohol have a predetermined biological effect on sexual activity? Or does it induce disinhibition only within the context and limits of a given culture? How do *our* cultural expectations influence the effects of the drug?

Actually receive

	Tonic water	Ethanol
Tonic water		
Ethanol		

Expect to receive

(A)

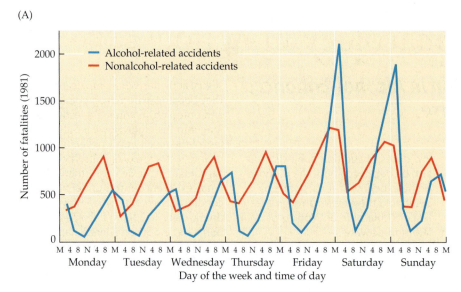

(B)

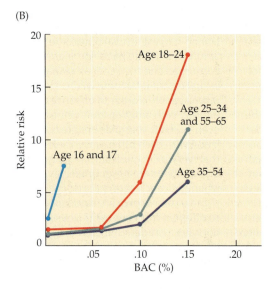

Figure 9.8 Relationship between alcohol use and traffic accidents
(A) The number of fatal auto accidents varies by day of the week, time of day, and alcohol involvement. Note that alcohol-related fatalities peak on Friday and Saturday night after midnight and that on other days the accidents involving alcohol are also most frequently late at night. Nonalcohol-related fatalities appear to be greatest during rush hours on weekdays and just before midnight on weekends. (B) The relationship between BAC and relative risk of auto accidents interacts with several factors, including age of the driver and years of driving experience. Notice that, in general, alcohol has a less detrimental effect on driving as drivers get older, but the 55-to-65-year age group is similar to the 25-to-34-year age group, which may indicate an interaction with age-related decreases in reaction time. The rapid rise in the number of accidents at BAC over 0.10% has prompted many states to reduce the definition of legal intoxication from 0.10% to 0.08%. (A after NIAAA, 1983; B after OECD, 1978.)

lent activities, although the direct pharmacological effect of alcohol is less clear. Box 9.3 looks at this relationship. Aggression and many of the other effects of alcohol on behavior are highly dependent on the environment, the user's mental set, and her expectations.

With increasing doses, mild sedation deepens and produces sleep. Alcohol suppresses REM (rapid eye movement) episodes (periods when the most dreaming occurs), and withdrawal following repeated use produces a rebound in REM sleep that may interfere with normal sleep patterns and produce nightmares. Higher doses produce unconsciousness and death. The blood alcohol level that is lethal in 50% of the population is in the range of 0.45%, which is only about five or six times the blood level (0.08%) that produces intoxication. Fortunately, most people do not reach a lethal blood level, because at around 0.15% vomiting may occur and a BAC of 0.35% usually causes unconsciousness, thereby preventing further drinking. However, if the alcohol is consumed very rapidly, as might occur in binge drinking, lethal blood levels may be reached before the individual passes out.

The usual symptoms of **alcohol poisoning** include unconsciousness; vomiting; slow and irregular breathing; and skin that is cold, clammy, and pale bluish in color. When death occurs from acute alcohol ingestion, it is due to depression of the respiratory control center in the brain stem. Once the respiratory mechanism is depressed, the drinker can sur-

related deaths (Figure 9.8A). In addition, there is a clear statistical relationship between BAC and the relative risk of an accident. At a BAC below 0.05%, the chances of having an accident are about the same as for nondrinking drivers, but between 0.05% and 0.10%, the curve rises steeply to seven times the nondrinking rate. It is this large increase that has prompted most states to change their blood level for legal intoxication from 0.10% to 0.08%. Beyond 0.10%, risk increases dramatically by 20 to 50 times. However, the relationship is complex, and BAC interacts with both age and driving experience (Figure 9.8B). Use Table 9.1 to estimate the amount of alcohol that you must consume in 1 hour to reach the BAC that increases risk.

In addition to involvement in automobile fatalities, alcohol use is also associated with homicide, rape, and other vio-

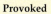

BOX 9.3   # Drugs and Society

Alcohol and Aggression

Alcohol is generally believed to elicit violence and aggression. Many reports show that the majority of individuals who commit violent offenses are under the influence of alcohol at the time of the crime. One 1997 survey reported that 42% of state prisoners and 25% of federal prisoners who were convicted of violent crimes including murder, rape, and assault had used alcohol at the time of the incident. In one-half to two-thirds of homicides, the offender, victim, or both were intoxicated. Overall, at least 50% of rape cases involve alcohol. In Pasadena, California, over a 2-week period, 50% of all arrests, 60% of rapes, and more than 50% of domestic assaults involved alcohol (Jung, 2001). In addition, alcohol intoxication is significant in many types of violent deaths including fire (46%), drowning (53%), and pedestrian deaths (27%).

Although these statistics are striking, keep in mind that such correlations do not constitute evidence that alcohol pharmacologically induces aggression. In our society, alcohol and violence frequently occur together, but as is true for all correlations, no cause-and-effect relationship can be assumed. After all, drinking alcohol may lead to aggression, but behaving aggressively may produce guilt or fear that causes drinking. Or, a third factor may be responsible for both behaviors. For instance, a personality factor such as impulsiveness or hyperactivity may lead one to be more aggressive and may also lead to greater alcohol consumption.

Laboratory studies measuring the tendency to "punish" an unseen individual generally show that alcohol increases aggression compared to controls. However, these situations are not readily generalizable to real-life situations where aggression is face-to-face and conducted in a complex setting. Furthermore, when balanced placebo designs are used, the role of expectancy (i.e., a subject's believing he received alcohol) on aggression in both provoked and unprovoked situations is more important than whether the individual actually receives alcohol (see figure). Finally, cross-cultural studies suggest that alcohol-induced aggression is not a universal occurrence and that, in contrast to other cultures, many Americans view being intoxicated as a legitimate occasion for aggressive and other socially inappropriate behaviors.

Chermack and Giancola (1997) provide a model to show the multiple factors that may interact with the pharmacological effect of alcohol consumption in determining the occurrence of violent behavior. Based on this model, early childhood experiences may set the stage for future aggressive acts. Psychiatric disorders, current mood, expectancies of alcohol's effects, and other variables interact with alcohol use and with the immediate situation that the individual finds himself in (threat, provocation, personal relationship). The reciprocal nature of these factors should be clear. For example, alcohol may lead to misinterpretation of social cues or remarks made in jest as threatening, which may influence aggression. But a threatening or provocative situation may also increase alcohol consumption.

We must conclude that there is no simple answer to the question of why alcohol use and violent behaviors are closely correlated in our society. In the meantime, alcohol use does not justify or condone illegal or violent behavior, nor does it diminish personal responsibility for one's actions.

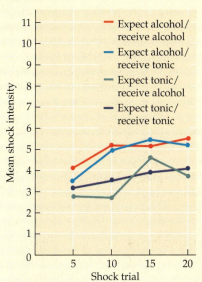

Provoked

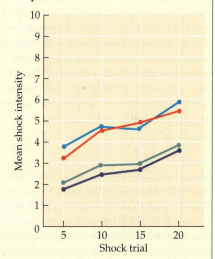

Unprovoked

Expectancy of alcohol increases aggression In both provoked and unprovoked situations, the subjects who expected to receive alcohol delivered stronger shocks to "punish" an unseen individual than those who expected tonic (regardless of what they actually received). (After Lang et al., 1975.)

TABLE 9.2 Blood Alcohol Concentration and Effects on Behavior

BAC	Effects on behavior
.02–.03	Minimal effects; slight relaxation; mild mood elevation
.05–.06	Decreased alertness; relaxed inhibitions; mildly impaired judgment
.08–.10	Loss of motor coordination; slower reaction times; less caution
.14–.16	Major impairment of mental and physical control; slurred speech; exaggerated emotions; blurred vision; serious loss of judgment; large increases in reaction time
.20–.25	Staggering; inability to walk or dress without help; tears or rage with little provocation; mental confusion; double vision
.30	Conscious but in a stupor; unaware of surroundings
.45	Coma; lethal for 50% of the population

vive for about 5 minutes, although brain damage from oxygen deprivation occurs. Some of the dose-dependent effects of alcohol are summarized in Table 9.2.

Brain damage   The brain damage that occurs after many years of heavy alcohol consumption is caused by the interaction of several factors, including high levels of alcohol, elevated acetaldehyde, liver deficiency, and inadequate nutrition. In particular, heavy alcohol use produces a serious deficiency in vitamin B$_1$ (thiamine) due to both a poor diet and failure to absorb that vitamin as well as other nutrients during digestion. Because thiamine is critical for brain glucose metabolism, its deficit causes cell death. One result is **Wernicke–Korsakoff syndrome,** which in its first stage is characterized by confusion and disorientation as well as tremors, poor coordination, and ataxia. In later stages the patient shows a significant memory disorder. Although the patient remembers the remote past, he remembers almost nothing of what goes on around him. He may read the same page over and over, repeatedly ask the same questions, or tell the same story. Although the syndrome is progressive, treatment with massive doses of vitamin B$_1$ can stop the degenerative process (if alcohol use stops), though it cannot reverse it. Wernicke–Korsakoff syndrome is characterized by bilateral cell loss in the medial thalamus and the mammillary bodies of the hypothalamus. Although nutritional deficits are not the sole cause of the disorder, the importance of thiamine to the degenerative process is evident in animal studies. Feeding animals with a thiamine-deficient diet or treating them with a thiamine antagonist produces lesions in the same brain areas and also impairs learning and memory (Langlais and Savage, 1995). In addition, selective brain lesions like those of Wernicke–Korsakoff syndrome are found in other individuals with severe nutritional deficiencies associated with gastrointestinal diseases, anorexia nervosa, or starvation.

Although thiamine deficiency causes the selective damage described in the previous paragraph, other brain areas also frequently show cell loss that seems to be unrelated to diet. The enlarged ventricles seen in the brains of alcoholics attest to the extensive shrinkage of brain tissue (Figure 9.9A). Exterior views of alcoholic brains compared to controls also show smaller brain mass (Figure 9.9B). Frontal lobes are the most affected, and this may be responsible for the personality changes, including apathy, disinhibition, and diminished executive functioning (ability to formulate strategies and make decisions) seen in alcoholics. The tissue shrinkage that occurs in medial temporal lobe structures, including the hippocampus and cholinergic cells in the basal forebrain, contribute to memory disturbances. Symptoms that implicate the hippocampus and basal forebrain include failure to remember recent events or form new memories. Cerebellar cell loss is correlated with ataxia and incoordination, particularly of the lower limbs. These brain changes are probably caused by multiple mechanisms, but the glutamate-induced hyperexcitability of neurons during abstinence (see the section on neurotransmitters later in the chapter) may play a central role (Fadda and Rossetti, 1998).

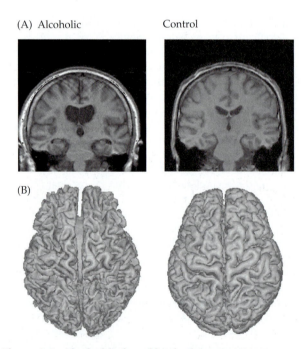

Figure 9.9 Alcohol-induced brain damage (A) Brain images of an alcholic male subject and a nonalcoholic male. Note the extreme difference in ventricle size, indicating tissue shrinkage in the alcoholic's brain. (B) Exterior views of the brains (from above). In the alcholic, the gyri are more narrow, and the sulci and fissure between the hemispheres are very enlarged, showing significant loss of tissue volume. (A from Pfefferbaum and Sullivan, 2004; B from Sullivan, 2000.)

Effects on other organ systems   Alcohol also has many effects on the body outside the CNS including the:

- cardiovascular system;
- renal–urinary system;
- reproductive system;
- gastrointestinal system; and
- liver.

One well-known cardiovascular effect of alcohol is the dilation of peripheral blood vessels, which brings them closer to the surface of the skin and makes an individual look flushed and feel warm. Of course, the vasodilation means that heat is actually being lost from the body rather than being retained. Although the myth of the Saint Bernard dog rescuing stranded skiers with a keg of brandy around his neck is widespread, in reality, drinking alcohol when you are truly cold produces an even more serious drop in body temperature. In cold climates, heavy drinkers who fall asleep outside risk death from hypothermia. Within the brain, vasodilation may help cognitive function in older adults. At the end of a 6-year period, researchers found that people 55 years and older who consumed one to three drinks a day were less than half as likely to have developed dementia linked to poor oxygen supply to the brain as those people who did not drink at all.

In addition to aiding circulation, low to moderate daily doses of alcohol (for example, less than three drinks) may reduce the risk of heart disease, because it increases the amount of "good" cholesterol in the blood while reducing the "bad" (Gaziano and Hennekens, 1995) and seems to reduce the incidence of blood clots and stroke. However, the beneficial effects are counteracted when consumption is higher. Alcoholism is associated with a higher-than-expected incidence of high blood pressure, stroke, and inflammation and enlargement of the heart muscle, which may be alcohol-induced or due to malnutrition and vitamin deficiency.

Alcohol's action on the renal–urinary system produces larger volumes of urine that is far more dilute than normal. The loss of fluids is caused by the reduced secretion of antidiuretic hormone. Although this is not normally of concern, alcohol consumption should be avoided by individuals involved in strenuous athletic activities in which fluids need to be maintained. Further, athletes should not try to rehydrate with any beverage containing alcohol.

The effect of alcohol on reproductive function is complex. Alcohol is widely believed to enhance sexual arousal and lower inhibitions. However, in Box 9.2 you saw that expectation plays a large part in alcohol's effects on sexual response. Furthermore, we need to distinguish between psychological arousal and physiological response. In one study, male college students consumed alcohol to achieve BACs of 0, 0.025, 0.050, or 0.075% while watching an erotic film (George and Norris, 1991). A plethysmograph was attached around the penis to measure degree of erection (both rate of tumescence and

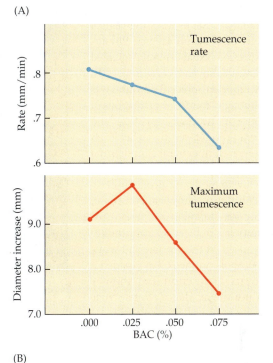

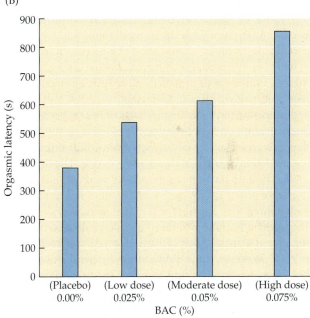

Figure 9.10 Effects of alcohol on sexual response (A) Changes in male sexual response occur after varying amounts of alcohol. With increasing concentrations of blood alcohol, both the rate of penile tumescence and the maximum size achieved decreased. (B) In women, increasing blood alcohol levels were directly proportional to orgasmic latency. (A after Farkas and Rosen, 1976; B after Blume, 1991.)

maximum achieved) during the film viewing. Figure 9.10A shows that low doses of alcohol enhanced the arousal to a small extent, but higher blood levels reduced the male sexual response. Parallel studies with college women measured sexual arousal by assessing vaginal blood pressure or orgasmic latency. Physiological measures of sexual arousal decreased with increasing alcohol levels (Figure 9.10B); however, the reported subjective arousal was increased. Although laboratory evaluations of sexual response are necessarily artificial and ethical restraint prohibits testing higher levels of alcohol, research in general supports the inverse nature of physiological and subjective arousal with low to moderate alcohol use.

When alcohol use is heavy and chronic, males may become impotent and show atrophy of the testicles, reduced sperm production, and shrinkage of the prostate and seminal vesicles. Alcoholic women often experience disrupted ovarian function and show a higher-than-normal incidence of menstrual disorders.

Alcohol alters gastrointestinal tract function in several ways. It increases salivation and secretion of gastric juices, which may explain its ability to increase appetite and aid digestion, although higher concentrations irritate the stomach lining and long-term chronic use produces inflammation of the stomach (gastritis) as well as of the esophagus. Heavy alcohol use causes diarrhea, inhibits utilization of proteins, and reduces absorption and metabolism of vitamins and minerals.

Among the most damaging effects of heavy chronic alcohol consumption is liver dysfunction. Three distinct disorders may develop. The first is **fatty liver,** which involves the accumulation of triglycerides inside liver cells. The liver normally takes up and metabolizes fatty acids as part of the digestive process; however, when alcohol is present, it is metabolized first, leaving the fat for storage. The condition produces no warning symptoms but is reversible, so if drinking stops, the liver begins to use the stored fat and returns to normal. However, some individuals who have abused alcohol for many years develop a serious and potentially lethal condition called **alcoholic hepatitis.** Liver cell damage is apparently caused by accumulation of high levels of acetaldehyde (a metabolite of alcohol formed in the liver). Symptoms include inflammation of the liver, fever, yellowing of the skin (jaundice), and pain. The death of liver cells stimulates the formation of scar tissue, which is characteristic of **alcoholic cirrhosis.** As the scar tissue develops, blood vessels carrying oxygen are cut off, leading to further cell death. Figure 9.11 compares pieces of normal liver, fatty liver, and cirrhotic liver from an alcoholic individual. Cirrhotic livers are usually firm or hard to the touch and develop nodules of tissue that give them a pebbly appearance. As cirrhosis continues, liver function decreases proportionately. Consumption of large quan-

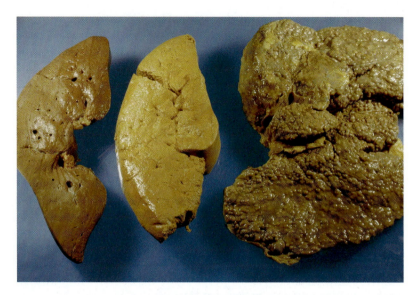

Figure 9.11 The effects of chronic alcohol use on the liver Portions of a healthy liver (left), fatty liver (center) and cirrhotic liver (right).

tities of alcohol over a prolonged period of time is necessary for the development of cirrhosis, and even among heavy drinkers, only 10 to 20% are likely to develop the disease. However, the incidence of alcoholic cirrhosis has increased over the last 10 years, and it is most common in men between 40 and 60 years of age. Although the liver damage is irreversible, cessation of drinking slows the rate of the damage. For severe liver damage, the most effective treatment is liver transplant surgery.

Section Summary

The unique physical properties of alcohol make it a drug that is readily absorbed from the GI tract and distributed to most cells of the body. Absorption, however, is highly variable from one person to another and from one occasion to another, depending on the amount of alcohol consumed and the individual's stomach contents and gender. Metabolism also varies significantly and depends on two metabolic pathways, one using alcohol dehydrogenase and the second, cytochrome P450. The most pronounced effects of alcohol involve alterations of nervous system function, causing reduced anxiety, disinhibition, intoxication, memory impairment, and sleep. Higher concentrations lead to anesthesia, coma, and death. Alcohol has effects on other organ systems as well, increasing blood circulation, enhancing fluid loss, diminishing physical sexual arousal while increasing subjective sexual arousal, and modifying digestion. Following chronic heavy alcohol use, significant brain damage occurs, leading to impaired learning, personality changes, reduced executive functioning, and poor coordination. Chronic alcoholism also impairs normal sexual function, damages the liver, and increases the chances of stroke and heart muscle enlargement.

Multiple forms of tolerance develop to chronic alcohol use, as does cross-tolerance with other sedative–hypnotic drugs. Physical dependence is manifested by an abstinence syndrome characterized by rebound anxiety, elevated heart rate and blood pressure, and nausea and vomiting. More severe withdrawal following higher doses may produce a potentially fatal hyperexcitability of the nervous system called delirium tremens.

Neurochemical Effects of Alcohol

The neurochemical effects of alcohol have proven more difficult to examine than some other drugs. One important reason is the chemical nature of the alcohol molecule that not only provides the means for easy penetration into the brain, but more importantly, influences the phospholipid bilayer of neurons. The latter action has a widespread impact on many normal cell functions and also modifies the action of many neurotransmitter systems. In addition, the initial effects of alcohol must be separated from the neuronal changes that occur after long-term drug use. For these and other reasons, research using animal experimentation is particularly important.

Animal models are vital to alcohol research

Animal models are particularly important in alcohol studies for several reasons. First, because research animals are maintained in controlled and healthful environments, they eliminate some of the common human correlates of heavy alcohol use: poor nutrition, liver damage, associated psychiatric disorders, and use of multiple drugs. Second, animal models allow us to use methods that are not appropriate for human subjects. For example, controlled chronic alcohol consumption can tell us about the long-term damaging effects on body functions and behavior and can model the effects of alcohol withdrawal. The effects of prenatal alcohol can be evaluated independently of issues such as maternal nutrition and substance abuse. Also, invasive procedures can be used to manipulate and measure the neurobiological correlates of intoxication, reinforcement, and behavioral effects of alcohol.

Third, genetic manipulations are possible. When large numbers of animals (usually mice or rats) are screened, a few will be found to voluntarily drink large quantities of alcohol rather than water, while most drink little of the ethanol solution. Two populations of animals can be developed by selectively breeding the heaviest drinkers and the abstainers

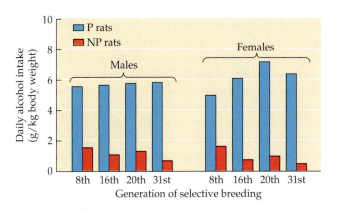

Figure 9.12 Average daily alcohol consumption for selected generations of rats bred for alcohol-preferring (P) or alcohol-nonpreferring (NP) behavior. Males and females show similar alcohol consumption. (After Stewart and Li, 1997.)

over several generations (Figure 9.12). Strains of alcohol-preferring or -nonpreferring animals may model human alcohol consumption and abuse and can be used to study behavioral, biochemical, and genetic differences. Animals can be bred for numerous alcohol-related characteristics including sensitivity to alcohol, intensity of withdrawal, and so forth. A second type of study uses genetically altered animals that fail to express a particular protein. These knockout animals are used to evaluate the role of one particular protein, for example, a specific receptor, in the effects of ethanol. Fourth, animal models serve as screening tools to evaluate treatment strategies. Several excellent reviews of animal models of various components of alcoholism, including adolescent onset, tolerance, abstinence, and relapse, are available for further study (Stewart and Li, 1997; McBride and Li, 1998).

The operant self-administration model used to evaluate the reinforcing effects of various drugs is described in Chapter 4. Self-administration procedures are more difficult with alcohol than with other drugs of abuse because most animals will not spontaneously consume enough alcohol to produce intoxication. However, one of several "training" methods can be used to get animals to self-administer alcohol. In the first, all dry food is presented once a day during the drinking session. Initially, water is available, but gradually increasing amounts of alcohol are added over a number of sessions. Finally, food presentation occurs at a different time, but the animals continue to consume the alcohol. Alternatively, after operant training to lever-press for a sucrose solution, the sucrose is gradually reduced in concentration and alcohol is gradually substituted until the animals are self-administering high levels of alcohol. These and other techniques using rats and nonhuman primates are described by Meisch and Stewart (1994).

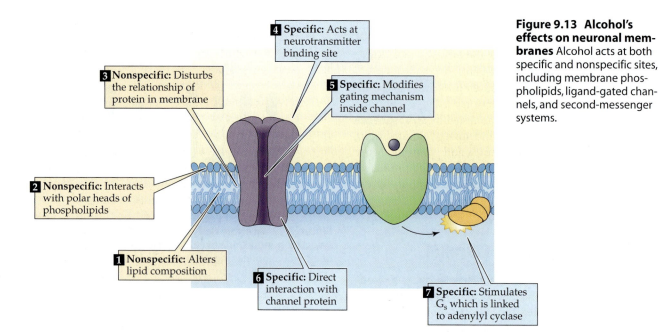

1 **Nonspecific:** Alters lipid composition

2 **Nonspecific:** Interacts with polar heads of phospholipids

3 **Nonspecific:** Disturbs the relationship of protein in membrane

4 **Specific:** Acts at neurotransmitter binding site

5 **Specific:** Modifies gating mechanism inside channel

6 **Specific:** Direct interaction with channel protein

7 **Specific:** Stimulates G_s which is linked to adenylyl cyclase

Figure 9.13 Alcohol's effects on neuronal membranes Alcohol acts at both specific and nonspecific sites, including membrane phospholipids, ligand-gated channels, and second-messenger systems.

Alcohol acts on multiple neurotransmitters

Because alcohol is such a simple molecule, it readily crosses cell membranes, including the blood–brain barrier, and can be detected in the brain within minutes after consumption. Alcohol has both specific and nonspecific actions. **Nonspecific actions** depend on its ability to move into membranes, changing the fluid character of the lipids that make up the membrane (Figure 9.13). As you might expect, the protein molecules that are embedded in that membrane are likely to function differently when their "environment" changes so dramatically and becomes less rigid. In contrast, at low to moderate doses, alcohol seems to interact with specific sites on particular proteins, and these **specific actions** are probably responsible for most of the acute effects of ethanol at intoxicating doses. Alcohol not only influences several ligand-gated channels but also directly alters second-messenger systems. For example, ethanol stimulates the G protein (G_s) that activates the cyclic adenosine monophosphate (cAMP) second-messenger system (Figure 9.13, step 7). Being able to identify specific sites of ethanol action means that ultimately new drugs will be found to compete with ethanol to prevent particular undesirable effects.

This section describes the acute effects of alcohol on several neurotransmitters, suggesting possible connections between the transmitter action and specific effects of alcohol. In addition, it examines the neuroadaptations that occur with repeated alcohol use as they link to tolerance and dependence. Throughout this discussion, keep in mind that no neurotransmitter system works in isolation; changes in each one certainly modify other neurotransmitters in an interdependent fashion.

Glutamate   As you may recall from Chapter 7, glutamate is a major excitatory neurotransmitter in the nervous system and has receptors on many cells in the CNS. Of the several subtypes of glutamate receptor, alcohol has its greatest effect on the NMDA (N-methyl-D-aspartate) receptor, which is a ligand-gated channel that allows positively charged ions (Ca^{2+} and Na^+) to enter and cause a localized depolarization. Glutamate action at NMDA receptors mediates associative learning (see Chapter 7) and also has a role in the damaging effects of excessive glutamate activity (excitotoxicity), as in the case of prolonged seizures or after stroke. Let's look at the role of NMDA receptors in several effects of alcohol: (1) memory loss associated with intoxication; (2) rebound hyperexcitability associated with the abstinence syndrome after long-term use; and (3) NMDA-mediated excitotoxicity associated with alcoholic brain damage.

Alcohol acutely inhibits glutamate neurotransmission by reducing the effectiveness of glutamate at the NMDA receptor. These effects occur at concentrations as low as 0.03%, blood levels normally achieved by social drinkers. Alcohol, like other glutamate antagonists, impairs learning and memory, as shown in studies of long-term potentiation (LTP) and conditioning (Fadda and Rossetti, 1998). In addition, alcohol significantly reduces glutamate release in many brain areas, including the hippocampus, as measured by microdialysis. Reduced glutamate release in the hippocampus is correlated with deficits in spatial memory. The combination of temporary inhibition of NMDA receptors by alcohol and reduced glutamate release may produce the amnesia that occurs for events that take place during intoxication (i.e., the blackouts so typical of heavy drinking) (Diamond and Gordon, 1997).

(A)

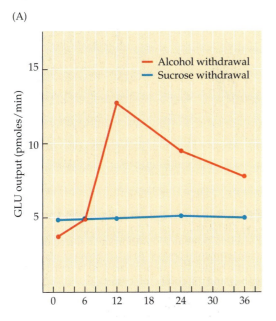

(B)

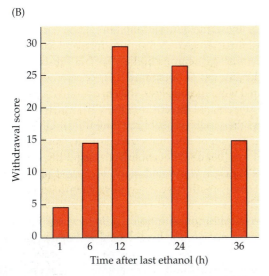

Figure 9.14 Relationship between alcohol withdrawal and glutamate release Withdrawal from chronic alcohol in dependent rats increases glutamate (GLU) release in the striatum (A) and behavioral rebound withdrawal hyperexcitability (B). The time course of the two withdrawal-related events is very similar. Experimental animals received intragastric delivery of ethanol at intoxicating concentrations (2–5g/kg) every 6 hours for 6 consecutive days. Control animals received an equally caloric sucrose solution. On day 7 the ethanol administration was terminated and behavioral testing of abstinence signs and simultaneous microdialysis collection began. (After Fadda and Rossetti, 1998.)

In the adult brain, repeated alcohol use leads to a neuroadaptive *increase* in the number of NMDA receptors (up-regulation) in response to the reduced glutamate activity.

The number of NMDA receptors in both the cerebral cortex and hippocampus is elevated in human alcoholics as well as in animal models of chronic alcohol exposure. In addition, in dependent rats, glutamate release, normally inhibited by alcohol, is dramatically increased at about 10 hours after withdrawal of alcohol. The time course (Figure 9.14A and B) of the CNS hyperexcitability and the seizures that are typical of the alcohol abstinence syndrome matches the pattern of increased glutamate release during withdrawal. Further, there is a strong positive correlation between the magnitude of glutamate output during withdrawal and the intensity of abstinence signs. This means that the increased glutamate acting on up-regulated NMDA receptors may be one neurochemical correlate of alcohol withdrawal. Additionally, the elevated glutamate activity during withdrawal causes excessive calcium influx, which contributes to cell death. Frequently experienced withdrawal may be responsible for some of the irreversible brain damage described earlier.

Additionally, studies with rats show that maternal BACs as low as 0.04% during the last trimester of pregnancy impair NMDA receptors and decrease glutamate release in the newborns. Unlike in the mature brain, inhibition of glutamate systems in the fetus may disrupt normal development and result in *reduced* NMDA receptors in the adult. It is reasonable to suspect that a reduction of NMDA receptors is related to subtle impairments in learning and memory in children born to alcoholic mothers, but further investigation is required.

GABA   GABA (γ-aminobutyric acid) is a major inhibitory amino acid neurotransmitter described in Chapter 7. It binds to the $GABA_A$ receptor complex and opens the chloride channel, allowing chloride to enter the cell to hyperpolarize the membrane. Many of the classic sedative–hypnotic drugs (see Chapter 17) such as the benzodiazepines (e.g., Valium) and the barbiturates (e.g., phenobarbital) are known to enhance the effects of GABA at the $GABA_A$ receptor by binding to their modulatory sites on the receptor complex. Since the drugs in this class and alcohol produce many of the same actions and show both cross-tolerance and cross dependence, it is not surprising to find that alcohol also modulates GABA function, although a specific modulatory site on the receptor has not been found.

What kinds of biochemical and electrophysiological evidence suggests that alcohol at intoxicating concentrations increases GABA-induced Cl⁻ flux and hyperpolarization? First, picrotoxin (which blocks the Cl⁻ channel) and bicuculline (which competes with GABA for its receptor) antagonize both the hyperpolarization and some of the behavioral effects of alcohol. This suggests that both Cl⁻ conductance and GABA binding to the receptor are necessary for alcohol's effect. Second, manipulations that increase GABA (for example, inhibiting its degradation) also increase alcohol-induced behavioral effects. Likewise, reducing GABA function with antagonists reduces signs of ethanol intoxication and its antianxiety effects (Grobin et al., 1998). Third, lines of mice bred for their sensitivity to some of the behavioral effects of alcohol show a relationship between the ability of ethanol to increase GABA-induced Cl⁻ entry and the intensity of their response to alcohol. Greater incoordination and loss of righting reflex in vivo corresponded to greater alcohol-induced Cl⁻ influx into the animals' brain preparations in vitro (Mihic and Harris, 1997).

In contrast to the acute GABA-enhancing effects of alcohol, repeated exposure to ethanol reduces $GABA_A$-mediated chloride flux. Also, chronic alcohol makes animals more sensitive to seizure-inducing doses of the GABA antagonist bicuculline. We might expect that result, since it should take less of the antagonist to reduce GABA function because it has already been *down-regulated* by chronic alcohol. This neuroadaptive mechanism apparently compensates for the initial GABA-enhancing effect of alcohol and may contribute to the appearance of tolerance and some of the signs of withdrawal such as hyperexcitability, seizures, and tremors. Because benzodiazepines also lose their GABA-enhancing effects at the receptor in mice treated chronically with ethanol, it may also be a mechanism for cross-tolerance with the other sedative–hypnotic drugs.

It seems appropriate to once again mention that neuronal excitability is due to a balance between excitation and inhibition. Since GABAergic neurons frequently have glutamate receptors and GABA frequently modulates glutamate release, the compensatory changes in each of the neurotransmitter systems may reflect an interaction of the two (Fadda and Rossetti, 1998).

Dopamine   Evidence from biochemical, electrophysiological, and behavioral studies suggests that the dopaminergic mesolimbic system plays a significant role in the reinforcement and motivational mechanisms underlying behaviors that are vital to survival (see Chapter 5). The pathway begins in the ventral tegmental area (VTA) of the midbrain and courses rostrally to innervate a number of limbic structures, including the nucleus accumbens (NA) and the central nucleus of the amygdala (Figure 9.15). The NA is particularly important because part of it (the shell) belongs to a network of structures called the extended amygdala, which is involved in integrating emotion with hormonal responses and sympathetic nervous system activity. The core of the NA is associated with the striatum, which modulates movement. The afferents to and efferents from the NA provide a means for combining motivational status, emotional content, and motor responses (DiChiara, 1997). Its role in substance abuse seems to be in supplying the primary reinforcing qualities that lead to repeated drug use and may help to explain why alcohol is so addictive for some people.

Increased dopaminergic transmission in the mesolimbic pathway occurs in response to the administration of most

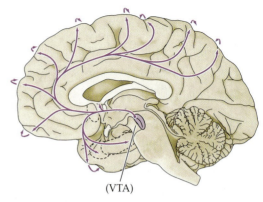

(VTA)

Figure 9.15 Dopaminergic mesolimbic and mesocortical pathways Midsagittal view of dopaminergic neurons involved in alcohol reinforcement and withdrawal-induced dysphoria. The ventral tegmental area (VTA) is the origin of neurons that innervate the nucleus accumbens, amygdala, hippocampus (mesolimbic), and the cortex (mesocortical).

drugs of abuse, including alcohol. In rats, alcohol consumption at intoxicating concentrations increases the firing rate of dopaminergic neurons in the VTA and subsequently elevates the amount of dopamine (DA) released in the NA, as measured with microdialysis. Rats in operant chambers self-administer ethanol directly into the VTA, which presumably activates those cells (probably by inhibiting inhibitory cells). Microinjection of dopamine receptor antagonists into the NA reduces (but does not abolish) the self-administration of ethanol in rats, as you would expect because alcohol-induced DA release is ineffective when postsynaptic receptors are blocked.

Since alcohol consumption clearly increases mesolimbic cell firing, we might ask how alcohol withdrawal affects the same reward pathway. In contrast to the acute effects, when animals have been allowed to consume alcohol in a chronic fashion, withdrawal of the drug dramatically reduces the firing rate of mesolimbic neurons and decreases DA release in the nucleus accumbens (Diana et al., 1993). Figure 9.16 shows the decrease in synaptic DA in the NA as well as the reduction in the DA metabolites 3,4-dihydroxyphenylacetic acid (DOPAC) and homovanillic acid (HVA), as measured by microdialysis at various times after the last injection of ethanol. The decrease began at approximately 5 hours after the last alcohol administration and reached a maximum at around 10 to 12 hours. The same animals showed behavioral signs of withdrawal that began at 8 to 10 hours and continued throughout the testing period. One might conclude that the behavioral signs, the reduced DA outflow, and the reduced mesolimbic cell firing, which were all reversed by a single administration of alcohol, may represent the neurobiological correlate of the dysphoria associated with the alcohol withdrawal syndrome.

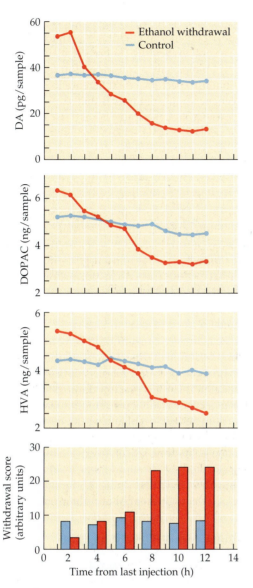

Figure 9.16 Dopamine turnover and alcohol withdrawal Microdialysis collection of DA and its major metabolites, DOPAC and HVA, in the nucleus accumbens of rats at varying times after ethanol withdrawal shows a significant reduction in DA turnover compared to control. The bottom graph shows the development of abstinence signs in the same animals. Note the similarity in time course of biochemical measures and occurrence of behavioral signs. The alcohol group received intoxicating doses of alcohol every 6 hours for 6 days before withdrawal. Control animals received sucrose of caloric value equal to the alcohol. The microdialysis collection of extracellular fluid and the behavioral measures of abstinence occurred at various times over the 12 hour period following ethanol withdrawal. Withdrawal scores were a composite of separate measures of tremor, vocalization on handling, bracing posture, rigidity, and others. (After Diana et al., 1993.)

mesolimbic firing indirectly secondary to its enhancement of other neurotransmitter action in the VTA such as GABA, acetylcholine, serotonin, or endorphins. Despite the apparent importance of the dopaminergic neurons, almost total destruction of the mesolimbic terminals with 6-hydroxy-dopamine (6-OHDA) does not abolish self-administration of alcohol, suggesting that other dopamine-independent mechanisms contribute to ethanol reinforcement. One such mechanism may be the opioid peptide transmitters.

Opioid systems   A family of neuropeptides (called the endorphins) that have opiate-like effects modulate pain, mood, feeding, reinforcement, and response to stress, among other things (see Chapter 10). The opioids also contribute to the reinforcing effects of alcohol. Support for this statement

The reduction in mesolimbic DA is also reflected in a rebound depression of reinforcement mechanisms, as shown by the elevation of threshold for intracranial stimulation. Elevated thresholds mean that more electrical current is needed to activate the reinforcing pathway (i.e., reinforcement is less rewarding than it was during the initial alcohol use). Figure 9.17 shows that the elevation of thresholds reached a maximum at 6 to 8 hours after abrupt withdrawal and disappeared by 72 hours. This down-regulation of the neuronal system that mediates reward may be the neuroadaptive mechanism that is responsible for the negative emotional signs (dysphoria and depression) characteristic of withdrawal from many abused substances, including psychostimulants and opiates as well as alcohol (Schulteis et al., 1995).

Although the release of DA in the NA may be instrumental in ethanol-induced reinforcement, alcohol may increase

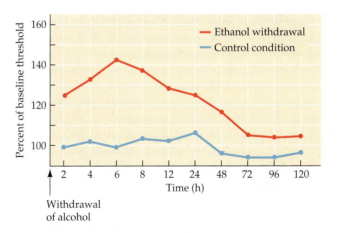

Figure 9.17 Rebound depression of reinforcement during withdrawal After alcohol withdrawal from dependent rats, a time-dependent increase in the current thresholds for electrical brain stimulation occurs, with maximum effect at 6 to 8 hours. The increase in threshold indicates that the animals need more stimulation to achieve reinforcement. Note that the x-axis is not a linear scale. (After Schulteis et al., 1995.)

comes from three types of studies (Froehlich, 1997). First, alcohol enhances endogenous opioid activity in both rodents and humans. Acute administration of alcohol increases endogenous opioid (endorphin and enkephalin) release from brain slices and pituitary gland in vitro and also increases blood levels of opioids in humans in vivo. Opioids are released into the blood from the pituitary gland. Acute alcohol administration also increases gene expression of both endorphin and enkephalin in selected brain areas of rats, which would increase the amount of peptides available. In contrast, *chronic* alcohol administration reduces gene expression, making less of the peptides available for release. In human subjects, chronic alcohol use also leads to reduced brain levels of endorphin. Since the release of DA in mesolimbic neurons is regulated by opioid cells in both the VTA and NA, the alcohol-induced opioid release may produce reinforcement by modulating dopamine (Herz, 1997). The reduced opioid levels may contribute to the dysphoria that accompanies chronic alcohol use and withdrawal.

Second, if alcohol-induced enhancement of opioid systems is at least partially responsible for reinforcement, then blocking opioid receptors should reduce alcohol consumption. Opioid receptor antagonists like naloxone and naltrexone, which compete for the endogenous opioid receptors, do significantly reduce alcohol self-administration in animals. Antagonists that act on specific subtypes (μ and δ) of opioid receptor (see Chapter 10) also reduce operant self-administration. Several clinical trials of opiate antagonists in alcoholic patients found reduced alcohol consumption, relapse, and craving as well as a reported decrease in the subjective "high." (Further discussion can be found in the section on alcoholism

treatment). Finally, μ-opioid receptor knockout mice fail to self-administer ethanol and in some experimental conditions show an aversion to the drug (Roberts et al., 2000).

Third, if opioids have a role in reinforcement, then perhaps we should expect to see a difference in the opioid systems of genetic strains of animals that show greater or less preference for alcohol. In rat strains that have been genetically bred for alcohol preference, endogenous opioid systems are generally more responsive to the effects of alcohol. For example, alcohol-preferring rats, when compared to alcohol-non-preferring rats, released significantly more β-endorphin from the hypothalamus when infused with alcohol in vitro and showed enhanced β-endorphin gene expression in the pituitary. The finding that alcohol-preferring rats have higher baseline levels of μ-opioid receptors in selected limbic areas, including the shell of the NA and amygdala, may indicate that those animals have a *lower*-than-normal opioid function (leading to the up-regulation of receptors). A deficit in opioid function might predispose animals to consume alcohol to compensate for those deficits and hence be "alcohol preferring." Indeed, alcohol consumption is reduced in animals after moderate and high doses of morphine, suggesting that alcohol may be compensating for ineffective opioid transmission (Herz, 1997). The fact that low doses of opioids increase rather than decrease alcohol consumption has been considered a "priming effect"—enhancing the motivation to use alcohol. However, why the opioid antagonists reduce alcohol consumption is far more difficult to explain using this model.

Other neurotransmitters   Table 9.3 summarizes some of the cellular effects of alcohol and their contribution to

TABLE 9.3 Role of Selected Neurotransmitters in Cellular and Behavioral Effects of Alcohol

Neurotransmitter	Acute cellular effects	Chronic cellular effects	Behavioral effects
Glutamate	Receptor antagonism and reduces release	—	Memory loss
	—	Up-regulation of receptors and rebound increase in release	Rebound hyperexcitability of the abstinence syndrome
	—	Extreme hyperexcitability and massive Ca^{2+} influx (rebound)	Brain damage
GABA	Acutely enhances GABA-induced Cl^- influx to hyperpolarize	—	Sedative effects: anxiety reduction, sedation, incoordination, memory impairment
	—	Neuroadaptive decrease in GABA function without change in receptor number	Tolerance and signs of hyperexcitability during withdrawal (seizures, tremors)
Dopamine	Acute increase in transmission in mesolimbic tract	—	Reinforcement
	—	Chronic effects show reduced firing rate, release, metabolism	Negative affect as a sign of withdrawal
Opioids	Acute increase in endogenous opioid synthesis and release	—	Reinforcement
	—	Neuroadaptive decrease in endorphin levels	Dysphoria

behavior. Both animal and human studies implicate many more interacting neurotransmitter systems in alcohol's action than we have had the space to discuss. The effects of acute and chronic alcohol administration on these receptors are responsible for the changes in cell signaling, both rapid ionotropic and slower metabotropic actions. Second messengers such as cAMP and their cascade of effects within the cell may be responsible for more long-term changes in cell function, including altered gene expression. Further discussion of the neurochemical effects is beyond the scope of this chapter, but details can be found in several reviews (Diamond and Gordon, 1997).

Section Summary

Animal models are a critical tool in evaluating the acute and chronic effects of alcohol on neurobiology. In addition, the inbred rodent strains and the gene knockout technique provide a springboard for human gene studies of alcohol abuse. You have just read about some of the ways that ethanol modifies synaptic function and contributes to the behavioral effects of intoxication, memory impairment, reinforcement, and dependence. Although most drugs impact the functioning of several neurotransmitter systems because no neuronal system operates in isolation, the multiple effects of alcohol are particularly dramatic. The multiple effects occur because the drug has both specific actions on receptor or channel proteins and also nonspecific effects on membrane fluidity. If you find it surprising that multiple neurotransmitters, including GABA, dopamine, glutamate, and opioids, affect reinforcement, consider the vital contribution of reward to the survival of a species. Certainly any function so significant must have multiple redundant circuits. In addition, abnormally low levels of reinforcing neurotransmitters in some individuals may be responsible for the appeal of alcohol and other abused substances.

Alcoholism

Alcoholism is a serious and complex phenomenon that consists of psychological, neurobiological, genetic, and sociocultural factors making it both difficult to define and treat. Regardless of the specific definition, it damages the health and well-being of the individual and those around him. Financial costs of alcoholism are huge and include medical treatment of alcohol-induced disease, loss associated with accidents on the road and at work, and financial disruption that accompanies the breakdown of families. Many volumes have been written about alcohol use and alcoholism from various points of view; some emotionally evocative, others based on theoretical models, or empirical research. The final section of this chapter represents a brief synopsis of some of the research findings.

Defining alcoholism and estimating its incidence prove difficult

Chapter 8 describes substance abuse and dependence in detail and identifies the criteria used by professionals to diagnose these conditions. In addition, the chapter provides multiple theoretical models of substance abuse and provides a critique of each. In this section we look specifically at **alcoholism,** a form of substance abuse that has been historically difficult to define because the drug is legal and is used by most individuals in a way that does not harm themselves or others. For the layman, a person with an "alcohol problem" may be anyone who drinks more than he or she does. However, it is hard to objectively define inappropriate amounts of alcohol because the frequency and pattern of use is as significant as the total amount. For example, consuming five alcoholic drinks over one week's time does not have the same physical and social consequences as five drinks in a row, which is the usual definition of **binge drinking.** An alcoholic does not necessarily have to start each day with a drink, nor does he necessarily drink all day long, but he may drink very heavily periodically. Instead of emphasizing quantity, diagnosis of alcoholism depends on identifying a cluster of behavioral, cognitive, and physical characteristics. For the clinician, the essential features of alcoholism are compulsive alcohol seeking and use despite damaging health and social consequences. The *Diagnostic and Statistical Manual of Mental Disorders (DSM-IV)* (American Psychiatric Association, 1994) emphasizes the *consequences* of drinking in its definition of **alcohol abuse,** which precedes **alcohol dependence** and is both less severe and more readily reversible (Table 9.4). Unfortunately, because other groups and government agencies use different criteria, there is still a great deal of vari-

TABLE 9.4 Diagnostic Criteria of Substance Abuse and Substance Dependence

Substance abuse occurs when the drug

impairs the ability of the individual to function at school, at work, or in the home.

causes legal problems like arrests for violence or driving under the influence.

is used in a dangerous manner.

is used despite legal, social, or medical problems.

Substance dependence occurs when the drug fulfills the criteria for abuse and also includes:

development of tolerance;

physiological or cognitive signs of withdrawal at abstinence;

frequent desire and effort to reduce drug use;

preoccupation with securing, consuming, and recovering from drug use so that most daily activity is directed by the drug.

Source: American Psychiatric Association, 1994.

ability in how professionals use the terms *addiction, misuse, abuse, dependency,* and *problem drinking.*

Many modern definitions are based on the work of Jellinek (1960), who made an early distinction between "chronic alcoholism," which includes the physical and behavioral consequences of long-term alcohol use, and "alcohol addiction," which is characterized by craving and lack of control. In addition, Jellinek was responsible for developing the disease model of addiction to replace the earlier moral model, which emphasized lack of willpower and personal weakness. His concept meant that alcoholism would be treated medically and nonjudgmentally, as is true for any other disease. Once the addiction is formed, the model suggests, the individual no longer has control over his drug-taking behavior. Although most treatment in the United States is based on this medical model, it does have many critics.

The disparities in the definition of alcoholism have led to equally large differences in estimated incidence. Although you may think of an alcoholic as a poor, aging, homeless individual living on the street, in reality there is no such thing as a typical alcoholic (Figure 9.18). Although many homeless individuals do suffer from a variety of psychiatric disorders and abuse both illicit drugs and alcohol at high rates, only 5% of alcoholics fit that category. Based on the U.S. government's annual survey of drug use, the most commonly accepted statistic is that approximately 10% of Americans have some problem with alcohol use and as many as 10.5 million adults are dependent on alcohol. Significant gender differences exist in alcohol use and abuse for all age groups. The 1998 National Household Survey of Drug Abuse found that more men (58.7%) than women (45.1%) consume alcohol to some extent. Heavy drinking was reported in 9.7% of men and 2.4% of women. Binge drinking was also higher in men (23.2%) compared to women (8.6%). Although the percentage of men declined on most drinking measures during their 30s, women had higher rates on some drinking indices between age 30 and 40. However, by age 60, the indicators of problem drinking fell into the single digits for both genders (Jung, 2000). Although problem drinking drops significantly in the elderly, the problems associated with drinking can be more serious because of drug interactions and medical complications.

A closer focus on the drinking patterns of college students might be appropriate, since there has been a great deal of public concern regarding student accidents and fatalities recently. Several large-scale studies are available to guide you in further research (Wechsler et al., 1995a, 1995b). Random sampling of students at both a small New England college

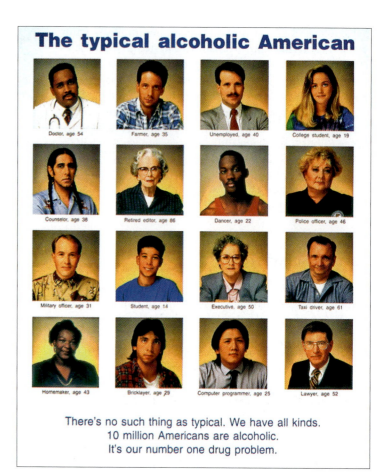

Figure 9.18 A wide variety of individuals are alcoholics. (Courtesy of the National Library of Medicine.)

and a large eastern public university found that overall drinking seems to have *declined* compared to 1979. About 20% of the sample reported alcohol abstinence, compared to only 4% in the earlier surveys. However, heavy drinking did not change, remaining at around 20%, and at least 25% of the population reported some damaging effects on academic performance.

Wechsler and colleagues examined binge drinking (i.e., consuming five drinks in a row) in a population of 17,592 students at 140 colleges and universities. Approximately 50% of the males and 39% of the females reported binge drinking, half of whom binged three or more times in a 2-week period. Although this group reported a significant number of alcohol-related problems (Table 9.5), only 1% felt they had a drinking problem. Significant variation occurred across campuses, and these differences were reflected in the impact of binge drinking on the welfare of other students. Students who were not heavy drinkers on campuses that had the highest rates of heavy drinkers reported significantly more negative experiences associated with other students'

TABLE 9.5 Percentage of Binge Drinkers Reporting Alcohol-Related Problems Since the Beginning of the School Year by Gender[a]

Alcohol-related problem	Percentage[b]	
	Women	Men
General disorientation		
Have a hangover	81%	82%
Do something you later regret	48%	50%
Forget what you did	38%	41%
Sexual activity		
Engage in unplanned sex	26%	33%
Not use protection before sex	15%	16%
Violence		
Argue with friends	29%	32%
Damage property	6%	24%
Disciplinary action		
Have trouble with campus/local police	4%	10%
Personal injury		
Get injured	14%	17%
Get medical treatment for overdose	<1%	1%
School performance		
Miss a class	42%	45%
Get behind in schoolwork	31%	34%

Source: Wechsler et al., 1995a.

[a] Women binge drinkers report having four or more drinks in a row at least once during the past 2 weeks. Men binge drinkers report having five or more drinks in a row.

[b] Percentage of binge drinkers who report that, since the beginning of the school year, their drinking has caused them to experience each problem one or more times.

drinking, including vandalism, violence, theft, and unwanted sexual advances. Jung (2001) provides a detailed discussion of student drug use with a strong research emphasis.

The causes of alcoholism are multimodal

There is no specific cause of alcoholism, but a variety of factors contribute to the vulnerability of any given individual. It is quite clear that multiple factors stem from three essential areas: (1) neurobiological; (2) psychological; and (3) sociocultural (Figure 9.19). Although we are forced to discuss them in a linear fashion, keep in mind that complex interactions exist among the areas. Because the literature is quite extensive, this section will provide an overview and suggest methods for research.

Psychological factors   Although no alcoholic personality has ever been defined, one vulnerability factor for alcoholism

is the response to stress. Both animal and human studies show an interaction between both acute and chronic stress and the initiation of alcohol use, maintenance of drug consumption, and relapse after withdrawal (Brady and Sonne, 1999). Some have used the term *symptomatic* drinking to describe the reinforcing effects of alcohol when stress and tension are relieved. The individual who no longer drinks as part of a social occasion but drinks each day after work to relieve tension is an example. Whether that individual escalates to alcoholism depends on multiple personal, environmental, and genetic factors.

Novelty seeking may also increase the risk for using alcohol and other drugs of abuse. Bardo and colleagues (1996) reviewed extensive literature to show that exposure to novel events activates the dopaminergic mesolimbic pathway in a manner similar to most abused substances. Individual differences in the need for novelty and drug-seeking behavior are under genetic control and may explain why some individuals experiment with drugs initially and also why some more readily become compulsive users. Differences in the need for stimulation have been applied to drug and alcohol prevention programs that use fast-paced, physiologically arousing, and unconventional message delivery to appeal to the target audience.

Neurobiological factors   One significant neurobiological factor in alcoholism is genetic vulnerability.

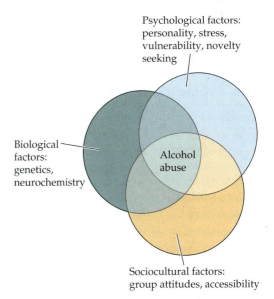

Figure 9.19 Three-factor vulnerability model Biological, psychological, and sociocultural influences contribute to the development of alcohol abuse.

Close relatives of alcoholics have a three to seven times greater risk for alcoholism than the general population. Both twin and adoption studies show that genetics is correlated with vulnerability, particularly for the more severe type of alcoholism. In adoption studies, the risk of alcoholism is higher in children of alcoholics even when they are adopted into nonalcoholic families. Alcoholism concordance rates are higher in monozygotic (54%) compared to dizygotic (28%) twins, demonstrating the influence of genes, although leaving significant variability to be explained by other factors. Overall, genetics explains 50 to 60% of the variance of risk for dependence in both men and women, although the percentage may be higher for some types of alcoholism than others. The heritability of alcohol abuse is less, at about 38%.

To help with genetic analysis, researchers try to establish subgroups of alcoholics based on a number of characteristics such as severity, occurrence of withdrawal, gender, and so forth. Cloninger (1987) and colleagues proposed a popular categorization called type I and type II alcoholics (Table 9.6). Type I generally begin drinking later in life and experience guilt and fear about their alcoholism. These individuals rarely have trouble with the law or display antisocial activities. Many drink to escape stress or unpleasant situations in their environment. Most female alcoholics are type I, although many men also fit this description. Type II alcoholics are almost always male and display thrill-seeking, antisocial, and perhaps criminal activities. They have lower cerebrospinal fluid levels of the serotonin 5-HT metabolite 5-HIAA, a result that matches the human and animal literature regarding impulsivity and suicide. Type II have a higher genetic vulnerability and initiate drinking at an early age.

To find genetic patterns in human alcoholics, several methods are available. One method, called **linkage studies**, examines the inheritance pattern of genes using DNA analysis and the occurrence of alcoholism in many members of a large number of families. Researchers look for easily identified genetic markers and determine which are most closely related to the alcohol-associated behaviors. One such evaluation of a Native American population identified two potential genes for alcoholism. One was on chromosome 11p close to the genes for the D_4 dopamine receptor and tyrosine hydroxylase. The second was on chromosome 4p near the gene for the $GABA_A$ receptor complex (Enoch and Goldman, 1999).

The **case-control method** compares the genes of unrelated, affected and unaffected individuals to see if the affected population have more of a particular form (allele) of genetic material. The gene does not necessarily have to be directly associated with the disorder but may be a marker associated with a characteristic that increases the risk of developing alcoholism. For example, specific genes control the manufacture of ALDH, the enzyme that converts the toxic metabolite acetaldehyde to acetic acid. Since individuals with the gene for the inactive form of the enzyme experience unpleasant effects when drinking alcohol, they have essentially no risk for alcoholism.

An additional risk factor that is genetically influenced (although no specific gene has been identified) is low sensitivity to alcohol. Alcoholics frequently report that early in their drinking, they experienced very little effect of alcohol unless they consumed large quantities. Schuckit (2000) measured subjective intoxication, "sway score" when balanced on a straight line, and hormonal response to alcohol in young sons of alcoholics compared to controls. The men who later developed alcoholism showed a reduced response to moderate levels of alcohol for each of the measures (Figure 9.20). More importantly, he found that the low response rate increased the risk for alcoholism fourfold *regardless of family history* when the men were evaluated 8 years later.

Other case-control studies have looked for variants in genes involved in neurotransmitter metabolism, such as receptor subtypes, synthesizing enzymes, and reuptake transporters. For example, a genetic variant of the 5-HT transporter is associated with anxiety and with low sensitivity to alcohol, which makes affected individuals more vulnerable to developing alcoholism.

Identifying an alcoholism gene in humans has not been very successful, because the disorder is complex and highly variable among individuals. Many researchers doubt that there is a gene specific to alcoholism and believe that the condition may share genes with other "compulsive" behaviors such as gambling, eating disorders, and substance abuse.

Rodent models are extremely important to the evaluation of the genetic contribution to isolated drinking behaviors. Researchers use selectively bred lines of animals that differ with respect to alcohol-related behaviors such as withdrawal sensitivity, alcohol consumption, and alcohol-induced

TABLE 9.6 Cloninger's Alcoholic Subtypes

Characteristics	Type I	Type II
Age of onset (years)	After 25	Before 25
Gender	Male and female	Male
Extent of genetic influence	Moderate	High
Environmental influence	High	Low
Alcohol used as escape	High	Low
Alcohol used to feel good	Low	High
Novelty-seeking personality	Low	High
Inability to control drinking	Infrequent	Frequent
Guilt and fear about alcohol	Frequent	Infrequent
Aggressive/antisocial action	Infrequent	Frequent
Inability to stop alcohol use	Infrequent	Frequent

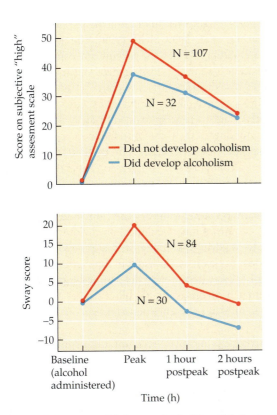

Figure 9.20 Low sensitivity to alcohol is a risk factor for alcoholism. Subjective assessment of "high" and sway scores following a moderate dose (0.75 ml/kg) of alcohol in men who later developed alcohol dependence and those who did not. Those vulnerable to alcoholism showed significantly less response to the same dose at peak blood level (1 hour) and 1 and 2 hours after the peak. N refers to number of subjects tested in each group. (After Schuckit, 1994.)

hypothermia to search for clusters of genes that are linked to several alcohol behaviors. A second technique uses gene knockout animals, in which a particular gene is selectively deleted, before evaluating the animal behaviors. For example, 5-HT$_{1B}$ receptor knockout mice self-administer twice as much alcohol but show less intoxication and less evidence of tolerance. They also self-administer cocaine more readily. When the dopamine D$_4$ receptor is knocked out, animals become supersensitive to alcohol as well as to cocaine and amphetamine.

Sociocultural factors Social and cultural factors mold the changing attitudes about drinking as well as the definition of problem drinking. Group attitudes also determine how much alcohol is available in a particular environment, for example, by controlling hours of sale, public consumption, and advertising. The examination of cultural influence on drinking was pioneered by Bales (1946), who suggested that cultures that abstain from alcohol use or restrict it to reli-

gious purposes have the lowest alcoholism rates. In contrast, societies that engage in social drinking in public settings and where drinking is condoned for personal reasons such as tension reduction have higher alcoholism rates. The importance of cultural influence is well demonstrated by the low alcoholism rate among Muslims and Mormons, two groups with religious prohibitions on alcohol use. A low rate of alcoholism also occurs in Jewish populations, who use alcohol in a religious ceremonial way among family and do not condone intoxication.

Levin (1989) contrasted attitudes in two Catholic countries, Italy and France, both of which produce and consume large quantities of alcohol. France has one of the highest alcoholism rates in the world, while Italy has only one-fifth the incidence as France. Among the differences of potential significance is that the French do not disapprove of drunkenness and consider refusal of alcohol as impolite. They also drink both wine and hard liquor, drink with meals and also in other contexts, and consume alcohol in the family setting and outside of it. The Italian culture disapproves of drunkenness and accepts abstinence. Their alcohol consumption is primarily wine taken with meals within the family. Further discussion of cultural influences on the vulnerability to alcoholism can be found in several sources, including McNeece and DiNitto (1998). An excellent pictorial article by Boyd Gibbons (1992) in *National Geographic* describes many cultural differences in alcohol use and abuse.

The most obvious conclusion to draw from our discussion of etiology is that multiple factors contribute to alcoholism. The neurochemical effects of alcohol and genetic predisposition to heavy drinking; the individual's personality, cognitive structure, and expectations; and social, cultural, and economic variables all affect the use of alcohol and vulnerability to alcohol dependence.

Multiple treatment options provide hope for rehabilitation

An increasing number of treatment programs for alcoholism have developed over the last few years, giving alcoholics more hope for recovery. One of the major hurdles in treating an alcoholic is getting the individual into a treatment program. **Denial** of a problem with alcohol is a significant characteristic of alcoholics, who often fail to recognize that alcohol is the source of their problems and not the cure for them. Denial by the alcoholic is often aided by family members and friends who repair the damage caused by the drinker and make excuses for his behavior. These people are called **enablers,** since they enable the alcoholic to function without getting treatment. The alcoholic frequently needs to be coerced into treatment by spouses threatening separation and loss of children, employers threatening loss of employment, and the legal system (arrests and jail time).

The first step in treatment is **detoxification,** because withdrawal symptoms are strong motivators and can also be physiologically dangerous. Under medical care, detoxification involves substituting a benzodiazepine such as chlordiazepoxide (Librium) or diazepam (Valium). These drugs prevent alcohol withdrawal, including seizures and DTs. The long-acting nature of the drugs stabilizes the individual, and as the dose is gradually reduced, withdrawal symptoms are minimized.

Psychosocial rehabilitation   After detoxification, **psychosocial rehabilitation** programs help the alcoholic to prevent relapse by abstinence or reduce the amount of alcohol consumed if relapse occurs (Fuller and Hiller-Sturmhofel, 1999). Several programs exist, but we provide only a cursory survey of a few of them. The three basic types include individual and group therapy to provide emotional support and address psychological and social problems associated with dependence, residential alcohol-free treatment settings, and self-help groups such as Alcoholics Anonymous (AA). All of these methods reduce alcohol use among patients, although the relapse rate is extremely high. Approximately 40 to 70% resume drinking after one year (Finney et al., 1996).

AA is an organization in which all members are alcoholics because an underlying assumption is that only a peer group is able to understand the alcoholic and help him accept his disorder and admit his powerlessness over it. The group's emphasis is a spiritual one in which the individual relies on a "higher power" to help him remain sober.

Other self-help groups vary dramatically from AA. Rational Recovery (RR), begun in 1990, is based on Albert Ellis's psychotherapeutic approach called rational–emotive therapy. The focus of the group is on helping the individual to get rid of irrational and harmful beliefs and emotions so that personal goals can be met and the use of alcohol becomes unnecessary. In this case, the alcoholic is considered in control of his own fate and needs neither spiritual guidance nor group support in the long run.

The Community Reinforcement Approach (CRA) is one of the top-ranked treatment methods (Wolfe and Meyers, 1999). CRA assumes that environmental contingencies (rewards and punishers) are powerful in encouraging drinking behavior but that they can be modified to become powerful reinforcers of nondrinking as well. If a nondrinking lifestyle is more appealing than a drinking one, the alcoholic will no longer turn to the drug. CRA focuses on the problems (e.g., job loss, marital issues) as perceived *by the alcoholic individual* and helps her set her own goals, enhances her motivation to achieve the goals, and teaches the skills needed to create the positive lifestyle she desires.

Pharmacotherapeutic approaches   Pharmacotherapeutic **treatment** for alcoholism includes two basic strategies: making

alcohol ingestion unpleasant or reducing its reinforcing qualities (Garbutt et al., 1999; Swift, 1999). The drug disulfiram (Antabuse) inhibits ALDH, the enzyme that converts acetaldehyde to acetic acid in the normal metabolism of alcohol. An individual who drinks as little as a quarter of an ounce of alcohol within a week of taking disulfiram experiences a sharp rise of blood acetaldehyde accompanied by facial flushing, tachycardia, pounding in the chest, drop in blood pressure, nausea, vomiting, and other symptoms. This method is clearly aimed at making alcohol ingestion unpleasant. Patients must be cautious about unknowingly consuming alcohol in beverages, foods, over-the-counter medications like cough syrup, or mouthwash. Because disulfiram can cause hepatitis, frequent liver function tests must be done. For obvious reasons, compliance to the drug-taking regimen is quite low. Disulfiram clearly does not treat alcoholism but may act as a motivational aid for those who are very determined to avoid alcohol. Unfortunately, rigorous double-blind studies show little difference in rates of abstinence between men on disulfiram and controls.

Naltrexone is an opiate receptor antagonist that reduces alcohol consumption and improves abstinence rates, according to a number of double-blind studies (Figure 9.21). Preclinical animal studies described earlier (in the section on opioid systems) showed that μ-opioid agonists increase alcohol consumption and μ-antagonists decrease it. It is assumed that naltrexone reduces the positive feelings and subjective "high" of alcohol by blocking the effects of alcohol-induced endorphin release. Social drinkers report more negative effects and greater sedation from a moderate amount of alcohol when taking naltrexone. The effectiveness of naltrexone

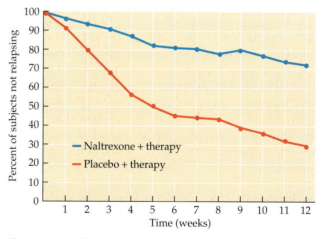

Figure 9.21 Effectiveness of naltrexone in alcoholism treatment Naltrexone along with coping skills therapy is more effective in preventing relapse than placebo and therapy over a 12-week period. At 12 weeks, relapse rates were approximately 65% for the placebo group compared to 30% for the naltrexone treatment group. (After O'Brien, 1994.)

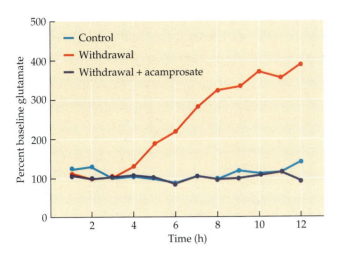

Figure 9.22 Acamprosate prevents withdrawal-induced glutamate release. The red line shows the rebound release of glutamate (measured by microdialysis) that occurs in the nucleus accumbens when alcohol is withdrawn from dependent rats. Alcohol-dependent animals who are withdrawn from alcohol but receive acamprosate (purple line) are no different in glutamate release from non-alcohol treated controls. (After Dahchour and DeWitte, 2000.)

is most pronounced when accompanied by counseling aimed at enhancing individual coping skills and relapse prevention.

Acamprosate is one of the newer agents available for the treatment of alcoholism. Several large, well-controlled studies have shown that acamprosate increases nondrinking days by 30 to 50% and approximately doubles the rate of abstinence, even though most patients ultimately return to drinking. The drug is safe and produces few side effects except for diarrhea. Acamprosate acts as a partial antagonist at the glutamate NMDA receptor and significantly blocks the glutamate increase that occurs during alcohol withdrawal in rats (Figure 9.22), which may explain its therapeutic effects. Acamprosate also has a chemical structure similar to GABA and returns basal GABA levels to normal in alcohol-dependent rats. Its ability to modify the functions of both GABA and glutamate in the nucleus accumbens may be the ultimate basis for its efficacy in preventing relapse.

Other available drugs have been tested in fewer well-controlled trials, but they have generally shown disappointing results. Serotonergic agents whose effectiveness is predicted by animal studies have not consistently been effective in humans, although results are often complicated by the presence of depression or anxiety disorders. The dopamine antagonist tiapride, sold only in Europe, reduces the symptoms of alcohol withdrawal and increases abstinence. However, in at least one clinical trial, compliance was an issue and only about half the subjects completed 1 month of treatment (Shaw et al., 1994).

Section Summary

Alcoholism is a significant substance abuse disorder characterized by compulsive alcohol seeking and continued use despite dangerous consequences. Approximately 10% of Americans have problems with alcohol use. Men are several times more likely to abuse alcohol than women, and also show greater incidence of binge drinking. Although alcohol consumption among college students has declined according to some statistics, the number of heavy drinkers and binge drinkers remains stable at 20%, although there is a good deal of variability depending on the type, location, and size of the school.

Biological factors such as genetic predisposition, psychological factors including vulnerability to stress and need for novelty, and sociocultural factors determining group attitudes and availability of alcohol all contribute to the vulnerability to alcoholism of a given individual. A variety of treatment facilities are needed to deal with the multimodal problem of alcoholism. Alcoholics Anonymous, Rational Recovery, and the Community Reinforcement Approach are three examples of psychosocial rehabilitation. Pharmacological treatments include disulfuram, which makes drinking unpleasant; naltrexone, which blocks opioid- and perhaps dopamine-mediated reinforcement; and acamprosate, which restores glutamate and GABA to normal. Overall, drug therapy, especially in conjunction with psychosocial therapy, seems to improve the outcome of alcoholism treatment, although total abstinence is unlikely.

Recommended Readings

Fadda, F., and Rossetti, Z. L. (1998). Chronic ethanol consumption: From neuroadaptation to neurodegeneration. *Prog. Neurobiol.*, 56, 385–431.

Gibbons, B. (1992). Alcohol: The legal drug. *Nat'l. Geogr.*, 181 (no. 2), 3–35.

Jung, J. (2001). *Psychology of Alcohol and Other Drugs: A Research Perspective*. Sage Publications, London.

Knapp, C. (1996). *Drinking: A Love Story*. Dell Publishing, New York.

Vallee, B. L. (1998). Alcohol in the western world. *Sci. Am.*, June, 80–85.

10

The Opiates

Moments after the arrival of the ambulance, a patient was rolled in on a stretcher to receive almost instant care by the emergency room staff. The patient was about 24 years old, Caucasian, and unconscious. Cardiac monitor leads were placed on his chest and oxygen was immediately provided. His pulse was weak and his blood pressure extremely low. Heart rate and respiration rate were also depressed. The neurological exam revealed extreme pinpoint pupils, failure to respond to pain, and no response to verbal instructions. Although he was rather thin, his appearance was otherwise unremarkable except that one rolled-up shirt sleeve exposed needle track marks indicating intravenous drug use. The triad of coma, pinpoint pupils, and depressed respiration is a strong indicator of opiate poisoning, and physical evidence of intravenous drug use further confirms the diagnosis.

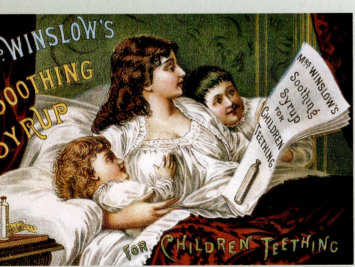

At the turn of the twentieth century, advertisements encouraged mothers to relieve their children's teething pain and restlessness with opium syrups.

To any bystander, death seemed imminent. Nevertheless, 0.8 mg of intravenous naloxone (Narcan) was ordered immediately. Within a minute or two respiratory rate had returned to normal, and soon after the young man was alert enough to respond to a few questions. Although capable of walking out of the emergency room, our patient was convinced to remain overnight for further observation since the half-life of naloxone is somewhat shorter than that of heroin and he might need a second naloxone infusion. How does a drug like heroin produce these potentially fatal effects? And what kind of miracle cure could reverse the condition so quickly? Chapter 10 tells you more about heroin and the other opiate drugs as well as the specific opiate receptor antagonist naloxone.

Narcotic Analgesics

The opiate drugs all belong to the class known as **narcotic analgesics.** These drugs reduce pain without producing unconsciousness, but do produce a sense of relaxation and sleep, and at high doses coma and death. As a class they are the very best painkillers known to man. In addition to inducing analgesia, opiates have a variety of side effects and also produce a sense of well-being and euphoria that may lead to increased use of the drugs. Continued use leads to tolerance and sometimes physical dependence. In contrast to analgesics, **anesthetics** reduce all sensations by depressing the central nervous system (CNS) and produce unconsciousness.

The opium poppy has a long history of use

Opium is an extract of the poppy plant and is the source of a family of drugs known as the opiates or sometimes opioids. Opium is prepared by drying and powdering the milky juice taken from the seed capsules of the opium poppy, *Papaver somniferum* (meaning "the poppy that causes sleep") just before ripening (Figure 10.1). When the capsules are sliced open, the juice leaks out and thickens into a red-brown syrupy material. In its crude state it is very dark in color and forms small balls, called "black tar." Cultivation of the opium

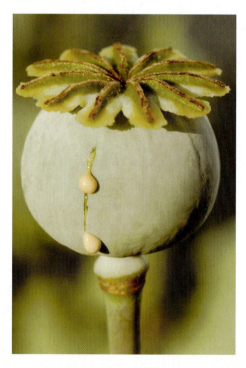

Figure 10.1 Preparing opium The unripe opium poppy capsule has been sliced and the crude opium is dripping from the incision.

poppy has been successful in the temperate zones as far north as England and Denmark, but the majority of the world's supply comes from Southeast Asia, India, China, Iran, Turkey, and southeastern Europe. The plant grows to about 3 or 4 feet in height and has large flowers in white, pink, red, or purple. This variety is the only poppy that has significant psychoactive effects.

The opiates have been used both as medicine and for recreational purposes for several thousand years. As early as 1500 B.C., the Egyptians described opiates' preparation and medicinal value. Archeological evidence from Cyprus dated as early as 1200 B.C. includes ceramic opium pipes and vases with poppy capsules for decoration. By the second century A.D., the famous Greek physician Galen prescribed opium for a wide variety of medical problems, including headache, deafness, asthma, coughs, shortness of breath, colic, and leprosy, among others. But the Greek author Homer, in *The Odyssey*, refers to the drug's recreational properties when he describes the plant as eliciting a feeling of warmth and well-being followed by sleep. More modern use began in Europe when news of the "miracle cure" was brought back by the religious crusaders from the Near East. Eating or smoking opium was accepted in Islamic countries such as Arabia, Turkey, and Iran, where it replaced the consumption of alcohol, which was prohibited. By 1680 an opium-based medicinal drink was introduced by the father of clinical medicine, the English physician Thomas Sydenham. His recipe for the drink called laudanum (meaning "something to be praised") included "2 ounces of strained opium, 1 ounce of saffron, and a dram of cinnamon and cloves dissolved in 1 pint of Canary wine." Drinking laudanum-laced wine was the accepted form of opium use in both Victorian England and America, especially among women, who considered it far more respectable than "common" alcohol use. Laudanum was also a common ingredient of many popular remedies for a wide variety of problems including teething pain and restlessness in infants, muscle aches and pains, and alcoholism. Right up to the turn of the twentieth century, opium-containing products with names such as "A Pennyworth of Peace," "Mrs. Winslow's Soothing Syrup," and "White Star Secret Liquor Cure" could be ordered through the Sears, Roebuck and Co. catalog for about $4 a pint (Figure 10.2).

In nineteenth-century America, neither the federal government nor individual states chose to control the availability and advertising of drugs such as opium and cocaine. There was clearly no significant concern about safety, long-term health issues, or dependence. Finally, in 1914, the Harrison Narcotics Act was passed, which required physicians to report their prescriptions for opiates. Only in the 1920s did the Supreme Court broadly interpret the Harrison Act to limit prescriptions to *medical* use, making it illegal to provide opiates for addicted individuals or recreational use.

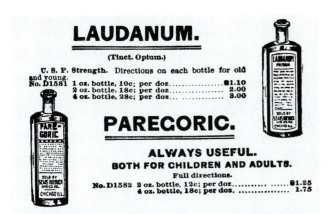

Figure 10.2 Mail order advertisement for opium preparations to treat pain and cough (laudanum) and diarrhea (paregoric) from the 1897 Sears, Roebuck and Co. catalog.

Minor differences in molecular structure determine behavioral effects

The principal active ingredient in opium was called morphine, after the Roman god of dreams, Morpheus, and it was first isolated in the early 1800s by a German chemist. In addition to morphine, opium contains other active ingredients including codeine, thebaine, narcotine, and others. Although morphine was isolated from opium in the early 1800s, the structure of morphine was not identified until 1925 (Figure 10.3). The nat-

urally occurring opiate codeine is identical in structure to morphine except for the substitution of a methoxy ($-OCH_3$) for a hydroxyl ($-OH$) group. This small molecular difference produces a drug that has less analgesic effect and fewer side effects than morphine but is still a potent cough suppressant. It was exciting for pharmacologists to discover that simple modifications to the morphine molecule produce great variations in potency, duration of action, and oral effectiveness. In many cases these differences are due to differences in pharmacokinetics rather than intrinsic activity. For example, heroin was manufactured by adding two acetyl groups onto the morphine molecule. This drug was developed by the Bayer Company to be more effective in relieving pain without the danger of addiction. Today we know that the pharmacological effects of morphine and heroin are essentially identical because heroin is converted to morphine in the brain. Heroin is, however, two to four times more potent when injected and faster-acting because the change in the molecule makes the drug more lipid soluble and allows it to get into the brain much more quickly to act on receptors there. When taken orally, morphine and heroin are approximately equal in potency. The very rapid action of heroin is apparently also responsible for the dramatic euphoric effects achieved with that drug.

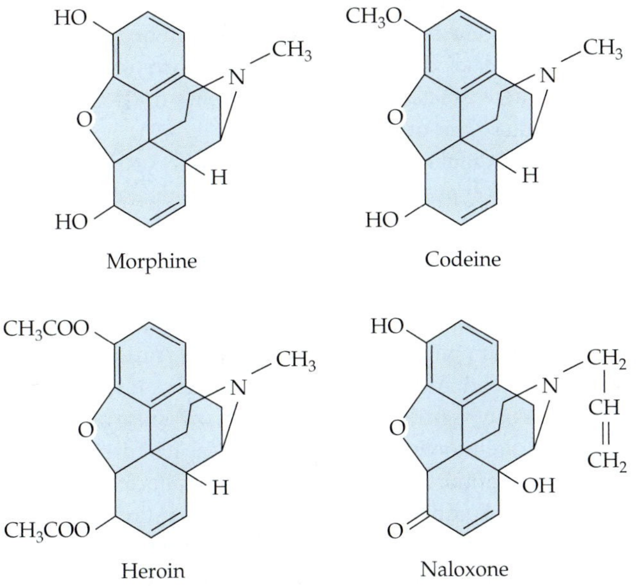

Some of the modifications to morphine's molecular structure produce **partial agonists,** which are drugs that bind readily to (i.e., have a high affinity for) the receptors but produce less biological effect (i.e., low efficacy). Therefore, when administered alone they produce partial opiate effects, but when given along with an opiate that has higher effectiveness they compete for the receptor and subsequently reduce the action of the more effective drug.

Other chemical modifications of the morphine molecule produce **pure antagonists** such as naloxone and nalorphine. These are drugs that have structures similar to those of the opiates but produce no pharmacological activity of their own (i.e., no efficacy). The receptor antagonists can prevent or reverse the effect of administered opiates because of their ability to occupy opiate receptor sites. As you saw in the opening paragraphs of this chapter, intravenously administered naloxone can revive an unconscious individual in a matter of seconds; it can reverse all of the opiate effects and save the lives of those brought to the emergency room after opiate overdose. Specific receptor antagonists are also important for understanding the mechanism of action of opiate analgesics (see the section on opiate receptors later in the chapter).

Some opioid drugs have the unusual characteristic of being **mixed agonist–antagonists.** That is, they are effective agonists at some opioid receptors but act as antagonists at others. As you will learn a bit later, the three principal types of opiate receptors (μ, δ, and κ) mediate different opiate actions. The prototypic agonist–antagonist is pentazocine (Talwin), but others in this category are nalbuphine

Figure 10.3 Molecular structure of morphine, codeine, heroin, and naloxone highlighting the similarities in structure. The minor differences contribute to effectiveness and side effects.

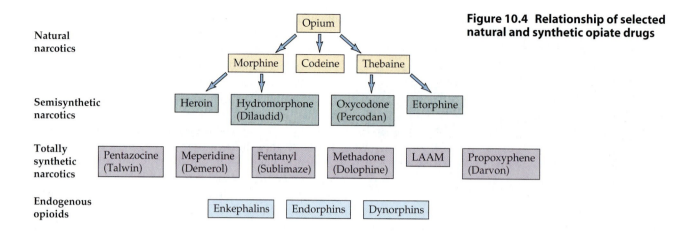

Figure 10.4 Relationship of selected natural and synthetic opiate drugs

(Nubain) and buprenorphine (Buprenex). Although as analgesics they are much less potent than morphine, they do not cause significant respiratory depression or constipation and they have a reduced risk for dependence. While some narcotic drugs are considered semisynthetic because they require chemical modifications of the natural opioids (e.g., hydromorphone [Dilaudid]), others are entirely synthetic and may have quite distinct structures (e.g., propoxyphene [Darvon], meperidine [Demerol]). The relationship of the major opiates and some of their derivatives as well as some of the synthetic opiates is shown in Figure 10.4.

Bioavailability predicts both physiological and behavioral effects

When morphine is administered for medical purposes, it is usually injected intramuscularly or given orally. Oral administration is convenient but produces more variable blood levels for the reasons discussed in Chapter 1. Recreational users often smoke opium for its rapid absorption from the lungs, although "snorting" heroin also leads to rapid absorption through the nasal mucosa. In addition, subcutaneous administration ("skin popping") may precede the more dangerous "mainlining" (intravenous injection).

Although morphine has pronounced psychoactive effects, only a small fraction of the drug is capable of crossing the blood–brain barrier to act on opiate receptors in the brain. Opiate distribution is fairly uniform in the rest of the body, and the drugs easily pass the placental barrier, exposing the unborn child to high levels. The newborn of an opiate-addicted mother suffers withdrawal symptoms within several hours after birth, which may have severe consequences for the infant, especially if the child is weak from inadequate prenatal nutrition. However, infants are readily stabilized with low doses of opiates to prevent abstinence signs, and the dose is gradually reduced. Following metabolism in the liver, most of the opiate metabolites are excreted in the urine within 24 hours.

Opioids have their most important effects on the CNS and on the gastrointestinal tract

The multiple effects of morphine and other opioids on the CNS are dose-related and also related to the rate of absorption. At low to moderate doses (5 to 10 mg), pain is relieved, respiration is somewhat depressed, and pupils are constricted. The principal subjective effects are drowsiness, decreased sensitivity to the environment, and impaired ability to concentrate, followed by a dreamy sleep. Because opiates have actions in the limbic system, some researchers suggest that the drugs relieve "psychological pain" including anxiety, feelings of inadequacy, and hostility, which may lead to increased drug use. Morphine also suppresses the cough reflex in a dose-dependent manner and has actions on the hypothalamus that lead to decreased appetite, drop in body temperature, reduced sex drive, and a variety of hormonal changes. Each of these effects can be associated with opiate receptors in particular areas of the CNS.

At slightly higher doses, particularly if the drug is administered intravenously or inhaled, the individual experiences an abnormal state of elation or euphoria, which is referred to as the "kick," "bang," or "rush" and is compared to a "whole-body orgasm." Nonaddicts describe it as a sudden flush of warmth located in the pit of the stomach. To achieve the maximum euphoria, very rapid penetration into the brain is needed. Although it is experienced as intense pleasure, the "rush" is not the principal basis for abuse but acts as a powerful reinforcer that encourages repeated drug use.

It is also important to know that the euphoric effect does not always accompany intravenous administration. For many individuals being medically treated, the drug may produce dysphoria, consisting of restlessness and anxiety. In addition, the nausea and vomiting that may accompany low doses of morphine is increased with higher doses. It is directly related to morphine's effect on the chemical trigger zone (the area postrema) in the brain stem that elicits vomiting. Although clearly unpleasant for most individuals, for the addict the nausea may become a "good sick" because it is closely associated with the drug-induced euphoria by classical conditioning.

At the highest doses, the opioids' sedative effects become stronger and may lead to unconsciousness. Body temperature and blood pressure fall. Pupils are now quite constricted and represent a clinical sign of opiate overdose in a comatose patient. Respiration is dangerously impaired due to morphine's action on the brain stem's respiratory center, which normally responds to high blood CO_2 levels by triggering increased respiration. Respiratory failure is the ultimate cause of death in overdose.

Apart from the CNS, the effects of morphine are greatest on the gastrointestinal tract. Opium was used for relief of diarrhea and dysentery even before it was used for analgesia. It remains one of the most important lifesaving drugs because of its ability to cause constipation and stop the life-threatening fluid loss associated with diarrhea that accompanies many bacterial and parasitic illnesses especially prevalent in developing countries. More modern treatment utilizes modified opiate molecules such as loperimide, which has been designed so that it cannot cross the blood–brain barrier. The major advantage is that it effectively slows gastrointestinal function but does not have any effect on the CNS. Unfortunately, when opiates are used for pain management, constipation is a common and disturbing side effect that does not diminish even after prolonged use.

Opioid Receptors and Endogenous Neuropeptides

The opiate drugs produce biobehavioral effects by binding to specific neuronal receptors. Since minor modifications of the morphine molecule produce significant changes in effect, analyses of the molecular structure of the drugs provides sufficient information to hypothesize definite structural features of the opiate receptor. Further, naloxone's blocking effects can be overcome by increasing concentrations of morphine, which demonstrates competition for the receptor. Not long after identifying opiate receptors, the natural neuropeptide ligands that act at the receptors were also characterized.

Receptor binding studies identified and localized opioid receptors

Although the existence of opiate receptors was evident, the initial attempts to label and locate these receptors in brain tissue using standard radioligand binding methods (see Chapter 4) proved to be a difficult task. Ultimately the opioid receptor was labeled (Pert and Snyder, 1973) by making several technical refinements in the assay and separation procedure, as well as having access to newer radioactive ligands

that had a greater amount of radioactivity per drug molecule. The receptors that they identified met the criteria described in Chapter 4. First, Figure 10.5A shows the classic

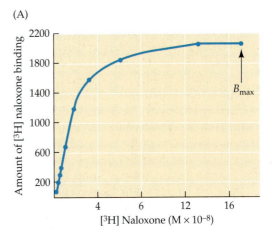

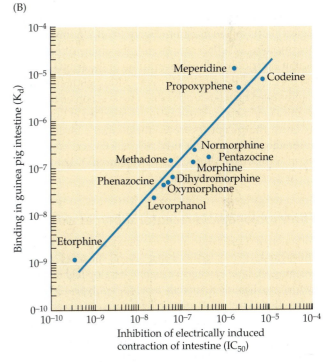

Figure 10.5 Opiate receptor binding (A) Binding of [^{3}H]naloxone to rat brain shows the saturation of opioid receptors. As the concentration of the opiate ligand (naloxone) increases, binding to the receptors increases linearly until the receptors are filled at B_{max}. (B) There is a strong positive correlation between the concentration of opiate drugs needed to inhibit electrically induced contraction of the intestine (IC$_{50}$) and the concentration needed to bind to opiate receptors in the same tissue. The results show clearly that drugs that bind readily at low concentrations of ligand (e.g., etorphine) also are effective in inhibiting the intestinal contraction at low doses. Drugs that bind less well (e.g., codeine) also require higher concentrations to inhibit the contraction.

binding curve, demonstrating that as the amount of radioactive opiate (in this case the antagonist naloxone) is increased, binding also increases in a linear fashion until the receptors are fully occupied. The leveling off of the binding curve at B_{max} shows that a finite number of receptors exists in a given amount of tissue. This saturation would not occur if the radioligand happened to be "sticky" and attached randomly to many cellular materials. Second, looking at the concentrations used in the assay, it is clear that the binding sites have a high affinity for the opiates. Third, the binding was shown to be reversible, with a time course that matches the loss of physiological effectiveness. Fourth, the concentrations needed in the binding assay are meaningfully related to the concentration of agonist needed to elicit a biological response.

But how do we know that these sites are those responsible for the opiates' pharmacological activity? Snyder (1977) and colleagues calculated binding affinity by measuring the ability of a number of nonradioactive opiates to compete with radioactive naloxone for the receptors. They found that the relative potency of various opiates in the competition experiments closely paralleled their relative potencies in pharmacological effects on the intestine (Figure 10.5B). In this case, the pharmacological effect measured is the ability of opiates to inhibit electrically induced contraction of the ileum (the lowest portion of the small intestine). Although many more-sophisticated methods are possible, opioid action on the ileum is considered a classic bioassay and is described in Box 10.1.

Once the receptors were labeled and characterized, autoradiography could be used to locate the receptors in the brain. Figure 10.6 shows a color-enhanced distribution of opiate receptors in rat brain.

Three major opioid receptor subtypes exist

Although the classic dose–response curves used by Martin and colleagues (1976) suggested that several subtypes of opiate receptors exist, researchers needed to develop highly *selective* radioactive ligands to directly label the subtypes. Selectivity means that a given molecule readily binds to one receptor subtype and has relatively low binding affinity for the others (Simon, 1991). The three most important subtypes have been called μ (mu), δ (delta), and κ (kappa). These receptor subtypes have distinct distributions in the brain and spinal cord, which suggests that they mediate a wide variety of effects.

The **μ-receptor** is the receptor that has a high affinity for morphine and related opiate drugs. The location of the μ-receptors has been mapped by autoradiography in several species (Mansour and Watson, 1993), including human brain postmortem (Quirion and Pilapil, 1991). Other researchers have performed in vivo mapping using positron emission tomography (PET) imaging (Mayberg and Frost, 1990). The results consistently show a wide distribution of μ-receptors in both the brain and spinal cord. The brain areas rich in μ-receptors support their role in morphine-induced analgesia

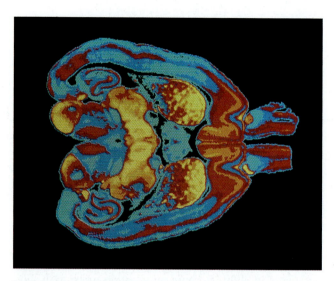

Figure 10.6 Distribution of opiate receptors in rat brain is shown in this autoradiogram. Higher densities, seen as warmer colors, occur in the striatum, medial thalamus, locus coeruleus, periaqueductal gray, and raphe nuclei. (Courtesy of Miles Herkenham, NIMH.)

(e.g., the medial thalamus, periaqueductal gray, median raphe, and clusters within the spinal cord). Other high-density areas suggest a role in positive reinforcement (nucleus accumbens), cardiovascular and respiratory depression, cough control, nausea and vomiting (brain stem), and sensorimotor integration (thalamus, striatum) (Mansour and Watson, 1993; Carvey, 1998). Figure 10.7A is an autoradiogram of μ-receptor binding in the rat CNS.

The **δ-receptors** have a distribution similar to that of μ-receptors (Figure 10.7B) but are more restricted. They are predominantly found in forebrain structures such as the neocortex, striatum, olfactory areas, substantia nigra, and nucleus accumbens. Many of these sites are consistent with a possible role for δ-receptors in modulating olfaction, motor integration, reinforcement, and cognitive function. Delta receptors in areas overlapping μ-receptors suggest modulation of both spinal and supraspinal analgesia.

The **κ-receptors** (Figure 10.7C) have a very distinct distribution compared to the μ- and δ-receptors. The κ-receptor was initially identified by high-affinity binding to ketocyclazocine, which is an opiate analog that produces hallucinations and dysphoria. This receptor is also found in the striatum and amygdala but additionally has a unique distribution in the hypothalamus and pituitary. These receptors may participate in the regulation of pain perception, gut motility, and dysphoria but also modulate water balance, feeding, temperature control, and neuroendocrine function.

Once the genetic material for each of the three receptor types was isolated, it was inserted into cells (a process called **transfection**) maintained in culture to produce large numbers of identical cells (cloning). The **receptor cloning** and

BOX 10.1 Pharmacology in Action

Opiate Bioassay

Bioassays are important and classic tools of pharmacology that provide relatively quick and inexpensive tests of agonist–receptor activity on a biological response. The assays generally measure a simple response in a tissue that is in its native functional state rather than a highly modified (e.g., homogenized cells) nonphysiological condition. Such measures are often used to demonstrate the biological relevance of a newly identified receptor protein. Under ideal conditions, receptor binding and biological response should be measured in the same simple, intact system before disruptive procedures are performed on the cells.

The most accurate bioassay to measure opioid activity was developed by a pioneer in opioid research, Hans Kosterlitz (Kosterlitz et al., 1970). The guinea pig intestinal muscle (ileum) and associated neuronal connections are dissected and maintained in a physiological solution. The muscle is fastened at each end to maintain a fixed tension, so that when the neurons are electrically stimulated, the muscle twitch can be recorded on a polygraph. The twitch is inhibited by opiate drugs, and this inhibition can be blocked by naloxone (Figure A), which shows that opiate receptors are involved. Further, the magnitude of the twitch inhibition is closely correlated with receptor binding potency. In addition, Kosterlitz and Waterfield (1975) showed that the naloxone-reversible

twitch inhibition is almost perfectly correlated with the potency of the opiates to relieve pain in humans (Figure B). Therefore, it is apparent that a correlation exists between analgesic effects in vivo, muscle-twitch inhibi-

tion in the bioassay in vitro, and the ability to bind to opiate receptors. Clearly the bioassay represents a simple and rapid means to screen opioid drugs.

(A)

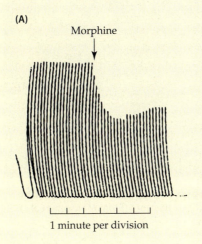

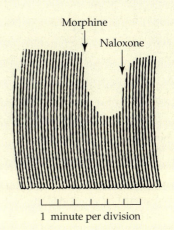

1 minute per division

1 minute per division

(B)

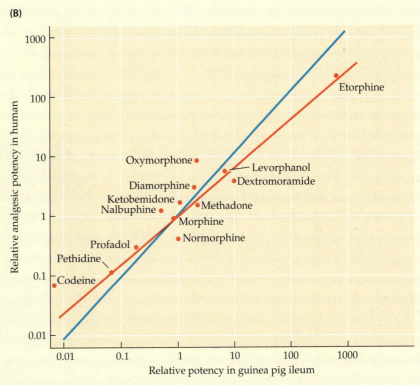

(B) A strong positive correlation (shown by the red line) exists between opiate inhibition of guinea pig ileum twitch and analgesic effects in humans. For comparison purposes, the blue line represents a perfect correlation. The values for potency were calculated relative to morphine (morphine = 1). (After Kosterlitz and Waterfield, 1975.)

(A) Mu   (B) Delta   (C) Kappa

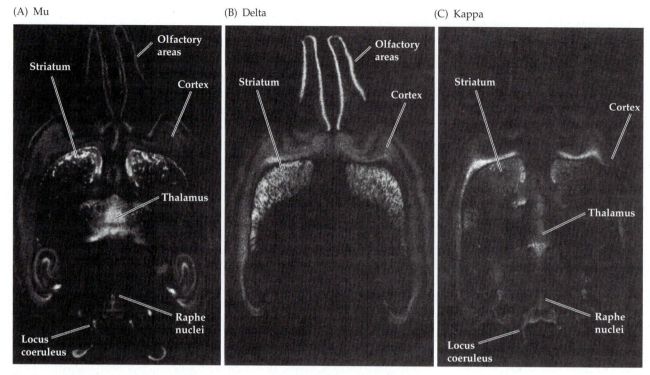

Figure 10.7 Autoradiograms of opiate receptor subtype binding in rat brain
Notice the distinct locations of (A) μ-, (B) δ-, and (C) κ-receptors. (From Mansour et al., 1988.)

molecular sequencing of the opiate receptor subtypes provided several key pieces of information:

1. For each of the receptors we now know the specific nucleic acid sequence making up the DNA that directs the synthesis of each receptor protein.

2. Using the nucleic acid sequence, the amino acids of the protein can be identified and compared with other families of receptor proteins.

3. The transfected cells can be used to study the intracellular changes induced by receptor agonists.

4. By radioactively labeling the genetic material, in situ hybridization makes it possible to visualize those cells in the brain that synthesize the receptor protein and more precisely localize the receptors themselves. (See Chapter 4 for a review of the techniques of molecular biology.)

Although the first opiate receptor to be successfully cloned was the δ-receptor (Evans et al., 1992; Kieffer et al., 1992), cloning of both μ- and κ-receptors was soon to follow. Each of the three receptors have between 370 and 400 amino acids and they bind with the ligands specific to each. All three of the protein receptors have a structure similar to the family of receptors that are linked to G proteins, which suggests that they mediate metabotropic (rather than ionotropic) responses. The structure of the δ-receptor, with the classic seven transmembrane portions, is shown in Figure 10.8.

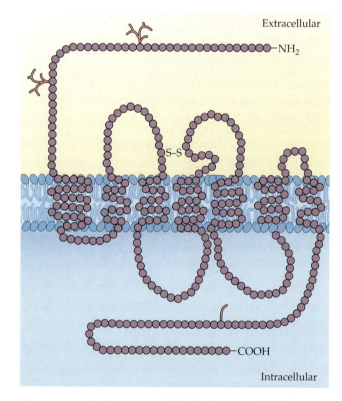

Figure 10.8 Proposed structure of the δ-opioid receptor
Each circle represents an identified amino acid. The seven regions spanning the cell membrane are typical for receptors that are coupled to G proteins.

Several families of naturally occurring opioid peptides bind to these receptors

Once the receptors were identified, researchers were quick to ask why the nervous system would have receptors for the derivatives of the opium poppy. It seemed more reasonable to hypothesize that an endogenous neurochemical must exist to act on opioid receptors. Since the distribution of the receptors failed to match the regional distribution of any known neurotransmitter, it was assumed that a novel neurochemical would be identified. A second rationale for searching for an endogenous opioid involved the analgesia produced by electrically stimulating specific areas of the CNS such as the periaqueductal gray. In many animal studies as well as human clinical trials, the analgesic effect could be partially antagonized by the opiate receptor antagonist naloxone, which suggested that opioids were involved. It is clear to us now that electrical stimulation causes the release of a natural ligand that acts on those opioid receptors.

Discovery   In 1974 two different laboratories identified a peptide in brain extracts and other tissues that mimicked opiate activity (electrophysiologically and in the ileum bioassay) and could also bind to opiate receptors (Terenius and Wahlstrom, 1974; Hughes, 1975). They named the first peptide enkephalin, meaning "in the brain." Soon a number of peptides were found to have these properties and were called endogenous opiates, or **endorphins** (from *endo*, signifying "endogenous," and -*orphin*, from "morphine"). The great similarity in structure among the peptides led researchers to conclude that there were several larger peptides, called propeptides (or precursor peptides), that are broken into smaller active opioids. Any confusion was resolved when molecular biologists found that there are three large propeptides and each is coded for by a separate gene. These large peptides are called **prodynorphin** (254 amino acids), **pro-opiomelanocortin or POMC** (267 amino acids), and **proenkephalin** (267 amino acids). Each of the three large peptides manufactured in the soma must be processed by enzymes (called proteases) that are packaged in the Golgi apparatus along with the peptide. The enzymes are responsible for chopping or cleaving the propeptide into individual peptide products that are stored in vesicles and further processed as they are transported down the axon to be released at the synapse. Each of the large propeptides produces a number of biologically active opioid and non-opioid peptides (Figure 10.9). More recently, Zadina and col-

leagues (1999) described a group of peptides with a distinct structure and distribution in the CNS. These peptides, called **endomorphins,** bind quite selectively to the μ-receptor and are as potent as morphine in relieving pain. Thus far, their propeptide has not been identified.

Localization   The mapping of the pathways utilizing the endogenous opioids was achieved by in situ hybridization to visualize propeptide mRNA, and immunohistochemistry was used to localize the propeptide itself (see Chapter 4). These propeptides are found in the brain, spinal cord, and peripheral autonomic nervous system, concentrated in areas related to pain modulation and mood. In addition, POMC is found in particularly high concentration in the pituitary gland, which releases a variety of hormones in response to hypothalamic releasing factors. The hypothalamus releases corticotropin-releasing factor (CRF) in response to stress, which in turn increases adrenocorticotropic hormone (ACTH) release from the pituitary and ultimately glucocorticoids from the adrenal cortex (Figure 10.10). CRF also causes a rapid increase in POMC mRNA and subsequent increases in release of β-endorphin from the pituitary. Since a variety of stressors, such as painful foot shock, restraint, and swim stress, increase both CRF mRNA and POMC mRNA, it is likely that this opioid provides a physiological link between pain and stress regulation (Young, 1993). Overall, the wide-

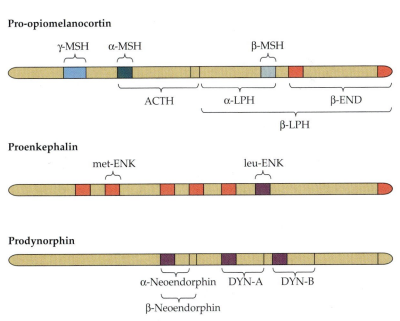

Figure 10.9 The three opioid propeptides and some of their possible products POMC is cleaved into β-endorphin (β-END) and a number of other peptides including γ- and α-melanocyte-stimulating hormone (MSH), adrenocorticotropic hormone (ACTH), and several forms of lipotropin (LPH). Proenkephalin cleavage produces several copies of met- and leu-enkephalin. Prodynorphin contains several endorphins (α- and β-neoendorphin) as well as dynorphin A and B. Note that the tiny enkephalin peptides are frequently found within the larger peptide fragments.

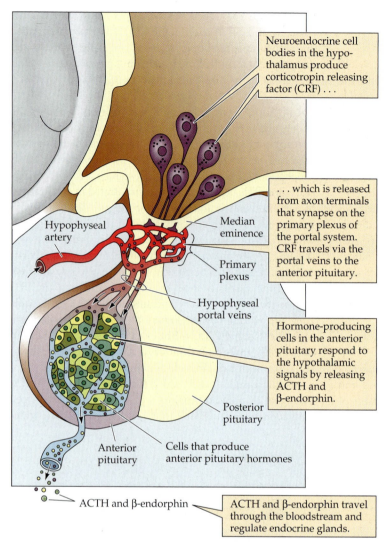

Neuroendocrine cell bodies in the hypothalamus produce corticotropin releasing factor (CRF) . . .

. . . which is released from axon terminals that synapse on the primary plexus of the portal system. CRF travels via the portal veins to the anterior pituitary.

Hormone-producing cells in the anterior pituitary respond to the hypothalamic signals by releasing ACTH and β-endorphin.

ACTH and β-endorphin travel through the bloodstream and regulate endocrine glands.

Hypophyseal artery

Median eminence

Primary plexus

Hypophyseal portal veins

Posterior pituitary

Anterior pituitary

Cells that produce anterior pituitary hormones

ACTH and β-endorphin

Figure 10.10 Hypothalamic control of ACTH and β-endorphin release The hypothalamus releases CRF, which causes the anterior pituitary to secrete ACTH, which in turn acts on the adrenal gland to prepare the individual to deal with stress. CRF also influences β-endorphin synthesis and release from the pituitary in response to stress. Notice in the previous figure that ACTH and β-endorphin come from the same propeptide, POMC.

spread locations of the peptides strongly implicates them in many functions including pain suppression, reward, motor coordination, endocrine function, feeding, body temperature and water regulation, and response to stress.

While some of the neurons containing the opioid propeptides have long projections, many more are small cells that form local circuits. Many of the peptides are co-localized with other neurotransmitters in the same neuron, including acetylcholine, GABA (γ-aminobutyric acid), serotonin, catecholamines, and other peptides. When peptides coexist with other neurotransmitters, they are likely to have a neuromodu-

latory role; that is, they modify the function of the neurotransmitter or produce changes in ion conductance and membrane potential.

Although we have three peptide families plus the endomorphins and three principal receptor subtypes, the peptides are not selective for a receptor type but show only a relative preference. The natural ligands for the δ-receptors are thought to be those derived from proenkephalin (enkephalins), and products from prodynorphin (dynorphin) are likely the natural κ-receptor agonists. The endomorphins bind preferentially to the μ-receptors, while POMC peptides (endorphins) bind readily to both μ- and δ-receptors. Table 10.1 summarizes receptor subtype location, function, and preference for endogenous opioids.

Opioid receptor–mediated cellular changes are inhibitory

You are already aware that each of the three opioid receptor types is linked to G proteins. You may recall from Chapter 3 that there are multiple forms of G proteins that have two principal actions. Some G proteins directly stimulate or inhibit the opening of ion channels (see Figure 3.11A) and others stimulate or inhibit enzymes to alter second-messenger production (see Figure 3.11B). Opioids work by both of those mechanisms to open K^+ channels, close Ca^{2+} channels, and inhibit adenylyl cyclase activity. The overall effects of opiates on nerve cell function include the reduction of membrane excitability and subsequent slowing of cell firing and the inhibition of neurotransmitter release.

There are three principal ways that endorphins reduce synaptic transmission: (1) postsynaptic inhibition; (2) axoaxonic inhibition; and (3) via presynaptic autoreceptors. First, opioid receptor–G protein activation opens K^+ channels, which increases K^+ conductance. Potassium exits the cell, forced by its concentration gradient, causing hyperpolarization. When the receptors are on the soma or dendrites of neurons, the hyperpolarization (IPSP) decreases the cell's firing rate (Figure 10.11A).

Second, opioids also produce an inhibitory effect by closing voltage-gated Ca^{2+} channels. In this case (Figure 10.11B), opioid receptors on the presynaptic terminal activate G proteins, which in turn close the Ca^{2+} channels. Reducing the amount of Ca^{2+} entering during an action potential proportionately decreases the amount of neurotransmitter released. For example, opioid-induced inhibition of norepinephrine and dopamine release has been found in many brain areas. As expected, this effect is prevented by the receptor antagonist naloxone. The inhibition of glutamate and substance P

TABLE 10.1 Location, Function, and Endogenous Ligand for Opioid Receptor Subtypes

Receptor subtype	Endogenous ligand (prohormone source)	Location (most dense)	Functions
μ	Endomorphins (unknown), endorphins (POMC)	Thalamus, periaqueductal gray, raphe nuclei, spinal cord, striatum, brain stem, nucleus accumbens, amygdala, hippocampus	Analgesia, reinforcement, cardiovascular and respiratory depression, antitussive, vomiting, sensorimotor integration
δ	Enkephalin (proenkephalin), endorphins (POMC)	Neocortex, striatum, olfactory areas, substantia nigra, nucleus accumbens, spinal cord	Analgesia, reinforcement, cognitive function, olfaction, motor integration
κ	Dynorphins (prodynorphin)	Pituitary, hypothalamus, amygdala, striatum, nucleus accumbens	Neuroendocrine function, water balance, feeding, temperature control, dysphoria, analgesia

release in the spinal cord is of particular significance because those neurotransmitters are released from the afferent sensory neurons that transmit pain signals from the periphery into the CNS (see the section on opioids and pain).

Third, opioid autoreceptors also produce inhibitory effects. Somatodendritic autoreceptors hyperpolarize cells in the locus coeruleus by enhancing K⁺ conductance and sub-sequently reducing cell firing (not shown in figure). Elsewhere, presynaptic autoreceptors reduce the release of co-localized neurotransmitters (Figure 10.11C). In summary, opioid effects on both K^+ and Ca^{2+} channels produce inhibitory effects and reduce neurotransmitter release. These actions in the appropriate circuitry are ultimately responsible for the analgesic effects (DiChiara and North, 1992).

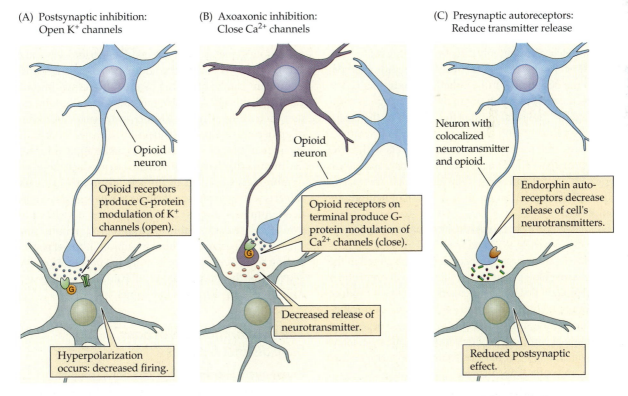

(A) Postsynaptic inhibition: Open K⁺ channels

Opioid neuron

Opioid receptors produce G-protein modulation of K⁺ channels (open).

Hyperpolarization occurs: decreased firing.

(B) Axoaxonic inhibition: Close Ca²⁺ channels

Opioid neuron

Opioid receptors on terminal produce G-protein modulation of Ca²⁺ channels (close).

Decreased release of neurotransmitter.

(C) Presynaptic autoreceptors: Reduce transmitter release

Neuron with colocalized neurotransmitter and opioid.

Endorphin autoreceptors decrease release of cell's neurotransmitters.

Reduced postsynaptic effect.

Figure 10.11 Inhibitory actions of endogenous opioids Opioids inhibit nerve activity in several ways. (A) Opioids bind to receptors that activate a G protein that opens K⁺ channels to hyperpolarize the postsynaptic cells, thereby reducing the rate of firing. (B) Opioid receptors on nerve terminals (axoaxonic) activate G proteins that close Ca²⁺ channels, reducing the release of the neurotransmitter. (C) Presynaptic autoreceptors activate G proteins and reduce the release of a co-localized neurotransmitter. The mechanism may involve closing Ca²⁺ channels or opening K⁺ channels that hyperpolarize the presynaptic cell.

All three types of opiate receptor are also coupled to inhibitory G proteins (called G_i) that inhibit adenylyl cyclase, which normally synthesizes the second messenger cyclic adenosine monophosphate (cAMP). The reduced cAMP and subsequent decreased function of cAMP-dependent protein kinase may in part be responsible for opiate-induced ion channel changes; however, the immediate effects of the inhibition on cell function is not entirely clear. Nevertheless, the cAMP cascade has been implicated in chronic effects of opioids including drug tolerance, dependence, and withdrawal. These topics are discussed in later sections.

Section Summary

The opiates are a class of drug originally derived from the opium poppy that relieve pain and produce a state of drowsiness and sleep. Under some conditions the drugs produce a sudden state of euphoria, although in other conditions dysphoria may occur. In addition, they cause pinpoint pupils, reduced concentration, suppression of the cough reflex, drop in body temperature, reduced appetite, and a variety of hormonal effects. Respiratory and cardiac depression may also occur, especially at higher doses. Repeated use produces tolerance to many of the drugs' effects as well as physical dependence. The many effects of opiate drugs are directly related to their action on opiate receptors (μ, δ, and κ), which are widely and unevenly distributed in the central and peripheral nervous systems. Discovery of receptor subtypes has led to the development of synthetic opioids designed to act on specific receptor subtypes to produce analgesia without causing the undesirable side effects. Each of the receptors has been isolated and cloned and found to be coupled to G proteins that induce metabotropic effects within the cell. The principal cellular activities include actions on ion channels (K^+, Ca^{2+}) and adenylyl cyclase, which are responsible for cell hyperpolarization and inhibition of neurotransmitter release.

The endogenous ligands (enkephalins) for the opiate receptors were discovered in 1975 and identified as small peptides that are cleaved from larger propeptides manufactured in the soma. Molecular biology has shown three distinct propeptides (prodynorphin, POMC, and proenkephalin), which produce a variety of opioid (e.g., endorphins, enkephalins, dynorphin) and non-opioid fragments. The location of these peptides in the brain, spinal cord, and pituitary implicates them in many functions, including water balance, feeding, body temperature regulation, and endocrine function.

Opioids and Pain

Although we all feel that we intuitively understand what pain is like, it is really far more complex than generally believed.

Since opioids are therapeutically best known as analgesics, a further discussion of pain and its neural circuitry is needed.

Pain is distinct from other sensory systems in that it can be caused by a variety of stimuli detected by several types of nociceptors (detectors of noxious stimuli). The nociceptors are networks of free nerve endings that are sensitive to intense pressure, extreme temperature including heat and cold, electrical impulses, cuts, chemical irritants, and inflammation. Pain varies not only in intensity but also in quality and may be described as "pricking," "stabbing," "burning," "aching," and so forth. Its perception is also highly subjective, and no single stimulus will be described as painful by all individuals nor perhaps even by the same individual under different circumstances. Pain is modified by a number of factors including strong emotion, environmental stimuli like stress, hypnosis, acupuncture, and opiate drugs.

Although we can get subjective reports of pain, quantification is difficult, particularly when testing analgesic drugs. In the laboratory, when methods such as the application of sudden pressure, pinpricks, or stabs are used to induce pain, most analgesic drugs show ineffective or inconsistent analgesic effects. The failure of these drugs to show a significant reduction in pain is probably because of the low emotional impact of those types of pain. More consistent results are obtained with the analgesics through the use of techniques that produce slowly developing or sustained pain. One technique used with human subjects is to stop blood flow to an exercising muscle with a tourniquet. With this method, the pain is slow in onset and is directly related to amount of exercise. Cutaneous pain in humans can be produced by the intradermal injection of various chemicals. A reliable method to test this kind of pain uses cantharidin to induce a blister, from which the outer layer of epidermis is removed to expose the blister base, on which small quantities of various agents can be applied for testing. Techniques that have been designed to produce more-intense or more-persistent pain are infrequently used because finding subjects willing to participate in such experiments is more difficult. Animal testing is overall more reliable, yielding conditions that are comparable to pathological pain in humans. This may be because the human subject in the experimental setting realizes that the pain stimulus poses no real threat, whereas for the animal subject, all pain is potentially serious. Animal tests are described in Chapter 4.

The two components of pain have distinct features

Pain is often described as having several components. "First," or early, pain represents the immediate sensory component and signals the onset of a noxious stimulus and its precise location to cause immediate withdrawal and escape from the damaging stimulus. "Second," or late, pain has a strong emotional component, that is, the unpleasantness of the sensation. Adaptation occurs more slowly to the secondary component, so it attracts our attention in prolonged fashion to motivate behaviors that limit further damage and aid recovery. Late pain is less localized and is often accompanied by autonomic responses such as sweating, fall in blood pressure, or nausea.

These distinct components of pain are in part explained by the types of neuron that carry the signal. Fibers called Aδ are larger in diameter and are myelinated, so they conduct action potentials more rapidly than the thin and unmyelinat-ed C fibers. The difference in speed explains why when you smash your finger in the car door, you first experience a sharp pain that is well localized but brief, followed by a dull aching that is a prolonged reminder of the damage your body has experienced. These neurons have their cell bodies in the dorsal root ganglia and terminate in the gray matter of the dorsal horn of the spinal cord, ending on projection neurons that transmit pain signals to higher brain centers (Figure 10.12).

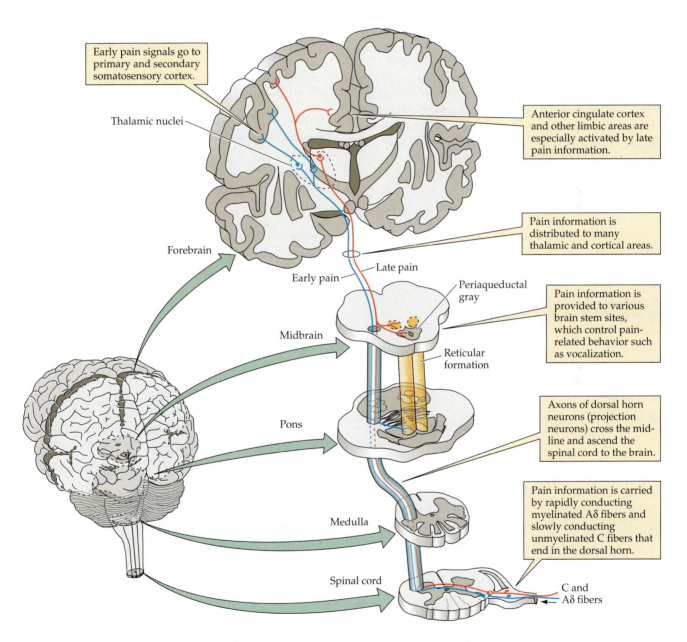

Figure 10.12 Ascending pain pathways Sensory neurons (Aδ and C fibers) activated by noxious stimuli enter the dorsal horn of the spinal cord. Dorsal horn neurons travel up the spinal cord on the contralateral side and ultimately reach various nuclei in the thalamus. Neurons transmitting "fast" (first pain) end first in the primary somatosensory cortex for well-localized sensory discrimination, before the information is transferred to the secondary somatosensory cortex, where pain recognition occurs. The slower-conducting neurons transmit information (second pain) to a variety of limbic areas including the anterior cingulate cortex, which is important for the emotional or suffering aspect of pain.

A second distinction between the two components of pain is their route and final destination in the brain. Early pain is transmitted from the spinal cord via the spinothalamic tract to the posteroventrolateral nucleus of the thalamus before going directly to the primary and then secondary somatosensory cortex. The primary somatosensory cortex provides sensory discrimination of pain, while the secondary cortex is involved in the recognition of pain and memory of past pain. Late pain also goes to the thalamus, but in addition gives off collaterals to a variety of limbic structures such as the hypothalamus and amygdala as well as the anterior cingulate cortex. The anterior cingulate has a role in pain affect, attention, and motor responses (Rainville, 2002).

For the first time, researchers have been able to demonstrate the temporal relationship between pain-evoked cortical activation and reported pain in human subjects. Ploner and colleagues (2002) subjected individuals to brief painful laser stimuli and continuously monitored the subjects' subjective pain rating while simultaneously recording faint magnetic fields on the surface of the skull using magnetoencephalogra-

phy (MEG). Although MEG is somewhat inaccurate in precisely locating brain activity, it is excellent at showing the neural changes over very small units of time (from one millisecond to another). In that way Ploner could trace a wave of brain activity from its origin to sequential brain areas during processing (Figure 10.13A). When the cortical activation was superimposed on magnetic resonance images (Figure 10.13B), they showed that first pain (pain recogntion), identified by subjects' ratings, was temporally related to activation of the primary somatosensory cortex, whereas second pain (identified by subjects' ratings of unpleasantness) was strongly associated with anterior cingulate activation. Both types of pain were associated with neural activity in the secondary somatosensory cortex.

Opioids inhibit pain transmission at spinal and supraspinal levels

By binding to opioid receptors, morphine and other opiate drugs mimic the inhibitory action of the endogenous opi-

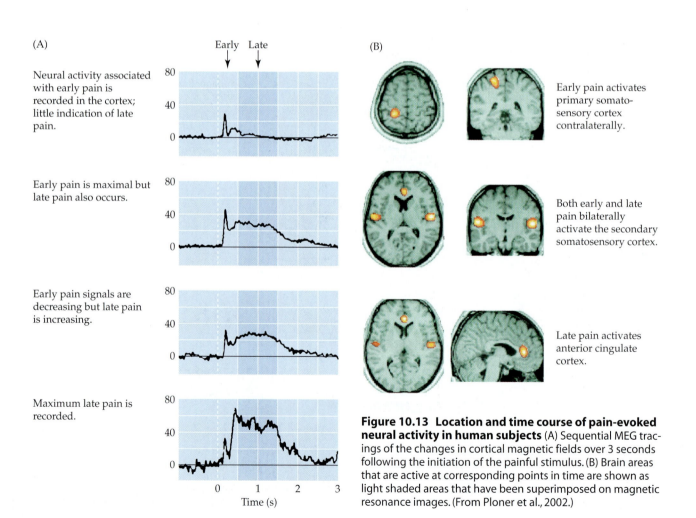

(A)

Neural activity associated with early pain is recorded in the cortex; little indication of late pain.

Early pain is maximal but late pain also occurs.

Early pain signals are decreasing but late pain is increasing.

Maximum late pain is recorded.

Time (s)

(B)

Early pain activates primary somatosensory cortex contralaterally.

Both early and late pain bilaterally activate the secondary somatosensory cortex.

Late pain activates anterior cingulate cortex.

Figure 10.13 Location and time course of pain-evoked neural activity in human subjects (A) Sequential MEG tracings of the changes in cortical magnetic fields over 3 seconds following the initiation of the painful stimulus. (B) Brain areas that are active at corresponding points in time are shown as light shaded areas that have been superimposed on magnetic resonance images. (From Ploner et al., 2002.)

oids at many stages of pain transmission within the spinal cord and brain. To simplify, we can say that opiates regulate pain in three ways:

1. Within the spinal cord by small inhibitory interneurons;
2. By two significant descending pathways originating in the periaqueductal gray (PAG); and
3. At many higher brain sites, which explains opioid effects on emotional and hormonal aspects of pain response.

As you know, information about pain, either from the surface or deep within the body cavity, is carried by neurons from the body into the spinal cord. Some of these primary afferent neurons end directly on projection neurons that transmit pain signals to higher brain centers (e.g., first to the thalamus and then to the somatosensory cortex) (Figure 10.14A). Others end on small excitatory interneurons (i.e., short neurons within the spinal cord) that in turn synapse onto the projection neurons (Figure 10.14B).

Opioids reduce the transmission of pain signals at the spinal cord in two ways. First, small inhibitory **spinal interneurons** release endorphins that inhibit the activation of the spinal projection neurons (Figure 10.14C). Morphine can act directly on those same opiate receptors to inhibit the transmission of the pain signal to higher brain centers that normally allow us to become aware of the sensory experience. Second, endorphins regulate several modulatory pathways that descend from the brain to inhibit spinal cord pain transmission either by directly inhibiting the projection neuron (A), or the excitatory interneuron (B), or exciting the inhibitory opioid neuron (C). These **descending modulatory pathways** (Figure 10.15) begin in the midbrain and modify the pain information carried by spinal cord neurons.

The most important descending pathways begin in the PAG. The PAG is a brain area rich in endogenous opioid peptides and high concentrations of opioid receptors, particularly μ and κ. Local electrical stimulation of the PAG produces analgesia but no change in the ability to detect temperature, touch, or pressure. Treatment of chronic pain in human patients with electrical stimulation of the PAG is frequently successful, although tolerance occurs with repeated use and cross-tolerance (see Chapter 1) with injected morphine also occurs. This phenomenon suggests that electrical stimulation releases a morphine-like substance onto the same postsynaptic receptor sites occupied by exogenous morphine. Partial blockade of stimulation-induced analgesia with the specific opioid antagonist naloxone further supports that idea.

The neurons beginning in the PAG end on cells in the medulla, including the serotonergic cell bodies of the nucleus of the raphe nuclei. Microinjection of opioids into the raphe produces significant analgesia. The serotonergic neu-

rons descend into the spinal cord to inhibit cell firing there and in that way reduce pain transmission.

Other cells originating in the PAG terminate in the brain stem in an area close to the locus coeruleus, an important cluster of noradrenergic cell bodies that also send axons to the spinal cord. Locus coeruleus cells increase their firing rate when noxious stimuli are applied. The same cells are hyperpolarized by μ-receptor agonists, which reduces their firing rate. Furthermore, neurotoxic lesions of the descending sero-

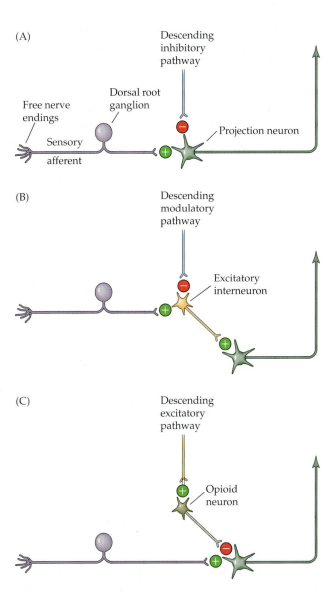

Figure 10.14 Pain transmission in the spinal cord is modified by descending modulatory neurons via (A) inhibition of the projection neuron; (B) inhibition of an excitatory interneuron; and (C) excitation of an inhibitory opioid interneuron. Opiate drugs can influence the activity of the descending pathways as well as acting directly on opioid receptors in the spinal cord.

tonergic and noradrenergic cells prevent systemic morphine-induced analgesia. Therefore, there are at least two major pathways that descend to the spinal cord to inhibit the projection of pain information to higher brain centers. However, the inhibitory action is direct in some cases, while at other times the inhibition occurs by acting on small spinal interneurons (as seen in Figure 10.15).

In summary, opioids modulate pain directly in the spinal cord and also by regulating the descending pain inhibitory pathways ending in the spinal cord. In addition, significant opioid action also occurs in other **supraspinal** (above the spinal cord) locations, including higher sensory areas and limbic structures as well as the hypothalamus and medial thalamus. A high concentration of endogenous opioids and the presence of opiate receptors suggest that these areas may be responsible for the emotional component of pain as well as autonomic and neuroendocrine responses. In a recent PET study, the endogenous activation of the μ-opioid system was evaluated during sustained pain. Zubieta and colleagues (2001) found a significant negative correlation between μ-opioid activity (measured as displacement of [^{11}C]carfentanil from μ-receptors) in the nucleus accumbens, amygdala, and thalamus and reported *sensory* pain scores (Figure 10.16). That is, the greater the μ-opioid activation, the lower was the individual's sensory pain score. The PAG also showed increased μ-receptor displacement, although it was not significant. When the scores on the *affective* component of pain were evaluated, increased μ-opioid activity was found in the bilateral anterior cingulate cortex, thalamus, and nucleus accumbens. These results indicate that endogenous μ-opioids modulate both the sensory and emotional components of pain and that morphine and other opiates likewise act at these sites. The existence of multiple circuits carrying pain information demonstrates the redundancy and diffuse nature of pain transmission, which reflects its tremendous evolutionary significance for survival.

Opioid Reinforcement, Tolerance, and Dependence

Although the opiates are the best pain reducing drugs presently available, their use continues to be problematic because of the potential for abuse. The drugs in this class are highly reinforcing, and despite strict legal controls they sometimes wind up in the hands of individuals who abuse these substances. Furthermore, chronic use leads to tolerance and ultimately to physical dependence.

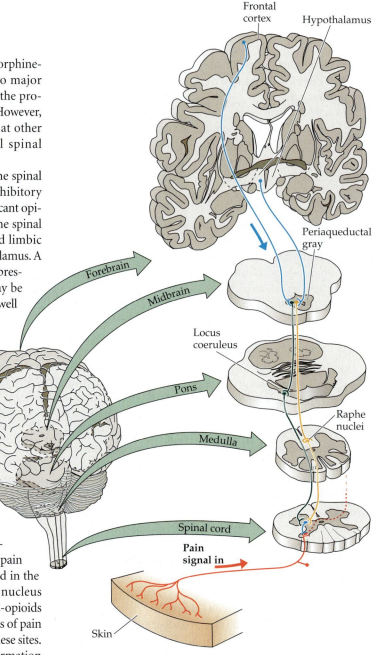

Figure 10.15 Descending pain modulation pathways
Neurons from the periaqueductal gray descend to the brain stem nucleus of the raphe and the locus coeruleus. Serotonergic and adrenergic neurons, respectively, descend to the spinal cord to modulate the transmission of the pain signal at that level.

Animal testing shows significant reinforcing properties

Experimental techniques used to demonstrate the reinforcement value of opiates are described in Chapter 4. Intracerebral electrical self-stimulation allows subjects to press a lever in order to self-administer a weak electric current to certain brain areas that constitute central reward pathways. When the animal presses the lever, electrical activation causes

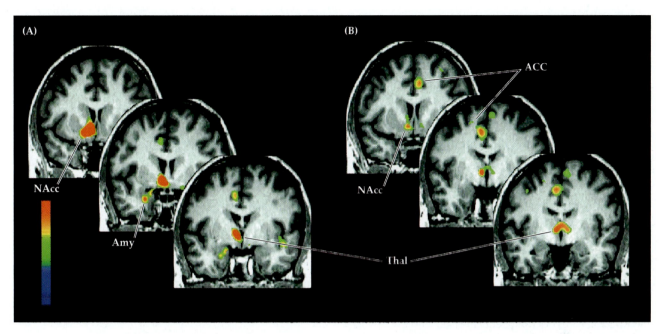

Figure 10.16 PET scans showing endogenous opioid activation during sustained pain In subjects injected with [^{11}C]carfentanil, endogenous opioid action is shown by the ability of the endogenous opioid to displace the radiolabeled μ-receptor ligand from the receptors. Pain was induced by continuous infusion of hypertonic saline in the masseter muscle and was compared to a control condition of isotonic saline infusion. (A) Activation of the μ-opioid system in the nucleus accumbens (NAcc), amygdala (Amy), and anterior thalamus (Thal) after the subjects were exposed to the prolonged noxious stimulus. These increases were negatively correlated with the subjects' *sensory* scores of pain. (B) μ-opioid activity in the bilateral anterior cingulate cortex (ACC) and anterior thalamus and unilaterally in the NAcc. These increases were negatively correlated with pain *affect* scores. Therefore, the greater the μ-opioid activation in these areas, the lower was the emotional component of pain. (Courtesy of Dr. Jon-Kar Zubieta.)

release of neurotransmitters from the nerve terminals in the region, which in turn mediate a rewarding effect. The fact that morphine and other opioids lower the electric current threshold for self-stimulation indicates that the drugs enhance the brain reward mechanism.

Using the drug self-administration technique, one striking finding is that the reinforcement value and the pattern of opioid use in animals are quite similar to those seen in humans. Self-injection gradually increases over time until the animals self-administer a stable and apparently optimal amount of drug. The ability of animals to maintain a stable blood level is demonstrated by pretreatment with morphine, codeine, or meperidine which subsequently reduces intravenous self-administration of morphine. In contrast, when some receptors are blocked with naloxone, the self-administration rate increases and matches that seen during morphine abstinence. It is evident from these studies that the animals learn to regulate with some accuracy the amount of morphine that they require. Dose–response curves can be used to compare the relative potencies of opiate drug reinforcement (Woods et al., 1993).

The endogenous opioid β-endorphin is also self-administered, which strongly suggests that it mediates opioid rein-forcement. Beta-endorphin self-administration is blocked by either μ- or δ-receptor antagonists. Thus, both types of receptor are involved in reward processes. In contrast, κ-agonists fail to produce self-injection and may induce aversive states, leading to avoidance behavior (Shippenberg, 1993).

Dopaminergic and nondopaminergic components contribute to opioid reinforcement

There are two important methods used to identify the neurobiology of opiate reinforcement. In one, self-administration of opioid ligands microinjected into discrete brain areas is evaluated. Second, selective lesions are used to identify the brain areas and neurotransmitter pathways that eliminate opiate-induced reinforcement.

Microinjection studies from many laboratories demonstrate the contribution of the dopaminergic mesolimbic pathway to opiate reinforcement. This pathway originates in the ventral tegmental area (VTA) of the midbrain and projects to limbic areas including the nucleus accumbens (NA). Return to Figure 5.7 to review the important dopamine (DA) pathways in the brain. Self-administration of morphine or endogenous peptides occurs when the microcannula is implanted near the dopamine cell bodies within the VTA. Intra-VTA microinjection of morphine or selective μ-agonists also produces conditioned place preference and reduces the threshold for intracranial electrical self-stimulation. Each of these results argues for a direct action of opiates on central reward mechanisms served by the mesolimbic pathway.

But what exactly happens to the cells in the VTA in the presence of opiates? First, both systemic opiates and opiates microinjected into the VTA increase dopaminergic cell firing, which subsequently increases the release of dopamine and its metabolites in the NA. Intraventricular β-endorphin produces similar enhancements of neuronal firing. In contrast, κ-agonists produce the opposite effects on mesolimbic neurons and reduce dopaminergic neuronal activity and subsequent DA turnover (release and metabolism). Since microinjected κ-agonists produce conditioned place *aversions,* it seems possible that the mesolimbic dopamine system may mediate aversive effects of opiates as well as their reinforcing properties (Shippenberg et al., 1991).

A model of the opposing effects of opioid neurons on mesolimbic dopaminergic cells is shown in Figure 10.17. Beta-endorphin and opiate drugs seem to increase VTA cell firing by inhibiting the GABA-inhibitory cells found in the VTA. They can decrease the release of GABA by opening K$^+$ channels or reducing Ca^{2+} influx on GABA terminals. This inhibition of inhibitory neurons leads to increased firing and greater DA release in the NA. The endogenous peptide dynorphin, which acts on κ-receptors on the terminals of the DA neurons, can reduce the release of DA by similar mechanisms.

How sure are we that mesolimbic DA is really important? DA receptor antagonists block the reinforcing effects of opiates when evaluated by each of the three behavioral measures. However, inducing lesions of dopaminergic neurons with the neurotoxin 6-hydroxydopamine (6-OHDA) reduces (but does *not* abolish) the reinforcement value. The fact that heroin self-administration is only *partially* reduced rather than eliminated by the lesion certainly suggests that other brain areas and other neurotransmitters in addition to dopamine are also involved. Although these studies clearly support earlier results showing that increased mesolimbic

firing is a common link in the actions of many self-administered drugs, including ethanol, nicotine, and psychostimulants (see Chapter 8), opiates do not have to release mesolimbic dopamine to be reinforcing (Gerrits and Vanree, 1996).

Further, the mesolimbic pathway may be more specifically involved in the salience (or significance) of events to an individual. What we mean is that the dopaminergic cell firing may tell an organism when some event is important or meaningful, regardless of whether it is appetitive (positive) or aversive (negative). We would therefore have incentive (or motivation) to approach (in the case of a reinforcer) or avoid (in the case of a noxious event) a particular significant stimulus. This idea has been developed in the "incentive–sensitization" hypothesis of addiction (see the section on long-term opiate use later in the chapter).

The consequences of long-term opiate use include tolerance, sensitization, and dependence

You have just read about the acutely rewarding effects of opiates, which increase the likelihood that the drug will be used again. Chronic use subsequently leads to neuroadaptive changes in the nervous system, which are responsible for tolerance, sensitization, and dependence.

Tolerance (see Chapter 1) refers to the diminishing effects of a drug with repeated use, and it occurs for all of the opioids, including the endorphins. Although tolerance to the opiates develops quite rapidly, tolerance does not occur for all of the pharmacological effects to the same extent or at the same rate. For example, tolerance to the analgesic effect occurs relatively rapidly, but the constipating effects and the pinpoint pupils persist even after prolonged opiate use.

Cross-tolerance among the opiates also exists. For this reason, when tolerance develops to one opiate drug, other chemically related drugs also show a reduced effectiveness. For instance, following chronic heroin use, treatment with codeine will elicit a smaller-than-normal response even if the individual has never used codeine before. Since we now know that at least three types of opiate receptors exist, we might wonder whether the receptor subtype plays a role in

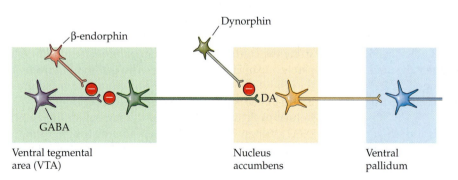

Figure 10.17 Model of the effects of opiates on mesolimbic dopaminergic cells The β-endorphin cell has an inhibitory effect on the normally inhibitory GABAergic cell, allowing the firing rate of the mesolimbic dopaminergic cells to increase and the cells to release more dopamine in the nucleus accumbens. In contrast, the dynorphin cell inhibits the release of dopamine from the mesolimbic cell by preventing calcium entry.

Dynorphin

β-endorphin

GABA

Ventral tegmental area (VTA)

DA

Nucleus accumbens

Ventral pallidum

cross-tolerance. Indeed, it seems that selective agonists for the μ-receptor reduce the effectiveness of other μ-receptor agonists, but only minimally reduce κ-agonists' activity. Likewise, repeated exposure to κ-agonists diminishes the effects of other κ-agonists but not μ-agonists.

As is true for many drugs, several mechanisms are responsible for the development of tolerance to the opioids. An increased rate of metabolism with repeated use (drug disposition tolerance) is responsible for some small portion of opioid tolerance. Classical conditioning processes also contribute to this phenomenon. However, most tolerance is based on changes in nerve cells that compensate for the presence of chronic opioids (pharmacodynamic tolerance). The cell mechanisms are discussed in more detail in the section on neurobiological adaptation and rebound.

Under some circumstances, repeated exposure to opiates produces **sensitization**. Sensitization refers to the increase in drug effects that occurs with repeated administration. Robinson and Berridge (2001) propose that in the case of substance abuse the motivation (incentive) to approach, better called craving or desire for the drug, undergoes sensitization. Meanwhile, the neural mechanism responsible for the high, or liking of the drug, remains unchanged or decreases as tolerance develops over repeated administration. Both the decrease in liking and increase in craving lead to further drug taking and may explain the intense compulsion to use a drug that no longer produces pleasurable effects.

The third consequence of chronic opioid use is the occurrence of **physical dependence** (see Chapter 8), which is a neuroadaptive state that occurs in response to the long-term occupation of opioid receptors. When the drug is no longer present, cell function not only returns to normal, but overshoots basal levels. The effects of drug withdrawal are a *rebound* in nature and are demonstrated by the occurrence of a pattern of physical disturbances called the **withdrawal** or **abstinence syndrome**. Since opiates in general depress CNS function, we consider opiate withdrawal to be a rebound hyperactivity (Table 10.2). You already know that opiate effects are due to drug action at various receptors in a variety of locations in the CNS and elsewhere in the body, so it should not be a surprise to learn that the abstinence signs reflect a loss of inhibitory opioid action at all of those same receptors as blood levels of the drug gradually decline. Withdrawal can also be produced by administering an opioid antagonist that competes with the drug molecules for the receptors and thus functionally mimics the termination of drug use. Note, however, that the withdrawal following antagonist administration is far more severe than that following drug cessation because the opiate receptors are more rapidly deprived of opiate.

Opiate withdrawal is not considered life-threatening, but the symptoms are extremely unpleasant and include pain and dysphoria, restlessness, and fearfulness, as well as several

TABLE 10.2 Acute Effects of Opioids and Rebound Withdrawal Symptoms

Acute action	Withdrawal sign
Analgesia	Pain and irritability
Respiratory depression	Panting and yawning
Euphoria	Dysphoria and depression
Relaxation and sleep	Restlessness and insomnia
Tranquilization	Fearfulness and hostility
Decreased blood pressure	Increased blood pressure
Constipation	Diarrhea
Pupil constriction	Pupil dilation
Hypothermia	Hyperthermia
Drying of secretions	Tearing, runny nose
Reduced sex drive	Spontaneous ejaculation
Flushed and warm skin	Chilliness and "gooseflesh"

symptoms that are flu-like in nature. How severe the symptoms are and how long they last depends on a number of factors: the particular drug used as well as the dose, frequency, and duration of drug use and the health and personality of the addict. To give an example, morphine withdrawal symptoms generally peak 36 to 48 hours after the last administration and disappear within 7 to 10 days. In contrast, methadone, which has a more gradual onset of action and is longer lasting, has a withdrawal syndrome that does not abruptly peak but increases to a gradual maximum after several days and decreases gradually over several weeks. Abstinence for the very long-acting opiate L-acetylmethadol (LAAM) is even more prolonged, but as is true for all of the longer-lasting opiates, the withdrawal signs are milder (Figure 10.18A and B). From this you should conclude that the longer the duration of action of the opiate, the more prolonged is the abstinence syndrome but the lower the intensity of the syndrome. At the point when abstinence signs end, the user is considered to be **detoxified**.

Readministering the opiate any time during withdrawal will dramatically eliminate all the symptoms. In addition, administering any other opiate drug will also stop or reduce the withdrawal symptoms because these agents show **cross dependence**. This characteristic plays an important part in drug abuse treatment and is discussed further later in the chapter.

It may be surprising to learn that although physical dependence commonly occurs following chronic opiate use, it does not necessarily lead to abuse or addiction. Patients treated with opiates for protracted pain (e.g., postsurgical or cancer-related pain) show both tolerance and physical dependence, although withdrawal signs can be minimized by gradually reducing the dose when pain relief is no longer needed. However, it is relatively rare to have a patient with

(A)

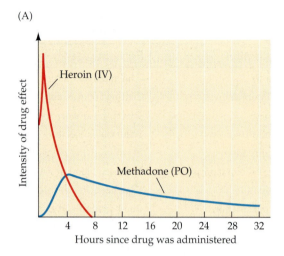

(B)

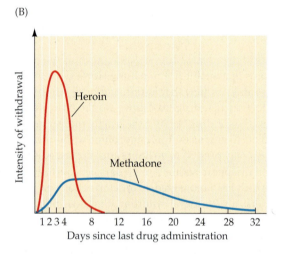

Figure 10.18 Relationship between acute effects and withdrawal (A) Time course showing the intensity and duration of the acute effects of intravenous heroin and oral methadone, and (B) the corresponding intensity and duration of withdrawal after chronic drug treatment.

chronic pain show addictive behaviors. Physicians' unfounded fears of such addiction have prevented many individuals from receiving the relief from severe pain that they require. Failure to use adequate painkilling treatment produces much more suffering and subsequently much slower healing than is warranted. Transdermal patches and patient-controlled drug delivery systems are drug administration techniques that provide more humane control of pain and more effective recovery.

Several brain areas contribute to the opioid abstinence syndrome

The signs of withdrawal represent the rebound hyperactivity in many different systems, including the gastrointestinal tract, the autonomic nervous system, and many sites within the brain and spinal cord. In order to identify which of the many brain areas are involved in the appearance of the particular signs of abstinence, an animal model is used. Pellets of opioid drugs are implanted under the skin so that the subcutaneous administration produces significant blood levels of drug over a week or more. After the animals have become physically dependent, selective intracerebral injection of an opiate antagonist produces distinctive and easily quantifiable signs of withdrawal. Withdrawal signs in rodents include jumping, rearing, "wet-dog" shakes, and increased locomotor behavior. Intracerebral injection of opiate antagonists into specific brain areas can help to identify which sites produce particular signs of abstinence. Based on these measures, no single brain area has been found to precipitate the entire withdrawal syndrome, but the locus coeruleus and the PAG are particularly sensitive to the antagonist in terms of precipitating withdrawal. As you will see in the next section, the locus coeruleus has become a neurochemical model for dependence.

In Chapter 8 you learned that the nucleus accumbens is a limbic structure that is particularly important for the reinforcement value of many abused substances. For this reason it is somewhat surprising that microinjection of opiate antagonists into this area is not very effective in eliciting bodily signs of withdrawal in a dependent animal. However, Koob and coworkers (1992) have suggested that the NA may be important in the aversive stimulus effects or motivational aspect of opiate withdrawal. This conclusion was based on a series of experiments in which opiate-dependent rats experienced naloxone-precipitated withdrawal in a novel environment. Under such conditions, the animals develop a place aversion for the novel location and remain in an adjacent compartment (see Figure 4.22). Koob and colleagues were interested in finding out which brain area, when microinjected with antagonist, is responsible for the place aversion. They found that the areas most sensitive to low doses of antagonist are the NA, followed by the amygdala and PAG. In conclusion, the brain areas implicated in the physiological response to opiate withdrawal are the PAG and locus coeruleus, which may also mediate withdrawal-induced anxiety, while the nucleus accumbens is likely responsible for the aversive qualities of withdrawal as well as some of the positive-reinforcing values of opiate use.

Neurobiological adaptation and rebound constitute tolerance and withdrawal

The classic hypothesis of opioid tolerance and dependence was first developed by Himmelsbach (1943) and is shown in Figure 10.19A. He suggested that acute administration of morphine disrupts the organism's homeostasis, but repeated

(A)

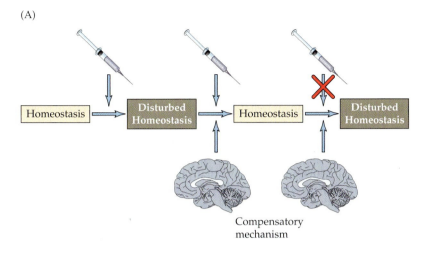

Compensatory
mechanism

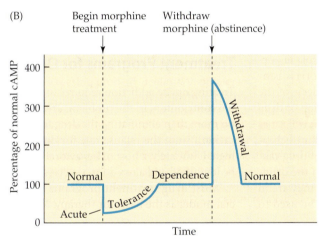

Figure 10.19 Model of tolerance and withdrawal (A) Himmelsbach's theoretical model suggests that the nervous system adapts to the disturbing presence of a drug, so tolerance develops; but if the drug is suddenly withdrawn, the adaptive mechanism continues to function, causing a rebound in physiological effects (withdrawal). (B) Morphine acutely inhibits the synthesis of cAMP, but the effect becomes less as tolerance develops and neural adaptation occurs. If morphine is suddenly withdrawn, a far larger than normal amount of cAMP is produced, suggesting that the adaptive mechanism is still operating. With time, the cells once again adapt, now to the absence of the drug.

administration of the drug initiates an adaptive mechanism that compensates for the original effects and returns to the normal homeostasis. At this point tolerance to the drug would have occurred, since the same dose of morphine no longer produces the original disturbance. When morphine administration is abruptly stopped, the drug's effects on the body are terminated but the adaptive mechanism remains active and overcompensates. The subsequent disruption of homeostasis is the withdrawal syndrome.

Although the Himmelsbach model was entirely theoretical, in the mid-1970s a physiological correlate was described

by Sharma and coworkers (1975). They used cells with opiate receptors and maintained them in cell culture. They found that the acute administration of morphine caused an inhibition of adenylyl cyclase, the enzyme that manufactures cAMP (Figure 10.19B). Himmelsbach would call this stage "disturbed homeostasis." However, when the cells were kept in the morphine solution for 2 days, they showed tolerance to the drug's inhibitory effect. That is, after 2 days they had levels of cAMP equal to control cells that had not been exposed to morphine. Apparently, the adaptive mechanism proposed by Himmelsbach became effective. When the opiate was abruptly removed from the cell culture solution or naloxone was added, the concentration of cAMP rose significantly above control levels. This rebound in cAMP levels corresponds with the withdrawal phenomenon and clearly represents disturbed homeostasis again. Other parts of the cAMP system such as cAMP-dependent protein kinase and phosphorylated neuronal proteins are also upregulated by the chronic use of opiates.

The relationship of cAMP to neural activity and the withdrawal syndrome is suggested by the parallel time course of changes in those three factors. Nestler and coworkers (1994) examined the electrophysiological effects of morphine on cells in the locus coeruleus. The acute effect of opioids acting at μ-receptors is hyperpolarization and reduced rate of firing. Repeated exposure to opiates produced a gradual increase in firing rates of locus coeruleus cells as tolerance developed. Administration of an opiate antagonist after chronic opiate treatment induced a significant rise in firing rate to levels well above pretreatment levels, reflecting a rebound withdrawal that gradually returned to normal. A similar time course occurred for the overshoot of cAMP synthesis and its return to control levels. Behavioral manifestations of abstinence also declined over the same 72-hour period.

Environmental cues have a role in tolerance, drug abuse, and relapse

We have already alluded to the idea that environmental factors can be classically conditioned to parts of the drug experience (see the section on behavioral tolerance in Chapter 1).

withdrawal for 24 to 36 hours. The time course of drug action means daily contact and interaction with clinical staff who can provide behavioral therapy, group and family counseling, and support in education or job training. In addition, medical care can be provided. Of particular significance is the prenatal care for pregnant addicts and treatment of diseases, such as HIV, hepatitis, and syphilis, that are common among addicted pregnant females. However, since methadone passes the placental barrier like other opiates, the infant at delivery will sometimes show withdrawal signs including tremors, twitching, seizures, vomiting, diarrhea, and poor feeding. These symptoms can be readily treated by low doses of opiates, which can then be tapered down until no drug is needed.

Fifth, methadone is considered medically safe even with long-term use and does not interfere with daily activities. Unfortunately, some side effects do not diminish with repeated use, so constipation, excessive sweating, reduced sex drive, and sexual dysfunction may persist during treatment for some individuals. It is noteworthy that long-term use of any opiate drug has few damaging effects on organ systems. The greatest dangers stem from poor living conditions including inadequate diet, lack of medical care, and homelessness; dangerous and unlawful behaviors required to secure the drugs; and potentially fatal side effects of using contaminated needles or impure sources of drug.

Two other opioids, the agonist **LAAM** (L-α-acetylmethadol [Orlamm]) and the agonist–antagonist **buprenorphine** (Buprenex), are used in the same manner as methadone and produce similar treatment results. Both of these drugs have a longer duration of action and so produce more even pharmacological effects and a milder withdrawal syndrome. The longer duration also means less frequent administration (one to three times a week), which significantly reduces the costs of the program and gives an extra measure of freedom to the addict who needs daily clinic visits for methadone. In addition, because buprenorphine does not produce more than a mild euphoria, the addict can get a supply of the drug rather than just a single dose. Fewer clinic visits also tends to improve the relationship with members of the surrounding community, who often object to high rates of addict visits to their neighborhood. It is to be hoped that greater use of this drug will reduce costs and make more treatment facilities available.

Use of narcotic antagonists   We have already described the utility of naloxone in reversing the effects of opiate toxicity. Antagonists also represent a component of some drug abuse treatment programs. After detoxification, antagonist treatment will block the effects of any self-administered opiate. Naltrexone (Trexan) is the most commonly used because it has a longer duration of action than naloxone and is effective when taken orally. It also has fewer side effects than

cyclazocine, which may produce irritability, delusions, hallucinations, and motor incoordination. Nalmefene (Revex) is a newer pure opiate antagonist and is similar to naltrexone but more potent and longer-lasting.

This method is effective for addicts who are highly motivated, have strong family support, and are involved in careers (e.g., addicted medical personnel). Reliable patients have taken naltrexone for 5 to 10 years without relapse to drug-taking behavior and with minimal adverse effects on appetite, sexual behavior, or endocrine function (O'Brien, 1993). Unfortunately, this method appeals to only about 10% of the addicted population because a great deal of motivation is needed to voluntarily substitute an antagonist for a drug with highly reinforcing properties. Since craving for the drug is not eliminated, most less-motivated addicts stop antagonist treatment and return to drug use. Only about 27% of addicts in these treatment programs complete a 12-week preliminary session (Osborn et al., 1986).

Counseling services   Most often, addicts benefit from a **multidimensional approach** that includes a combination of detoxification, pharmacological support, and group or individual counseling. Counseling frequently is used to help addicts identify the environmental cues that trigger relapse for the individual. Having identified his "triggers," the addict must then design a behavioral response to those cues to prevent relapse. Furthermore, job training, educational counseling, and family therapy may be useful. Box 10.3 describes one program that utilizes group support after detoxification has occurred. Based on a model program for alcohol abuse treatment, Narcotics Anonymous is another option for motivated drug abusers to achieve drug abstinence.

Section Summary

The ability of opiates (both endogenous and exogenous) to relieve pain depends on a complex and highly redundant set of neuronal pathways at both the spinal cord level and supraspinal sites. Small endorphin neurons in the spinal cord act on receptors to decrease the conduction of pain signals from the spinal cord to higher brain centers. Descending neurons originating in the periaqueductal gray give rise to two pathways that further impede pain signals in the spinal cord. The pathways begin in the locus coeruleus (noradrenergic) and the nucleus of the raphe (serotonergic). In addition, opiate receptors in the neocortex modulate the emotional component of pain to relieve the sense of suffering.

As is true for many other abused substances, opiate drugs increase dopamine release in the nucleus accumbens. This effect occurs because opiates inhibit the inhibitory GABA cells in the ventral tegmental area, hence increasing mesolimbic cell firing. However, since the DA release in the NA is not

BOX 10.3   # Clinical Applications

Narcotics Anonymous

For many addicts, social support is a significant factor in preventing relapse. Based on the model of Alcoholics Anonymous, the Twelve Steps of the program of Narcotics Anonymous are designed to aid the addict in remaining drug free after completing either inpatient or outpatient treatment for narcotics abuse. According to its website (www.na.org), the nonprofit fellowship was started in 1947 and presently runs weekly meetings in 70 countries around the world. Its meetings are open to any individual who wants to be drug free regardless of the drug and regardless of the addict's race, gender, religion, or social class. Membership is entirely voluntary, and there are no dues or fees.

NA views addiction as a disease that can be "arrested" but not "cured." If left untreated, addiction has physically damaging effects similar to those of disease. The official position of the group is that relapse is a sometimes necessary part of the overall recovery process. As such, relapse is not shameful but is seen as an opportunity to learn from the experience and move on.

NA has no therapists or clinics. There is no vocational, legal, medical, or psychiatric service rendered. In their regular meetings, members share personal experiences with others who are seeking help. The addicts share support for current problems as well as dealing with their difficult past.

Although the group has no religious affiliation, it emphasizes a "spiritual awakening" and has a distinctly spiritual orientation and a theistic bent to most of its literature. Emphasizing self-appraisal and making amends, the Twelve Steps for self-development are presented below.

The Twelve Steps

1. We admitted that we were powerless over our addiction—that our lives had become unmanageable.
2. We came to believe that a Power greater than ourselves could restore us to sanity.
3. We made a decision to turn our will and our lives over to the care of God as we understood Him.
4. We made a searching and fearless moral inventory of ourselves.
5. We admitted to God, to ourselves, and to another human being the exact nature of our wrongs.
6. We were entirely ready to have God remove all these defects of character.
7. We humbly asked Him to remove our shortcomings.
8. We made a list of all persons we had harmed and became willing to make amends to them all.
9. We made direct amends to such people wherever possible, except when to do so would injure them or others.
10. We continued to take personal inventory and when we were wrong, promptly admitted it.
11. We sought through prayer and meditation to improve our conscious contact with God as we understood Him, praying only for knowledge of His will for us and the power to carry that out.
12. Having had a spiritual awakening as a result of these steps, we tried to carry this message to addicts and to practice these principles in all our affairs.

necessary for the reinforcing effects, other nondopaminergic mechanisms must also play a part.

Opioid drugs demonstrate tolerance to many of the drug effects and cross tolerance with other drugs in the same class as well as with endogenous opioids. Prolonged use produces physical dependence, which is characterized by a classic rebound withdrawal syndrome that includes many flu-like symptoms, insomnia, depression, and irritability. Cross dependence means that any drug in the opioid family can abruptly stop withdrawal symptoms. The physiological mechanism for tolerance and dependence may depend on the compensatory response of cells in the locus coeruleus to the acute inhibition of adenylyl cyclase. The increased activity of adenylyl cyclase and the subsequent cellular effects are kept in check as long as the exogenous drug is administered.

However, if drug use is discontinued, the now noninhibited adenylyl cyclase precipitates withdrawal symptoms.

Classical conditioning of environmental cues associated with components of drug use is important in the development of tolerance and in maintaining the drug habit. Conditioned craving is significant in producing relapse in the detoxified addict.

Opiate abuse treatment programs include the substitution of one opiate, such as methadone, buprenorphine, or LAAM, for the abused drug. These substitutes, when given orally, produce no euphoria but eliminate craving for heroin and the need to engage in criminal activity to supply the drug habit. Elimination of disease-carrying injection equipment reduces exposure to HIV and hepatitis. The long-acting opioids stabilize the physiological effects and encourage contact with support staff who provide medical and psychological support as well as education and job training.

A second pharmacological treatment option is the use of antagonists. Opioid antagonists are effective in blocking the opiate receptors so that self-administered narcotics have no effect. Addicts who are highly motivated following detoxification may benefit from the reassurance that if they relapse, no reinforcing euphoria will occur. Group therapy and support groups like Narcotics Anonymous also provide alternate ways to treat addiction. The most successful approaches are typically multidimensional ones.

Recommended Readings

Musto, D. F. (1991). Opium, cocaine, and marijuana in American history. *Sci. Amer.,* 265, 40–47.

Petrovic, P., Kalso, E., Pettersson, K. M., and Ingvar, M. (2002). Placebo and opioid analgesia: Imaging a shared neuronal network. *Science,* 295, 1737–1740.

Yeomans, M. R., and Gray, R. W. (2002). Opioid peptides and the control of human ingestive behaviour. *Neurosci. Biobehav. Rev.,* 26, 713–728.

11 Psychomotor Stimulants: Cocaine and the Amphetamines

"The psychic effect ... consists of exhilaration and lasting euphoria, which does not differ in any way from the normal euphoria of a healthy person. ... One senses an increase of self-control and feels more vigorous and more capable of work. ... Long-lasting, intensive mental or physical work can be performed without fatigue; it is as though the need for food and sleep, which otherwise makes itself felt peremptorily at certain times of the day, were completely banished. ... Opinion is unanimous that the euphoria ... is not followed by any feeling of lassitude or other state of depression."

Any substance having the marvelous properties just described should be a boon to humankind. What is this miracle drug, then? The answer, unfortunately, is cocaine, and the nearly rapturous description quoted above comes from the writings of Sigmund Freud (*Über Coca;* reprinted in Byck, 1974, pp. 60–62).

Cocaine, amphetamine, and related compounds belong to a class of drugs called **psychomotor stimulants.** This term refers to the marked sensorimotor activation that occurs in response to drug administration. Indeed, psychomotor stimulants are characterized by their ability to increase alertness, heighten arousal, and cause behavioral excitement. This chapter considers the behavioral and physiological effects of these stimulants, their mechanisms of action, and their potential for producing abuse and dependence. Chapter 12 covers nicotine and caffeine, two less potent but more widely used stimulants.

ÜBER COCA.

Von

DR. SIGM. FREUD

Secundararzt im k. k. Allgemeinen Krankenhause in Wien.

Neu durchgesehener und vermehrter Separat-Abdruck aus dem „Centralblatt für die gesammte Therapie".

WIEN, 1885.
VERLAG VON MORITZ PERLES

The title page of *Über Coca,* Freud's tribute to the virtues of cocaine.

Cocaine

Background and History

Cocaine is an alkaloid found in the leaves of the shrub *Erythroxylon coca.* The coca shrub is native to South America and is particularly cultivated in the northern and central Andes Mountains extending from Colombia into Peru and Bolivia (Figure 11.1). The inhabitants of these regions consume cocaine by chewing the leaves, a practice thought to have begun at least 2000 and perhaps as many as 5000 years ago, according to archeological evidence. Because cocaine is a weak base, coca chewers also include some lime or ash to make the pH of the saliva more alkaline (Figure 11.2). This decreases ionization of the cocaine and promotes absorption across the mucous membranes of the oral cavity.

Coca chewing was an important feature of ceremonial or religious occasions in the Incan civilization, and use of the drug was ordinarily restricted to the ruling classes up to the time of the Spanish conquest. After the fall of the Incan empire, coca chewing became more widespread and com-

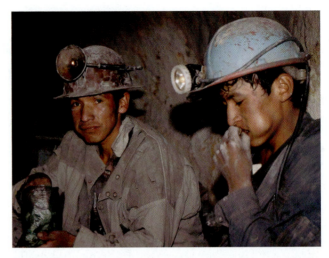

Figure 11.2 Coca chewing is still practiced by some Bolivian miners to help them work long hours in the mines. The miner on the right is chewing coca, while his partner consumes a snack.

monplace, and there are even reports that coca was used as a medium of exchange. Over time, many Spanish missionaries and churchmen argued that coca chewing was idolatrous and interfered with conversion of the natives to Catholicism. The practice was consequently discouraged and even banned in some areas. The Spaniards soon discovered, however, that without the stimulating and hunger-reducing effects of coca, Incan workers lacked the endurance necessary to work long hours in the mines and fields at high altitudes and with little food. Thus coca cultivation and chewing were restored with the blessing of the Spanish rulers and the church.

Although coca leaves were brought back to Europe, coca chewing never caught on, possibly due to degradation of the active ingredient during the long sea voyage. But travelers to the New World had occasion to sample the leaf, and several came back with glowing reports of its beneficial effects. By the late 1850s, German chemists had isolated pure cocaine and characterized it chemically. Over the next 30 years, cocaine became tremendously popular as many notable scientists and physicians lauded its properties. A chemist named Angelo Mariani concocted an infamous mixture of cocaine and wine (*Vin Mariani*), while the Italian neurologist Paolo Mantegazza wrote, "I would rather have a life span of ten years with coca than one of 1,000,000 centuries without coca" (Petersen, 1977). The most famous cocaine user of all, though, was Sigmund Freud. In 1885, Freud published the monograph *Über Coca* ("On Coca"), which extolled the drug's virtues and recommended its use in the treatment of alcoholism, morphine addiction, depression, digestive disorders, and a variety of other ailments. Freud also performed the first recorded psychopharmacological experiments on cocaine and published the results in a paper entitled "Con-

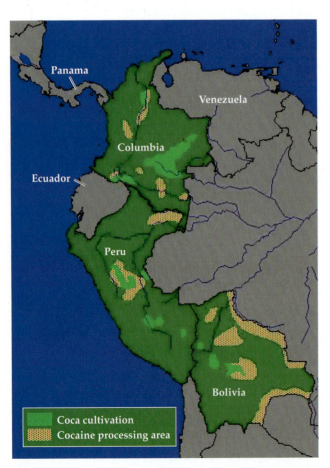

Figure 11.1 Map of principal coca-growing regions of South America (Courtesy of Rosemary Mosher and Michael Steinberg.)

tribution to the Knowledge of the Effect of Cocaine." In his last written comments about cocaine in 1887, Freud acknowledged its danger when used to treat morphine addiction, although he continued to maintain that the drug was nonaddictive under other circumstances.* Others, however, were more perceptive. The harshest critic was the German psychiatrist A. Erlenmeyer, who labeled cocaine the "third scourge of the human race," after alcohol and opium.

Despite the warning signs emanating from Europe, cocaine's popularity grew in the United States during the late nineteenth and early twentieth centuries. By 1885, Parke Davis & Co. pharmaceuticals was manufacturing 15 different forms of cocaine and coca, including cigarettes, cheroots (a type of cigar), and inhalants. One year later, a Georgia pharmacist named John Pemberton introduced a new beverage, "Coca Cola," that contained cocaine from coca leaves and caffeine from cola nuts. Coca Cola and similar concoctions were marketed as suitable alternatives to alcoholic drinks because of the growing strength of the alcohol temperance movement at that time (Figure 11.3).† Cocaine-containing tooth drops were even given to infants to relieve the discomfort of teething (the local anesthetic effects of cocaine are discussed further in the section on mechanisms of action). Not surprisingly, widespread cocaine abuse began to appear across the United States until President Taft declared cocaine to be "public enemy number one" in 1910. Congress then passed the 1914 Harrison Narcotic Act prohibiting the inclusion of cocaine (as well as opium) in patent medicines and specifying other restrictions on its import and sale (see Chapter 8). Subsequent state and federal laws, of course, placed even tighter regulations on cocaine distribution and use.

From the 1920s to the 1960s, cocaine use continued primarily among a relatively small group of avant-garde artists, musicians, and other performers. Beginning in the 1970s, however, we have seen two successive waves of increasing cocaine use in the United States. The first involved an escalation of cocaine use by snorting or intravenous (IV) injection, whereas the most recent epidemic of cocaine use has been driven by the smoking of "crack" cocaine.

According to estimates derived from the 2002 National Survey on Drug Use and Health, approximately 2 million people aged 12 or older (0.9% of the population) were current users of cocaine at that time. By "current user," we mean that the individual had used cocaine at least once during the previous month. A larger number of individuals (about 6

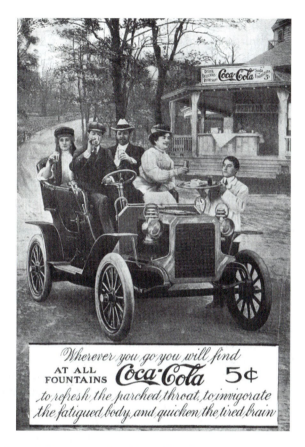

Figure 11.3 Coca-cola ad from 1906

million) had used cocaine during the previous year, whereas the number who had used the drug at least once during their lifetime was reported to be almost 34 million. This represents over 14% of the total U.S. population.

Basic Pharmacology of Cocaine

Figure 11.4 presents the chemical structure of alkaloidal cocaine, which is its naturally occurring form. The molecule contains two rings, the six-carbon phenyl ring shown on the right and the unusual nitrogen (N)-containing ring shown on the left. Both are necessary for the drug's biological activity. Other features of the molecule have been manipulated with interesting results. For example, Figure 11.4 also depicts the structures of two synthetic cocainelike drugs, WIN 35,428 (also known as CFT) and RTI-55 (also called β-CIT). Notice that both compounds lack the ester (—O—CO—) linkage between the rings, and they both possess a halogen (fluorine [F] or iodine [I]) atom on the phenyl ring. WIN 35,428 and RTI-55 are more potent than cocaine, and they presumably would be highly addictive if available on the

---

*In fairness to Freud, it should be noted that he normally took cocaine orally, a route of administration with less abuse potential than intravenous injection, smoking, or even snorting.

†Although caffeine still persists in regular Coca Cola, the cocaine was eliminated in 1906.

neurotransmitter levels in the synaptic cleft and a corresponding increase in transmission at the affected synapses.

Cocaine does not affect all monoamine transporters equally. Based on in vitro studies using rat brain tissue, cocaine binds most strongly (with highest affinity) to the 5-HT transporter, followed by the DA transporter and then the NE transporter (Ritz et al., 1990). On the other hand, later in this chapter we will see that blockade of DA reuptake appears to be most important for cocaine's stimulating, reinforcing, and addictive properties. Indeed, many drugs used in the treatment of depression block the 5-HT and/or the NE transporter (see Chapter 16). Yet these agents do not have the strong arousing effect produced by cocaine in nondepressed individuals, nor do they have any abuse potential. Nevertheless, 5-HT and NE must also be taken into account, as alterations in the DA system do not explain all of cocaine's effects.

At relatively high concentrations, cocaine additionally inhibits voltage-gated sodium (Na^+) channels in nerve cell axons. As these channels are necessary for neurons to generate action potentials, this action of cocaine causes a block of nerve conduction. Thus, when cocaine is applied locally to a tissue, it acts as a local anesthetic by preventing transmission of nerve signals along sensory nerves. Indeed, two synthetic local anesthetics that are widely used in medical and dental practice, procaine (Novocain) and lidocaine (Xylocaine), were developed from the structure of cocaine.

Section Summary

Cocaine is an alkaloid derived from the leaves of the shrub *Erythroxylon coca,* which is indigenous to the northern and central Andes Mountains of South America. Although the peoples of that region have been chewing coca leaves for perhaps 5000 years, cocaine use did not become popular in Western cultures until after the pure compound was isolated in the late 1850s. Freud was one of many notable cocaine users in nineteenth-century Europe. In the United States, cocaine was a constituent of numerous popular beverages and over-the-counter pharmaceutical products in the late nineteenth and early twentieth centuries until its nonprescription use was banned by the Harrison Narcotic Act of 1914. Cocaine then went "underground" until the 1970s, at which time the first of two waves of increased cocaine use began in this country. Household survey data indicate that more than 14% of residents of the United States have used cocaine at least once during their lifetime, whereas a much smaller but still significant percentage are current users.

Cocaine HCl is water soluble and therefore can be taken orally, intranasally, or by IV injection. On the other hand, cocaine base (including crack cocaine) is the chemical form most suitable for smoking. The most rapid absorption and distribution of cocaine occur following IV injection and smoking, which may account for the highly addictive properties of these routes of consumption. One of the main cocaine metabolites is benzoylecgonine, whereas a compound called cocaethylene is also formed when alcohol is ingested along with cocaine.

At typical doses, cocaine acts mainly to block synaptic uptake of DA, 5-HT, and NE by binding to their respective membrane transporters. This enhances transmission at monoaminergic synapses by increasing the synaptic concentrations of each transmitter. At higher concentrations, cocaine also blocks voltage-gated Na^+ channels, which leads to a local anesthetic effect.

Acute Behavioral and Physiological Effects of Cocaine

Cocaine stimulates mood and behavior

Cocaine is used and abused for the "high" and the "rush" produced by the drug. Typical aspects of the cocaine "high" are feelings of exhilaration and euphoria, a sense of well-being, enhanced alertness, heightened energy and diminished fatigue, and great self-confidence. Taken by IV injection or by smoking, cocaine also produces a brief "rush," described by some users as involving a sense of great pleasure and power and by others as being like an intense orgasm. At low and moderate doses, cocaine often increases sociability and talkativeness. There are also reports of heightened sexual interest and performance under cocaine's influence, although the drug's legendary ability to enhance sexual prowess is highly exaggerated. Cocaine can apparently also increase aggressive behavior, which suggests that some of the street violence associated with cocaine might be attributable to a direct effect of the drug.

The major subjective and behavioral effects of cocaine and other psychostimulants are summarized in Table 11.1. Effects listed in the "mild to moderate" category are generally produced by single, low to moderate doses of cocaine in either naive subjects or in users who have not yet progressed to heavy, chronic patterns of drug intake. "Severe" effects are most likely to be seen with high-dose use, particularly in individuals with long-standing patterns of chronic intake. It is easy to see that many of the positive characteristics of cocaine that may contribute to its powerful reinforcing properties become negative or aversive with escalation of dose and duration. Some of these aversive effects (e.g., irritability) are present in most high-dose users, whereas others mainly occur in cases of cocaine-induced psychosis (e.g., incoherence or delusions; see the discussion on health consequences later in the chapter).

Cocaine and other psychomotor stimulants also cause profound behavioral activation in rats, mice, and other animals used in psychopharmacological studies. At low doses, such acti-

TABLE 11.1 Mild to Moderate versus Severe Behavioral and Subjective Effects of Cocaine and Other Psychostimulants in Humans[a]

Mild to moderate effects	Severe effects
Mood amplification; both euphoria and dysphoria	Irritability, hostility, anxiety, fear, withdrawal
Heightened energy	Extreme energy or exhaustion
Sleep disturbance, insomnia	Total insomnia
Motor excitement, restlessness	Compulsive motor stereotypies
Talkativeness, pressure of speech	Rambling, incoherent speech
Hyperactive ideation	Disjointed flight of ideas
Increased sexual interest	Decreased sexual interest
Anger, verbal aggression	Possible extreme violence
Mild to moderate anorexia	Total anorexia
Inflated self-esteem	Delusions of grandiosity

Source: After Post and Contel, 1983.

[a]The actual effects observed show individual variability and depend on the dose, route of administration, pattern and duration of use, and environmental context.

vation takes the form of increased locomotion, rearing, and mild sniffing behavior. As the dose is increased, these behaviors are replaced by **focused stereotypies** (repetitive, seemingly aimless behaviors performed in a relatively invariant manner) confined to a small area of the cage floor. Psychostimulant stereotypies vary according to species and other factors. In rats and mice, one observes intense sniffing, continuous head and limb movements, and licking and biting. Humans using large amounts of cocaine occasionally also exhibit motor stereotypies such as repetitive picking and scratching.

All species tested thus far readily learn to self-administer cocaine intravenously. Marilyn Carroll and her colleagues (1990) were also able to train monkeys to smoke cocaine freebase. Furthermore, as discussed in Chapter 8, unlimited access to cocaine leads to heavy self-administration, gradual debilitation of the animals, and a high rate of mortality. These findings underscore the drug's powerful reinforcing properties in animals and its high abuse potential in humans. On the other hand, it is important to recognize that such compulsivity is not observed under all circumstances. When cocaine is pitted against an alternative reinforcer under controlled laboratory conditions, preference for the drug in both monkeys and humans depends on the relative magnitude of each reinforcer.

Animals can also learn to discriminate cocaine from vehicle treatment. Subjects initially trained on cocaine readily generalize to amphetamine, indicating a fundamental similarity in the cue properties of these two drugs. In contrast, there is much less generalization to caffeine, which is a weaker stimulant and which exerts its behavioral effects by a different mechanism than cocaine or amphetamine (see Chapter 12).

Cocaine's physiological effects are mediated by the sympathetic nervous system

Cocaine is considered a **sympathomimetic** drug, which means that it produces symptoms of sympathetic nervous system activation. The physiological consequences of acute cocaine administration include increased heart rate, vasoconstriction (narrowing of blood vessels) and hypertension (increased blood pressure), and hyperthermia (elevated body temperature). At low doses, these physiological changes are usually not harmful to the individual. High doses of cocaine, however, can be toxic or even fatal. Some of the potential adverse consequences of heavy cocaine use are seizures, heart failure, stroke, or intracranial hemorrhage (Figure 11.8).

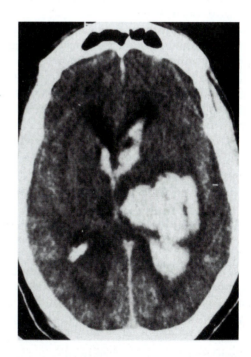

Figure 11.8 Computerized tomographic (CT) scan of a thalamic hemorrhage in a crack cocaine smoker The patient was a 45-year-old man who had smoked an unknown amount of crack and was found unconscious several hours later. The hemorrhage can be seen as the large, irregularly shaped white area on the middle-to-lower right side of the scan. (From Jacobs et al., 1989.)

Dopamine plays a key role in the subjective and behavioral effects of cocaine and other psychostimulants

There is overwhelming evidence that DA plays a central role in the behavioral responses of animals to cocaine, amphetamine, and related psychostimulant drugs (Gold et al., 1989). Of special importance are the dopaminergic projections from the midbrain (substantia nigra and ventral tegmental area) to the striatum and nucleus accumbens that were first described in Chapter 5. Table 11.2 summarizes the results of numerous microinjection and lesion studies concerning the involvement of these DA systems in the behavioral effects of psychostimulants. For example, psychostimulants elicit a locomotor response when microinjected directly into the nucleus accumbens. Injection into the striatum instead leads to a pattern of stereotyped behavior. Another approach has been to lesion DA nerve terminals in either the accumbens or striatum using the catecholamine neurotoxin 6-hydroxydopamine (6-OHDA). Such lesions cause a profound reduction of both DA and its transporter in the affected area, thereby preventing activation of dopaminergic transmission by psychostimulants. 6-OHDA lesions of the nucleus accumbens blunt psychostimulant-induced locomotion, whereas similar lesions of the striatum antagonize the stereotypies associated with higher drug doses.

The mesolimbic DA pathway to the nucleus accumbens also plays a key role in the reinforcing effects of cocaine and amphetamine in animals. Thus 6-OHDA lesions of the accumbens reduce the reinforcing properties of systemically administered cocaine or amphetamine. Moreover, rats will self-administer amphetamine directly into the nucleus accumbens (Hoebel et al., 1983). Surprisingly, however, attempts to demonstrate cocaine self-administration into this area were not successful (Goeders and Smith, 1983). One neurochemical difference between cocaine and amphetamine is that cocaine only blocks DA uptake, whereas amphetamine not only blocks uptake but also stimulates DA release (refer to the section on amphetamines). In addition, cocaine but not amphetamine has local anesthetic effects. However, we don't know whether these differences explain the lack of cocaine self-administration into the nucleus accumbens.

More recently, the neurochemical mechanisms of cocaine action have been studied using genetic knockout mice. We saw in Chapter 5 that mutant mice lacking the DA transporter (DAT) fail to show hyperactivity following psychostimulant treatment. Most investigators expected that the rewarding effects of psychostimulants would similarly be lost in the absence of DAT. Therefore, it was surprising to psychopharmacologists when two separate research groups, one using drug self-administration and the other using conditioned place preference, reported that cocaine reward* was still present in DAT knockout mice (Rocha et al., 1998; Sora et al., 1998) (Figure 11.9). It is critical to recognize that while these findings raise important questions, they do not invalidate all of the previous pharmacological results (for example, with receptor antagonists or 6-OHDA lesions) that have pointed to a key role for DA in psychostimulant reward and reinforcement. It is possible that the rewarding and reinforcing effects of cocaine depend not only on inhibition of DA uptake by DAT but also an interaction of the drug with one or more additional molecular targets. Alternatively, adaptations may occur in the DAT knockout mice that provide an alternate route for cocaine reward that is not present in normal animals. Like most mouse genetic engineering studies that have been performed up to now, the DAT knockout experiments involved changes in gene expression beginning in early embryonic development and continuing throughout the life of the animal. We now know that over the course of

---

*In the discussion that follows, we will sometimes use the term *reward* instead of or in addition to *reinforcement* because unlike the self-administration paradigm, the place conditioning procedure does not directly test drug reinforcement (see Chapter 4).

TABLE 11.2 Dopaminergic Projections to the Striatum and Nucleus Accumbens: Role in Psychostimulant-Induced Behaviors in Animals

Experimental manipulation	Brain area	Behavioral effect
Psychostimulant microinjection	Nucleus accumbens	Increased locomotor behavior
Psychostimulant microinjection	Striatum	Increased stereotyped behaviors
6-OHDA lesion	Nucleus accumbens	Decreased locomotor response following systemic administration of a low-dose psychostimulant
6-OHDA lesion	Striatum	Decreased stereotyped behaviors following systemic administration of a high-dose psychostimulant
6-OHDA lesion	Nucleus accumbens	Decreased reinforcing effectiveness of systemically administered psychostimulants
Amphetamine microinjection	Nucleus accumbens	Reinforcing to the animal
Cocaine microinjection	Nucleus accumbens	Not reinforcing to the animal

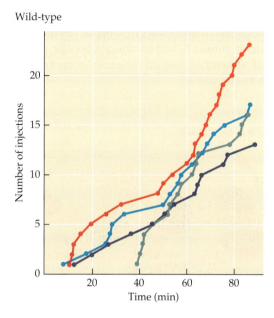

Wild-type

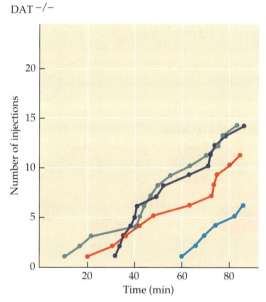

DAT −/−

Figure 11.9 Cocaine self-administration in individual wild-type and DAT knockout (DAT−/−) mice Mice received cocaine (0.5 mg/kg per infusion) on a fixed-ratio 2 (FR-2) reinforcement schedule. The graphs illustrate the cumulative number of drug injections over a 90-minute test session for four mice in each group, with each data point depicting an injection. Cocaine was clearly self-administered by the DAT−/− mice, although these animals generally did not obtain as many doses as the wild-type animals over the test period. (After Rocha et al., 1998.)

time, various biochemical adaptations occur in the brain following the loss of an important gene such as the one coding for DAT. Consequently, such adaptations must be taken into consideration when interpreting the results of any standard gene knockout study.

Following the initial studies with DAT knockout mice, cocaine place conditioning was examined in mice either with a single knockout of the 5-HT or NE transporter or with double knockouts of two different transporter genes in the same animals (Uhl et al., 2002; Rocha, 2003). Particularly interesting are the results involving the 5-HT transporter (abbreviated SERT, for *serotonin transporter*). As in the case of DAT, inactivation of SERT did not eliminate cocaine's ability to produce a conditioned place preference (Sora et al., 1998, 2001). In fact, SERT knockout mice show even stronger cocaine place conditioning than wild-type controls. However, no place conditioning could be obtained in mice with a double deletion of DAT and SERT (Sora et al., 2001). In addition, fluoxetine, which selectively blocks SERT, was found to be rewarding in DAT knockout but not wild-type mice. These and other studies led Uhl and colleagues (2002) to suggest that the enhancement of serotonergic transmission caused by SERT blockade produces a combination of rewarding and aversive effects that are presumably mediated by various 5-HT receptors in different neural circuits. If we assume that these opposing effects tend to counterbalance each other in genetically intact organisms, then it follows that DAT blockade is still the critical factor in cocaine reward under normal circumstances. Such an assumption is also consistent with the observations that fluoxetine is not rewarding in wild-type mice and is not usually abused by humans (fluoxetine and other selective 5-HT reuptake inhibitors are widely prescribed as antidepressant medications; see Chapter 16). Uhl and his colleagues further proposed that in mice lacking DAT, the balance of serotonergic effects (i.e., reward vs. aversion) shifts to favor reward. Because of this shift, blockade of SERT by either cocaine or fluoxetine has a net rewarding effect in DAT knockout mice, but this effect is absent in double knockouts lacking both transporters.

Mateo and her coworkers (2004) recently discovered an unexpected adaptation in DAT knockout mice that seems to be consistent with the hypothesis of Uhl et al. In DAT knockout but not wild-type mice, SERT blockade by cocaine, fluoxetine, or citalopram (another 5-HT reuptake inhibitor) was found to act in the ventral tegmental area to stimulate nucleus accumbens DA release. The increased release added more DA to the already high extracellular levels that were present due to the lack of a functional DA uptake system. Further studies are needed to determine whether this adaptation underlies the rewarding effects of cocaine or fluoxetine in DAT knockout mice.

Brain imaging allows researchers to explore the neural mechanisms of psychostimulant action in human subjects

Given the critical role of DA in the rewarding and reinforcing effects of psychostimulants, are the mood-altering properties

stereotyped behaviors. Cocaine can function as a discriminative stimulus, and it exhibits powerful reinforcing effects in standard self-administration paradigms. Physiologically, cocaine produces sympathomimetic effects such as increased heart rate, vasoconstriction, hypertension, and hyperthermia. High doses can be toxic or even fatal due to seizures, heart failure, stroke, or intracranial hemorrhage.

Most of the subjective and behavioral effects of cocaine have been attributed to DAT inhibition and the resulting activation of dopaminergic transmission, particularly in the nucleus accumbens and striatum. On the other hand, studies of DAT knockout mice as well as combined DAT and SERT knockouts suggest that 5-HT may also play a role in cocaine reward and reinforcement. D_1, D_3, and to a lesser extent D_2 receptors appear to mediate the dopaminergic component of cocaine's behavioral effects.

Cocaine Abuse and the Effects of Chronic Cocaine Exposure

Experimental cocaine use may escalate over time to a pattern of cocaine abuse and dependence

Cocaine users give many different reasons for their initial decision to use the drug. Some of these reasons are to satisfy their curiosity; to facilitate social interactions; to relieve feelings of depression, anxiety, or guilt; to have fun and celebrate; or simply to get "high." Cocaine users typically describe early experimentation with both legal (e.g., alcohol) and illegal drugs, often beginning by 13 or 14 years of age. Early use of other substances may therefore be an important risk factor for the initiation of cocaine use.

People usually begin taking cocaine via the intranasal route, that is, by snorting it. Most individuals who try cocaine do not progress to a pattern of abuse. Some report a strong anxiety response as their initial reaction to cocaine and are thereby dissuaded from further experimentation. Other factors may likewise mitigate against the development of a long-term abuse pattern, including unavailability of the drug, the cost of maintaining a steady supply, the social and legal consequences of illicit drug use, and the very real fear of losing control over one's drug-taking behavior. These factors often lead to a termination of cocaine use, though there are some intranasal users who maintain long-term periodic and controlled cocaine consumption.

Surveys performed by the National Institute on Drug Abuse suggest that approximately 10 to 15% of initial intranasal users eventually become cocaine abusers. The details of this transition process certainly vary for different individuals, yet a few factors have been identified that may generally be important. The stimulating, euphoric, and con-fidence-enhancing effects described earlier provide a powerful reinforcing effect during the early stages of cocaine use. Furthermore, these aspects of cocaine reinforcement may be augmented by social responses from friends and acquaintances who respond positively to the user's newfound energy and enthusiasm. Over time, cocaine use escalates as the individual discovers that higher doses produce a more powerful euphoric effect. Even more importantly, the user may switch from intranasal administration to crack smoking, freebasing, or IV injection. For many, this is a significant event in their drug history because of the greater abuse potential of these latter routes of administration. Moreover, some individuals develop a pattern of **cocaine binges,** which are episodic bouts of repeated use lasting from hours to days with little or no sleep. During these periods, nothing is important to the user except maintaining the "high," and all available supplies of cocaine are consumed in this pursuit. A 3-day freebasing binge may involve the consumption of as much as 150 g of cocaine, which is an enormous amount. Many individuals who abuse cocaine also suffer from other psychiatric disorders, such as depression, anxiety disorders, or personality disorders. A comorbid psychiatric disorder may precede the individual's cocaine use and predispose him to begin taking the drug (see the self-medication hypothesis in Chapter 8), or the disorder may be induced as a consequence of the chronic cocaine exposure.

Chronic psychostimulant exposure can give rise to tolerance or sensitization

As with many drugs, chronic exposure to psychostimulants can lead to reduced responsiveness, or tolerance. Yet the reverse effect, namely sensitization, is also often seen with psychostimulants. One of the amazing aspects of sensitization is that just a few exposures to cocaine or amphetamine can produce an increased responsiveness that lasts for weeks, months, or even longer.

How can psychostimulants produce both tolerance and sensitization? Various studies have shown that which kind of change you observe depends on the pattern of drug exposure, the response that's being measured, and the time interval that has elapsed since the last dose. For example, continuous cocaine infusion into rats causes tolerance to the drug's locomotor-stimulating effect (Figure 11.12A), whereas once-daily cocaine injections lead to behavioral sensitization, as shown by enhanced stereotyped behaviors (Figure 11.12B). Sensitization can actually increase in strength after the last drug dose (that is, during the period of withdrawal) due to ongoing neurochemical changes in the brain.

Under some conditions, researchers have observed a short-lasting acute tolerance to psychostimulants along with a longer-term sensitization. This combination of effects was found in an experiment in which extracellular DA levels in

(A)

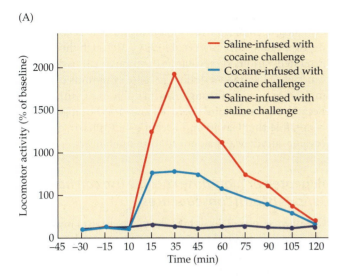

(B)

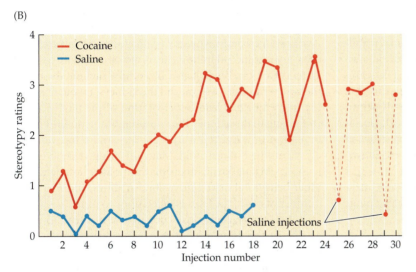

Figure 11.12 Chronic cocaine administration can produce tolerance or sensitization, depending on the pattern of administration. (A) Rats were given a continuous intravenous infusion of either saline or 60 mg/kg cocaine per day for 11 or 12 days. One day after the end of the infusion, the animals were given a saline injection or challenged with cocaine (20 mg/kg intraperitoneally), and they were then tested for locomotor activity. The previously cocaine-exposed animals showed tolerance, as indicated by a decreased locomotor response to the challenge dose. (B) Rats given once-daily cocaine injections (10 mg/kg intraperitoneally) showed a progressive increase in stereotyped behavior (sensitization) compared with saline-treated controls. The behavior patterns observed in these animals consisted of repetitive corner-to-corner locomotion, vertical rearing and nose poking, and head bobbing. Saline test injections on days 25 and 29 showed that the high levels of stereotypy seen on the other days were due to the cocaine injections on those days and were not a residual effect of the prior treatments. (A after Inada et al., 1992; B after Post and Contel, 1983.)

the striatum were measured in monkeys repeatedly self-administering cocaine over a period of 6 months (Bradberry, 2000). When animals gave themselves two doses of cocaine within a single session, the DA response to the second dose was usually lower than the response to the first dose (acute tolerance). However, when the response to the first dose within each session was examined over the entire 6-month period, there was a gradual escalation in cocaine's effectiveness in elevating extracellular DA levels (long-term sensitization). These findings are important because they may help explain both the development of psychostimulant dependence and the drug-taking patterns of dependent individuals. Some researchers believe that a sensitization-like mechanism underlies the increased drug craving experienced by cocaine or amphetamine users who are in the process of developing a dependence on these substances. Moreover, users report that during a cocaine or amphetamine binge, they need more

drug later in the binge to obtain the same "high" as they felt at the beginning. Such reports suggest the development of a short-term tolerance that may wear off if sufficient time elapses between successive binges.

Sensitization can be divided into two phases: **induction,** which means the process by which sensitization is established, and **expression,** which refers to the process by which the sensitized response is manifested. Somewhat different neurochemical mechanisms underlie these two phases (Vanderschuren and Kalivas, 2000). Activation of glutamate NMDA receptors and (in the case of amphetamine) dopamine D_1 receptors is necessary for the induction of sensitization. Expression of sensitization is dependent at least partly on enhanced reactivity of dopaminergic nerve terminals in the nucleus accumbens. That is, a given psychostimulant dose causes a greater increase in accumbens extracellular DA levels in sensitized compared to nonsensitized animals.

Binge cocaine use has been linked to a specific abstinence syndrome

Until the early 1980s, cocaine was not believed to produce a syndrome of dependence and withdrawal, and hence the drug was not considered addictive by classical criteria. For example, cocaine dependence was not listed as a substance abuse disorder in the 1980 version of the *Diagnostic and Statistical Manual of Mental Disorders (DSM-III)*. This situation began to change, however, when Frank Gawin and Herbert Kleber (then at Yale University School of Medicine) described a pattern of withdrawal symptoms (abstinence syndrome) hypothesized to occur following a cocaine binge (Gawin and Kleber, 1986, 1988). Based on a combination of clinical observations and patient interviews, the investigators concluded that the cocaine abstinence syndrome occurred in three phases that they called crash, withdrawal, and extinction. During the crash, the user feels exhausted and suffers from a depressed mood. Later, during the withdrawal phase, some of the important symptoms include anhedonia (inability to experience normal pleasures), anergia (a lack of energy), anxiety, and a growing craving for cocaine that increases the risk of relapse. Symptoms subside during the extinction phase, although relapse to cocaine use may still occur. Around the same time as Gawin and Kleber's report, Dackis and Gold (1985) proposed that the negative mood state and craving associated with cocaine withdrawal stem from temporarily decreased synaptic levels of DA (Figure 11.13). This hypothesis needs to be tested using appropriate brain imaging techniques during the various phases of a cocaine binge and withdrawal.

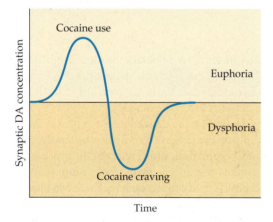

Figure 11.13 Hypothetical relationship between cocaine use, synaptic DA levels, and mood Cocaine use acutely elevates DA concentrations, which is thought to play a critical role in the euphoric effects of the drug. After use has ended, synaptic DA concentrations may decrease below normal levels, thus leading to cocaine craving and a dysphoric mood. (After Dackis and Gold, 1985.)

Other investigators have studied the pattern of withdrawal in long-term cocaine users following hospitalization (Weddington et al., 1990; Satel et al., 1991). Although the subjects exhibited various symptoms at the time of admission, they experienced a gradual decline in these symptoms over time instead of passing through distinct phases of withdrawal. Because these individuals were not known to be binge users, it is possible that Gawin and Kleber's multiphasic model of cocaine withdrawal does not apply to nonbingers.

Repeated or high-dose cocaine use can have serious health consequences

Cocaine use, especially at high doses, can have many adverse physiological and behavioral consequences. With respect to the brain, for example, a single dose of cocaine may trigger a stroke or seizure. Effects of chronic use on the brain are discussed in Box 11.1. Complications associated with the heart range from chest pains to cardiac arrhythmias (irregular heart rate), cardiac myopathy (damaged heart muscle), and even myocardial infarction (heart attack). Other organs or systems that can be damaged by cocaine include the lungs, the gastrointestinal system, and the kidneys. Frequent snorting of cocaine can lead to perforation of the nasal septum (the tissue that separates the two sides of the nose). Finally, ingestion of cocaine by a pregnant woman has variable effects on the unborn child. Many offspring seem to escape without obvious harm; others may show attention deficits or other behavioral or cognitive abnormalities; and in a small number of cases, the fetus is killed prior to birth.

Behaviorally, high-dose cocaine use can lead to panic attacks or the development of a temporary paranoid psychosis with delusions and hallucinations. One particularly frightening type of hallucination is called "cocaine bugs," which refers to the sensation of tiny creatures crawling over the user's skin. More than 100 years ago, some of Freud's colleagues were already seeing patients with these kinds of psychotic reactions. Cocaine psychosis occurs more frequently with repeated use, which is consistent with a growing sensitization to the drug.

Pharmacological, behavioral, and psychosocial methods are used to treat cocaine abuse and dependence

Pharmacotherapies High rates of cocaine abuse in our society have spurred a great deal of interest in developing effective therapies for cocaine users. At present, the most widely used agent is probably desipramine, which is a tricyclic antidepressant that mainly inhibits NE uptake. This compound seems to be most helpful as an adjunct therapy in treating patients diagnosed with cocaine abuse (rather than the more severe cocaine dependence) who additionally suffer from depression. Interestingly, the 5-HT reuptake inhibitor fluoxetine (trade name Prozac) seems to be less effective than desipramine in cocaine users.

The National Institute on Drug Abuse is currently directing an active program to identify and test pharmacological agents that might reduce cocaine's euphoric effects and/or the craving that ensues during cocaine withdrawal. Because of the well-known role of DA in cocaine reinforcement in animal models and its presumed involvement in human cocaine addiction, much attention has been directed to various dopaminergic drugs, including receptor agonists, antagonists, and uptake inhibitors, that might compete with cocaine for access to the DA transporter (Platt et al., 2002).

At this time, the most promising compounds appear to be DA receptor partial agonists, particularly those that bind to D_1 or D_3 receptors. Partial agonists would compete with DA for access to the receptors, thereby possibly blunting the euphoric effects of cocaine-induced dopaminergic stimulation. They would have much less abuse potential than cocaine, however, because of their lower efficacy at the receptors. BP 897, the D_3 receptor partial agonist previously mentioned for its ability to reduce cocaine-seeking behavior in rats, is currently in phase 2 clinical trials. We hope that BP 897 or other D_3 selective agents will prove to be more efficacious against cocaine abuse than compounds currently in use.

BOX 11.1 — Pharmacology in Action

Your Brain on Cocaine

In 1987, the Partnership for a Drug-Free America unveiled a national ad campaign depicting an egg frying in a skillet and stating ominously that "This is your brain on drugs." Well, obviously drugs don't literally fry your brain, but can they cause serious damage? Later in this chapter we will see that certain amphetamine analogs do cause damage to specific neurotransmitter systems in experimental animals and probably also in high-dose human users. The situation is less clear for cocaine. Nevertheless, there is substantial evidence that chronic cocaine exposure can lead to biochemical, physiological, and structural abnormalities in the brain, as well as neurological deficits.

Several research groups have looked for changes in the DA system in chronic cocaine users. This has been accomplished by means of both brain imaging methods in living subjects and postmortem brain studies, including some instances in which the subjects died from drug overdose. A number of changes in dopaminergic functioning have been reported, although the results are not entirely

consistent. Such discrepancies are probably due to differences in subject populations and experimental methodology.

In one important study, Volkow and her colleagues used PET imaging with [^{18}F]N-methylspiroperidol to determine D_2 receptor availability in cocaine-dependent freebase or crack users (Volkow et al., 1993). Receptor availability in the cocaine group was significantly decreased compared to normal controls, and this difference persisted even in subjects who were retested following 3 months of cocaine abstinence. This finding could reflect either reduced D_2 receptor density or increased levels of DA competing with the radiolabeled drug for access to the receptors. Volkow and coworkers (1997) subsequently examined the DA response to methylphenidate, a drug that increases synaptic DA levels by blocking reuptake. Two PET scans were performed, the first under baseline conditions and the second after methylphenidate administration. The drug was given by IV injection, which is noteworthy because unlike standard oral dosing, this route of methylphenidate administration produces a subjective high. D_2 receptors were again imaged, but this time with [^{11}C]raclopride, a drug that is particu-

larly known to be sensitive to changes in synaptic levels of DA. Consequently, the reduction in radiolabeled raclopride binding in the second scan compared to the first was taken as a measure of the methylphenidate-induced increase in DA. Compared with controls, the cocaine-dependent subjects showed a lower response to methylphenidate in the striatum, and they also reported a less intense drug high. In contrast, a greater methylphenidate response occurred in the thalamus, which was statistically correlated with self-reported cocaine craving. These results indicate that chronic cocaine use is associated with alterations in DA availability that vary with brain region.

Other kinds of imaging techniques have enabled researchers to look for possible abnormalities in regional cerebral blood flow, utilization of glucose (the brain's primary metabolic fuel), brain volume, and gray-matter density in chronic cocaine users. Although such measures do not tell us about neurotransmitter systems, they do provide important information about the structural and functional integrity of the brain areas being scanned. Therefore, it is noteworthy that several research groups

(continued on next page)

In the following discussion, amphetamine and methamphetamine are presented together because of their similar neurochemical and behavioral effects. MDMA, MDA, and MDE are covered in a separate section at the end of the chapter because they differ in important ways from the other amphetamines.

Basic Pharmacology of Amphetamine

Amphetamine is typically taken either orally or by IV or subcutaneous injection (the latter is sometimes called "skin popping"). Street names for amphetamine include "uppers," "bennies," "dexies," "black beauties," and "diet pills." Because absorption from the gastrointestinal tract is relatively slow, it may take up to 30 minutes for behavioral effects to be experienced after a typical oral dose of 5 to 15 mg. In contrast, IV injection provides a much more rapid and intense "high" than oral consumption and has much greater abuse potential.

Methamphetamine is more potent than amphetamine in its effects on the central nervous system and is therefore favored by substance abusers when it is available. Typical street names for methamphetamine are "meth," "speed," "crank," "zip," and "go." The drug can be taken orally, snorted, injected intravenously, or smoked. Smoking methamphetamine can be accomplished either using a glass pipe or by heating the compound on a piece of aluminum foil (a practice sometimes called "chasing the dragon"). Methamphetamine hydrochloride in a crystalline form particularly suitable for smoking (called "ice" or "crystal" on the street) began showing up Hawaii in the 1980s. This material has since spread to many parts of the country, particularly in the West, South, and Midwest. Because "ice" is inexpensive to make and highly addictive, it poses a serious risk for society's attempts to control and reduce the incidence of stimulant abuse.

Some amphetamine or methamphetamine users (called "speed freaks") go on binges, or "runs," of repeated IV injections to experience recurrent highs. During a run, the drug is typically injected approximately every 2 hours for a period as long as 3 to 6 days or more. Little sleep or eating occurs during a run. The user finally becomes exhausted, ends the run, and goes to sleep for many hours. Barbiturates or other depressant drugs are sometimes used either to "take the edge off" during a run or to assist in sleeping following the run. Yet another approach is to moderate the extreme stimulatory effect of IV amphetamine or methamphetamine by combining it with heroin to yield a so-called "speedball."

Amphetamine and methamphetamine are metabolized by the liver, though at a slow rate. Metabolites, as well as some unmetabolized drug molecules, are mainly excreted in the urine. The elimination half-life of amphetamine ranges from 7 to more than 30 hours depending on the pH of the urine. Because of this long half-life, users obtain a much longer-lasting "high" from a single dose of amphetamine or methamphetamine than they can get from a dose of cocaine.

Mechanisms of Amphetamine Action

Amphetamine and methamphetamine are indirect agonists of the catecholaminergic systems. Unlike cocaine, which only blocks catecholamine reuptake, amphetamine and methamphetamine also release catecholamines from nerve terminals. At very high doses, these compounds can even inhibit catecholamine metabolism by monoamine oxidase.

Studies on the mechanism of catecholamine release by amphetamine have particularly focused on DA. The results of this research suggest that two related drug actions are involved. One action is to cause DA molecules to be released from inside the vesicles into the cytoplasm of the nerve terminal. These DA molecules are subsequently transported outside of the terminal by a reversal of the DAT (Figure 11.17). The result is a massive increase in synaptic DA concentrations and an associated stimulation of dopaminergic transmission.

In animals, amphetamine- or methamphetamine-stimulated DA release has been demonstrated using techniques

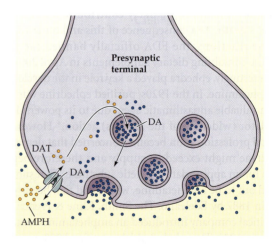

Figure 11.17 Mechanisms of amphetamine-stimulated DA release Amphetamine (AMPH) molecules enter DA nerve terminals partly due to uptake by DAT. Once inside the terminal, the drug provokes DA release from the synaptic vesicles into the cytoplasm. In addition, DAT functions in a reverse direction to release DA from the cytoplasm into the extracellular fluid. The combined effect of these processes is a massive increase in synaptic DA levels.

such as in vivo microdialysis. Brain imaging studies have likewise provided evidence for DA release in humans following IV amphetamine injection in the laboratory (Drevets et al., 2001). It is important to recognize that the NE-releasing effects of amphetamines occur not only in the brain but also in the sympathetic nervous system. Consequently, these compounds exert potent sympathomimetic actions similar to those seen with cocaine.

Behavioral and Neural Effects of Amphetamine

Amphetamine is a psychostimulant that has therapeutic uses

Like cocaine, amphetamine causes heightened alertness, increased confidence, feelings of exhilaration, reduced fatigue, and a generalized sense of well-being in human users. A number of other effects have also been observed, including improved performance on simple, repetitive psychomotor tasks; a delay in sleep onset; and a reduction in sleep time, particularly with respect to REM (rapid eye movement) sleep. Indeed, amphetamine permits sustained physical effort without rest or sleep, which accounts for its distribution to military personnel during World War II as well as its occasional use by truck drivers and other workers desirous of foregoing sleep for extended periods of time. The drug can also enhance athletic performance and is therefore one of the many banned substances in athletic competitions. In rodents and other animals, amphetamine elicits behavioral activation (locomotor stimulation and stereotypy) similar to that seen with cocaine. It is also highly reinforcing, as shown by numerous studies involving drug self-administration or place conditioning.

Although amphetamine is a controlled substance, it does have a few medical uses. As mentioned earlier, one such use is in the treatment of narcolepsy. Narcolepsy typically involves recurring and irresistible attacks of sleepiness during the daytime hours, although other symptoms may also be present. Amphetamine and particularly methylphenidate are even more widely used in treating children with ADHD. This disorder is discussed further in Box 11.2.

High doses or chronic use of amphetamine or methamphetamine can cause psychotic reactions as well as brain damage

Psychotic reactions   More than 30 years ago, several research groups first described in some high-dose amphetamine users a psychotic reaction consisting of visual and/or auditory hallucinations, behavioral disorganization, and the development of a paranoid state with delusions of persecu-

tion. Users may experience the same hallucination of a parasitic skin infestation described earlier for cocaine. These reactions to amphetamine usually do not occur upon first exposure to the drug, but only after a chronic abuse pattern has developed. Furthermore, in at least one study the paranoia and hallucinations did not typically begin until the second or third day of a "speed run."

With the increasing use of methamphetamine, the incidence of psychotic reactions to this substance is growing. Anecdotal reports suggest that high-dose methamphetamine use can also lead to violent behavior. Finally, some methamphetamine users who had an earlier psychotic reaction may undergo spontaneous recurrences known as "flashbacks" even while abstinent from the drug. These flashbacks can be triggered by stressful events and may reflect heightened stress sensitivity in former psychostimulant users.

Neurotoxicity   There is a special danger to methamphetamine users due to the neurotoxic properties of this substance. Investigators have known for many years that administration of multiple doses of methamphetamine to animals causes long-lasting reductions in the levels of DA, tyrosine hydroxylase (the key enzyme in DA synthesis), and the DAT in the striatum (McCann and Ruacarte, 2004). These changes are indicative of damage to DA axons and terminals, which has been confirmed by histological experiments showing the presence of degenerating fibers. Methamphetamine also produces damage to serotonergic fibers in several parts of the brain, including the neocortex, hippocampus, and striatum.

Until recently, no one knew whether human methamphetamine users suffer the same consequences as methamphetamine-treated experimental animals. Now, however, there are at least two different imaging studies reporting reduced DAT density in the striatum of methamphetamine users, even in individuals who had been abstinent from the drug for many months or longer (McCann et al., 1998; Volkow et al., 2001a). Several PET scans from one of these studies are shown in Figure 11.18. Decreases in neurotransmitter transporters sometimes reflect loss of the corresponding (in this case, DA) nerve fibers, since the transporters are located on the membrane of these fibers. Note, for example, the large reduction in DAT in the striatum of a Parkinson's disease patient, where the dopaminergic innervation of the striatum is known to be severely compromised. At this point, we can't be certain that the reduced DA transporter density in methamphetamine users is a sign of DA neurotoxicity, although such an interpretation is consistent with the animal studies. Moreover, since there appears to be a progressive loss of dopaminergic neurons and fibers during normal human aging, even a modest amount of damage to this system early in life could predispose the individual to developing Parkinson's disease later on.

exhilaration. Sleep is delayed, and performance of simple, repetitive tasks is improved. Therapeutically, amphetamine is used in the treatment of narcolepsy. Both amphetamine and another stimulant, methylphenidate, are also widely prescribed for children suffering from attention-deficit/hyperactivity disorder (ADHD). At relatively low doses, these stimulants produce calming and attention-enhancing effects that differ from the typical responses found in adults taking higher drug doses. In experimental animals, amphetamine acts much like cocaine. It elicits dose-dependent stimulation of locomotion and stereotyped behaviors, and it is highly reinforcing in self-administration and place conditioning paradigms.

Heavy use of amphetamine or methamphetamine can lead to the development of a psychotic state that closely resembles paranoid schizophrenia. Psychotic reactions may recur as flashbacks even after the user has been abstinent from the drug for a prolonged period. There is also substantial evidence from animal studies that methamphetamine can have neurotoxic effects on the dopaminergic and serotonergic systems. Recent results from brain imaging studies suggest that DA neurotoxicity may also occur in humans, which raises the possibility of increased vulnerability to Parkinson's disease as the affected individuals grow older.

MDMA and the related drugs MDA and MDE differ in several ways from amphetamine and methamphetamine. MDMA has been called an entactogen due to its reported ability to increase emotional openness and empathy in a psychotherapeutic context. This compound is used recreationally at dances called raves, where it causes feelings of euphoria, heightened sensory awareness, increased energy, enhanced well-being and self-confidence, and greater sociability. Physiologically, MDMA leads to elevated body temperature and fluid loss, which can be potentially dangerous at a dance or other situation involving physical exertion. Neurochemically, MDMA acutely stimulates 5-HT release, inhibits 5-HT reuptake, and also has some DA-releasing effects. In experimental animals, repeated MDMA treatment leads to a depletion in 5-HT and a pruning of serotonergic fibers in the cortex and hippocampus. Monkey studies have shown long-lasting serotonergic deficits following MDMA exposure.

Studies of human MDMA users have been controversial due to issues around dose levels, subject selection, and control for use of illicit drugs other than MDMA. Nevertheless, the findings to date strongly support the existence of serotonergic deficits and cognitive (particularly memory) problems in heavy MDMA users. Consequently, it is prudent to avoid regular use of MDMA or related substances.

Recommended Readings

Higgins, S. T., and Katz, J. L. (eds.). (1998). *Cocaine Abuse: Behavior, Pharmacology, and Clinical Applications.* Academic Press, San Diego.

Platt, J. (1995). *Cocaine Addiction: Theory, Research, and Treatment.* Harvard University Press, Cambridge, Massachusetts.

Quinones-Jenab, V. (ed.). (2001). *The Biological Basis of Cocaine Addiction.* Ann. N. Y. Acad. Sci., Vol. 937.

levels of nicotine across the day, since each dose builds on the residual nicotine left over from that day's previous cigarettes. However, this does not cause greater and greater effects, because of tolerance that has also developed over the same time period. Mild nicotine withdrawal emerges during the overnight period while the smoker is sleeping, yet at the same time the nicotine tolerance built up over the previous day partially dissipates. Because of these two processes, the individual awakens the next morning with a strong craving for a cigarette but also may experience the strongest or best response that she will have all day.

Mechanisms of Action

Nicotine works mainly by activating **nicotinic cholinergic receptors (nAChRs),** one of the two basic subtypes of acetylcholine (ACh) receptor (see Chapter 6). You will recall that nAChRs are ionotropic receptors comprising five separate protein subunits, and that these subunits are somewhat different when we compare neuronal nicotinic receptors to those found on muscle cells. Although the makeup of brain nicotinic receptors is complex, we can provide a few generalizations. First, these receptors contain only α- and β-subunits, and several different varieties of each subunit are present in the brain. Second, despite the fact that all of these receptors are considered nicotinic because of their basic structure and function, some of them bind nicotine with a much higher affinity than others. High-affinity nAChRs are found in many parts of the brain, including the cerebral cortex, thalamus, striatum, hippocampus, and monoamine-containing nuclei such as the substantia nigra, ventral tegmental area (VTA), locus coeruleus, and the raphe nuclei. Peripherally, such receptors are found in the ganglia of the autonomic (parasympathetic and sympathetic) nervous system. Finally, the high-affinity nAChRs are commonly thought to possess two α- and three β-subunits, and within this general category the most common type of receptor contains a mixture of α_4- and β_2-subunits (Figure 12.4).

When nicotine binds to a nicotinic receptor, it opens a channel that allows sodium (Na^+) ions to flow into the cell across the plasma membrane. This depolarizes the cell membrane, leading to a fast excitatory response by the cell. Some nAChRs also allow significant amounts of calcium (Ca^{2+}) to enter the cell, thereby stimulating Ca^{2+}-dependent second-messenger functions. Also note that some nAChRs are located presynaptically, that is, on nerve terminals. At this location, the receptors function by enhancing neurotransmitter release from the terminal.

High doses of nicotine lead to a persistent activation of nicotinic receptors and a continuous depolarization of the postsynaptic cell. As we saw in Chapter 6, this causes a depolarization block, and the cell cannot fire again until the nicotine is removed. In this way, a high dose of nicotine exerts a

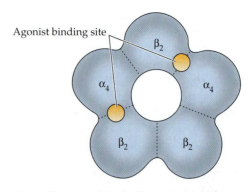

Figure 12.4 The nicotinic cholinergic receptor A top-down view of the proposed structure of the high-affinity nicotinic cholinergic receptor containing a combination of α_4- and β_2-subunits. The five subunits form a central ion channel that opens in response to agonist (for example, acetylcholine or nicotine) binding at the two sites shown on the diagram. (Adapted from Cordero-Erausquin et al., 2000.)

biphasic effect that begins with stimulation of nicotinic cholinergic functions but then turns to a nicotinic receptor blockade. This biphasic action accounts for the features of nicotine poisoning discussed later.

Section Summary

Nicotine is an alkaloid found in tobacco leaves. Tobacco plants are native to North and South America, and these plants were domesticated several thousand years ago by Native Americans. When tobacco was first brought back to Europe from the New World, use of this substance was primarily by means of pipe smoking, cigar smoking, and chewing. Snorting finely powdered tobacco leaves (snuff) later became popular. Cigarettes were first introduced in the mid-nineteenth century, and cigarette smoking subsequently increased due to improved methods of curing the tobacco leaves as well as the advent of modern cigarette manufacturing machines.

Although a typical cigarette contains 6–11 mg of nicotine, only about 1–3 mg actually reaches the smoker's bloodstream. Nicotine is vaporized by the high temperature at the tip of the burning cigarette and enters the smoker's lungs on tiny particles called tar. Once in the lungs, the nicotine is readily absorbed into the blood and quickly reaches the brain. The rapid delivery of a small burst of nicotine to the brain following each puff on the cigarette is believed to be a powerful reinforcer of smoking behavior. Arterial rather than venous levels of nicotine are considered to be the best indicator of the amount of nicotine being delivered to the brain.

Nicotine is metabolized primarily to cotinine by the liver enzyme CYP2A6. The cotinine and other nicotine metabolites are then excreted mainly in the urine. People who metabolize nicotine inefficiently due to a genetically determined low CYP2A6 activity seem to be less vulnerable to cigarette smoking than efficient metabolizers. The elimination half-life of nicotine is typically around 2 hours. Nicotine clearance from the body is an important reason why most smokers smoke throughout the day. Tolerance to at least some of nicotine's effects occurs during this period, but during sleep this tolerance partially dissipates and the smokers awaken in a state of mild withdrawal.

The principle mechanism of nicotine action is to stimulate nicotinic cholinergic receptors in the brain and the autonomic nervous system. In particular, there are high-affinity nAChRs that comprise two α- and three β-subunits, the most common of which contains a mixture of α_4- and β_2-subunits. The opening of nAChR channels permits Na^+ to flow across the cell membrane, thereby causing membrane depolarization and a fast excitatory response. Certain nAChRs also permit Ca^{2+} ions to enter the cell, thereby stimulating Ca^{2+}-dependent second-messenger functions. In some brain areas, nAChRs are located presynaptically and function to enhance neurotransmitter release. High doses of nicotine can cause persistent activation of nicotinic receptors, leading to a temporary depolarization block of the postsynaptic cell.

Behavioral and Physiological Effects

Nicotine elicits different mood changes in smokers compared to nonsmokers

If one wishes to determine the pharmacological effects of nicotine itself, separated from the complex behavioral aspects of smoking, it is necessary to give subjects the pure drug. This is routinely accomplished through the use of nicotine injections, nicotine patches, or nicotine-containing gum. Nevertheless, many studies still suffer from a significant methodological problem due to the use of current smokers, who are required to refrain from smoking for a specified period of time, typically ranging from 8 to 24 hours. Because nicotine abstinence produces withdrawal symptoms in dependent individuals, it is often difficult to determine whether nicotine-induced changes represent true differences from "normal" or simply reversal of withdrawal symptoms. Fortunately, researchers have more recently begun to study subjects who have never smoked, thereby permitting us to compare the findings of those studies with the results from abstinent smokers.

With respect to mood states, nicotine is usually found to increase calmness and relaxation in abstinent smokers. This fits well with numerous self-reports of smokers that smoking a cigarette has a relaxing, tension-reducing effect. However, it seems likely that these mood changes are significantly related to relief from nicotine withdrawal symptoms, because nicotine administration to nonsmokers tends to elic-

it feelings of heightened tension or arousal along with lightheadedness, dizziness, and even nausea (Kalman, 2002). If you either smoke now or have ever smoked in the past, you may recall having experienced some of these same effects when you tried your first cigarette.

Nicotine enhances cognitive function

We saw in Chapter 6 that ACh plays an important role in certain aspects of cognitive functioning. Although this is mediated in large part by the muscarinic cholinergic receptors, nicotinic receptors could also be involved. Based on this hypothesis, a number of studies have examined the effects of nicotine on cognitive function.

Abstinent smokers given nicotine show enhanced performance on many kinds of cognitive tasks, particularly those involving attentional demands (Sherwood, 1993). As in the case of mood effects, much of this enhancement appears to be due to alleviation of withdrawal-related deficits. Yet there is some indication that nicotine has positive effects on cognitive performance even in nonsmokers. One example is shown in Figure 12.5, where nicotine injection decreased reaction times of both smokers and non-

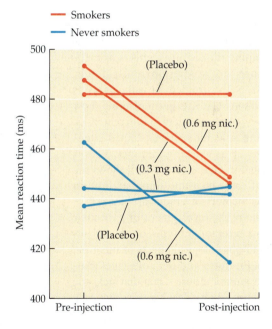

Figure 12.5 Nicotine-induced reduction of reaction time in a rapid visual information processing task The subjects were tested using a computer screen on which numerical digits were displayed one at a time at a rate of 100 per minute for a total of 10 minutes. Each subject was instructed to respond as quickly as possible when he or she detected three consecutive digits that were all either even or odd. Both doses of nicotine improved reaction time in regular smokers; however, only the higher dose had a similar effect in subjects who had never smoked. (From Foulds et al., 1996.)

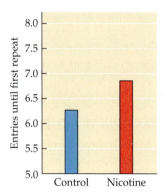

Figure 12.6 Nicotine-induced enhancement of working memory in the radial arm maze Rats received an acute injection of either nicotine (0.2 mg/kg) or placebo and then were tested for their performance in the radial arm maze. The nicotine-treated animals showed better working memory as indicated by a greater number of arm entries before they committed their first error (going into a previously entered arm). (After Levin, 1996.)

smokers in a task requiring sustained visual attention (Foulds et al., 1996). Cognitive enhancement by nicotine is also indicated by the drug's effects on electroencephalogram (EEG) activity. In both smokers and non-smokers, administration of nicotine transdermally (i.e., by skin patch) produces cortical EEG changes consistent with increased arousal and attention (Griesar et al., 2002; Knott et al., 1999). The ability of nicotine to improve cognitive function has led to considerable interest in the possible use of nicotinic receptor agonists in the treatment of Alzheimer's disease (see Chapter 6).

Animal studies have also been useful in determining the cognitive effects of nicotine, since such studies obviously do not suffer from the problem of using subjects who are smokers. Rats given nicotine show improvement on a variety of different tasks, including tasks requiring sustained attention as well as working memory. This is illustrated in Figure 12.6, which shows the effect of acute nicotine administration on working memory in a radial arm maze.*

To study the involvement of particular nicotinic receptor subtypes on the behavioral and physiological effects of nicotine, Marina Picciotto and her colleagues produced a mutant mouse strain that lacks the β_2-receptor subunit. Wild-type (genetically

normal) mice showed enhanced retention of a one-trial passive avoidance task when given a low dose of nicotine immediately after the learning trial. However, nicotine had absolutely no effect on memory in the β_2 knockout mice (Picciotto et al., 1997; Figure 12.7A and B). Since the β_2-subunit is most commonly found along with α_4, this finding raises the possibility that $\alpha_4\beta_2$ receptors may be critical for the memory-enhancing effects of nicotine.

(A)

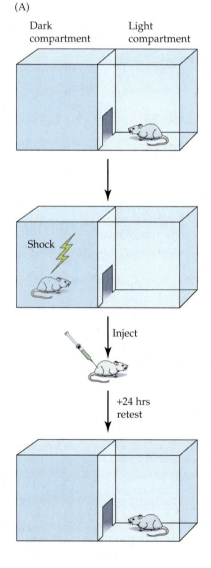

Dark compartment Light compartment

Shock

Inject

+24 hrs retest

(B)

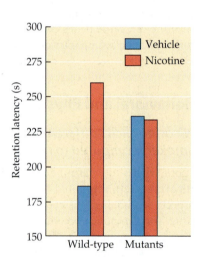

Figure 12.7 Failure of nicotine to increase retention of a one-trial passive avoidance task in mutant mice lacking the nicotinic receptor β_2-subunit (A) Mice were given one trial of passive avoidance learning, injected immediately afterwards with either 10 μg/kg nicotine or vehicle, and then tested for retention of the avoidance response 24 hours later. (B) Compared to vehicle treatment, nicotine produced increased retention in the wild-type mice as indicated by greater latency to enter the dark compartment. No such effect was observed in the mutant (β_2-subunit knockout) mice. (From Picciotto et al., 1997.)

---

*Working memory (formerly called short-term memory) involves information specific to the current trial on a task that is necessary for making the correct response(s) on that trial. In a radial arm maze, for example, working memory entails the retention of which arms of the maze have already been entered during the current trial.

Nicotine's reinforcing effects are mediated by activation of the mesolimbic dopamine system

Within a certain dose range, cigarette smokers will self-administer pure nicotine by intravenous injection (Harvey et al., 2004). This shows that nicotine by itself is reinforcing at the right dose (the drug is actually aversive at higher doses due to various side effects). On the other hand, it is clear that the reinforcement provided by smoking is much more complex than simply the delivery of nicotine to the individual. In a later section, we will discuss the relative contributions of nicotine versus other aspects of smoking in the reinforcing properties of this behavior.

Nicotine self-administration has also been investigated in laboratory animals. Although nicotine is not sought after as avidly as cocaine, amphetamine, or opioid drugs, nicotine self-administration has been demonstrated in rats, mice, dogs, and primates. Interestingly, Levin et al. (2003) recently reported that female rats self-administered significantly greater amounts of nicotine when drug exposure began during adolescence compared to adulthood (Figure 12.8). When extrapolated to humans, this finding suggests that adolescence may represent a particularly vulnerable period for the development of nicotine (tobacco) addiction.

As in the case of cocaine and amphetamine, the mesolimbic dopamine (DA) pathway from the VTA to the nucleus accumbens plays a key role in nicotine's reinforcing effects. High-affinity nicotinic receptors located in the VTA stimulate the firing of dopaminergic neurons, which causes increased DA release in the nucleus accumbens. Nicotine-induced activation

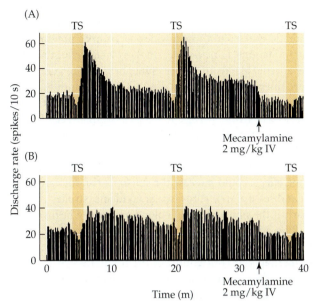

Figure 12.9 Activation of midbrain dopamine neuron by tobacco smoke Rats were connected to an artificial respirator through which tobacco smoke (TS) could be delivered. Smoke containing approximately 100 µg of nicotine was inhaled several times for 2 minutes during each trial (shaded area). Firing rates of a representative neuron in the VTA (A) and another neuron in the substantia nigra (B) are shown by the amplitude of the rate histogram. Tobacco smoke caused a substantial increase in VTA neuronal firing that returned to baseline within a few minutes. A smaller but still noticeable effect also occurred for cells in the substantia nigra. Note that prior intravenous (IV) infusion of the selective nicotinic receptor antagonist mecamylamine (lower right-hand part of each graph) completely blocked the effects of tobacco smoke on dopaminergic neuron firing, demonstrating that these effects are mediated by nicotinic cholinergic receptors. (From Fà et al., 2000.)

of DA neurons has usually been investigated using injection of the drug; however, a group of Italian researchers recently found the same phenomenon when rats inhaled cigarette smoke (Fà et al., 2000; Figure 12.9). The importance of accumbens DA for nicotine reinforcement was demonstrated by Corrigall and his coworkers (1992), who showed that lesioning the dopaminergic innervation of this area with 6-hydroxydopamine (6-OHDA) significantly attenuated nicotine self-administration. Several subtypes of nicotinic receptors are probably involved in the activation of DA neurons and the elicitation of behavioral reinforcement. Among these may be receptors that contain the β_2-subunit, since β_2 knockout mice show little self-administration of nicotine (Picciotto et al., 1998).

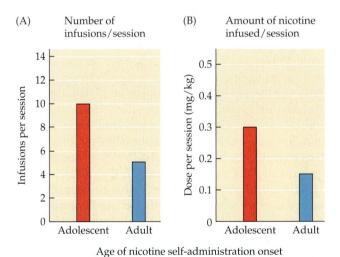

Figure 12.8 Increased nicotine self-administration in rats first exposed to the drug during adolescence versus adulthood Female rats were trained to self-administer nicotine intravenously over a 4-week period, beginning either at 54 days of age (late adolescence) or at 84 days of age (adulthood). The animals in which training was begun during adolescence administered more infusions (A) and more nicotine (B) per test session. (After Levin et al., 2003.)

Nicotine produces a wide range of physiological effects

We mentioned earlier that nicotinic receptors are abundantly expressed in autonomic ganglia. Consequently, nicotine can activate elements of both the sympathetic and parasympathetic systems to cause a wide spectrum of physiological manifestations. For example, smoking a cigarette stimulates the adrenal glands to release epinephrine (adrenaline) and norepinephrine (noradrenaline). These hormones, along with direct nicotine-induced activation of sympathetic ganglia, lead to symptoms of physiological arousal such as tachycardia (increased heart rate) and elevated blood pressure. This mild physiological arousal is thought to contribute to the reinforcing features of smoking. On the other hand, the same effects could increase the smoker's risk for cardiovascular disease and cerebrovascular accidents (strokes), particularly if the smoker has high blood pressure to begin with.

The action of nicotine on parasympathetic ganglia increases hydrochloric acid secretion in the stomach, which exacerbates or contributes to the formation of stomach ulcers. There is also increased muscle contraction in the bowel, which sometimes leads to chronic diarrhea that is especially harmful to individuals vulnerable to colitis, a chronic irritability of the colon. Together, these autonomic nervous system effects contribute to the deleterious consequences of heavy and prolonged use of tobacco products (see the section on smoking-related illness).

One consequence that many cigarette smokers find desirable is the constraining effect of nicotine on body weight. Cigarette smokers weigh an average of 8–10 pounds less than gender- and age-matched nonsmokers, and quitting smoking usually results in weight gain. This effect of nicotine has been attributed to an increase in metabolic rate combined with appetite suppression. Nevertheless, no one would recommend smoking for weight control because the terrible health consequences of smoking far outweigh the modest benefit derived from losing a little weight.

Nicotine is a toxic substance that can be fatal at high doses

Nicotine is quite toxic; as little as 60 mg can be fatal to an adult. If you do the math based on the nicotine content of a typical cigarette, you will see that a single pack contains several lethal doses of the drug. Of course, cigarettes are only smoked one at a time, and most of the nicotine is not taken in due to burning of the tobacco and loss of sidestream smoke (smoke not inhaled by the smoker). Cases of nicotine poisoning can occur through accidental swallowing of tobacco (usually by children), by absorption of excessive nicotine through the skin when field workers are harvesting wet tobacco leaves,* or by exposure to pure nicotine used in certain insecticides, as described in the opening part of this chapter (also see Box 12.1). When tobacco is swallowed, the

nicotine is less toxic than would be expected due to slow absorption of the drug from the stomach, first-pass metabolism in the liver, and possible regurgitation of the tobacco remaining in the stomach due to nicotine activation of the chemical trigger zone (vomiting center) in the medulla. Consequently, most cases of severe nicotine poisoning have been associated with nicotine-based insecticides.

The symptoms of nicotine poisoning include nausea, excessive salivation, abdominal pain, vomiting, diarrhea, cold sweat, headache, dizziness, disturbed hearing and vision, mental confusion, and marked weakness. This is quickly followed by fainting and prostration; falling blood pressure; difficulty in breathing; weakening of the pulse, which becomes rapid and irregular; and collapse. Left untreated, a fatal dose ends with convulsions followed shortly by respiratory failure due to depolarization block of the muscles of breathing. The treatment of nicotine poisoning involves inducing vomiting if the poison has been swallowed, placing adsorptive charcoal in the stomach, giving artificial respiration, and treating for shock.

Chronic exposure to nicotine induces tolerance and dependence

Repeated exposure to nicotine leads to a complex pattern of tolerance and, in some instances, sensitization. It is useful to distinguish between acute and chronic nicotine tolerance. For example, acute tolerance can be studied by pretreating subjects (for instance, by injection or by nasal spray) with either nicotine or vehicle and then testing their responses to a subsequent nicotine challenge. In both smokers and nonsmokers, many behavioral and physiological responses are attenuated by nicotine pretreatment, indicating the occurrence of tolerance. In much the same way, cigarette smokers undergo a significant degree of nicotine tolerance during the course of the day. This tolerance may be related to the fact that daytime nicotine levels in the bloodstream of regular smokers are sufficient to desensitize (and therefore temporarily inactivate) a high proportion of the nicotinic receptors, including the ones that mediate nicotine reinforcement by activating DA neurons in the VTA (Pidoplichko et al., 1997). Acute tolerance is short-lived; after an overnight period of abstinence, smokers awake the next morning more sensitive to nicotine than at the end of the previous day. This neurobiological mechanism helps explain why smokers often report that the first cigarette of the day is the most pleasurable one.

Long-term exposure to nicotine causes chronic tolerance. This chronic tolerance is superimposed on the acute within-a-day tolerance, and, of course, it is only present in smokers and others who use tobacco frequently. An early clue to the existence of chronic nicotine tolerance was the observation that green-tobacco illness occurred much more frequently

---

*This is sometimes called "green-tobacco sickness" by harvesters.

| BOX 12.1 | Pharmacology in Action |

Why Do Tobacco Plants Make Nicotine?

Growing up, we all learned that the dried leaves burned in cigarettes and cigars come from the tobacco plant and that people smoke this material at least partly because they obtain a substance from it called nicotine. As children or teenagers, most of us were more interested in trying out this forbidden activity called smoking than in thinking about why tobacco plants make nicotine in the first place. Yet if you consider it a bit, you realize that it's quite a legitimate question. Nicotine production certainly didn't evolve in tobacco plants to enable human beings to manufacture cigarettes, so it must help the plant in some way. However, the role of this substance is not immediately obvious. Unlike chlorophyll, nicotine plays no role in photosynthesis. Nor does it help the tobacco plant in pollination or in energy storage.

The best clue as to the biological function of nicotine is its toxicity. As mentioned in the text, nicotine is toxic not only to vertebrates but also to a wide range of insects. When insects absorb nicotine through direct con-

tact, the result is a paralysis similar to the paralytic effect of large doses of nicotine in humans. This effect of nicotine has been known for well over 200 years and has been exploited in a variety of both commercial and homemade insecticidal agents. Two common nicotine-based insecticides in the United States were Black Leaf 40, which was a 40% water-based solution of nicotine sulfate (see chapter opening image), and Nico-Fume Liquid, which was a 40% solution of free nicotine. These potent and highly toxic liquids were diluted and then sprayed on common garden plants, on agricultural crops, and even around chicken coops to control insect pests. Although manufacture of these nicotine concentrates has been discontinued, one can still obtain a formulation called Nico Soap that contains 7.35% nicotine in a surfactant (surface tension-lowering) soap that helps the solution cover and penetrate into the insect. Chemical companies have also developed and marketed a number of synthetic nicotine-like insecticides (called nicotinoids) such as imidacloprid and thiacloprid that are generally safer to use than nicotine itself.

The insecticidal properties of pure nicotine very likely represent at least

one purpose it serves for the tobacco plant. Nicotine is just one of many different kinds of alkaloids (nitrogen-containing compounds) made by various species of plants. These alkaloids are often toxic to animals, birds, or insects that may try to eat the plant. Botanists believe that plants evolved such alkaloids as a defense against being eaten. For example, cocaine, which is another plant alkaloid, has been shown to exert a deterrent effect on insects. Because of their chemical reactivity, some of these alkaloids, such as nicotine, cocaine, or morphine, happen to interact with nerve cells and thus produce psychoactive and even addictive effects.

To summarize, nicotine is a plant alkaloid that is highly toxic to insects as well as humans and animals. This toxicity serves as a defense against being eaten and is therefore probably responsible for the evolution of nicotine production by tobacco plants. The insecticidal properties of nicotine have been exploited for many years by farmers and gardeners, but caution must be used because of the dangers of nicotine poisoning. Somewhat safer synthetic substances called nicotinoids have largely replaced nicotine for purposes of insect control.

among harvesters who didn't smoke than among smokers (Gehlbach et al., 1974). Laboratory studies have similarly found that many effects of nicotine administration are attenuated in smokers compared to non-smokers. For example, a study by Foulds and his coworkers (1997) showed that subcutaneous injection of a high dose of nicotine elicited an aversive reaction consisting of at least some symptoms of mild nicotine toxicity (nausea, dizziness, sweating, headache, palpitations, stomachache, or clammy hands) in nonsmokers, but no such reaction in smokers (Figure 12.10). This not only demonstrates the presence of chronic nicotine tolerance in smokers, but it also raises the possibility that tolerance to these aversive effects must occur before individuals can fully experience nicotine's reinforcing effects.

Studies of nicotine responses in rats and mice have found evidence for both tolerance and sensitization. For example, rats given a single high dose of nicotine typically show an initial decrease in locomotor activity compared to saline treatment. However, when the animals are given daily nicotine injections, the locomotor suppression is gradually eliminated and replaced by locomotor activation (Domino, 2001). This pattern is sometimes considered to reflect a combination of tolerance to nicotine's locomotor suppressant effect and sensitization to the drug's activating effect.

Nicotine dependence in smokers is discussed later in the chapter. However, laboratory animals such as rats can also be made dependent on nicotine by giving them continuous exposure to the drug. This is usually accomplished by

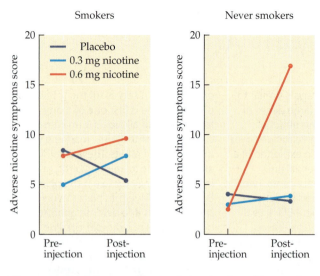

Smokers   **Never smokers**

Figure 12.10 Adverse effects of nicotine in subjects who never smoked compared to smokers Subjects rated the following symptoms that have been associated with adverse nicotine reactions: cold hands, dizziness, headache, nausea and upset stomach, palpitations, and sweating. Overall symptom ratings were obtained prior to nicotine administration (preinjection) and then 15 minutes after receiving a subcutaneous injection of either placebo, 0.3 mg of nicotine, or 0.6 mg of nicotine. Although smokers showed no significant increase in symptoms in response to either dose of nicotine, subjects who had never smoked exhibited a substantial adverse reaction to the higher dose. (After Foulds et al., 1997.)

implanting a small device known as an **osmotic minipump** under the skin of the animal. The minipump is filled with a nicotine solution and slowly infuses the solution subcutaneously at a constant rate for a set period of time such as 1 or 2 weeks. Some withdrawal symptoms (abstinence syndrome) can be observed when the nicotine clears the animal's system when the pump either runs out of solution or is removed by the experimenter. However, a stronger reaction can be triggered by administering a nicotinic receptor antagonist such as **mecamylamine,** thereby blocking the action of any residual nicotine still present in the animal. In rats, typical nicotine withdrawal symptoms include gasps, shakes or tremors, teeth chatter, ptosis (drooping eyelids), reduced locomotor activity, and increased startle reactivity (Helton et al., 1993; Hildebrand et al., 1997). Brain reward function (as indicated by the threshold for intracranial electrical self-stimulation) is also significantly reduced during nicotine withdrawal (Epping-Jordan et al., 1998), an effect seen during withdrawal from other abused drugs as well. A decreased ability to experience rewarding stimuli might also be present during tobacco withdrawal in smokers and might contribute to the well-known difficulty in stopping smoking.

Current evidence suggests that the nicotine abstinence syndrome is mediated by a combination of central (that is, within the brain) and peripheral (outside of the brain) nicotinic receptors (Hildebrand et al., 1997). The peripheral receptors might be those located within autonomic ganglia, whereas the central component of nicotine withdrawal may involve receptors in the VTA. Recall that when these VTA nicotinic receptors are activated, they stimulate DA cell firing and DA release in the nucleus accumbens. Recent studies found that when rats are subjected to mecamylamine-precipitated nicotine withdrawal, accumbens DA release actually falls to a level below normal (Hildebrand et al., 1998). Furthermore, injections of mecamylamine directly into the VTA of nicotine-dependent rats produces both reduced DA release in the accumbens and withdrawal symptoms (Hildebrand et al., 1999). Thus it appears that nicotinic receptors in the VTA play a significant role in nicotine withdrawal and that this role at least partially involves changes in accumbens DA release.

Section Summary

The mood-altering effects of nicotine depend on whether the subject is an abstinent smoker or a nonsmoker. In temporarily abstinent smokers, administration of pure nicotine usually increases calmness and relaxation. This effect is likely due to relief from nicotine withdrawal symptoms, because nicotine given to nonsmokers more often elicits feelings of tension, arousal, lightheadedness or dizziness, and sometimes nausea. Administration of nicotine to abstinent smokers also leads to enhanced performance on various cognitive tasks, particularly those involving attentional demands. In this case, however, some nicotine-related functional enhancement has also been reported for nonsmokers. Thus nicotine may produce certain positive effects in addition to its ability to alleviate withdrawal-related deficits.

Animal studies have found that nicotine improves performance on tasks requiring sustained attention and working memory. The memory-enhancing effects of nicotine may depend on high-affinity $\alpha_4\beta_2$ nicotinic receptors, as nicotine has no influence on retention of a one-trial passive avoidance task in knockout mice lacking the β_2-subunit of the nicotinic receptor.

Within a certain dose range, pure nicotine is reinforcing to both humans and experimental animals. However, nicotine self-administration is blunted in mice lacking the β_2-subunit of the nicotinic receptor, again pointing to the importance of receptor complexes bearing this subunit. The reinforcing properties of nicotine are believed to involve activation of high-affinity receptors located in the VTA that stimulate the firing of DA neurons and increase DA release in the nucleus accumbens. Indeed, the mesolimbic DA pathway from the VTA to the nucleus accumbens seems to be necessary for nicotine's reinforcing effects.

Nicotine additionally produces a variety of peripheral physiological effects. These include release of epinephrine and norepinephrine from the adrenal glands, tachycardia, and elevated blood pressure, all of which contribute to the arousing effects of the drug. Nicotine also increases hydrochloric acid secretion in the stomach and muscle contraction in the bowel, both of which can adversely affect the gastrointestinal tract. Finally, nicotine modestly increases metabolic rate and suppresses appetite, which accounts for why smokers typically gain weight after quitting.

Nicotine is a toxic substance that can cause dangerous symptoms such as nausea, salivation, abdominal pain, vomiting and diarrhea, confusion, and weakness. If a sufficient dose has been ingested, death may occur from respiratory failure. Treatment involves an attempt to remove the nicotine from the victim's stomach (if the nicotine has been swallowed), administration of artificial respiration, and dealing with drug-induced shock.

Repeated exposure to nicotine can lead to tolerance and, in some cases, sensitization. Single doses of nicotine cause a rapid but transient form of acute tolerance. Long-term nicotine exposure is associated with chronic tolerance. Consequently, smokers do not exhibit the adverse reactions to high doses of nicotine that are observed in nonsmokers. In animals given repeated nicotine injections, there develops a tolerance to the drug's locomotor suppressant effect accompanied by an emerging locomotor activation that is interpreted as sensitization.

When rats are made dependent on nicotine by giving them continuous exposure to the drug, withdrawal symptoms can be observed if the dependent animals are administered a nicotinic receptor antagonist such as mecamylamine. Both peripheral and central nicotinic receptors are thought to be involved in this abstinence syndrome, with at least part of the central component located in the VTA. DA release in the nucleus accumbens is inhibited during mecamylamine-precipitated nicotine withdrawal, and withdrawal symptoms can be elicited by injecting mecamylamine directly into the VTA of nicotine-dependent rats.

Cigarette Smoking

How many people smoke, and who are they?

The amount of cigarette smoking in the United States has varied tremendously over the past 100 years. As illustrated in

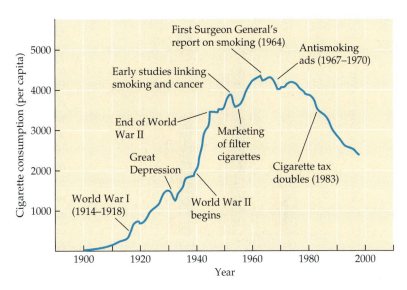

Figure 12.11 Yearly per capita cigarette consumption in the United States from 1900 to 1998 for individuals 18 years of age or older. (After Smith and Fiore, 1999.)

Figure 12.11, yearly per capita cigarette consumption was quite low at the beginning of the twentieth century but then rose steeply until the mid-1950s. There was a brief dip in cigarette consumption following publication of the first studies linking smoking with lung cancer, but consumption rose again with the marketing of filtered cigarettes. The decline in cigarette consumption since the 1960s coincides with the Surgeon General's reports on the health consequences of smoking, the appearance of antismoking ads, large increases in cigarette taxes, and general disapproval of smoking in many parts of society.

Despite the trend shown in the previous figure, a large number of people in this country continue to smoke. The 2002 National Survey on Drug Use and Health found that more than 70 million Americans were current tobacco users at that time (Substance Abuse and Mental Health Services Administration, 2003). This figure corresponds to approximately 30% of the population age 12 years or older. Of course, the majority of these are cigarette smokers. Tobacco use varies significantly by age, with the highest incidence in the 18-to-25-year age range (Figure 12.12). Other differentiating factors are gender, ethnicity, and educational attainment. Males are generally more likely to smoke than females, although it can be seen from the figure that this gender difference is not present within the 12-to-17-year age group. Across different ethnic groups, the highest rate of smoking occurs in Native Americans, followed by whites, Hispanics and African Americans, and then Asians. Finally, the prevalence of cigarette smoking is inversely related to level of education. For individuals 18 years or older, about 14% of college graduates are smokers, compared to 32% of

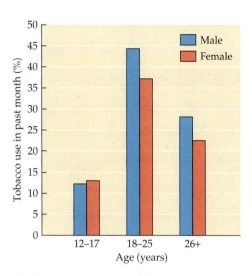

Figure 12.12 Percentage of subjects reporting current (in the past month) tobacco use according to age and gender. (After Substance Abuse and Mental Health Services Administration, 2003.)

high school graduates and 35% of people without a high school diploma.

In addition to the gender difference in smoking prevalence, there is emerging evidence that women tend to differ from men in the characteristics of their smoking behavior and in the determinants of smoking. Women typically smoke fewer cigarettes per day than men, they may prefer cigarettes with less nicotine, and they generally don't inhale as deeply. Some studies have also found that women are more influenced than men by the nonnicotine aspects of smoking (for example, sensory or social factors) compared to reinforcement from nicotine, and women find it more difficult to quit smoking, even when given nicotine replacement therapy (Perkins et al., 1999). We don't yet understand the reasons for these significant gender differences.

Cigarette smokers progress through a series of stages in their smoking behavior

Most smokers pick up the habit during adolescence. Looked at another way, early smoking greatly increases the chances that one will smoke as an adult. For this reason, teenage smoking has received a lot of attention from researchers as well as from policy makers interested in reducing the prevalence of this behavior in our society. There are many theories about why teenagers take up smoking. Some of the hypothesized reasons include establishing feelings of independence and maturity (by defying parental wishes or societal norms), improving self-image and enhancing social acceptance (assuming that one's friends are already smokers), counteracting stress and/or boredom, and simple curiosity. Moreover, young people tend to emphasize the positive elements of smoking while disregarding or denying the negative aspects, including the health consequences.

Most investigators agree that smokers pass through several different stages on their way to eventual nicotine dependence. Kathryn Mayhew and her colleagues have proposed a sequence of stages that is summarized in Table 12.1 (Mayhew et al., 2000). Just as we saw in Chapter 8 for drug addiction generally, there can be movement in both directions along the continuum from occasional to regular smoking. However, unless an individual is actively attempting to quit, stage changes are usually toward heavier cigarette use.

Why do smokers smoke?

Smoking and stress Smokers routinely report that smoking causes relaxation, alleviation of stress, and increased ability to concentrate. Consequently, some researchers have hypothesized that smoking (presumably through the delivery of nicotine) provides two specific advantages to the smoker: greater mood control (specifically with respect to stress reduction) and enhancement of concentration. This has been termed the **nicotine resource model.** An alternative model, sometimes called the **deprivation reversal**

TABLE 12.1 Stages in the Development of a Smoking Habit

Stage	Definition
1a. Nonsmoking—precontemplation	Nonsmoker and doesn't intend to start smoking
1b. Nonsmoking—contemplation or preparation	Nonsmoker but is thinking about starting
2. Initiation or tried	Has smoked a few cigarettes only
3. Experimentation	Smokes occasionally/experimentally; not yet committed to smoking
4. Regular smoker	Smokes on a regular basis (for example, on weekends or at parties), but not too frequently and not daily
5. Established smoker	Smokes daily or almost daily, sometimes heavily; nicotine-dependent

Source: Adapted from Mayhew et al., 2000.

model, suggests that the positive effects of smoking actually represent the alleviation of irritability, stress, and poor concentration experienced by smokers between cigarettes. This model, therefore, proposes that having a smoking habit increases overall stress, which then must be countered by repeated smoking.

Researchers have debated these two ideas for many years and there are still proponents of both. However, recent studies by the British psychologist Andrew Parrott argue strongly for the idea of deprivation reversal (Parrott, 1999; Parrott and Kaye, 1999). It seems that the "relaxing" effect of smoking merely brings the smoker to the same state as a typical nonsmoker, rather than producing a higher level of relaxation.

The role of nicotine in smoking Delivery of nicotine is obviously one of the key factors in smoking. As mentioned earlier, nicotine is intravenously self-administered by animals as well as by humans under the appropriate conditions. Other evidence for an involvement of nicotine comes from smoking behavior itself. Cigarettes devoid of nicotine (for example, lettuce-based cigarettes) have never been commercially successful. Furthermore, it is well established that smoking intensity is increased when smokers of regular cigarettes switch to a brand that is low in nicotine and tar. This change in smoking behavior increases nicotine yields well beyond those specified by the Federal Trade Commission (FTC), which are based on standardized smoking by a machine.

Finally, withdrawal from regular tobacco use leads to significant abstinence symptoms that are thought to result primarily from removal of nicotine from the person's system. For habitual smokers who meet the criteria for nicotine dependence, even a brief abstinence of a few hours leads to craving and a growing urge to smoke. These feelings correlate with a drop in nicotine levels in the individual's bloodstream. The much longer abstinence that occurs when people try to quit smoking leads to a more complex abstinence syndrome characterized not only by tobacco craving but also by irritability, impatience, restlessness, anxiety, insomnia, difficulty concentrating, and hunger and weight gain. Figure 12.13 presents the results from one study that examined the time course of withdrawal symptoms as well as the ability of nicotine gum to prevent such symptoms (Hughes et al., 1991).

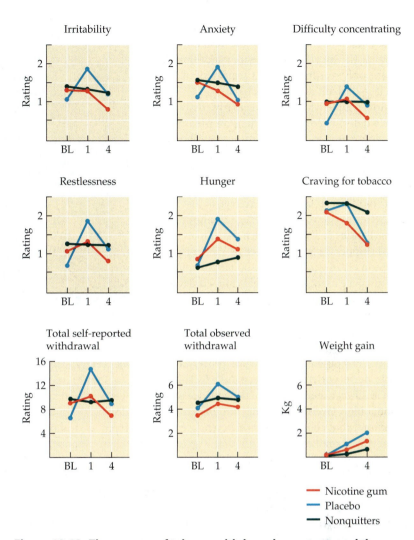

Figure 12.13 Time course of tobacco withdrawal symptoms and the effects of nicotine replacement therapy Regular smokers who wanted to quit smoking were randomly assigned to either a nicotine gum or placebo gum group. Symptom ratings were obtained before the beginning of treatment (baseline, BL) and then again 1 and 4 weeks later. The figure illustrates data for those subjects who were abstinent at the 4-week test point compared to those who failed to quit during the study. (After Hughes et al., 1991.)

We can see that the abstinence syndrome was still present at 1 week postcessation, but except for hunger and weight gain, the average levels of most symptoms were at or near baseline at 4 weeks. These group data suggest that the abstinence syndrome from tobacco is relatively short-lasting. Nevertheless, the investigators found that about 20 to 25% of the subjects still reported significant symptoms at the 4-week time point. Nicotine gum clearly prevented almost all of the withdrawal symptoms except for hunger and weight gain, supporting the conclusion that most of these symptoms are due to nicotine dependence. Not shown in this figure, however, is the fact that even with the nicotine gum, more than two-thirds of the subjects were back smoking at a 6-month follow-up test despite lacking the typical withdrawal symptoms. These and other experimental results indicate that the nicotine abstinence syndrome is not the only reason that most regular smokers find it so difficult to quit their habit.

Most people who smoke regularly (daily or nearly daily) become dependent on nicotine. However, there is a small percentage of long-term smokers who smoke regularly but smoke only a few cigarettes each day and do not become dependent. In one recent study, the nondependent smokers had smoked an average of just 3.4 cigarettes per day for an average of about 14 years (Perkins et al., 2001). Such individuals are called **chippers,** a term first used by Zinberg and Jacobson (1976) to describe a similar phenomenon in opiate users. Interestingly, chippers develop tolerance to nicotine despite their limited exposure (Perkins et al., 2001). The finding that nicotine dependence and tolerance can be separated from each together suggests that they are produced by different physiological processes. It would be very useful to understand why some individuals can avoid nicotine dependence and maintain low levels of smoking, but unfortunately we don't yet know what characteristics differentiate chippers from more typical smokers.

The role of other factors in smoking   Even though most of us think "nicotine" when we think about smoking, it cannot be the only factor responsible for maintaining this behavior. Indeed, we discussed earlier that the nicotinic receptors responsible for stimulating DA release in the nucleus accumbens are probably desensitized for most of the day in regular smokers. Why, then, do such individuals continue to smoke throughout the day in the presumed absence of direct nicotine reinforcement? One reason, of course, is because they are nicotine-dependent and want to avoid nicotine withdrawal symptoms. However, it is also likely that sensory stimuli associated with the act of smoking, such as the taste and smell of inhaling cigarette smoke, become conditioned to the reinforcing effects of nicotine and are thus able to function as secondary reinforcers themselves (Balfour et al., 2000). Recall that each puff on a cigarette delivers a small burst of nicotine to the brain. Assuming 30 cigarettes per day and 10 puffs per cigarette, a 10-year smoker has had over 1 million "learning trials" in which a mouthful of cigarette smoke was paired with one of those bursts of nicotine. Consider further that in a nonsmoker who has not developed such an association, the sensory qualities of cigarette smoke are harsh and unpleasant. For these reasons, it is likely that the sensory aspects of smoking help maintain this behavior under conditions where direct nicotine reinforcement is minimal due to receptor desensitization.

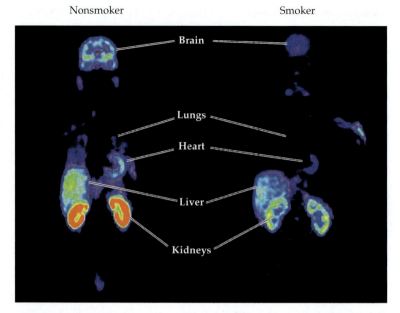

Figure 12.14   Whole-body PET scans illustrating reduced MAO-B activity in various organs of a smoker compared to a nonsmoker. (From Fowler et al., 2003b.)

One additional factor to be mentioned is a pharmacological one unrelated to nicotine. Brain imaging studies using positron emission tomography (PET) found a large reduction in the activities of both monoamine oxidase A (MAO-A) and MAO-B in smokers compared to nonsmokers (Fowler et al., 2003a). This effect is not produced by administration of pure nicotine and therefore must be caused by other substances present in cigarette smoke (Castagnoli et al., 2002). Furthermore, MAO inhibition seems to require repeated cigarette use, since it is not found after the smoking of a single cigarette (Fowler et al., 1999). Since MAO is an enzyme that plays a critical role in metabolizing the neurotransmitter DA, it is possible that smoking not only causes DA release (via nicotine) but also slows its breakdown in the brain. Both of these influences on the DA system could contribute to smoking-related reinforcement. Subsequent work involving whole-body PET imaging found that MAO-B activity in smokers was decreased not only in the brain but also in various peripheral organs such as the heart, lungs, and kidneys (Fowler et al., 2003b; Figure 12.14). As these organs are exposed to catecholamines via the circulation as well as from sympathetic nerve endings, a deficiency in MAO-B could result in adverse consequences due to augmented catecholamine activity throughout the body.

Smoking is a major cause of illness and premature death

It has been estimated that one-third to one-half of smokers die prematurely due to their exposure to tobacco. According to government statistics, cigarette smoking is the major preventable cause of death among Americans, with more than 440,000 people dying each year from tobacco-related causes (Centers for Disease Control and Prevention, 2004). The medical costs associated with smoking-related illnesses are thought to exceed $75 billion a year.

Cigarette smoking increases the risk for many life-threatening illnesses, including several kinds of cancer as well as cardiovascular disease. The deleterious effects of smoking stem from a combination of factors, including tar, carbon monoxide gas that is produced by the burning of tobacco, and possibly also nicotine. Tar contains a number of identified carcinogens, and the strong association between cigarette smoking and lung cancer has been known for well over 30 years. Smoking can also lead to other respiratory diseases such as emphysema and chronic bronchitis. Although there is less public recognition of the relationship between smoking and cardiovascular disease, this relationship is actually quite strong. Smokers are at increased risk for heart attack, stroke, and atherosclerosis. Finally, pregnant smokers in particular should try to stop or at least cut back on their smoking habit. Smoking during pregnancy is the leading cause of low birth weight, which delays the infant's development and puts him at risk for other complications.

Behavioral and pharmacological strategies are used to treat tobacco dependence

Surveys indicate that 70 to 75% of current smokers in the United States would like to quit smoking, and about 40 to 45% of daily smokers actually attempt to quit each year. However, addiction to nicotine is so powerful that the success rate is very low. As was the case for one of the authors (JM) many years ago, the smoking habit can be overcome but the process is difficult and usually requires multiple attempts to quit.

We will consider a variety of behavioral and pharmacological approaches for treating tobacco dependence. It is important to recognize that the success rate of any treatment approach is influenced by numerous variables, such as the duration of smoking behavior and number of cigarettes smoked daily, the intensity of the abstinence syndrome, the motivation to quit, whether or not the smoker lives and/or works in a smoking environment, and so on. Furthermore, even if a given therapeutic program claims a high success rate for its clients, such claims are meaningless unless there is careful follow-up for months and years to ascertain long-term abstinence.

Behavioral interventions   A number of strategies are directed toward discouraging young people from beginning tobacco use or giving it up if it is already habitually used. For example, various state and federal agencies sponsor antismoking appeals in the media, and the Surgeon General's

office has mandated health warnings on cigarette packages for many years. Another approach is the levying of high taxes on tobacco products. This may not prevent people from starting to use these products, but it does reduce the amount of use.

Many smokers attempt to quit by using various self-help programs involving books or manuals. While such programs are generally inexpensive, they don't appear to offer much benefit to the smoker. A bit more successful are individual or group counseling programs provided by health professionals, particularly those that provide social support and/or coping-skills training to their clients.

Pharmacological interventions   The most common pharmacological intervention for smoking cessation is **nicotine replacement**. This approach is based on several premises: (1) that the difficulty associated with smoking cessation is significantly related to nicotine withdrawal symptoms; (2) that blocking (or at least reducing) these symptoms by maintaining a certain circulating level of nicotine can assist in terminating smoking; and (3) that there are safer ways for individuals to obtain nicotine than by smoking.

Nicotine replacement was first accomplished by formulating a special nicotine-containing chewing gum (nicotine polacrilex), which has the advantage that nicotine can be absorbed by the buccal mucosa (mucous membranes lining the mouth) rather than the gastrointestinal tract, where absorption is minimal and there is substantial first-pass metabolism in the liver. Nicotine gum was approved as a pharmacotherapeutic aid in the treatment of cigarette dependence in 1984 under the trade name Nicorette. This was later followed by the transdermal nicotine patch (Nicoderm, Habitrol, Nicotrol), nicotine nasal spray (Nicotrol NS), nicotine inhaler (Nicotrol Inhaler), and nicotine lozenges (Commit Lozenges). The nasal spray and inhaler require a doctor's prescription, whereas nicotine gum, patches, and lozenges can be obtained over-the-counter (OTC). Making at least some nicotine medications available OTC was a significant advance in the battle against smoking, because some smokers are reluctant or unable financially to enter a formal treatment program yet may still be willing to try something they can obtain at a drug store without a prescription.

With all these choices available, which kind of nicotine replacement therapy should a smoker choose? Table 12.2 lists some of the advantages and disadvantages of each nicotine delivery vehicle. Two other points should also be noted with respect to nicotine replacement therapy. First, combination treatments such as nicotine gum plus the patch or the nicotine inhaler plus the patch may be more effective than either treatment alone in helping some smokers quit their habit (George and O'Malley, 2004). Second, a number of studies have shown that success rates are increased when behavioral or psychosocial (supportive) therapy is provided along with nicotine replacement. Given the complex nature of nicotine addiction and the smoking habit, it should not be surprising

TABLE 12.2 Advantages and Disadvantages of Different Kinds of Nicotine Replacement Therapy

Treatment	Advantages	Disadvantages
Nicotine polacrilex (gum)	Easy to use; flexible dosing; OTC availability; rapid nicotine delivery	Frequent dosing needed; side effects such as jaw pain or mouth soreness
Nicotine lozenge	Easy to use, flexible dosing; OTC availability; rapid nicotine delivery	Frequent dosing needed; side effects such as heartburn or indigestion if lozenges consumed too rapidly
Transdermal nicotine patch	Easy to use; OTC availability; morning craving reduced with overnight use; few side effects except for possible skin irritation	Less flexible dosing and slower delivery of nicotine than with other treatments; overnight use may cause insomnia
Nicotine nasal spray	Flexible dosing; fastest nicotine delivery and reduction of cravings	Frequent dosing needed; initial side effects such as nose and eye irritation, sneezing, and coughing
Nicotine inhaler	Flexible dosing; use mimics the hand-to-mouth feature of smoking; few side effects except for mild throat irritation and coughing	Frequent dosing needed

that a combined therapeutic approach gives the smoker the best chance of quitting.

Although nicotine replacement therapy continues to be refined and improved, another valuable drug for smoking cessation was discovered serendipitously by staff working at a Veterans Administration hospital clinic in California. Some of their depressed patients were undergoing treatment with bupropion, an unusual antidepressant medication thought to act by inhibiting DA and norepinephrine reuptake. Depressed patients often smoke, yet some of the smokers given bupropion reported reduced cigarette cravings and were able to quit smoking without additional therapeutic intervention. Formal studies confirmed the efficacy of bupropion, and the drug is now available for smoking cessation in the form of a sustained-release preparation (trade name Zyban). Figure 12.15A and B show that sustained-release bupropion is as effective as the nicotine patch in reducing nicotine withdrawal symptoms in newly abstinent smokers (Jorenby et al., 1999). However, the combination of bupropion and the patch did not reduce symptoms below the level achieved with either treatment alone.

Finally, you may recall that in the last chapter we discussed efforts by researchers to develop a vaccine against cocaine. Similar work is being carried out with nicotine. In fact, at the time of this writing a nicotine vaccine (trade name NicVAX) is currently undergoing human clinical trials to determine whether it is effective in reducing the incidence of smoking (Kantak, 2003). Because the vaccine does not completely prevent nicotine from reaching the brain, it will probably be combined with existing treatment approaches

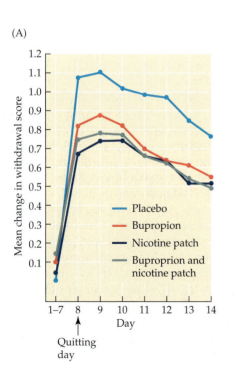

(A)

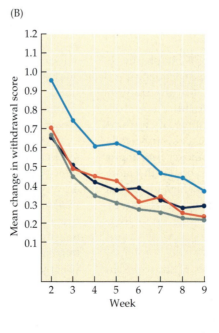

(B)

Figure 12.15 Efficacy of bupropion treatment in reducing symptoms of smoking withdrawal Subjects were enrolled in a smoking cessation program in which they received bupropion alone, nicotine patch alone, bupropion plus nicotine patch, or placebo. The intensity of withdrawal symptoms was rated and compared to baseline (pretreatment) scores for the first 6 days after quitting (A), and then at weekly intervals for a total of 9 weeks (B). All treatment groups showed reduced withdrawal symptoms compared to the placebo group. (From Jorenby et al., 1999.)

such as bupropion (to reduce withdrawal symptoms) and counseling.

Section Summary

There are more than 70 million smokers in this country, according to the 2002 National Household Survey on Drug Use and Health. There are fewer female than male smokers, and women also differ from men in their smoking habits. Smokers typically begin during adolescence, and many different reasons have been given for teenage smoking.

Because smokers commonly report that smoking causes relaxation, a reduction in stress, and increased concentration, some researchers have proposed a nicotine resource model hypothesizing that the nicotine obtained through smoking has the beneficial effects of increasing mood control (in relation to stress reduction) and enhancing concentration. However, accumulated evidence favors an alternative model, the deprivation reversal model, which argues that the positive effects experienced when smoking actually constitute the alleviation of withdrawal effects such as irritability, anxiety, and poor concentration. These and other symptoms are components of a well-established abstinence syndrome seen in nicotine-dependent smokers who try to quit. It is interesting that some individuals, called chippers, can smoke small numbers of cigarettes regularly without becoming dependent. Chippers do develop tolerance, however, which demonstrates a separation between the processes underlying nicotine tolerance and dependence.

Although withdrawal symptoms undoubtedly play an important role in maintaining the smoking habit in dependent smokers, other factors also contribute to this habit. One factor is the sensory aspects of smoking, namely the taste and smell of cigarette smoke. Researchers have also recently discovered that some component of cigarette smoke other than nicotine inhibits MAO activity in the brain and in other organs. As this enzyme plays a key role in DA metabolism, MAO inhibition as well as direct stimulation of DA release may both be involved in the neurochemical mechanisms underlying nicotine reinforcement.

Chronic use of tobacco results in many adverse health consequences, including cancer, emphysema and bronchitis, and cardiovascular disease. For this reason, many different treatment strategies have been developed to assist smokers in quitting. These include behavioral as well as pharmacological interventions. Nicotine replacement for the alleviation of withdrawal symptoms can be accomplished by means of nicotine gum, lozenges, patches, nasal spray, or inhaler. Also useful is a sustained-release preparation of the antidepressant bupropion (Zyban), which reduces nicotine craving. Finally, a nicotine vaccine (NicVAX) that reduces nicotine availability to the brain is undergoing clinical testing. Despite all of these treatment options, overall success rates are still low, and thus more-effective treatment programs must continue to be sought. Breaking the smoking habit is almost always a difficult proposition, so it is much better never to become dependent in the first place.

Caffeine

Background

If you are like most people living in Western societies, you probably had at least one cup of coffee (or perhaps tea) this morning, possibly followed up by additional cups as the day progressed. Whether you like the taste of coffee (which is bitter when taken black) or not, you are probably consuming it at least partly for its pharmacological properties as a stimulant. This, of course, brings us to the subject of caffeine, the principal psychoactive ingredient in coffee.

The major source of caffeine is coffee beans, which are the seeds of the plant *Coffea arabica*. Tea leaves contain significant amounts of both caffeine and a related compound called theophylline (which is Greek for "divine leaf") (Figure 12.16). Caffeine is one of the most widely used drugs in the world. In the United States, for example, it is estimated that 80 to 90% of adults regularly drink caffeinated beverages. The typical caffeine content of various foodstuffs and over-the-counter drugs is shown in Table 12.3. Taking these various sources together, the average adult caffeine intake in the United States has been estimated at 200 to 400 mg per day. As discussed later in the chapter, individuals who are compulsive users can greatly exceed this dose. Children may also ingest considerable amounts of caffeine through consumption of caffeinated soft drinks and chocolate.

Basic Pharmacology of Caffeine

Caffeine is normally consumed orally through the beverages in which it is present. Under this condition, it is virtually completely absorbed from the gastrointestinal tract within 30 to 60 minutes. Caffeine absorption begins in the stomach but takes place mainly within the small intestine. The plasma half-life of caffeine varies substantially from one person to another, but the average value is about 4 hours. Conse-

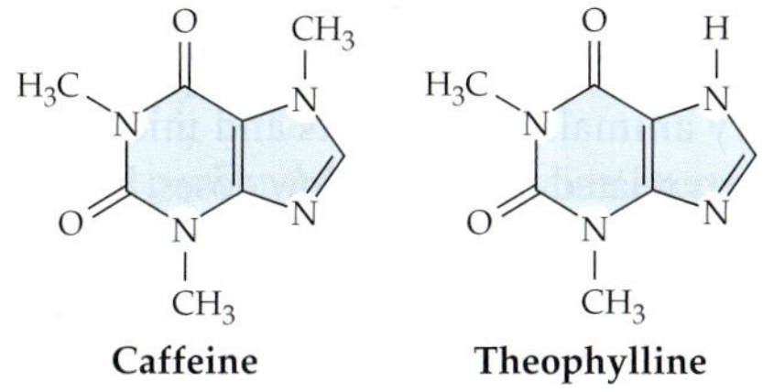

Figure 12.16 Chemical structures of caffeine and theophylline

Section Summary

Caffeine is contained in a number of foods, especially coffee and tea. When consumed orally, it is readily absorbed from the gastrointestinal tract and is gradually metabolized and excreted with a typical half-life of approximately 4 hours. In rodents, caffeine has locomotor stimulant effects at low doses but actually reduces activity at high doses. Humans generally experience heightened arousal, reduced fatigue, and reduced sleep in response to normal amounts of caffeine. Higher doses can lead to feelings of tension and anxiety. Laboratory studies have also demonstrated enhanced psychomotor performance following caffeine administration; however, it is not clear whether these findings represent a true positive effect of the substance or an alleviation of caffeine withdrawal. Caffeine produces various physiological effects, such as increased blood pressure and respiration rate, diuresis, and increased catecholamine release. It has several clinical uses, including relief of mild headache and the treatment of newborn infants with apnea.

Regular caffeine use leads to tolerance and physical dependence. Symptoms of caffeine withdrawal include headache, drowsiness, fatigue, impaired concentration, and reduced psychomotor performance. The ability of caffeine to produce dependence and withdrawal accounts for the anecdotal observations of those who insist that they cannot "get started" in the morning without a cup of coffee. Although most users consume caffeine at low to moderate doses, a small number of individuals consume extremely high amounts that can lead to adverse psychological and physiological consequences (caffeinism). In addition to the obvious problems associated with caffeinism, even more modest caffeine consumption has been associated with a heightened risk for coronary heart disease and low infant birth weight (when the drug is taken by pregnant women).

Although caffeine has a number of biochemical effects on the brain, its psychological and behavioral properties are thought to be mediated primarily by its ability to block A_1 and A_{2A} adenosine receptors. There is growing evidence from animal studies that adenosine is a sleep- or drowsiness-inducing factor released after a period of waking. This may explain why caffeine use in humans causes increased alertness and suppression of sleep.

Recommended Readings

Gately, I. (2003). *Tobacco: A Cultural History of How an Exotic Plant Seduced Civilization.* Grove Press, New York.

Laviolette, S. R., and van der Kooy, D. (2004). The neurobiology of nicotine addiction: Bridging the gap from molecules to behaviour. *Nat. Rev. Neurosci.,* 5, 55–65.

Lorist, M. M., and Tops, M. (2003). Caffeine, fatigue, and cognition. *Brain Cogn.,* 53, 82–94.

Weinberg, B. A., and Bealer, B. K. (2002). *The World of Caffeine: The Science and Culture of the World's Most Popular Drug.* Routledge, New York.

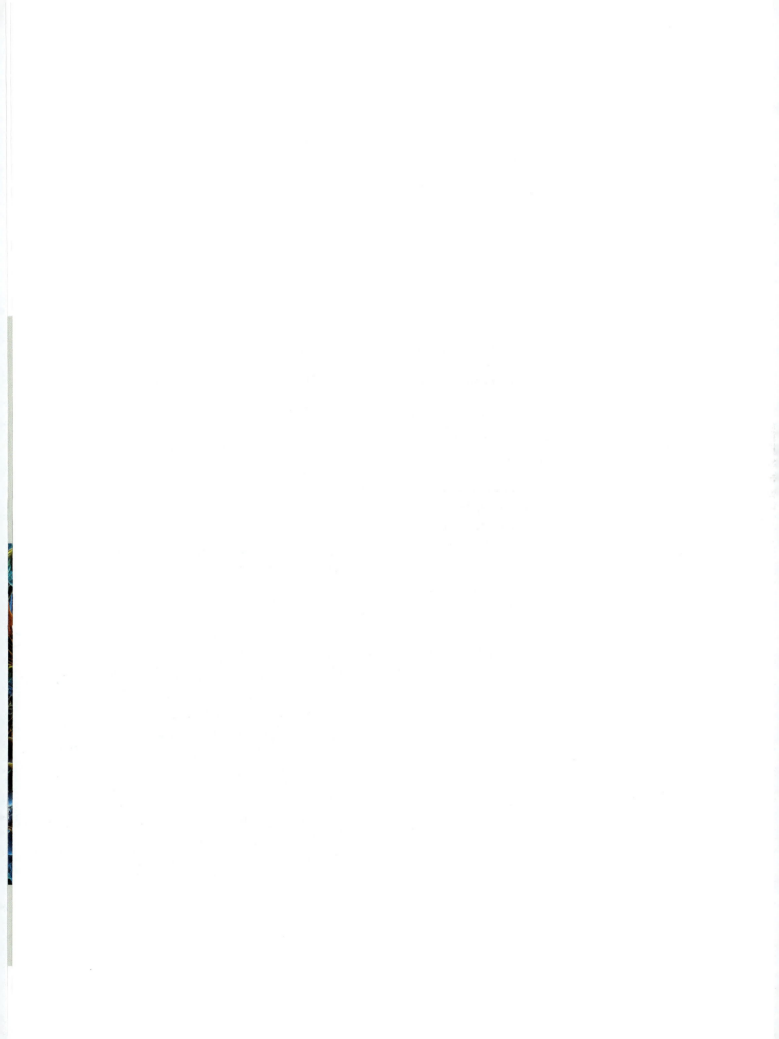

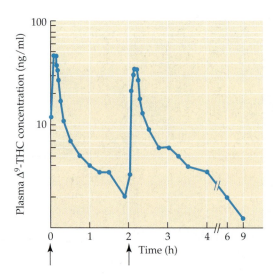

Figure 13.5 Chemical structure of Δ⁹-tetrahydro-cannabinol (THC)

A typical hand-rolled marijuana cigarette ("joint") consists of around 0.5 to 1 gram of cannabis. If the THC content is 4% (though it can be even higher depending on the strain and growing conditions), then a 1-gram joint contains 40 mg of active ingredient that is available to the smoker. As in the case of nicotine in tobacco leaves (see Chapter 12), burning of the marijuana causes the THC to vaporize and to enter the smoker's lungs in small particles. But due to a variety of factors, only about 20% of the original THC content is absorbed in the lungs. In practice, the amount of THC absorbed is affected not only by the initial amount of plant material used and the potency of this material but also by the pattern of smoking. Experienced marijuana users adjust their puff volumes and puff frequency to carefully regulate the behavioral effects of the drug. Another widely used technique is to hold the smoke in one's lungs for the purpose of enhancing the drug's effectiveness. Most experimental studies involving controlled marijuana smoking have surprisingly failed to show that breathhold duration influences the subjective "high." However, Block and coworkers (1998) found a modest but statistically significant increase in the reported "high" with a breathhold duration of 15 seconds compared to 7 seconds. Consequently, it is possible that longer breathholds may have at least some influence on the smoker's response to the marijuana.

THC is readily absorbed through the lungs, resulting in rapidly rising levels in the blood plasma of the smoker (Figure 13.6). After peak levels are reached, plasma THC concentrations begin to decline due to a combination of metabolism in the liver and accumulation of the drug in the body's fat stores. In contrast, oral consumption of marijuana leads to prolonged but poor absorption of THC, thus resulting in low and variable plasma concentrations. The reduced bioavailability of THC following oral consumption compared to smoking probably results from both degradation in the stomach and first-pass hepatic metabolism. That is, once orally ingested THC has been absorbed from the gastrointestinal tract, it must pass through the liver, where much of it is metabolized before it can enter the general circulation.

THC is converted into several metabolites, notably 11-hydroxy-THC and 11-nor-carboxy-THC (THC-COOH). These substances as well as various minor metabolites are

Figure 13.6 Mean time course of plasma THC concentrations in subjects who smoked a marijuana cigarette containing approximately 9 mg of THC at the two time points indicated by the arrows. (After Agurell et al., 1986.)

excreted primarily in the feces (about two-thirds of the administered dose) and the urine (about one-third of the administered dose). Even though THC levels in the bloodstream decline fairly rapidly after one smokes marijuana, complete elimination from the body is much slower due to persistence of the drug in fat tissue. Consequently, the elimination rate, or half-life ($t_{1/2}$), of THC is generally estimated at around 20 to 30 hours. Furthermore, the gradual movement of THC and fat-soluble metabolites back out of fat stores means that sensitive urine screening tests for THC-COOH can detect the presence of this metabolite more than 2 weeks following a single marijuana use.

Section Summary

Cannabis sativa, the flowering hemp plant, exudes a resin containing a number of unique compounds known as cannabinoids. Cannabis can be obtained in several different types of preparations, including marijuana and hashish, both of which may be smoked or taken orally. The consumption of cannabis for its intoxicating effects is thought to date back thousands of years in Eastern cultures. The practice of marijuana smoking was introduced into the United States in the early 1900s by Mexican and West Indian immigrants.

The most important naturally occurring cannabinoid is Δ⁹-tetrahydrocannabinol (THC). Inhaled THC is rapidly absorbed from the lungs into the circulation, where it is almost completely bound to plasma proteins. Oral THC consumption yields slower absorption and a lower plasma peak than occurs following smoking. THC is extensively metabolized in the liver, and the metabolites are excreted mainly in the feces and urine. Following a single dose of THC, total clearance of the drug and its metabolites may take days because of sequestration of these compounds in fat tissue.

Mechanisms of Action

Cannabinoid effects are mediated by cannabinoid receptors

For many years, researchers interested in how THC and other cannabinoids work in the brain were hampered by the lack of an identified cellular receptor for these compounds. In 1988, however, pharmacological characterization of a central nervous system (CNS) **cannabinoid receptor** was announced by a group of researchers that included William Devane and Allyn Howlett at St. Louis University and Lawrence Melvin and M. Ross Johnson at the Pfizer pharmaceutical company (Devane et al., 1988). This initial characterization was quickly followed by other studies showing significant expression of cannabinoid receptors in many brain areas such as the basal ganglia (including the striatum, globus pallidus, entopeduncular nucleus, and substantia nigra pars reticularis), cerebellum, hippocampus, and cerebral cortex (Figure 13.7). As discussed later, localization of cannabinoid receptors in these areas is consistent with the recognized behav-

ioral effects of these compounds on locomotor activity, coordination, and memory.

Around the same time that the St. Louis University and Pfizer researchers were first characterizing the cannabinoid receptor pharmacologically, another group of scientists at the National Institute of Mental Health (NIMH) including Lisa Matsuda and Tom Bonner cloned a novel gene from rat cerebral cortex that coded for a membrane protein with the characteristics of a G protein-coupled receptor. Further studies revealed that these investigators, who were working on an unrelated problem, had actually cloned the gene for the rat brain cannabinoid receptor (Matsuda et al., 1990). This is a good example of an approach that is sometimes called reverse pharmacology, namely the cloning of a novel receptor gene, the identity of which must then be determined by more classical pharmacological methods. The CNS cannabinoid receptor is currently designated **CB$_1$.** An additional cannabinoid receptor, **CB$_2$,** was discovered later; however, this receptor will not be discussed further because it is found primarily in the immune system and does not seem to be expressed in the brain.

CB$_1$ receptors belong to the broad family of metabotropic receptors. The CB$_1$ receptors exert a variety of cellular effects, the most important of which involve inhibition of cyclic adenosine monophosphate (cAMP) formation, inhibition of voltage-sensitive Ca^{2+} channels, and activation of K$^+$ channel opening. Electron microscopy in conjunction with antibodies against the CB$_1$ receptor have been used to determine the location of these receptors within the synapse. In most instances, CB$_1$ receptors have been shown to exist on the axon terminal instead of the postsynaptic cell. By activating these presynaptic receptors, cannabinoids can inhibit the release of many different neurotransmitters including acetylcholine, dopamine, norepinephrine, serotonin, glutamate, and GABA (γ-aminobutyric acid) (Iversen, 2003).

A complete understanding of any receptor requires the development and testing of selective antagonists in addition to agonists at that receptor. Although THC, the classical cannabinoid receptor agonist, was isolated 40 years ago, it wasn't until 1994 that the first useful antagonist was introduced. This compound, called **SR 141716** (also known as **rimonabant**), was developed by a team of scientists at the French pharmaceutical firm Sanofi Recherche. Not only is SR 141716 a potent and selective antagonist at CB$_1$ receptors, it is also orally active, which means that it can readily be administered to humans. Later we shall see how this compound has helped researchers clarify the behavioral and physiological functions mediated by CB$_1$ receptors.

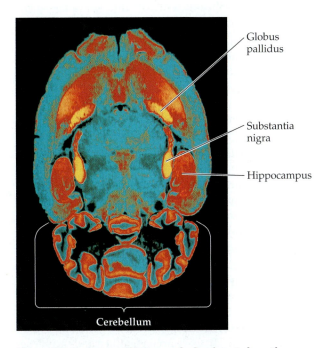

Globus pallidus

Substantia nigra

Hippocampus

Cerebellum

Figure 13.7 Autoradiogram of a horizontal section through a rat brain showing the distribution of CB$_1$ cannabinoid receptors. Color coding of receptor density: yellow > orange > red > blue. (Courtesy of Miles Herkenham, National Institute of Mental Health.)

Endocannabinoids are cannabinoid agonists synthesized by the brain

The discovery and characterization of cannabinoid receptors finally enabled pharmacologists to study the cellular mechanisms by which marijuana produces its behavioral effects. Yet why should our brain possess receptors for substances made by a plant? This situation is reminiscent of the quandary faced by opiate researchers when opioid receptors were first identified as mediating the actions of morphine, which comes from a poppy plant (see Chapter 10). Accordingly, the same assumption was made that there must be an endogenous neurotransmitter-like substance that acts on the newly discovered receptors. Within a few years, a group headed by Raphael Mechoulam, the same Israeli scientist involved in the discovery of THC almost 30 years earlier, announced that they had isolated a substance with cannabinoid-like activity from pig brain (Devane et al., 1992). Chemical analysis revealed the substance to be a lipid with a structure similar to that of arachidonic acid. The formal chemical name of this substance is **arachidonoyl ethanolamide,** but the researchers gave it the additional name **anandamide,** from the Indian Sanskrit word *ananda,* meaning "bringer of inner bliss and tranquility" (Felder and Glass, 1998, p. 186). Later studies demonstrated the existence of other arachidonic derivatives such as **2-arachidonoylglycerol (2-AG)** that also bind to and activate CB_1 receptors (Figure 13.8). Together, these substances have come to be known as **endocannabinoids,** meaning endogenous cannabinoids.

The endocannabinoids are generated from arachidonic acid, a fatty acid commonly found in membrane phospholipids. Unlike the classical neurotransmitters, however, they are too lipid soluble to be stored in vesicles since they would just pass right through the vesicle membrane. Thus researchers believe that endocannabinoids are made and released when needed. One mechanism for triggering endocannabinoid release is a rise in intracellular Ca^{2+} levels, which follows from the fact that some of the enzymes involved in the generation of these compounds are Ca^{2+} sensitive.

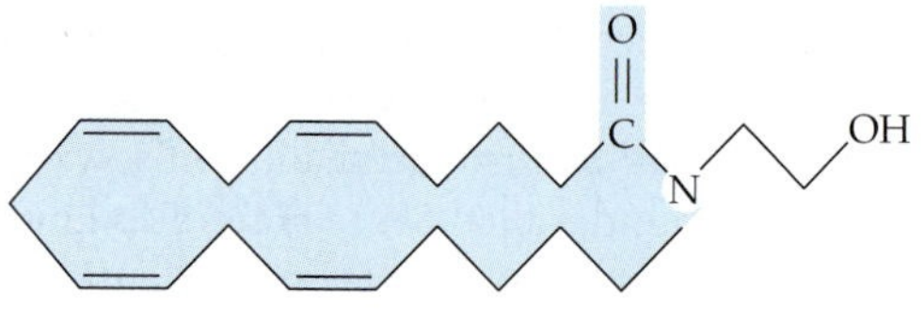

After being released, endocannabinoids are taken up from the extracellular fluid by a specific transport protein. This process appears to be important in terminating the biological action of these substances, as inhibition of the transporter by a drug called *N*-(4-hydroxyphenyl)arachidonylamide (AM 404) enhanced the effects of anandamide both in animals and in a cell culture system (Beltramo et al., 1997). Once inside the cell, endocannabinoids can be metabolized by several enzymes, the best known of which is **fatty acid amide hydrolase (FAAH).** Cravatt and colleagues (2001) demonstrated an important role for FAAH in anandamide breakdown by showing that genetic knockout mice lacking this enzyme had greatly elevated anandamide levels in the brain.

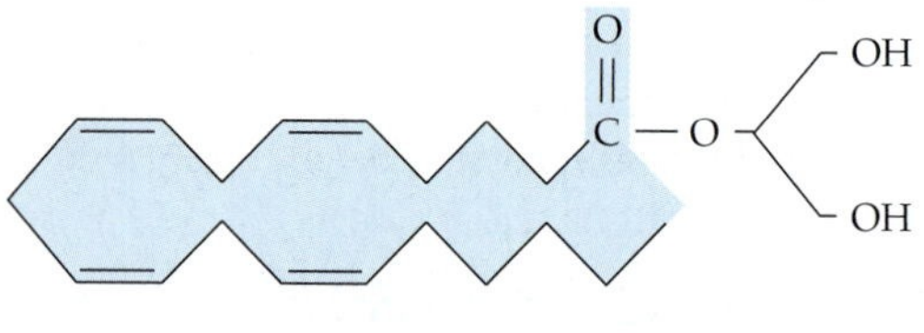

Based on the discovery that many cannabinoid receptors are localized presynaptically, we might suspect that endocannabinoids are often released from postsynaptic cells to act on nearby nerve terminals. When a signaling molecule carries information in the opposite direction from normal (that is, postsynaptic to presynaptic), it is called a **retrograde messenger.** One such retrograde messenger discussed in Chapter 3 is the gas nitric oxide. Researchers now hypothesize that endocannabinoids are also retrograde messengers at specific synapses in the hippocampus and cerebellum (Piomelli, 2003; Wilson and Nicoll, 2002). These substances are synthesized and released in response to depolarization of the postsynaptic cell due to the influx of Ca^{2+} through voltage-gated Ca^{2+} channels. Following their release, the endocannabinoids cross the synaptic cleft, activate CB_1 receptors on the nerve terminal, and inhibit Ca^{2+}-mediated neurotransmitter release from the terminal. In the hippocampus, for example, the endocannabinoids are generated by the pyramidal neurons, which are the principal output neurons of the hippocampus. The endocannabinoids diffuse to the nearby terminals of GABAergic interneurons that normally suppress the firing of the pyramidal cells. The resulting inhibition of GABA release temporarily permits the pyramidal cells to fire more rapidly (Figure 13.9). Given the widespread distribution of cannabinoid receptors in the brain, it is possible that many more examples of retrograde signaling by endocannabinoids will be discovered in future studies.

Anandamide

2-Arachidonylglycerol (2-AG)

Figure 13.8 Chemical structures of the endocannabinoids anandamide and 2-arachidonylglycerol (2-AG)

Section Summary

Significant progress has been made in our understanding of the mechanisms of cannabinoid action. Two cannabinoid receptors, CB_1 and CB_2, have been identified and their genes cloned. Only the CB_1 receptor is found in the brain, where it is expressed at a high density in the basal ganglia, cerebellum, hippocampus, and cerebral cortex. Cannabinoid receptors belong to the G protein-coupled receptor superfamily.

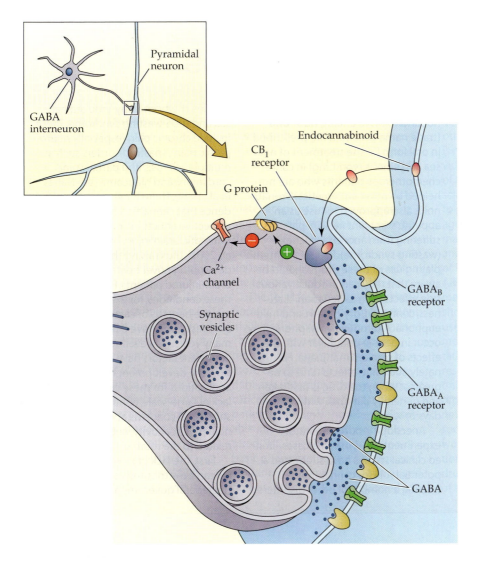

Figure 13.9 Retrograde signaling by endocannabinoids reduces GABAergic inhibition of pyramidal neurons in the hippocampus. Endocannabinoids released by the pyramidal neurons are thought to diffuse back to the nerve terminals of GABAergic interneurons that normally inhibit the pyramidal cells. The endocannabinoids activate presynaptic CB_1 receptors, which in turn suppress Ca^{2+} channel opening through a G protein-mediated mechanism. The resulting decrease in Ca^{2+} influx into the terminals reduces GABA release and allows the pyramidal cells to fire more readily.

Receptor activation can inhibit cAMP formation, inhibit voltage-sensitive Ca^{2+} channels, and activate K^+ channels. Many CB_1 receptors are located on axon terminals, where they act to inhibit the release of many different neurotransmitters. Studies on the function of CB_1 receptors have been aided by the development of a selective antagonist, SR 141716.

The brain synthesizes several substances, called endocannabinoids, that are neurotransmitter-like agonists at cannabinoid receptors. Anandamide was the first endo-

cannabinoid to be discovered, and it is the best characterized member of the group. Endocannabinoids are generated on demand from arachidonic acid and released from the cell by a process that does not involve synaptic vesicles. They are removed from the extracellular space by an uptake process and they are degraded by several enzymes, including fatty acid amide hydrolase. In certain populations of synapses in the hippocampus and cerebellum, endocannabinoids function as important retrograde messengers. They are released from postsynaptic cells in a Ca^{2+}-dependent manner, travel to nearby nerve terminals that carry CB_1 receptors, and inhibit neurotransmitter release from the terminals.

Acute Behavioral and Physiological Effects of Cannabinoids

Cannabis consumption produces a dose-dependent state of intoxication in humans

The earliest recorded clinical studies on the intoxicating properties of cannabis were performed by Moreau, the French physician mentioned earlier who introduced hashish to nineteenth-century Parisian literary society. Moreau, who is sometimes called the "father of psychopharmacology," became interested in the possible relationship between hashish intoxication and the characteristics of mental illness. Consequently, he and his students meticulously recorded their subjective experiences after consuming varying amounts of hashish. Due to the potency of their preparation, these individuals reported profound personality changes and perceptual distortions, even frank hallucinations.* Hallu-

*Moreau's work culminated in a book entitled *Du Hachich et de l'aliénation mentale (Hashish and Mental Alienation)*, major excerpts of which can be found in Nahas (1975).

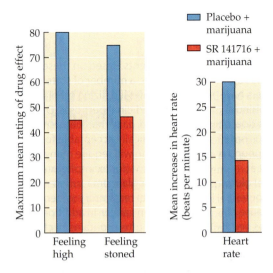

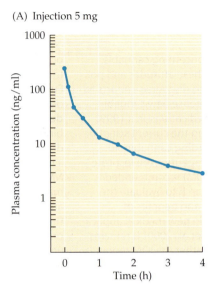

(A) Injection 5 mg

Figure 13.10 Reduction in the subjective and physiological effects of smoked marijuana by pretreatment with the CB$_1$ cannabinoid receptor antagonist SR 141716
Subjects received 90 mg of SR 141716 or a placebo orally, after which they smoked either an active (2.64% THC content) or a placebo marijuana cigarette. Self-reported subjective effects and heart rate were measured over the next 65 minutes. The data shown represent the maximum mean effects of the active marijuana cigarette in the presence or absence of the receptor antagonist. (After Huestis et al., 2001.)

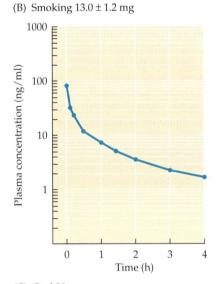

(B) Smoking 13.0 ± 1.2 mg

effects of actual cannabinoid administration, but it also elicited a more positive reaction when the subjects were given placebo instead.

Plasma THC levels peak much more rapidly following intravenous THC injection or marijuana smoking than after oral ingestion (Figure 13.11). Consequently, users reach the peak "high" sooner with the first two routes of administration. Nevertheless, users who are smoking marijuana do not reach this peak until some time after the cigarette has been finished. This delay means that the maximum level of intoxication occurs when plasma THC concentrations are already declining, suggesting that the brain and plasma THC concentrations are not yet equilibrated at the time when the plasma level is peaking. Another possible factor is the contribution of active THC metabolites (whose peak does not coincide with that of THC itself) to the psychoactive properties of marijuana.

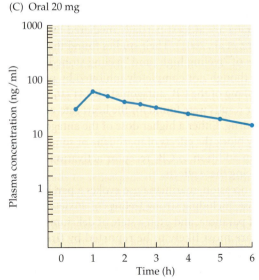

(C) Oral 20 mg

Figure 13.11 Time course of plasma THC concentrations as a function of route of THC administration. (After Agurell et al., 1986.)

Marijuana use can lead to deficits in cognition and psychomotor performance

Clinical accounts of marijuana intoxication have often noted deficits in thought processes and in verbal behavior. These may include illogical or disordered thinking, fragmented speech, and difficulty in remaining focused on a given topic of conversation. The early descriptive work later gave rise to quantitative experimental assessments of marijuana's effects on learning, memory, and other cognitive processes. Marijuana or THC administration does not appear to impair subjects' ability to recall simple, "real-world" information. On the other hand, drug-induced performance decrements have been noted for a variety of verbal, spatial, time estimation, and reaction time tasks. For example, Valerie Curran and her colleagues at University College of London recently demonstrated dose-dependent deficits in two different verbal memory tasks at 2 and 6 hours following oral THC administration to infrequent cannabis users (Curran et al., 2002; Figure 13.12). It is interesting to note that significant prior marijuana usage may reduce the adverse cognitive effects of acute marijuana exposure, which has led to the hypothesis that behavioral ("cognitive") tolerance develops in heavy marijuana smokers (Hart et al., 2001).

In addition to its deleterious effects on cognitive functioning, marijuana can also negatively influence psychomotor performance. This has been demonstrated not only under controlled laboratory conditions but also in real-world tasks such as driving an automobile. Low doses of marijuana generally produce relatively few psychomotor effects, particularly in subjects who have previous experience with the substance. However, even regular users show impaired psychomotor functioning under demanding task conditions (including driving) following a moderate or high dose of marijuana or when a low dose of marijuana is combined with alcohol. It is not surprising, then, that recent (shortly prior to driving) use of cannabis with or without alcohol has been implicated as a risk factor in automobile accidents (Ramaekers et al., 2004). Based on these results, it is prudent for individuals to avoid driving or other activities requiring operation of heavy machinery for a significant period of time after smoking marijuana.

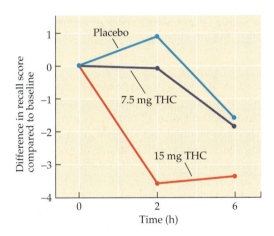

Figure 13.12 Oral THC produces a dose-dependent impairment in explicit memory. Subjects were tested on a variety of cognitive tasks either before or after oral consumption of 7.5 mg or 15 mg THC (dronabinol) or a placebo. Each subject was tested under all three conditions using a double-blind crossover design. Explicit memory, which involves the recall of specific information or events, was examined using a prose recall task in which the subjects listened to a short passage of prose and were then tested on their ability to remember details of the story 45 minutes later. Testing occurred 1 hour before drug or placebo administration (0 time point = baseline) and again at 2 and 6 hours after treatment. The results shown in the figure represent the differences in recall scores at the 2- and 6-hour time points compared to baseline. The high dose of THC led to a significant decrement in prose recall at 2 hours, which corresponds to the approximate time of peak plasma drug levels following oral administration. The lower dose of THC did not differ significantly from the placebo condition. (After Curran et al., 2002.)

Animals show a variety of behavioral and physiological responses to cannabinoid administration

Following the identification in 1964 of THC as the major biologically active constituent of cannabis, researchers began to examine the effects of this drug on unconditioned behaviors in various animal species. Such early studies quickly showed that THC produced motor impairment, catalepsy (lack of voluntary movement), hypothermia, and analgesia in mice and/or rats. At low doses, THC actually elicits a mixture of excitatory and depressant effects. At higher doses, the drug produces a more uniform motor depression and catalepsy, although hyperactivity may be seen initially as the plasma drug concentration rises. Most of the behavioral effects of THC are abolished in CB_1 receptor knockout mice, thereby confirming that these effects are mediated by CB_1 receptor activation (Ledent et al., 1999; Zimmer et al., 1999).

Given the adverse effects of cannabinoids on human cognitive function, researchers have sought to determine whether these drugs also influence learning or memory in laboratory animals. The results of this work indicate that cannabinoids disrupt memory in several different kinds of learning tasks, including the radial arm maze, Morris water maze, and delayed non-match-to-position task (see Chapter 4). Moreover, cannabinoids can impair radial arm maze performance when injected directly into the hippocampus (Lichtman et al., 1995), a structure that is critical for spatial learning and that is also rich in CB_1 receptors. Activation of these receptors decreases hippocampal synaptic transmission and interferes with long-term potentiation, an important form of synaptic plasticity thought to underlie at least some forms of learning (see Chapter 7). Thus it is possible that many of the acute cognitive effects of marijuana smoking in humans are attributable to actions of THC within the hippocampus.

The discovery of anandamide and the other endocannabinoids has raised interesting questions about whether this signaling system might be involved in the normal regulation of the same behavioral and physiological functions influenced by exogenous cannabinoids such as THC. One way to address this question is to examine the effects of administering the antagonist SR 141716 in the absence of an exogenous cannabinoid agonist. Several studies using this approach reported cannabinoid antagonist-induced **hyperalgesia** (increased pain sensitivity), thereby raising the possibility that release of endocannabinoids may decrease responsiveness to certain types of painful stimuli (Calignano et al., 1998;

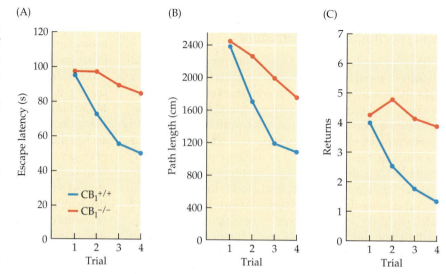

Figure 13.13 CB$_1$ receptor knockout mice show impaired reversal learning in the Morris water maze. Knockout (CB$_1^{-/-}$) and wild-type (CB$_1^{+/+}$) mice were first trained to swim to a hidden platform in the Morris water maze. The groups did not differ with respect to acquisition of this task. Then a reversal procedure was instituted in which the platform was moved to the opposite side of the tank. The figure shows the results obtained over four trials under reversal conditions. The CB$_1^{-/-}$ mice were significantly impaired in learning the new platform location as shown by (A) longer latencies to reach the platform, (B) greater swimming path lengths, and (C) a greater number of returns to the previous location of the hidden platform. (After Varvel and Lichtman, 2002.)

Richardson et al., 1998). SR 141716 administration also reduces food consumption in both experimental animals and human subjects, suggesting a role for endogenous cannabinoids in provoking eating behavior (Black, 2004). These findings help explain why our appetite is stimulated by exposure to exogenous cannabinoids either through smoked marijuana or through orally ingested THC. They have also led to the clinical testing of SR 141716 as a possible antiobesity agent. If the clinical trials show a positive outcome, then this compound will join a growing list of novel agents under development to treat the obesity problem.

Potential endocannabinoid involvement in learning and memory has been investigated by comparing the performance of CB$_1$ knockout mice to their wild-type counterparts. Particularly intriguing are two recent papers suggesting that endocannabinoids may participate in processes of forgetting or extinction. First, Varvel and Lichtman (2002) found that whereas CB$_1$ knockout mice exhibited normal acquisition of a Morris water maze task, the mice performed extremely poorly in a reversal phase in which the hidden platform was moved to the opposite side of the tank. The animals persisted in returning to the original platform location, which could be interpreted as a deficit in eliminating the memory of their previously learned response (Figure 13.13A–C). The second study, performed by Marsicano and colleagues (2002), examined the possible involvement of endocannabinoids in acquisition and extinction of an auditory fear-con-

ditioning task in mice. In this type of task, an auditory stimulus such as a tone is paired with foot shock during the acquisition (conditioning) phase. As a result, the tone becomes a conditioned fear stimulus that elicits freezing behavior, which is the typical response of mice and rats to a fearful situation. Extinction of conditioned fear can be examined by conducting repeated trials in which the tone alone is presented. Freezing behavior should decrease under these conditions if extinction mechanisms are operating properly. Marsicano et al. found that the acquisition of conditioned fear was normal in CB$_1$ knockout mice. However, extinction of the fear response was impaired not only in the knockout mice but also in wild-type mice treated with SR 141716. Moreover, presentation of the conditioned stimulus stimulated endocannabinoid release in the basolateral amygdala, a brain area thought to be involved in the extinction of aversively motivated responses. Although more work needs to be done before definite conclusions can be drawn, the results of these two studies support a significant role for endocannabinoids in extinction or forgetting.

Cannabinoids are reinforcing to both humans and animals

Cannabinoids are obviously reinforcing to users who smoke marijuana recreationally or consume cannabis by other means. However, cannabinoid reinforcement in humans has also been studied under controlled laboratory conditions. For example, Chait and Zacny (1992) found that regular marijuana users could discriminate THC-containing marijuana cigarettes from placebo cigarettes containing no THC, and that all subjects preferred the marijuana with THC when given a choice. In the same study, pure THC taken orally in capsule form was also preferred over a placebo. Chait and Burke (1994) subsequently related marijuana preference to THC content, as users reliably selected marijuana with a 1.95% THC content over marijuana containing only 0.63% THC.

As we have seen in earlier chapters, the rewarding and reinforcing properties of drugs can also be studied in animals using the techniques of drug-induced place conditioning and intravenous drug self-administration. Although most drugs that are abused by humans are rewarding or reinforcing in these experimental paradigms, cannabinoids were thought to be among the exceptions to this general principle until fairly recently. However, it now appears that the early negative studies were compromised by several factors, particularly the presence of aversive reactions that can result from initial cannabinoid exposure, particularly at high doses.

In one set of studies conducted by researchers at the National Institute on Drug Abuse, squirrel monkeys were shown to reliably self-administer THC (Justinova et al., 2003; Tanda et al., 2000). The key factor in these experiments was the use of low drug doses that are within the range of estimated human THC intake from a single puff on a typical marijuana cigarette (Figure 13.14). Lever pressing for THC was completely blocked by pretreatment with SR 141716,

indicating that the reinforcing effect was dependent on CB$_1$ receptor activation. Other studies have also found that THC can produce a conditioned place preference in mice (Valjent and Maldonado, 2000), and that rats and mice will self-administer low doses of the synthetic CB$_1$ receptor agonist WIN 55,212-2 (Fattore et al., 2001; Martellotta et al., 1998). It is interesting to note that in the place-conditioning study, the rewarding properties of THC could be demonstrated only in mice that had been preexposed once to the drug in their home cage. This was interpreted by the authors to mean that first exposure to THC involves aversive responses that mask its rewarding effects. Preexposure outside of the experimental apparatus presumably reduces the occurrence of these responses when the THC is subsequently administered during the conditioning trials.

Now that cannabinoids have been shown to be reinforcing under the appropriate conditions, researchers have begun to investigate the mechanisms underlying the reinforcing effects. One factor in cannabinoid reinforcement may be activation of the mesolimbic dopamine (DA) system, as cannabinoids have been found to stimulate the firing of DA neurons in the ventral tegmental area (VTA) and to enhance DA release in the nucleus accumbens. More surprisingly, there is growing evidence for close interactions between the cannabinoid and opioid systems that play a critical role in both cannabinoid and opioid reward and reinforcement. For example, systemic administration of the general opioid receptor antagonist naltrexone reduced THC self-administration in squirrel monkeys (Justinova et al., 2004). Furthermore, the conditioned place preference produced by a low dose of THC was abolished in μ-opioid receptor knockout mice, whereas the conditioned place aversion produced by a higher THC dose was abolished in mutant mice lacking κ-opioid receptors (Ghozland et al., 2002). Finally, microinfusion of the μ$_1$-opioid receptor antagonist naloxonazine directly into the VTA of rats blocked not only heroin-induced DA release in the nucleus accumbens but also DA release associated with THC administration (Tanda et al., 1997). Together, these findings suggest that μ-opioid receptors, particularly of the μ$_1$ subtype, mediate the rewarding and reinforcing effects of cannabinoids, whereas the aversive effects may be due to κ-opioid receptor activation. Nevertheless, we must be cautious in extrapolating the results to human users, as Haney and coworkers (2003) recently reported that the opioid antagonist naltrexone increased rather than decreased the positive subjective effects of oral THC in regular heavy marijuana smokers.

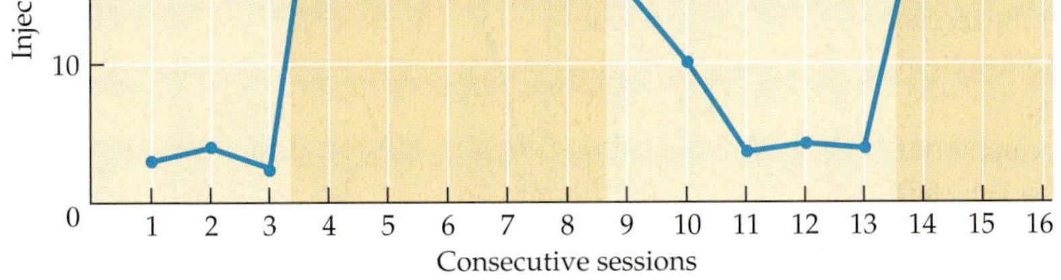

Figure 13.14 Acquisition of THC self-administration by squirrel monkeys Monkeys were initially trained in drug self-administration on a fixed-ratio (FR) 10 schedule using cocaine as the reinforcer (not shown). They were then switched to saline, which led to a nearly complete elimination of lever-pressing behavior. When THC (2.0 μg/kg/injection) was substituted for saline, lever pressing immediately increased to an amount sufficient to deliver approximately 30 drug injections per 1-hour session. Substitution with the vehicle again reduced operant responding until the active drug was made available once again. (After Tanda et al., 2000.)

This section has focused on the rewarding and reinforcing properties of cannabinoids themselves. However, over the past few years a number of studies have examined the effects of either genetic deletion of CB_1 receptors or administration of the cannabinoid antagonist SR 141716 on responses to *other* drugs of abuse. The results of these studies suggest that the endocannabinoid system may play a significant role in the processes of reinforcement, dependence, and/or relapse for a number of other drugs, including ethanol (Naassila et al., 2004; Racz et al., 2003), opioids (De Vries et al., 2003; Ledent et al., 1999; Navarro et al., 2001), cocaine (De Vries et al., 2001), and nicotine (Castañé et al., 2002). This "cross-talk" between the endocannabinoid system and the neurochemical systems associated with other drugs of abuse has implications not only for our understanding of the cellular mechanisms underlying drug addiction but also for the development of novel treatment approaches.

Section Summary

The subjective characteristics of cannabis intoxication include feelings of euphoria, disinhibition, relaxation, altered sensations, and increased appetite. The euphoric effects produced by smoking marijuana appear to be mediated at least partly by CB_1 receptors. Psychopathological reactions can occur, particularly at high doses or in the case of inexperienced users. Cannabis adversely affects memory, psychomotor performance, and other cognitive functions. However, there are accepted therapeutic uses for orally administered dronabinol (synthetic THC) and the THC analog nabilone in treating nausea and vomiting in cancer chemotherapy patients as well as the wasting syndrome in AIDS sufferers.

Laboratory animals have also been used in the study of cannabinoid pharmacology. In rodents, THC produces changes in motor activity (which can involve both excitatory and depressant components), catalepsy, hypothermia, and analgesia. Cannabinoids disrupt memory in several kinds of learning tasks, an effect thought to be related to activation of CB_1 receptors in the hippocampus. Studies involving either SR 141716 administration or genetic deletion of CB_1 receptors suggest an involvement of the endocannabinoid system in pain modulation and in extinction or forgetting.

Although early studies failed to demonstrate cannabinoid reward or reinforcement, more recent work has shown that THC can support self-administration in squirrel monkeys and formation of a conditioned place preference in mice. Rats and mice will also self-administer low doses of the synthetic CB_1 agonist WIN 55,212-2. Cannabinoid reinforcement has been shown to depend on both CB_1 receptor and μ-opioid receptor activation. Dopamine may also be involved, since cannabinoids stimulate the firing of DA neurons in the VTA and enhance DA release in the nucleus accumbens.

Cannabis Abuse and the Effects of Chronic Cannabis Exposure

Marijuana is the most widely used illicit drug in the United States. According to the 2002 National Household Survey on Drug Use and Health, more than 14 million Americans aged 12 or older were current marijuana users at the time of the survey (Substance Abuse and Mental Health Services Administration, 2003). Frequency of use is very high in some cases, with an estimated 3 million individuals using marijuana on a daily or near daily basis (≥ 300 days) during the year surveyed. Trends in the initiation of drug use are also important for several reasons, including potential health implications as well as social policy decisions. Thus it is noteworthy that the number of new marijuana users per year has remained fairly steady from 1995 to 2001, the most recent year reported for drug use initiation. These findings suggest that government efforts to dissuade young people from trying marijuana have not been particularly successful.

Cannabis use typically begins in adolescence and peaks during young adulthood

Initial marijuana use typically occurs in adolescence. If an individual has not yet tried marijuana by his or her mid-twenties, he or she is unlikely to begin at a later age. This is shown in Figure 13.15, which is derived from a longitudinal study of 976 subjects drawn from upstate New York. In this cohort, the peak age for initiating marijuana use was 17, although a few children began as early 10 or 11 years of age. It is also the case that the prevalence of illicit drug use (including marijuana) declines with age. In the 2002 National Household Survey, for example, the percentage of responders who were current users of at least one illicit drug (typically marijuana) was 22.5% at 18 to 20 years of age, 8.8% at 30 to 34 years of age, and only 0.8% at 65 years or older.

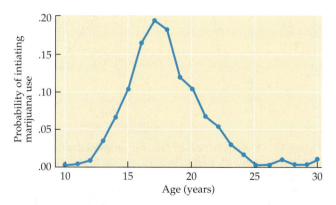

Figure 13.15 Probability of initiating marijuana use as a function of age (After Brooks et al., 1999.)

Most adolescents have prior experience with alcohol and/or cigarettes before trying marijuana. For this reason, alcohol and tobacco have been hypothesized as "gateway" drugs to marijuana use. Some evidence exists that marijuana, in turn, may serve as a gateway to other illicit drugs (e.g., cocaine) or to prescribed psychoactive drugs such as sedatives. However, it is difficult to determine whether marijuana actually facilitates the progression to "hard drugs" or whether certain users are already predisposed to seek out these more dangerous substances due to some combination of personality traits, life circumstances, or other factors independent of their exposure to marijuana (see the discussion of the gateway theory in Chapter 8).

A further issue to consider is the progression from initial to regular (that is, daily or near daily) marijuana use. Risk factors in the development of heavy marijuana use by adolescents include emotional problems in the family, heavy drug use in the household and/or by peers, dislike of school and poor school performance, and an early age of first use of marijuana (Gruber and Pope, 2002). On the other hand, rates of marijuana use tend to be lower among adolescents from stable families with close parental supervision, as well as those who have strong career aspirations or assume adult responsibilities such as marriage and parenthood. Another important factor may be the degree to which the young person experiences positive reactions to his or her early use of cannabis. Researchers in New Zealand examined the relationship between the subjective responses to early cannabis use at 14 to 16 years of age and the likelihood of becoming cannabis-dependent by the age of 21, according to criteria of the *Diagnostic and Statistical Manual of Mental Illness (DSM-IV)* (Fergusson et al., 2003b). Individuals who reported more positive responses (that is, feeling happy, feeling relaxed, laughing a lot, doing silly things, or getting very "high") to their early experience with cannabis were at greater risk of later dependence than those who reported fewer of these positive reactions.

Tolerance and dependence can develop from chronic cannabinoid exposure

For many drugs of abuse, regular heavy use leads to powerful tolerance as well as physical and/or psychological dependence. Is this also the case for marijuana? We will first consider studies of cannabinoid tolerance in humans and animals.

Tolerance The human literature on cannabis tolerance is somewhat variable. Although some investigators have observed tolerance following repeated administration of marijuana or pure THC to subjects (Compton et al., 1990), there are also reports that the "high" produced by a given dose of THC is similar in heavy or frequent marijuana users compared to light or infrequent users (Kirk and de Wit, 1999; Lindgren et al., 1981). It appears that further studies

are needed to determine the conditions under which cannabinoid tolerance occurs in humans.

In contrast to the results just described, there are consistent findings over many years showing that animals exposed repeatedly to THC develop a profound tolerance to the drug's behavioral and physiological effects. This tolerance appears to be largely pharmacodynamic in nature. Research by Breivogel and coworkers (1999) found that rats given daily THC injections (10 mg/kg) over a 3-week period showed gradual reductions both in regional CB_1 receptor density and in cannabinoid agonist-mediated receptor activation (Figure 13.16). In some brain areas, the cannabinoid receptors were almost entirely desensitized following 3 weeks of THC exposure.

Dependence and withdrawal During the 1990s, investigators began to recognize the existence of cannabis dependence in some users. Such dependence is manifested as a difficulty in stopping one's use, a craving for marijuana, and unpleasant withdrawal symptoms that are triggered by abstinence. Controlled studies of abstinence in long-term heavy marijuana users have reported a number of withdrawal symptoms including irritability, increased anxiety, depressed mood, sleep disturbances, heightened aggressiveness, and decreased appetite (Budney et al., 2003; Kouri et al., 1999; Kouri and Pope, 2000). These withdrawal symptoms resemble those seen with several other drugs of abuse, most notably nicotine. Overall symptomatology is greatest during the first 1 to 2 weeks of withdrawal (Figure 13.17), but some symptoms may persist for a month or longer.

Early experimental studies in which animals were administered THC chronically and then examined after the treatment was stopped found few if any signs of withdrawal. Although these results may seem to be at odds with reports of an abstinence syndrome in humans, researchers recognized that the absence of withdrawal symptoms might have been due to THC's long elimination half-life, which causes the cannabinoid receptors to remain partially occupied for a significant period of time even after termination of drug treatment. Once the CB_1 receptor antagonist SR 141716 was developed, it could be used to test for dependence and withdrawal, since administration of the antagonist would abruptly block the receptors despite the continued presence of THC in the animal. In two initial studies using this approach, which is called **precipitated withdrawal,** rats were given chronic THC either by twice-daily injections or by infusion, and they were then challenged with SR 141716 at the same time that THC administration was terminated. The challenged animals displayed an abstinence syndrome characterized by wet-dog shakes, increased grooming behaviors (facial rubbing, licking, and scratching), and other symptoms of hyperactivity (Aceto et al., 1996; Tsou et al., 1995). These and other studies have convincingly shown that chronic THC treatment produces physical dependence in animals,

Figure 13.16 Desensitization of cannabinoid receptors produced by chronic THC exposure Rats were treated daily with 10 mg/kg THC or vehicle for 3 to 21 days, after which their brains were obtained and horizontal sections were prepared for autoradiography. Some sections were incubated with the synthetic cannabinoid agonist [³H]WIN 55,212-2 to determine the density of cannabinoid receptors in different brain areas. Other sections were incubated with [³⁵S]GTPγS in the presence of unlabeled WIN 55,212-2. This procedure allows the measurement of receptor-mediated G protein activation in each area. The autoradiograms show that chronic THC administration led to progressive reductions in both receptor density (lower sections) and receptor-mediated G protein activation (upper sections) throughout the brain. (Images courtesy of Steven Childers.)

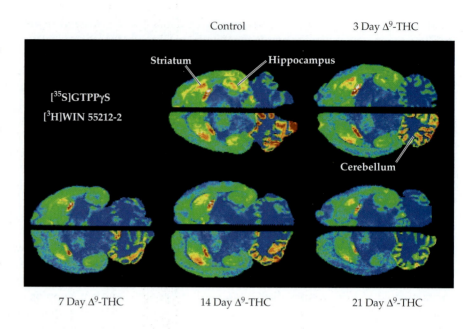

although such dependence generally requires antagonist treatment to provoke the withdrawal symptoms.

The possible neurochemical basis for a marijuana abstinence syndrome has been investigated using the precipitated withdrawal model in cannabinoid-dependent rats. Using this model, researchers have demonstrated decreased DA cell firing in the VTA (Diana et al., 1998) and increased corticotropin-releasing factor (CRF) release in the central nucleus of the amygdala (de Fonseca et al., 1997). Together, these alterations could contribute to the mood reduction, irritability, and stress experienced by dependent cannabis users during periods of abstinence. Moreover, similar responses have been reported to occur during withdrawal from cocaine, alcohol, and opiates, thereby linking cannabinoids with substances generally considered to have greater abuse potential.

Treatment of cannabis dependence The 2002 National Household Survey estimated that approximately 4.3 million people were suffering from cannabis abuse or dependence at that time (Substance Abuse and Mental Health Services Administration, 2003). This figure represents a 23% increase over the previous year's survey results, which indicates a growing need for treatment services. Dependent marijuana users seeking treatment are typically entered into an outpatient program that may involve cognitive behavior therapy, relapse prevention training, and/or motivational enhancement therapy* (McRae et al., 2003). These approaches can also be combined with an incentive program in which participants who submit cannabinoid-negative urine samples earn vouchers redeemable for various goods and services (Budney et al., 2000). Although these different treatment programs have met with some success, patients are highly vulnerable to relapse even after an initial period of abstinence (Figure 13.18; Moore and Budney, 2003). Thus, marijuana appears to be similar to other drugs of abuse with regard to the difficulty in achieving long-term treatment success in dependent individuals.

The idea of pharmacotherapy for cannabis dependence is still relatively new. Several compounds that have been tested,

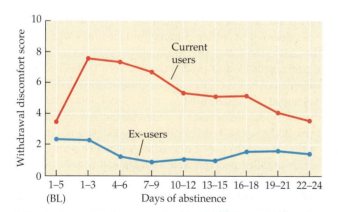

Figure 13.17 Time course of overall withdrawal discomfort in heavy marijuana users undergoing abstinence Current marijuana users were compared to ex-users on a battery of 15 possible self-reported withdrawal symptoms over a 5-day baseline period (BL) during which marijuana use was permitted and then during a 45-day period of abstinence. Data shown represent the mean composite withdrawal scores (up to a possible maximum of 36) during baseline and the first 24 days of abstinence. (After Budney et al., 2003.)

---

*Motivational enhancement therapy is a type of psychotherapy that seeks to elicit a desire for behavioral change on the part of the patient.

including the antidepressants bupropion and nefazadone and the mood stabilizer divalproex (an antiepileptic medication also used to treat bipolar disorder), have shown only a limited ability, if any, to reduce marijuana withdrawal symptoms or to promote abstinence. On the other hand, Haney et al. (2004) recently reported that oral THC could reduce marijuana craving and other withdrawal symptoms in heavy users who were undergoing abstinence. These results raise the possibility that oral THC treatment could be useful in assisting cannabis-dependent patients to get through the initial period of withdrawal, although long-term abstinence might still be difficult to achieve.

Chronic cannabis use may lead to adverse behavioral and health effects

It is not unusual for dedicated cannabis users to consume the drug on a regular, even daily, basis for many years. Concern naturally has arisen over whether such lengthy periods of chronic drug exposure might lead to adverse psychological or physiological effects. Evidence for such effects is discussed in this final section of the chapter.

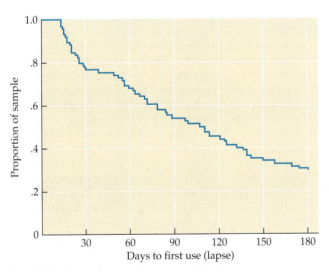

Figure 13.18 Time to first marijuana use following 2 weeks of abstinence in patients undergoing outpatient treatment for marijuana dependence. Patients received one of the following four different treatments: motivational enhancement therapy, motivational enhancement combined with behavioral coping-skills training (MBT), MBT plus a voucher-based program with regular urine screening, and the voucher program alone. All treatment programs were carried out for 14 weeks. Forty-six percent of the patients failed to achieve at least 2 weeks of continuous abstinence, and their data are not shown. The figure illustrates the proportion of the remaining patients who had not yet lapsed (used marijuana for the first time) as a function of time since their initial 2-week abstinence period. Note the steady decrease in the line as more and more patients suffered a lapse in their attempt to remain abstinent. (After Moore and Budney, 2003.)

Psychological and neurological effects   Survey studies indicate that the amount of cannabis use by young people is inversely related to educational performance. That is, greater use is associated with poorer grades, more negative attitudes about school, and increased absenteeism (Lynskey and Hall, 2000). Furthermore, prospective longitudinal studies suggest that regular cannabis use beginning relatively early in life is a significant risk factor for poor performance in school and even dropping out (Fergusson et al., 2003a; Lynskey et al., 2003).

At the present time, we do not know whether there is a causal relationship between amount of cannabis use and educational achievement. Even if there is, the direction of causation would still need to be established. Does early cannabis use cause a lack of success in school, or does a lack of success early in one's academic career cause an increase in cannabis use? One hypothesis is that heavy cannabis use leads to persistent cognitive deficits, thereby impairing school performance. The existence of such impairment is currently a matter of controversy (Box 13.2). Another possibility involves drug-related motivational changes that would have a negative impact on performance in the classroom. Indeed, research going back more than 30 years has found evidence for apathy, aimlessness, loss of achievement motivation, lack of long-range planning, and decreased productivity in chronic marijuana users. Together, these symptoms have been termed the **amotivational syndrome** (Lynskey and Hall, 2000). We cannot rule out the possibility that some users experience a loss of drive and achievement motivation as a result of chronic, heavy exposure to cannabis. However, one could argue just as plausibly that such personality characteristics are a cause, rather than a consequence, of adopting a marijuana-centered lifestyle.

It is possible that students who use cannabis heavily over a long period of time could perform poorly in school due to the cognitive impairment described in Box 13.2. However, at this time there is little evidence linking the cognitive deficits measured under laboratory conditions to the actual school performance of cannabis users. Instead, researchers have hypothesized that the social context surrounding heavy cannabis use at a relatively early age promotes the rejection of mainstream social values such as educational achievement in favor of a more unconventional lifestyle (Fergusson et al., 2003a; Lynskey et al., 2003). This hypothesis could explain why heavy users perform poorly in school without postulating a direct effect of cannabis on their performance.

Health effects   In considering the potential health consequences of cannabis use, there is both good and bad news. The good news is that there is no published report of anyone dying as a result of cannabis overdose. This means that the use of this substance has a margin of safety that is lacking with many other substances of abuse such as heroin, cocaine, and sedative–hypnotic drugs. The bad news is that the lack of fatal overdosing does not mean that cannabis use, particularly in large amounts or for long periods of time, is without risk.

The Cutting Edge

Does Chronic Cannabis Use Cause Persistent Cognitive Deficits?

Earlier in this chapter we learned that memory and other cognitive functions are impaired shortly after smoking marijuana. Few people, however, smoke marijuana while they're at work, in class, or at other times when a high level of functioning is required. If marijuana is used only during recreational times (for example, evenings and weekends) and drug-related cognitive deficits do not outlast the period of use, then one could argue that such deficits are harmless. On the other hand, is it possible that heavy recreational use over a long period of time somehow compromises brain function such that cognitive problems persist even after drug use is stopped?

The question of residual cognitive deficits from heavy marijuana use is a controversial one. Research in this area has suffered from two major limitations: (1) possible preexisting differences in cognitive functioning between the users and control subjects and (2) the potential influence on test performance of either ongoing drug effects due to the slow rate of THC elimination or withdrawal symptoms associated with abstinence. Some studies have attempted to control the first problem either by matching the groups in terms of ver-

bal IQ or by controlling statistically for IQ differences between the groups. These approaches assume that IQ is relatively unaffected by marijuana use and is therefore a reasonable indicator of cognitive function prior to the beginning of such use. The second problem can be addressed either by comparing the performance of subjects at different times during withdrawal or by studying ex-users who have been abstinent for a long period of time.

Some of the best work in this area has been carried out by two research groups, one headed by Harrison Pope and the other by Nadia Solowij. Interestingly, both groups have reported cognitive deficits in long-term heavy marijuana users subjected to standard neuropsychological tests of learning, memory, and attention (Pope et al., 2001a, 2001b; Solowij et al., 2002). These effects were present for at least 1 day and possibly up to a week following the most recent drug exposure, suggesting that heavy marijuana users can experience some performance decrements that carry over beyond the periods of actual use. However, there is a major disagreement about the persistence of such decrements. Pope and his coworkers (2001a) found no differences between the heavy users and control subjects following 28 days of abstinence. Consequently, these investigators concluded that the cognitive deficits associated with heavy marijuana use are linked to recent exposure to the substance and are reversible over time. Contrasting results were

obtained by Solowij (1998) in an earlier study that examined attentional performance and event-related potentials (ERPs) in current cannabis users, former users who had used regularly for at least 5 years but who had been abstinent for an average of 2 years, and control subjects. ERPs are electrophysiological responses of the brain that are time-locked to a specific sensory stimulus such as a tone and that can provide insight into sensory processing and attention. On both the behavioral and ERP measures, control subjects showed the best results, current users showed the worst results, and former users were in-between. Furthermore, Solowij and her colleagues have also found evidence for a relationship between the duration of cannabis use and the degree of cognitive impairment (Solowij, 1998; Solowij et al., 2002). Taken together, these results have led them to hypothesize that heavy, long-term cannabis use leads to progressive deficits in attentional function that only partially recover, even after a significant period of abstinence.

At the present time, we cannot determine who is right about the possibility of lingering effects of long-term marijuana use that might persist for months, if not years. Given the difficulties inherent in trying to answer this question, the current uncertainty may not be resolved any time soon. In the meantime, marijuana users should be aware that heavy, long-term use has been associated with at least temporary deficits in learning, memory, and attention.

Because cannabis is almost always consumed by smoking, the possibility of lung damage is one obvious area of concern. Although marijuana joints and tobacco cigarettes contain different psychoactive ingredients (cannabinoids vs. nicotine), the smoke they produce has the same kinds of irritants and carcinogens. Tar from cannabis smoke actually contains higher concentrations of certain carcinogens known as benzanthracenes and benzpyrenes. Even so, one might think that marijuana smoking is not harmful because users typically smoke only one or a few joints a day, compared to the one or more packs of cigarettes smoked by regular tobacco users. Unfortunately, it appears that the amounts of tar and carbon monoxide taken in *per cigarette* are much greater for marijuana joints than for tobacco cigarettes (Wu et al.,

1988). It is not surprising, therefore, that regular marijuana smoking is associated with an increased risk for bronchitis, the symptoms of which are chronic cough and phlegm production. Furthermore, microscopic examination of bronchial biopsies from marijuana users has revealed several kinds of cellular abnormalities, some of which are considered precancerous (Tashkin et al., 2002). Researchers have not yet established a relationship between long-term marijuana smoking and lung cancer. Nevertheless, heavy use has definite risks for the respiratory system, and future studies may show that development of lung cancer is one such risk.

Evidence has also been accumulating that cannabinoids influence the immune system. Numerous laboratory studies have demonstrated that THC can suppress immune function and impair an organism's resistance to bacterial and viral infections (Cabral and Pettit, 1998). We don't yet know, however, whether marijuana use leads to an increased incidence of infectious disease under real-life conditions.

Lastly, there has been some debate in the literature about the effects of cannabis on reproductive function. For example, marijuana smoking by women can acutely suppress the release of luteinizing hormone (LH), an important reproductive hormone secreted by the pituitary gland. But this effect was not observed in regular users, suggesting that tolerance may develop to this action of the drug. Studies of male marijuana users in a controlled inpatient setting found significant reductions in sperm counts. However, this occurred under conditions of extremely heavy use (10 joints per day for 4 weeks), and the effect dissipated within 3 to 4 weeks of abstention from marijuana (see Smith and Asch, 1987). Thus there is no convincing evidence at this time of reproductive problems stemming from cannabis use.

Section Summary

Marijuana is the most heavily used illicit drug in the United States. Initial exposure to marijuana usually occurs during adolescence, after the individual has already had experience with alcohol and/or cigarettes. Some investigators have hypothesized that alcohol and tobacco are "gateway" drugs to marijuana, which then serves as a potential gateway to other illicit drugs. However, it is difficult to determine whether marijuana actually facilitates the progression to these more dangerous substances.

In humans, tolerance may occur following prolonged consumption of large amounts of marijuana or purified THC, but current findings are inconsistent. In contrast, there is growing evidence for the occurrence of cannabis dependence and withdrawal in heavy users. Withdrawal symptoms include heightened irritability, anxiety, aggressiveness, depressed mood state, sleep disturbances, reduced appetite, and craving for marijuana.

Chronic THC exposure in laboratory animals causes the development of behavioral and physiological tolerance. This is related to a gradual down-regulation and desensitization of brain CB_1 receptors. Animals chronically exposed to cannabinoids also develop physical dependence, although such dependence can only be demonstrated by means of precipitated withdrawal using SR 141716. Neurochemical studies of cannabinoid-dependent rats indicate that reduced DA cell firing and increased CRF release could contribute to some of the symptoms of cannabis withdrawal in human users.

The increasing prevalence of cannabis dependence has led to a growth in treatment programs. Some success has been achieved with various kinds of psychotherapeutic interventions, and additional improvement in outcome has been reported by adding a voucher-based incentive program to the standard treatment approach. Nevertheless, most dependent individuals find it difficult to maintain long-term abstinence. Pharmacotherapeutic approaches to the treatment of cannabis dependence are now being investigated. Oral THC has been shown to reduce withdrawal symptoms in heavy marijuana users, but this approach has not yet been incorporated into any established treatment programs.

Concerns have been raised over possible adverse consequences of chronic cannabis consumption. There is a negative association between the amount of cannabis use by young people and their educational performance, although it is not yet known whether this association is causal. It is possible that heavy cannabis use can produce persistent cognitive deficits and/or an amotivational syndrome characterized by apathy, loss of achievement motivation, and decreased productivity. Long-term use has been associated with at least temporary decrements in cognitive function, although the degree of persistence of these effects has been disputed. Because there is also little evidence in favor of an amotivational syndrome, researchers currently favor the hypothesis that early cannabis use is linked to the adoption of an unconventional lifestyle that devalues educational striving and achievement. Finally, there are health risks associated with marijuana smoking that involve respiratory problems along with possible deleterious effects on immune function.

Recommended Readings

Iverson, L. L. (2000). *The Science of Marijuana*. Oxford University Press, New York.

Solowij, N. (1998). *Cannabis and Cognitive Functioning*. Cambridge University Press, Cambridge.

Sullivan, J. M. (2000). Cellular and molecular mechanisms underlying learning and memory impairments produced by cannabinoids. *Learn. Mem.*, (7), 132–139.

Tanda, G., and Goldberg, S. R. (2003). Cannabinoids: Reward, dependence, and underlying neurochemical mechanisms—a review of recent preclinical data. *Psychopharmacology*, (169), 115–134.

14 Hallucinogens, PCP, and Ketamine

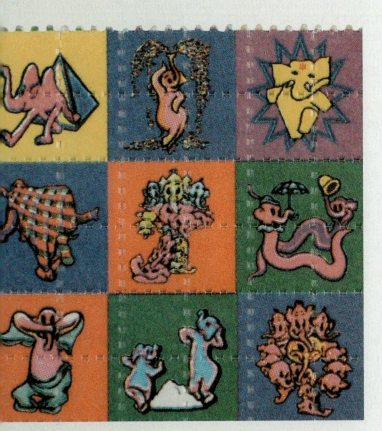

A typical "blotter" used to disseminate LSD.

Rob is invited to go dancing at a club on Saturday night. While at the club, a friend gives him a small, square piece of paper with a cartoonish-looking character inscribed on it. The friend tells Rob that if he swallows the paper he'll have an interesting experience. He does as suggested, but nothing happens for a while. After about 45 minutes, however, Rob begins to experience strange visual sensations. The colors of his girlfriend's dress become more vivid. He can see moving patterns when he closes his eyes. As time goes on, Rob's reactions become more intense. Everyday objects like tables and chairs take on grotesque forms. People's bodies become distorted and misshapen. Rob becomes frightened, because he doesn't know what's happening to him. The effects finally wear off after a number of hours, leaving Rob confused and exhausted.

In reading this passage, you probably recognized that Rob was given LSD by his friend. In his naiveté, Rob didn't know what to expect when he ate the drug-laced piece of paper. As we will see in the first section of this chapter, hallucinogenic substances like LSD have powerful effects on perceptual and conscious processes. Where do these substances come from, and how do they produce their effects? We will also cover PCP and ketamine, two other drugs also known for their mind-altering properties but that act through a different neurochemical mechanism than LSD.

Hallucinogenic Drugs

Some substances are valued primarily for the unusual perceptual and cognitive distortions they produce. Users may find such distortions novel, stimulating, or even spiritually uplifting. Among the substances categorized in this way are **lysergic acid diethylamide (LSD), mescaline, psilocybin, dimethyltryptamine (DMT), and 5-methoxy-dimethyltryptamine (5-MeO-DMT).** Over the years, many different names have been given to this drug class, including **psychotomimetic** (psychosis-mimicking), **psychedelic** (mind-opening), and **hallucinogenic** (hallucination-producing). The term *psychotomimetic* is now rarely used in this context because most researchers no longer consider these compounds to be useful models of psychosis. Of the two remaining alternatives, the term *psychedelic* is often preferred by recreational users and by those who take such drugs in a quest for spiritual or mystical experiences. The modern pharmacological literature, however, strongly favors the term *hallucinogenic,* and we will follow that practice here. Specifically, we will define hallucinogens as substances whose primary effect is to cause perceptual and cognitive distortions without producing a state of toxic delirium.

Mescaline

Mescaline is obtained from the peyote cactus

Many hallucinogenic drugs are either synthesized by plants or are based on plant-derived compounds. Mescaline, for example, is found in several species of cactus, such as the **peyote cactus** *(Lophophor williamsii)* (Figure 14.1). When the crown (top part) of this small spineless cactus is cut off and dried, it is known as a **mescal button** or **peyote button.**

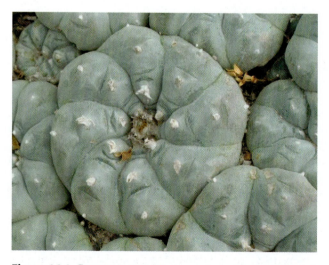

Figure 14.1 Peyote cactus (Photo courtesy of Gerhard Köhres.)

These buttons can be chewed raw or cooked and then eaten in order to obtain their psychoactive effects. Alternatively, the mescaline can be extracted from the cactus and consumed as a relatively pure powder. The peyote cactus is native to the southwestern United States and northern parts of Mexico, and archeological evidence suggests that the inhabitants of these regions used peyote for at least a few thousand years before invasion by the Spanish. Indeed, Bruhn and colleagues (2002) recently reported an analysis of mescaline-containing peyote buttons from Mexico that were radiocarbon dated to be 5700 years old. Peyote was used by Native Americans for religious and healing rituals, and such rituals continue to take place under the auspices of the Native American Church of the United States and Canada, which was founded in 1918.

Pure mescaline was first isolated from peyote in 1896 by Arthur Heffter and later synthesized in 1919 by Ernst Spath. However, the drug did not enter mainstream American culture until the famous novelist Aldous Huxley tried mescaline in 1953 and subsequently described his experience in a book entitled *The Doors of Perception.* Publication of this book and its sequel, *Heaven and Hell,* were among the seminal events that spawned a major rise in hallucinogenic drug use in the United States in the 1960s. At present, however, mescaline is not as readily available as various other hallucinogens, due to its relatively high cost of synthesis and the lack of a large market for the drug.

Psilocybin, DMT, and 5-MeO-DMT

"Magic mushrooms" are the source of psilocybin and other hallucinogens

Numerous species of mushrooms manufacture alkaloids with hallucinogenic properties. These fungi, which are sometimes called "magic mushrooms" or simply "shrooms," include members of the genera *Conocybe, Copelandia, Panaeolus, Psilocybe,* and *Stropharia,* which are found in many places around the world (Figure 14.2). Depending on the species, users take 1 to 5 g of dried mushrooms to obtain the desired effects. The dried material may be eaten raw, boiled in water to make tea, or cooked with other foods to cover its bitter flavor. The major ingredients of these mushrooms are psilocybin and the related compound **psilocin.** After ingestion, the psilocybin is enzymatically converted to psilocin, which is the actual psychoactive agent. A different species of mushroom, *Amanita muscaria* (fly agaric), produces a state of delirium that also includes hallucinations, but its primary active agents are muscimol and ibotenic acid.

The use of hallucinogenic mushrooms probably goes back at least as far historically as peyote use. There are two spectacular rock cave paintings in Algeria, dated at least to 3500 B.C., depicting people holding mushrooms in their hands and danc-

Figure 14.2 Psilocybe mushrooms

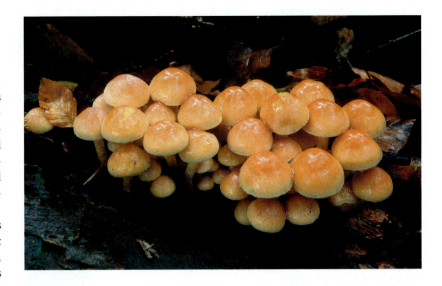

ing. The more famous of the two paintings shows a single man (possibly a shaman*) with a beelike head and mushrooms sprouting from his entire body. In Mexico and Central America, the Aztec and Mayan civilizations developed religious rituals around the eating of psilocybin-containing mushrooms.

After defeating the Aztecs, the Spaniards soon learned of their use of hallucinogenic mushrooms, which they called *teonanácatl*, meaning "flesh of the gods." The conquerors brutally suppressed mushroom eating along with other aspects of the Aztec religion, but they were unable to completely wipe it out. Nevertheless, the existence of hallucinogenic mushrooms in the New World was largely ignored until 1938, when Richard Schultes of the Harvard Botanical Museum traveled to Oaxaca, Mexico, and collected specimens of several different types of mushrooms being used in sacred rituals by the Mazatec people of that region. The publication of Schultes' findings ultimately led Gordon Wasson, a wealthy investment banker and amateur mycologist (someone who studies fungi), to visit Oaxaca in 1953 and again in 1955. During the second visit, Wasson and a photographer friend became the first known Westerners to participate in a Native American mushroom eating ritual, which was led by a Mazatec curandera, or shaman, named María Sabina (Figure 14.3). In a 1957 *Life* magazine article entitled "Seeking the Magic Mushroom,"[†] Wasson describes his reaction as follows:

> We lay down on the mat that had been spread for us, but no one had any wish to sleep except the children, to whom mushrooms are not served. We were never more wide awake, and the visions came whether our eyes were opened or closed. They emerged from the center of the field of vision, opening up as they came, now rushing, now slowly, at the pace that our will chose. They were in vivid color, always harmonious. They began with art motifs. . . . Then they evolved into palaces with courts, arcades, gardens. . . . Then I saw a mythological beast drawing a regal chariot. Later it was as though the walls of our house had dissolved, and my spirit had flown forth, and I was suspended in mid-air viewing landscapes of mountains, with camel caravans advancing slowly across the slopes, the mountains rising tier above tier to the very heavens. . . . For the first time the word ecstasy took on real meaning. For the first time it did not mean someone else's state of mind. (Wasson, 1957, pp. 102, 103, 109)

---

*In ancient cultures, shamans were people thought to possess special abilities to contact the spirit world.

[†]The title of this article is generally considered to be the first use of the term "magic mushroom."

Among those who read Wasson's account was Timothy Leary, a young clinical psychologist pursuing a mainstream academic career. But after gaining a lectureship at Harvard in late 1959, Leary began to have reservations about his chosen career path. Then while vacationing in Mexico the following summer, Leary ate a handful of "magic mushrooms" and underwent the same kind of transforming experience reported by Huxley several years earlier with mescaline. Leary returned to work, where he founded the Harvard Psy-

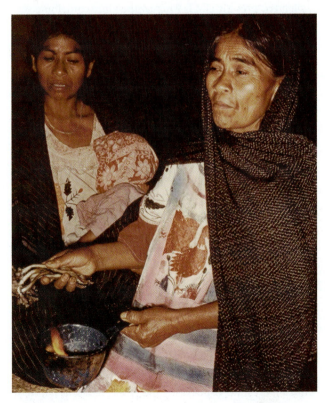

Figure 14.3 María Sabina engaged in the mushroom eating ritual

chedelic Drug Research Program. In his own words, the purpose of this program was "to teach individuals how to self-administer psychoactive drugs in order to free their psyches without reliance upon doctors or institutions" (Leary, 1984, p. 35). Over the next few years, Leary and his colleague Richard Alpert (later known as Ram Dass) gave psilocybin to many graduate students and faculty members, as well as to notable artists, writers, and musicians. He also began experimenting with LSD, having taken the drug for the first time in 1962. Leary and Alpert's work became increasingly controversial, and they were dismissed from Harvard in 1963, but they continued their activities privately and went on to become leaders of the psychedelic movement.

Other naturally occurring hallucinogens include DMT and 5-MeO-DMT

DMT and 5-MeO-DMT are found in a number of plants that are indigenous to South America. Native tribes in Brazil, Colombia, Peru, and Venezuela make hallucinogenic snuffs from plants containing these compounds. From the Amazonian rain forest also comes a strong reddish-brown drink called ayahuasca, which is a Quechua Indian word meaning "vine of the soul." This potent hallucinogenic brew requires at least two different kinds of plants, typically stalks from the *Banisteriopsis caapi* vine as well as leaves from *Psychotria viridis* and/or *Diplopteris cabrerena*. *Psychotria* and *Diplopteris* provide DMT, whereas the vines contribute several alkaloids called β-carbolines, which are known to inhibit the enzyme monoamine oxidase. It is interesting to note that DMT is usually devoid of psychoactivity when taken orally, but this is not the case when people drink ayahuasca. Some researchers have hypothesized that the β-carbolines block DMT breakdown by monoamine oxidase, thereby permitting the substance to reach the brain and exert its hallucinogenic effects. Recreational users in this country occasionally brew their own homemade version of ayahuasca, but more typically DMT is sold in powdered form and taken by smoking.

Recently, two orally active synthetic DMT analogs have been gaining in popularity. These are α-methyltryptamine (AMT) and 5-methoxy-diisopropyltryptamine. The latter compound is known on the street as "Foxy Methoxy" or simply "Foxy." One type of foxy tablet is shown in Figure 14.4.

LSD

LSD is a synthetic compound based on ergot alkaloids

Unlike mescaline, psilocybin, and DMT, LSD is a synthetic compound, although its structure is based on a family of

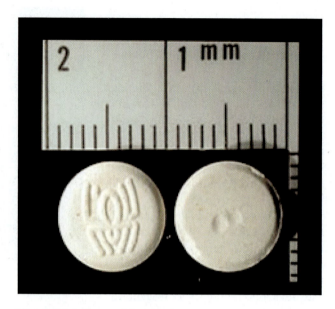

Figure 14.4 Foxy tablets

fungal alkaloids. The famous story about the synthesis of LSD and the discovery of its astonishing psychoactive potency is presented in Box 14.1. Once LSD was made available to psychiatrists and medical researchers in the late 1940s and early 1950s, the drug began to be intensively studied. Indeed, there were only six published papers on LSD before 1951, but from 1951 to 1962 more than 1000 LSD-related articles appeared in the scientific literature (U.S. Department of Health, Education, and Welfare, 1968). During this period, researchers were first beginning to appreciate that nerve cells in the brain communicate with each other chemically by means of neurotransmitters like serotonin. When LSD was reported to alter serotonergic activity (see the section below on the pharmacology of hallucinogenic drugs), the finding generated tremendous excitement about the possibility of understanding human mental activity and behavior at a chemical and physiological level.

Some researchers approached LSD as a psychotomimetic drug that would help reveal the biochemical underpinnings of schizophrenia. However, the LSD model proved to be inadequate in a number of ways, and it subsequently gave way to a PCP/ketamine model that is discussed later in the chapter. Others believed that LSD could be a valuable tool in psychotherapy or psychoanalysis. One way of using LSD was in **psycholytic therapy,** which was mainly practiced in continental Europe. This therapeutic method was based on the concept of drug-induced "psycholysis," meaning psychic loosening or opening. It involved giving LSD in low but gradually increasing doses to promote the release of repressed memories and enhance communication with the analyst. British, Canadian, and American psychiatrists, on the

BOX 14.1

History of Psychopharmacology

The Discovery of LSD

LSD was first synthesized in 1938 by Albert Hofmann, a chemist working for the Sandoz pharmaceutical company in Switzerland. Sandoz was interested in alkaloids obtained from **ergot,** a substance produced by the parasitic fungus *Claviceps purpurea* that can infest rye and wheat (see the figure). Ergot is an extremely toxic material, and consumption of ergot-contaminated grain can cause a serious illness known as **ergotism.**

Although no outbreak of ergotism has occurred in recent years, the disease was quite common in the Middle Ages and is thought to have caused the death of as many as 40,000 people in the year 944. Nevertheless, ergot came to have medicinal value because it produces powerful contractions of the uterus that can help trigger labor and reduce postbirth uterine hemorrhage.

Hofmann began to combine **lysergic acid,** which is the core structure in all ergot alkaloids, with other compounds to see what would emerge. The twenty-fifth different substance synthesized in the course of this research was d-lysergic acid diethylamide, which Hofmann abbreviated LSD-25 (from the German name LysergSäure-Diäthylamid). Hofmann's purpose in making this compound was to generate a new circulatory and respiratory stimulant (such drugs are sometimes called **analeptics**). This expectation was based on the structural similarity of LSD to nicotinic acid diethylamide, a known analeptic drug. However, LSD failed to show any analeptic activity, so the compound was temporarily abandoned.

Five years later, Hofmann decided to reexamine LSD, thinking that it might have useful pharmacological properties not recognized during initial testing. In the final stages of synthesizing a new batch of the compound, he was overcome by a series of strange sensations that prevented him from continuing in the lab. The following famous passage is taken from Hofmann's report to Sandoz, which describes the world's first LSD "trip":

> Last Friday, April 16, 1943, I was forced to interrupt my work in the laboratory in the middle of the afternoon and proceed home, being affected by a remarkable restlessness, combined with a slight dizziness. At home I lay down and sank into a not unpleasant intoxicated-like condition, characterized by an extremely stimulated imagination. In a dreamlike state, with eyes closed (I found the daylight to be unpleasantly glaring), I perceived an uninterrupted stream of fantastic pictures, extraordinary shapes with intense, kaleidoscopic play of colors. After some two hours this condition faded away. (Hofmann, 1979, p. 58).

Hofmann suspected that this amazing experience had come from accidentally ingesting a small amount of the newly synthesized LSD. Therefore, the following Monday he carefully measured out a minute amount of the drug, 250 micrograms (1/4000 of a gram), dissolved it in a small volume of water, and drank it. Hofmann soon underwent an even more intense experience than before. He somehow managed to ride his bicycle home with the help of a lab assistant, and his hallucinations took a threatening form that later passed, leaving him the next day with a profound sense of well-being and a temporarily heightened perceptual awareness.

Hofmann's colleagues at Sandoz initially did not believe that LSD could be as potent as he claimed, but when they took minute quantities themselves they were able to confirm Hofmann's result. Sandoz first marketed LSD in 1947 under the name Delysid for the purpose of helping neurotic patients uncover repressed thoughts and feelings. The company also suggested that psychiatrists self-administer the drug in order to better understand the perceptual distortions and hallucinations suffered by patients with schizophrenia. Remarkably, even now, over 60 years after LSD's discovery, we still don't know what accounts for the tremendous potency of this fascinating compound.

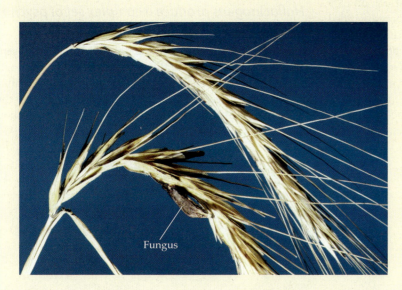

Fungus

other hand, tended to prefer **psychedelic therapy,** in which the patient was typically given a single high dose of LSD with the hope of gaining insight into his or her problems through a drug-induced spiritual experience. During the 1950s and 1960s, a number of studies were performed using this technique to treat alcoholic patients (Mangini, 1998). Unfortunately, these studies were marred by poor experimental control and inconsistent findings, leading to a cessation of this work by the early 1970s.

Interestingly, at the same time that LSD was being investigated as a possible aid to psychotherapy, it was also being considered by the United States government as a potential psychological weapon. In the early 1950s, the Central Intelligence Agency (CIA) began a top secret program called MK-ULTRA that was designed to investigate the possible use of LSD as a mind control agent (Lee and Shlain, 1992). In one particularly disgraceful part of this program, CIA operatives administered LSD to unsuspecting members of the public in order to observe their behavioral reactions. According to Lee and Shlain (1992), Fidel Castro and then Egyptian president Gamal Abdel Nasser were among the foreign leaders targeted for LSD "attacks," although it appears that no such attacks were actually carried out before the program was eventually disbanded.

LSD's popularity exploded with the hippie culture of the 1960s. As part of their nonconformist, anti-Establishment attitudes, hippies openly sought mind expansion through the use of psychedelic drugs, especially LSD. However, the inevitable backlash soon occurred amid growing anecdotal accounts as well as scientific reports of LSD-related problems. A 1965 federal law greatly restricted new research on LSD, and soon thereafter Sandoz stopped distributing LSD for research purposes and recalled all of the existing drug that had previously been supplied to investigators. After a long period of inactivity, however, clinical research on LSD has begun to make a slow comeback. An organization called MAPS (Multidisciplinary Association for Psychedelic Studies) has been promoting new research on the potential psychotherapeutic applications of hallucinogens (see the MAPS Web site at www.maps.org). Nevertheless, given the general cultural and governmental attitudes toward LSD and other hallucinogenic drugs, it seems unlikely that these compounds will enter mainstream psychiatric practice any time soon.

Recreational use of LSD was banned nationwide in 1967. Of course, LSD didn't disappear, it merely went underground. Indeed, in recent years hallucinogenic drug use has increased as a new generation of young people has rediscovered these substances. LSD is active orally, and that is the standard mode of administration. As we read in Box 14.1, the drug is so potent that a single dose in crystalline form is barely visible to the naked eye. Consequently, larger amounts of LSD representing many doses are usually dissolved in water and then droplets containing single-dose units are applied to a sheet of paper (a "blotter") and dried. The paper is subsequently divided into individual squares, often decorated with fanciful designs, and sold as single-dose "tabs" to be swallowed by the user (see chapter opening photograph).

Pharmacology of Hallucinogenic Drugs

Different hallucinogenic drugs vary in potency but have a similar time course of action

One way of comparing the potency of various hallucinogenic drugs is to consider the typical doses taken by recreational users. Common dose ranges for LSD, psilocybin, mescaline, and DMT are presented in Table 14.1. You can see that these compounds vary widely in their potency, ranging from LSD as the most potent to mescaline as the least potent. All of the hallucinogens that are taken orally have a fairly similar time course of action. Depending on the dose and when the user last ate, the psychedelic effects of these substances generally begin within 30 to 90 minutes following ingestion. An LSD or mescaline "trip" typically lasts for 6 to 12 hours or even longer, whereas the effects of psilocybin-containing mushrooms may dissipate a bit sooner. DMT, however, presents a very different picture, at least partly due to its route of administration. The effects of smoked DMT are felt within seconds, reach a peak by 5 to 20 minutes, and are over within an hour or less. For this reason, the DMT experience is sometimes referred to as the "businessman's trip."

Hallucinogens produce a complex set of psychological and physiological responses

Since LSD is considered to be the prototypical hallucinogen, we will focus primarily on the psychological and physiological responses associated with this compound. Other hallucinogens may have slightly different response profiles, but the core effects are similar across drugs. The state of intoxication

TABLE 14.1 Route of Administration and Potency of Various Hallucinogenic Drugs

Drug	Usual route of administration	Typical dose range
LSD	Oral	50–100 µg (0.05–0.10 mg)
Psilocybin	Oral	10–20 mg
Mescaline	Oral	200–500 mg
DMT	Smoking	20–50 mg

produced by LSD and other hallucinogens is usually called a "trip," presumably because the user is taking a mental journey to a place different than his normal conscious awareness. The LSD trip can be divided into four phases: (1) onset; (2) plateau; (3) peak; and (4) "come-down." Trip onset occurs about 30 minutes to an hour after one takes LSD. Visual effects begin to occur, with an intensification of colors and the appearance of geometric patterns or strange objects that can be seen with one's eyes closed. The next 2 hours of the trip represent the plateau phase. The subjective sense of time begins to slow and the visual effects become more intense during this period. The peak phase generally begins after about 3 hours and lasts for another 2 or 3 hours. During this phase, the user feels like he's in another world in which time has been suspended. He sees a continuous stream of bizarre, distorted images that may be either beautiful or menacing. The user may experience **synesthesia,** a crossing-over of sensations in which, for example, colors are "heard" and sounds are "felt." The peak is followed by the come-down, a phase lasting for 2 hours or more depending on the dose. Most of the drug effects are gone by the end of the come-down, although the user may still not feel completely normal until the following day. In addition to the sensory–perceptual effects just described, hallucinogenic drugs produce a wide variety of other psychological changes. These include feelings of depersonalization, emotional shifts to a euphoric or to an anxious and fearful state, and a disruption of logical thought.

A hallucinogenic trip as a whole may be experienced either as mystical and spiritually enlightening (a "good trip") or as disturbing and frightening (a "bad trip"). Whether the user has a good or bad trip depends in part on the dose; the individual's personality, expectations, and previous drug experiences; and the physical and social setting. But even in the best of circumstances, one cannot predict in advance the outcome of an LSD trip.

Besides their psychological effects, hallucinogens also give rise to various physiological responses. In the case of LSD, these responses reflect activation of the sympathetic nervous system and include pupil dilation and small increases in heart rate, blood pressure, and body temperature. LSD use can also lead to dizziness, nausea, and vomiting, although such reactions are more likely to occur after consumption of peyote or psilocybin-containing mushrooms.

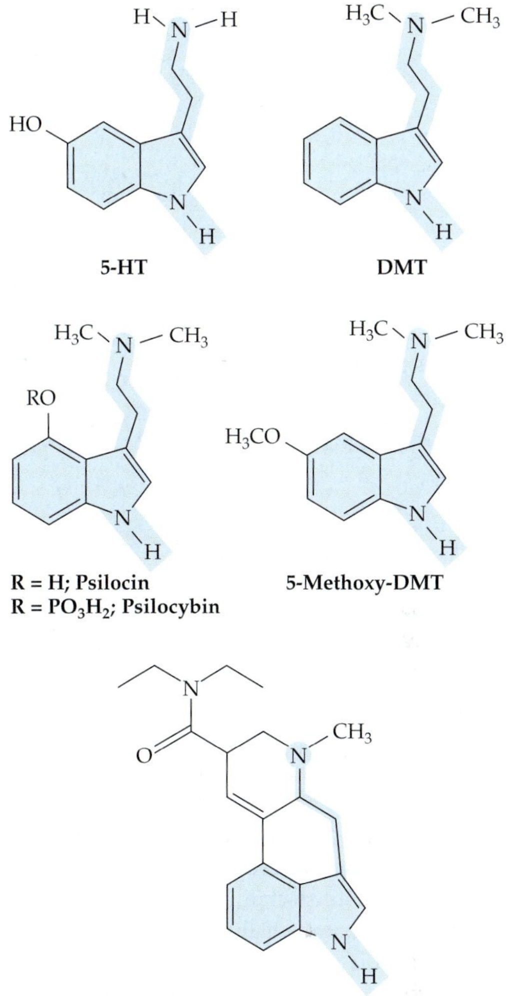

Hallucinogenic drugs share a common indoleamine or phenethylamine structure

Most hallucinogenic drugs have either a serotonin-like or a catecholamine-like structure. The serotonin-like, or **indoleamine,** hallucinogens include LSD, psilocybin, psilocin, DMT, 5-MeO-DMT, and the synthetic tryptamines mentioned earlier. When the serotonin (5-HT) molecule is oriented in the proper manner, it is easy to see how its basic

Figure 14.5 Structures of 5-HT and the indoleamine hallucinogens The core indoleamine structure in each compound is highlighted.

structure is incorporated into the structures of these hallucinogenic compounds (Figure 14.5). Important studies in the early 1950s by John Gaddum in Scotland and by Edward Wooley and David Shaw in the United States led these investigators to conclude that LSD works by antagonizing the action of 5-HT in the brain. We shall see in the next section that LSD can be understood more as an agonist than as an antagonist in the serotonergic system. Nevertheless, the linking of 5-HT with such a powerful psychoactive drug as LSD brought this recently discovered neurotransmitter into the forefront of behavioral and psychiatric research, a place that it continues to hold to the present day.

Of the hallucinogens covered in this chapter, the only one that is catecholamine-like is mescaline. As shown in Figure 14.6, mescaline has structural similarities to the neurotrans-

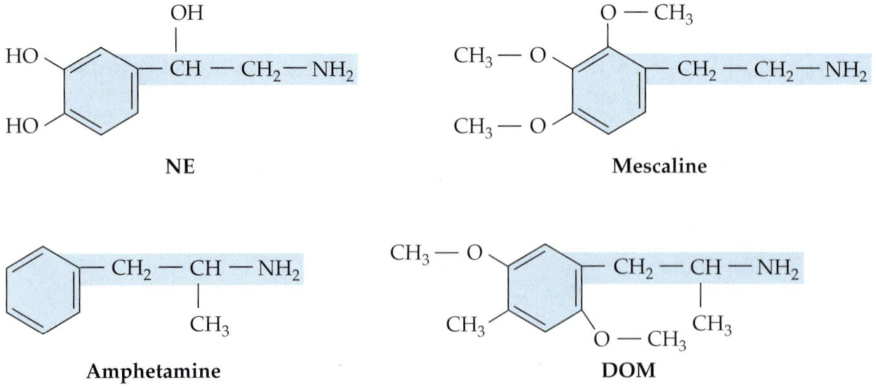

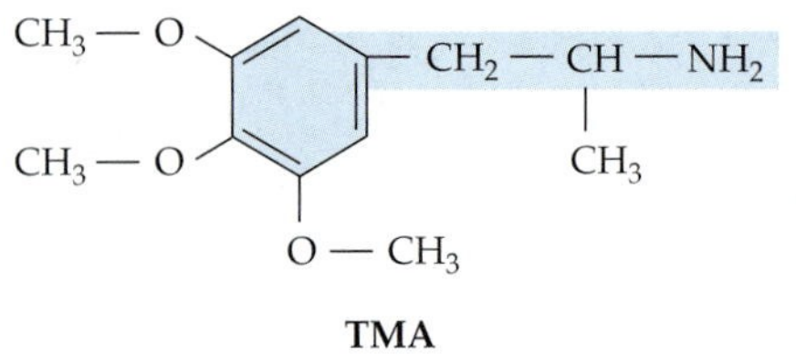

Figure 14.6 Structures of NE and the phenethylamine hallucinogens The core phenethylamine structure in each compound is highlighted.

mitter norepinephrine (NE) as well as to the psychostimulant amphetamine. Indeed, amphetamine can produce hallucinogenic effects with prolonged administration of high doses, and several amphetamine analogs such as 2,5-dimethoxy-4-methylamphetamine (DOM, also known as "STP") and 3,4,5-trimethoxyamphetamine (TMA) possess even greater hallucinogenic properties. Together with mescaline, these NE- and amphetamine-related compounds are known as **phenethylamine** hallucinogens.

Hallucinogens are 5-HT₂ receptor agonists

Although we still don't completely understand how hallucinogens produce their dramatic perceptual and cognitive effects, some progress has been made. Over time it has become clear that the serotonergic system is intimately involved in this process, but that still leaves a number of additional questions. Which serotonergic receptors are targeted by hallucinogenic drugs? Do other neurotransmitters also play a role? Do the phenethylamine hallucinogens such as mescaline work by the same mechanism as indoleamine hallucinogens like LSD, psilocybin/psilocin, and DMT? Finally, what brain circuits are activated by hallucinogenic drugs?

Beginning our exploration of hallucinogenic action with LSD, we can immediately see that this is a very complicated substance with respect to its potential effects on the serotonergic system. LSD binds with relatively high affinity to at least eight different serotonergic receptor subtypes: $5\text{-}HT_{1A}$, $5\text{-}HT_{1B}$, $5\text{-}HT_{1D}$, $5\text{-}HT_{2A}$, $5\text{-}HT_{2C}$, $5\text{-}HT_{5A}$, $5\text{-}HT_6$, and $5\text{-}HT_7$ (Nichols, 2004). There are several approaches we can take toward understanding which of these receptor interactions are important for basic hallucinogenic drug action. One

approach is to compare the receptor binding properties of indoleamine hallucinogens such as LSD with those of the phenylethylamine hallucinogens. As shown in Table 14.2, such a comparison reveals that the only known common sites of interaction for both classes of compounds are the $5\text{-}HT_{2A}$ and $5\text{-}HT_{2C}$ receptor subtypes (Aghajanian and Marek, 1999). Moreover, the potencies of various phenethylamine hallucinogens in humans are closely correlated with their affinities for both of these subtypes (Nelson et al., 1999). Together, these findings suggest that $5\text{-}HT_{2A}$ and/or $5\text{-}HT_{2C}$ receptors might play a key role in the subjective and behavioral effects of hallucinogenic drugs.

Receptor binding data alone cannot determine the mechanism of action of a psychoactive drug. Behavioral studies are also needed. There is little work on the neurochemistry of LSD action in humans due to current restrictions on clinical research with this compound. However, Vollenweider

TABLE 14.2 Known Interactions of LSD and Phenethylamine Hallucinogens with Specific 5-HT Receptor Subtypes[a]

Receptor subtype	LSD	Phenethylamines
$5\text{-}HT_1$ family	+	−
$5\text{-}HT_{2A}$	+	+
$5\text{-}HT_{2C}$	+	+
$5\text{-}HT_3$	−	−
$5\text{-}HT_4$	−	?
$5\text{-}HT_{5A}$	+	−
$5\text{-}HT_6$	+	?
$5\text{-}HT_7$	+	−

Source: After Aghajanian and Marek, 1999.
[a] +, significant affinity for that receptor subtype; −, low affinity for that subtype; ?, no currently available data.

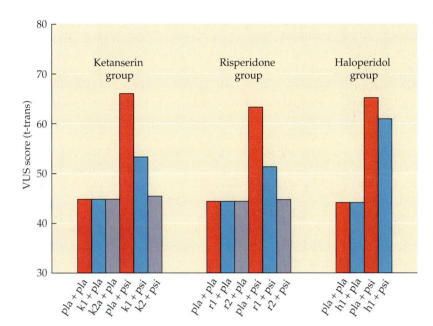

Figure 14.7 Blockade of psilocybin-induced visual illusions and hallucinations by 5-HT$_{2A}$ receptor antagonists Subjects received 0.25 mg/kg of oral psilocybin (psi) or placebo (pla), and then 80 minutes later they completed the Altered State of Consciousness (APZ-OAV) rating scale. The subjects were also pretreated either with placebo, oral ketanserin (k1 = 20 mg, k2 = 40 mg), oral risperidone (r1 = 0.5 mg, r2 = 1.0 mg), or intravenous haloperidol (h1 = 0.021 mg/kg). The data shown are for the VUS (visionary restructuralization) subscale, which assesses hallucinatory phenomena, visual illusions, and other perceptual changes. In all cases, psilocybin increased VUS scores compared to placebo (pla + psi vs. pla + pla). These increases were dose-dependently blocked by ketanserin (k1 + psi and k2 + psi vs. pla + psi) and by risperidone (r1 + psi and r2 + psi vs. pla + psi) but not by haloperidol (h1 + psi vs. pla + psi). (After Vollenweider et al., 1998.)

and his coworkers (1998) studied the indoleamine hallucinogen psilocybin and showed that drug-induced visual illusions and hallucinations were dose-dependently blocked by ketanserin and risperidone, two compounds that antagonize 5-HT$_{2A}$ receptors. Because risperidone also blocks D$_2$ receptors for dopamine (DA), it is important to note that haloperidol, an antagonist at D$_2$ but not 5-HT$_{2A}$ receptors, completely failed to prevent the hallucinogenic effects of psilocybin (Figure 14.7). Thus the limited human data available at this time suggest an important role for 5-HT$_{2A}$ receptors in the mediation of drug-induced hallucinations.

Due to the scarcity of human experimental research on hallucinogens, animal studies have been extremely important in helping us understand how these drugs work. Studies using the drug-discrimination procedure (see Chapter 4) have been particularly useful in this regard. Figure 14.8 presents an example from the work of James Appel of the University of South Carolina and his collaborators (Appel et al., 2004). The researchers first trained rats to press one lever in a Skinner box when they received an injection of LSD and a different lever when they received saline. Figure 14.8A shows

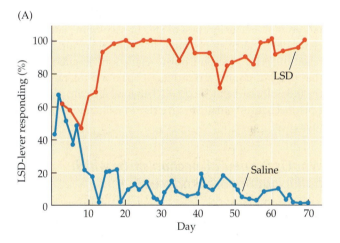

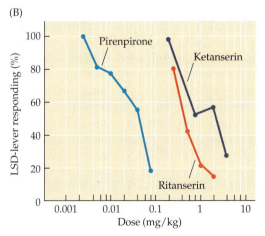

Figure 14.8 Acquisition of an LSD/saline discrimination and attenuation of the drug stimulus cue by 5-HT$_{2A}$ receptor antagonists (A) Rats readily learned to discriminate LSD (0.08 mg/kg intraperitoneally) from saline, as shown by the progressive increase in responding on the correct lever over days. (B) In rats previously trained to discriminate this dose of LSD from saline, responding on the LSD-appropriate lever was dose-dependently reduced by pretreatment with the 5-HT$_{2A}$ receptor antagonists ritanserin, pirenperone, and ketanserin. (After Appel et al., 2004.)

that the discriminative stimulus properties of the drug as measured by responding on the appropriate lever were acquired within about 2 weeks. Once the animals had been trained, some were given varying doses of a 5-HT$_{2A}$ receptor antagonist such as ritanserin, pirenperone, or ketanserin 1 hour prior to administration of LSD. In Figure 14.8B you can see that all three compounds dose-dependently reduced responding on the LSD-appropriate lever, presumably because the interoceptive cue produced by LSD was blocked by the antagonist pretreatment. Indeed, other work by Winter et al. (1999) has shown a strong correlation between the affinity of various serotonergic antagonists for the 5-HT$_{2A}$ receptor and their potency in blocking the LSD stimulus cue. Based on these and other findings, it appears that the discriminative stimulus procedure is consistent with the other experimental approaches discussed earlier in this section that point to the 5-HT$_{2A}$ receptor as a key mediator of hallucinogenic drug action.

Most hallucinogenic drugs, with the possible exception of DMT, produce rapid tolerance with repeated use. Early studies involving LSD administration to human subjects found that over a 4-day period of daily dosing, nearly complete tolerance was observed by the fourth day (Nichols, 1997). One likely mechanism underlying this tolerance is a down-regulation of 5-HT$_{2A}$ receptors, which has been demonstrated in rats given several daily doses of LSD or psilocybin (Buckholtz et al., 1990). Surprisingly, mescaline administration did not result in 5-HT$_{2A}$ receptor down-regulation, despite the fact that this compound can produce behavioral tolerance like the indoleamine hallucinogens. Therefore, there may be multiple mechanisms that can give rise to hallucinogenic drug tolerance.

What is the neural mechanism by which hallucinations are produced?

Although the above-mentioned studies have helped identify *which* 5-HT receptor is most important for hallucinogenic drug effects, they do not tell us *where* the critical receptors are located or *how* the activation of these receptors produces the sensory and cognitive distortions experienced during a "trip." Due to a lack of relevant human studies, these questions have thus far been addressed mainly by various experimental approaches using animals. For example, electrophysiological studies by George Aghajanian and his colleagues have suggested an important role for the locus coeruleus (LC), a dense cluster of norepinephrine-containing neurons in the pons that is responsible for most of the noradrenergic projections to the forebrain (see Chapter 5). A key feature of the LC is that it receives and integrates input from all of the major sensory systems and sends information to all areas of the cortex including the sensory cortex. Aghajanian's group found that LSD, DOM, and mescaline all decreased the spontaneous fir-

ing of rat LC neurons but paradoxically enhanced the excitation of these cells by sensory stimulation (Aghajanian and Marek, 1999). This effect is caused by drug-induced activation of 5-HT$_{2A}$ receptors, although the receptors in question are not located directly on the LC neurons but rather on other cells that modulate LC activity. A reduction in spontaneous neuronal firing with a simultaneous enhancement of sensory responsiveness means that in the presence of hallucinogenic drugs, the LC is more sensitive to sensory input. This may be one of the key factors leading to the genesis of hallucinations, although Aghajanian and Marek discuss additional processes that may also play important roles.

Franz Vollenweider and Mark Geyer (2001) have proposed an alternative hypothesis, in which they suggest that hallucinogenic effects are produced by a disruption of normal information processing in a circuit that includes the prefrontal cortex, striatum, and thalamus. This hypothesis argues that hallucinogenic drugs interfere with the normal "gating," or screening, of sensory information passing through this circuit, thereby resulting in information overload at the cortical level. Vollenweider and Geyer further argue that such a mechanism accounts not only for the perceptual distortions associated with hallucinogenic drug use but also for simultaneous disturbances in cognition that these investigators consider to be psychotic-like.

Hallucinogenic drugs cause problems for some users

Hallucinogens are not thought to be addictive in the standard sense. Users do not binge on these substances, and it is rare for people to experience the kind of cravings seen with drugs such as opiates, cocaine, ethanol, and nicotine. Furthermore, hallucinogens do not produce physical dependence or withdrawal. Finally, these compounds are not effective reinforcers in animal tests such as the self-administration paradigm.

Despite this lack of addictive potential, hallucinogens can still cause serious problems for some users. As mentioned earlier, the user may have a "bad trip" in which he or she experiences an acute anxiety or panic reaction in response to the drug's effects (Figure 14.9). Although we don't understand the exact cause of these reactions, they are probably related to an interaction between the drug, the individual's emotional state going into the trip, and the external environment. In most cases, friends will talk the person through the ordeal. However, if this is unsuccessful, then it may be necessary to take the person to the hospital emergency room for treatment. The incidence of bad trips is not known, but existing data from older clinical studies of LSD administration suggest that they are rare when users are prescreened for emotional stability and the environmental conditions are carefully controlled.

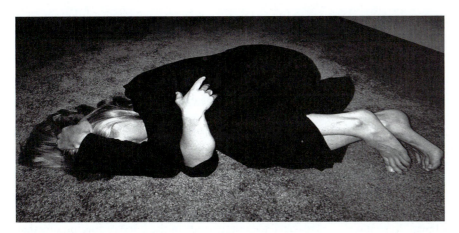

Figure 14.9 LSD users sometimes experience acute panic or anxiety reactions to the drug (a "bad trip").

A second potential complication of hallucinogen use is the occurrence of **flashbacks.** This term is defined in the *Diagnostic and Statistical Manual of Mental Disorders (DSM-IV)* as "the reexperiencing, following cessation of use of a hallucinogen, of one or more of the perceptual symptoms that were experienced while intoxicated with the hallucinogen" (American Psychiatric Association, 1994, p. 234). When flashbacks occur a long time after prior drug use and are sufficiently intense to cause major disturbance or impairment, then the individual is considered to be suffering from hallucinogen persisting perception disorder (HPPD). Halpern and Pope (2003) recently reviewed the literature on flashbacks and HPPD. They concluded that although some LSD users do suffer from HPPD, the prevalence of this disorder may not be very high considering the relatively few documented cases of HPPD in relation to the large number of people who have taken LSD over the years. The neural mechanisms responsible for flashbacks have not yet been studied, although it is interesting to note that the use of other psychoactive drugs such as marijuana seems to trigger flashbacks in some cases.

The most severe adverse reaction to LSD is a psychotic breakdown. At one time, LSD opponents argued that this was a major risk factor in using this substance. However, it now seems clear that prolonged psychotic episodes following LSD use almost invariably involve individuals who had already been diagnosed with a psychotic disorder such as schizophrenia or who had manifested prepsychotic symptoms before taking the drug.

Section Summary

Hallucinogens are substances that cause perceptual and cognitive distortions in the absence of delirium. Many hallu-

cinogens such as mescaline, psilocybin, DMT, and 5-MeO-DMT are plant compounds that were used for hundreds or thousands of years in spiritual or religious ceremonies before their discovery by Western culture. In contrast, LSD is a synthetic drug, although it is based on a series of alkaloids found in ergot fungus.

Recognition of the powerful mind-altering properties of hallucinogenic drugs led to both clinical and recreational use beginning in the late 1950s and early 1960s. Some psychiatrists gave patients LSD in the course of psycholytic or psychedelic therapy. LSD became readily available on the street despite a federal ban on recreational use in 1967. Most hallucinogenic drugs are orally active, with a slow onset of action and a long time course of action. One exception is DMT, which is usually smoked, thereby leading to rapid drug effects and a much shorter duration of action. Of the commonly used hallucinogens, LSD is the most potent and mescaline is the least potent, based on the range of doses taken by users.

An LSD "trip" is sometimes divided into four phases: onset, plateau, peak, and come-down. During the trip, the user experiences vivid visual hallucinations, a slowing of the subjective sense of time, feelings of depersonalization, strong emotional reactions, and a disruption of logical thought. There are also physiological reactions such as pupil dilation and increased heart rate, blood pressure, and body temperature. A number of factors determine whether the user has a "good trip" or a "bad trip."

Hallucinogenic drugs are classified chemically as either indoleamines or phenethylamines. The indoleamines are related structurally to 5-HT, whereas the phenethylamines instead share a common structure with NE. Both classes of drugs are agonists at 5-HT$_2$ receptors, which is believed to be an essential component of their hallucinogenic properties. Activation of 5-HT$_{2A}$ receptors may be particularly important for hallucinogenic activity. Repeated exposure to hallucinogens leads to rapid tolerance, possibly through down-regulation of these receptors in key target cells. The specific brain areas responsible for the production of hallucinogenic drug effects have not yet been identified, but hypotheses have been proposed that focus either on the locus coeruleus or on the cortical–striatal–thalamic circuit.

Hallucinogens are not considered to be dependence forming or addictive. However, they can lead to other adverse effects such as "bad trips" and flashbacks. People who suffer from severe flashbacks long after discontinuing hallucinogenic drug use are diagnosed as having hallucinogen persisting perception disorder. At the present time, little is known about the causes or treatment of HPPD.

PCP and Ketamine

Background and History

This section of the chapter deals with two closely related compounds: **phencyclidine** and **ketamine.** Phencyclidine is usually abbreviated **PCP,** which comes from the drug's full chemical name, 1-(1-*p*henyl*c*yclohexyl)*p*iperidine (Figure 14.10). PCP (trade name Sernyl) was first tested in the mid-1950s by Parke, Davis and Company as a potential anesthetic agent. However, early studies revealed that the drug produced an unusual kind of anesthesia. Although subjects given PCP showed no responsiveness to nociceptive (painful) stimuli, they were not in the typical state of relaxed unconsciousness seen with traditional anesthetics like barbiturates. Instead, the subjects exhibited a trancelike or catatonic-like state characterized by a vacant facial expression, fixed and staring eyes, and a maintenance of muscle tone. Indeed, it was not unusual for individuals to develop either rigidity or waxy flexibility, motor symptoms often observed in catatonic schizophrenics.

PCP was initially thought to be clinically promising because it did not produce the respiratory depression associated with barbiturate anesthesia and thus possessed a high therapeutic index (see Chapter 1). However, early enthusiasm was soon tempered by reports of problematic reactions in many patients. In a few cases, this took the form of marked agitation rather than quieting during the drug-induced state. In other instances, PCP induced postoperative reactions ranging from blurred vision, dizziness, and mild disorientation to much more serious reactions involving hallucinations, severe agitation, and even violence. These problems caused the clinical use of PCP to be terminated in 1965.

Of course, the abandonment of PCP as a medication did not prevent it from coming into illicit use. In 1967, PCP found its way onto the streets of several cities including San Francisco, where it was dubbed the "PeaCe Pill" by the drug culture protesting the Vietnam War. By the mid-1970s, PCP use and abuse under new street names such as "angel dust" and "hog" had become much more widespread across the country. Yet the popularity of this drug never rivaled that of marijuana or even cocaine or heroin, and the incidence of PCP use subsequently declined to the rather low level seen at the present time.

Ketamine came into being as a safer alternative to PCP. Even before PCP was withdrawn, Parke, Davis had begun to screen related compounds in the hope of finding one that would be less toxic in its behavioral effects. One such compound, designated CI-581, was synthesized in 1962 and first tested in humans 2 years later. CI-581, later renamed ketamine, was less potent and shorter acting than PCP. Ketamine was soon found to be a valuable anesthetic for certain medical procedures, particularly in children, and it is also widely used as a general sedating and immobilizing agent by veterinarians. It is currently marketed legally as a prescription medication under the trade names Ketalar, Ketaset, and Vetalar. Despite its lower potency, ketamine can still cause adverse emergence reactions in human patients similar to those seen with PCP. Fortunately, techniques have been developed to minimize the frequency of such reactions.

Pharmacology of PCP and Ketamine

PCP and ketamine produce a state of dissociation

PCP is generally obtained in powdered or pill form, and the drug can be ingested by virtually any common route. It can be taken orally, administered intranasally (i.e., snorted), or injected intravenously or intramuscularly. Many PCP users apply the drug to tobacco, marijuana, or parsley cigarettes for purposes of smoking. Illicitly used ketamine typically comes from the diversion or theft of medical- or veterinary-grade material. Ketamine is marketed commercially as an injectable liquid, but street sellers commonly evaporate the liquid to yield a powder that is either snorted directly or compressed into pill form (Figure 14.11). It is sold on the street under such names as "K," "special K," or "cat Valium." Users who don't wish to become too intoxicated often snort small lines or piles of ketamine called "bumps." However, initial snorting of ketamine can escalate over time to intramuscular or even intravenous injection of the liquid solution as the user becomes tolerant to the drug or seeks a more powerful effect.

The first studies on the subjective effects of PCP were conducted in the late 1950s and early 1960s. When given a

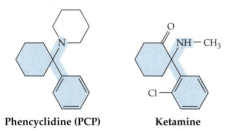

Phencyclidine (PCP)   **Ketamine**

Figure 14.10 Chemical structures of PCP and ketamine

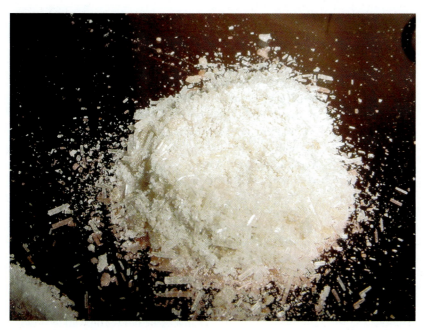

Figure 14.11 Ketamine crystals

subanesthetic dose of PCP, subjects reported feeling detached from their body, sensations of vertigo or of floating, numbness, and sometimes a dreamlike state. They also experienced a variety of affective reactions including drowsiness and apathy, loneliness, negativism or hostility toward the experimenters, or, alternatively, euphoria and inebriation toward them. Finally, all of the treated subjects exhibited a marked cognitive disorganization manifested by difficulty in maintaining concentration or focus, deficiencies in abstract thinking, and halting speech.

Edward Domino and his colleagues at the University of Michigan published the first study of ketamine's pharmacological effects in 1965. Low doses of ketamine yielded reactions similar to those mentioned in the previous paragraph for low-dose PCP administration. However, when subjects received doses in the anesthetic range (at least 1 mg/kg intravenously), the investigators observed a remarkable phenomenon. The subjects appeared to lose all mental contact with their environment for up to 10 minutes or more, despite the fact that their eyes remained open and they retained significant muscle tone. When Domino described to his wife how the ketamine-treated subjects seemed to be disconnected from their environment, she proposed the term **dissociative anesthesia** to describe this unique state of detachment (E. F. Domino, personal communication). This term was subsequently applied to both ketamine and PCP.

More recent studies have documented the subjective experiences reported by ketamine users while in the dissociated state (Table 14.3). As noted in the table, the individual may feel separated from his body, perhaps floating above and looking down at himself. Some have described this as a "near-death" experience (Jansen, 2000, 2001), even though the person is not actually dying. This state of being, which is called the "K-hole," can be either spiritually uplifting or terrifying. As one user put it, "A K-hole can be anything from going to hell and meeting Satan to going to heaven and meeting God" (quote from Time Out, 2000, p. 20).

PCP and ketamine exhibit potent reinforcing effects

Both PCP and ketamine are highly reinforcing in several different species of animals, as shown by drug self-administration. Interestingly, early studies on rhesus monkeys that self-administered high doses of PCP found that the animals took in sufficient quantities of the drug to be intoxicated almost continuously (Balster and Woolverton, 1980, 1981). Under the influence of PCP, the subjects could not support themselves on four legs, but instead were typically found near the response lever either in an awkward sitting position or lying on the cage floor. The ability to elicit self-intoxication in animals is not unique to PCP, but has also been observed with cocaine, amphetamine, opiates, and in some cases alcohol.

TABLE 14.3 Subjective Experiences Reported by Ketamine Users

Sensations of light coming through the body and/or of colorful visions
Complete loss of time sense
Bizarre distortions of body shape or size
Altered perception of body consistency (e.g., feeling as though one is made of a strange material such as rubber, plastic, or wood)
Sensations of floating or hovering weightlessly in space
Feelings of leaving one's body
Sudden insights into the mysteries of existence or of the self
Experiences of being "at one" with the universe
Visions of spiritual or supernatural beings

Source: After Dalgarno and Shewan, 1996.

(A)

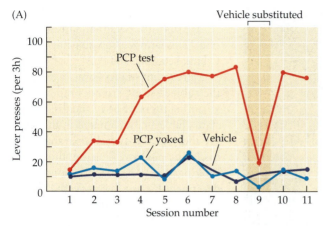

(B)

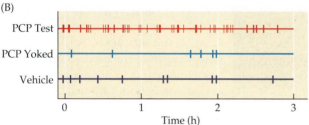

Figure 14.12 Self-administration of PCP into the nucleus accumbens shell by rats Rats in the PCP test group were trained to lever-press for administration of 12 nmol of PCP directly into the shell of the nucleus accumbens, a brain region known to be important for the rewarding effects of many abused drugs. The rats were tested for 3-hour sessions on a continuous reinforcement schedule, which means that every lever-pressing response resulted in drug infusion. Each animal in the PCP-yoked group was paired with an animal in the PCP test group. These yoked control animals received a PCP infusion each time their counterpart pressed its lever. The vehicle group received an intra-accumbens infusion of the vehicle solution for each response. (A) shows that the PCP test group readily self-administered PCP into the nucleus accumbens shell, as shown by their increasing lever-pressing behavior across test sessions. When vehicle was substituted for PCP during session 9, responding dropped to the same low level exhibited by the PCP-yoked and vehicle control groups. (B) shows the pattern of lever pressing during session 8 for representative animals from each group. (After Carlezon and Wise, 1996.)

PCP and ketamine activate midbrain DA cell firing and stimulate DA release, particularly in the prefrontal cortex. This enhancement of dopaminergic neurotransmission could contribute to PCP's and ketamine's reinforcing effects. On the other hand, rats will also self-administer PCP directly into the nucleus accumbens (Figure 14.12), and this local reinforcing effect appears to be DA-independent (Carlezon and Wise, 1996). Thus it seems likely that there are both dopaminergic and nondopaminergic mechanisms underlying PCP and ketamine reinforcement.

PCP and ketamine are noncompetitive antagonists of NMDA receptors

The principal molecular target for both PCP and ketamine is the NMDA (*N*-methyl-D-aspartate) receptor. To review briefly, the NMDA receptor is an important ionotropic receptor for the excitatory amino acid neurotransmitter glutamate. PCP and ketamine are both noncompetitive antagonists at the NMDA receptor complex; that is, they block the receptor at a site different than the site at which glutamate or NMDA binds. In fact, as we saw in Chapter 7, the PCP/ketamine binding site is found inside of the receptor's ion channel (see Figure 7.5). NMDA receptors are widely distributed in the brain and play a key role in glutamate signaling. The cerebral cortex and hippocampus contain significant numbers of NMDA receptors, and blockade of the receptors in these areas presumably contributes to the cognitive deficits produced by PCP and ketamine. Other behavioral and subjective effects of these substances are also thought to be mediated by NMDA receptor antagonism, although the exact mechanisms are not yet fully understood.

Dextromethorphan, a common ingredient in over-the-counter cough and cold medications, is another noncompetitive NMDA receptor antagonist with abuse potential. This compound is discussed in Box 14.2

Ketamine is an increasingly popular drug of abuse

Data from the National Survey on Drug Use and Health indicate that the prevalence of PCP use is much lower than that of major abused drugs like alcohol, marijuana, cocaine, and heroin. There are currently no comparable statistics for ketamine, but the use of this substance is believed to be on the rise primarily due to its popularity at raves.

Although ketamine has only recently come to the attention of the popular media, illicit use and abuse of this substance actually dates back many years. Some abusers were, and continue to be, medical or veterinary practitioners who have easy access to ketamine in the course of their work. Ketamine was also favored by some intellectuals as a mind-expanding drug in the tradition of LSD. Two of the most famous ketamine users were Marcia Moore, a well-known astrologer and author of the 1970s, and Dr. John Lilly, a physician and researcher known for his groundbreaking studies on interspecies communication (for example, with dolphins) and on the psychological effects of sensory isolation. Both Moore and Lilly became heavily dependent on ketamine, and both developed psychotic reactions as a result.*

*In Moore's case, the consequences were especially tragic when she left her home on a cold, wintry night in 1979, climbed a tree, gave herself a ketamine injection, and froze to death while in a state of drug intoxication.

BOX 14.2   Pharmacology in Action

Getting High on Cough Syrup

One of the most annoying features of a bad cold is the persistent cough that it may bring on. That is why **antitussives,** medications that suppress the cough reflex, are big sellers in pharmacies across the country. The active ingredient in most of these over-the-counter products is an opioid-like compound called **dextromethorphan.** For example, dextromethorphan is the antitussive agent in Robitussin-DM cough syrup as well as in Coricidin HBP Cough & Cold tablets. Unlike codeine, an opioid agonist typically found in prescription cough medications, dextromethorphan does not directly stimulate opioid receptors. Instead, it is known to be a noncompetitive NMDA receptor antagonist, much like PCP and ketamine.

Cough medications based on dextromethorphan have been on the market for many years. The first one was Romilar, a dextromethorphan-containing tablet that was introduced in the 1960s. Romilar was meant to be a replacement for codeine-containing medications, since the latter were already being abused. However, it did not take long before users discovered the psychoactive properties of Romilar and began abusing it as well. The drug was eventually withdrawn from the market and later replaced with a codeine-containing, prescription-only version. Pharmaceutical companies subsequently decided to put dextromethorphan into a cough syrup, presumably to discourage recreational use by requiring the ingestion of large amounts of the syrup in order to obtain a psychoactive effect. However, this has not prevented users, typically adolescents or young adults, from continuing to experiment with this substance.

Dextromethorphan is typically taken orally in the form of cough syrup or tablet. On the street it goes by names like "DXM," "DM," or "Robo." The standard dose of dextromethorphan for cough suppression is 15 to 30 mg, but recreational users take doses that are at least 10 times higher. This requires drinking half or more of a typical 8-oz. bottle of cough syrup. There are even reports of heavy users ingesting three or four entire bottles in one day. Drinking this much cough syrup usually causes nausea and vomiting due to the effects of guaifenesin, an expectorant (agent that facilitates expulsion of phlegm from the throat or airways) found in most cough syrups. Some users have tried to avoid this unpleasant side effect by taking large amounts of dextromethorphan-containing Coricidin tablets. However, this is a very dangerous, even potentially fatal, practice due to the presence of chlorpheniramine in these tablets. Chorpheniramine is an antihistamine/anticholinergic agent that not only produces serious reactions by itself at high doses but also intensifies the effects of dextromethorphan by inhibiting its metabolism in the liver. Given the limitations associated with dextromethorphan use via standard cough medications, enterprising users have discovered methods for extracting the substance from cough syrup. As a result, dextromethorphan has become available on the street in repackaged pills or capsules for oral administration and even in powdered form for intranasal use (snorting). Indeed, tablets sold as "Ecstasy" occasionally contain dextromethorphan instead of the expected MDMA.

Users report that the subjective effects of dextromethorphan occur as a series of four dose-related "plateaus." Low doses (approximately 2 oz. of cough syrup) produce the first plateau, during which the user feels a mild euphoria and intoxication and may also experience slight perceptual effects. The second plateau is the most commonly sought after and requires a dose of about 4 oz., containing more than 200 mg of dextromethorphan. At this stage, the user becomes ataxic, experiences visual hallucinations when he closes his eyes, and is significantly more intoxicated than at the first plateau. The third and fourth plateaus occur at doses ranging from 400 to 1000 mg or more of dextromethorphan. At these doses, the drug produces powerful dissociative effects resembling those seen with PCP and ketamine.

As mentioned earlier, the principal molecular target of dextromethorphan is believed to be the NMDA receptor. This is supported not only by in vitro receptor binding and electrophysiological studies but also by the demonstration that both dextromethorphan and its bioactive metabolite **dextrorphan** exert PCP-like discriminative stimulus effects in both rats and monkeys (Nicholson et al., 1999). The dissociative effects of dextromethorphan at high doses in human users are also consistent with a mechanism involving NMDA receptor blockade.

We do not have good statistics at this time on the prevalence of recreational dextromethorphan abuse across the population. However, recent informal school surveys (Noonan et al., 2000) as well as hospital reports (Banerji and Anderson, 2001) indicate that dextromethorphan-containing medications are being abused by school-age children. Several deaths among dextromethorphan abusers have also been recorded. Therefore, it is particularly important for parents to become more knowledgeable about this substance and for educators to inform young people about the potential dangers associated with the recreational use of cough syrups and tablets.

Development of ketamine tolerance and dependence can be seen not only in the extreme cases of Marcia Moore and John Lilly but also in the self-reports of other heavy users. Accounts of dose escalation and compulsive use are presented by Karl Jansen, a British psychiatrist who has investigated ketamine use for many years (Jansen, 2001; Jansen and Darracot-Cankovic, 2001). Interestingly, many of the ketamine-dependent subjects studied by Jansen are described as being highly intelligent, even Ph.D. students. One straight-A Ph.D. candidate said that overcoming his ketamine problem was "harder than heroin" (Jansen, 2001, p. 167).

PCP and ketamine have provided new insights into the neurochemistry of schizophrenia

There is growing interest in the idea that PCP and ketamine may help us understand the biological underpinnings of severe psychopathology, particularly schizophrenia. This is based on two related findings: first, that acute PCP or ketamine exposure causes perceptual, cognitive, and affective responses closely resembling many of the symptoms associated with schizophrenia (see Chapter 18); and second, that administration of either drug to patients with schizophrenia exacerbates their psychotic symptoms.

The psychiatric effects of a subanesthetic ketamine infusion in healthy volunteers are shown in Figure 14.13 (Newcomer et al., 1998). Although the figure depicts total symptom scores, it is worth noting that the subjects experienced

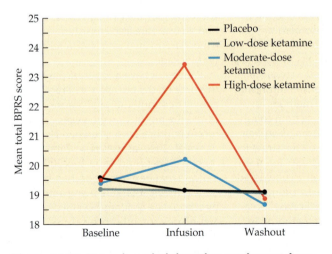

Figure 14.13 Ketamine administration produces a dose-dependent increase in psychotic-like symptoms. Subjects were given an intravenous infusion of ketamine at one of three doses designed to achieve very low, moderate, or high plasma drug concentrations. Psychotic-like symptoms were assessed using the Brief Psychiatric Rating Scale (BPRS) before (baseline), during (infusion), and after (washout) the drug treatment. The high dose of ketamine produced a marked increase in BPRS scores. (After Newcomer et al., 1998.)

both positive symptoms (hallucinatory responses, conceptual disorganization, and bizarre thought content) and negative symptoms (blunted affect, emotional withdrawal, and motor retardation) when given the high dose of ketamine. In this study, the psychotic-like reaction disappeared after drug administration was terminated. However, a subsequent study of recreational ketamine users by Curran and Morgan (2000) found that dissociative and schizotypal symptoms (perceptual distortion, magical ideation, and thought disorder) were still present 3 days after the most recent use.

PCP and ketamine have also been used by some investigators in searching for an animal model of schizophrenia. One experimental approach has been to examine the neurochemical and behavioral effects of administering one or just a few doses of the compound. In contrast, a research group headed by Robert Roth at Yale University has proposed that long-term PCP administration may provide a better model, particularly of the severe cognitive deficits seen in schizophrenic patients (Jentsch et al., 1997; Jentsch et al., 2000). One advantage of this procedure is that the animals can be studied without the drug "on board" to determine whether the prior treatment has produced lingering behavioral effects. These researchers found that 2 weeks of twice-daily PCP administration to vervet monkeys caused severe deficits in an "object retrieval with a detour" task when the animals were tested 1 week after the last drug dose. This is an important finding because the detour task involves the prefrontal cortex, which is believed to be dysfunctional in patients with schizophrenia (see Chapter 18). Moreover, repeated PCP treatment also led to a significant reduction in DA utilization in the prefrontal cortex, and DA hypofunction in this area is also thought to occur in schizophrenia. In conclusion, chronic PCP administration to nonhuman primates is an intriguing model of schizophrenia that may help us understand at least some of the mechanisms underlying this tragic disorder.

Section Summary

PCP and ketamine belong to the class of drugs known as dissociative anesthetics. PCP was withdrawn from clinical use due to its prominent adverse side effects, but ketamine, which is less potent than PCP, has significant applications in both human and veterinary medicine. The acute effects of these compounds include sensory distortions and altered body image, cognitive disorganization, and various affective changes. High doses of ketamine give rise to a state called the "K-hole" in which the user feels separated from his body, perhaps in the manner of a near-death experience.

Both PCP and ketamine are reinforcing to animals, as indicated by drug self-administration. These reinforcing effects may be mediated by both dopaminergic and non-dopaminergic mechanisms. Regardless of the role of DA in

PCP or ketamine reinforcement, the direct molecular target of these compounds is the glutamate NMDA receptor. PCP and ketamine bind to a site within the receptor channel, thereby acting as noncompetitive NMDA receptor antagonists. Blockade of glutamate action at these receptors is thought to be responsible for the subjective and behavioral effects of PCP and ketamine. Dextromethorphan is an opioid-like compound found in cough medications that also acts as a noncompetitive NMDA receptor antagonist and can produce PCP- or ketamine-like dissociative effects at high doses.

Although illicit use of ketamine has occurred for many years, the popularity of this compound may be on the rise. Heavy ketamine users show dose escalation and compulsive use, which indicates the development of tolerance and dependence on the drug.

Recent studies suggest that PCP and ketamine may help us understand the neurochemical processes underlying schizophrenia. Acute PCP or ketamine exposure mimics many of the symptoms of schizophrenia. Moreover, administration of either compound to schizophrenic patients exacerbates their psychotic symptoms. Animal models involving PCP or ketamine treatment, particularly those based on nonhuman primates, may also provide important insights into the neurochemistry of severe psychopathology.

Recommended Readings

Aghajanian, G. K., and Marek, G. J. (1999). Serotonin and hallucinogens. *Neuropsychopharmacology*, 21, 16S–23S.

Hoffman, A. (1979). How LSD originated. *J. Psychoactive Drugs,* 11, 53–60.

Jansen, K. L. R. (2001). *Ketamine: Dreams and Realities.* Multidisciplinary Association for Psychedelic Studies, Sarasota, Florida.

Lee, M. A., and Shlain, B. (1992). *Acid Dreams. The Complete Social History of LSD: The CIA, the Sixties, and Beyond.* Grove Press, New York.

Ulrich, R. F., and Patten, B. M. (1991). The rise, decline, and fall of LSD. *Perspect. Biol. Med.,* 34, 561–578.

15 Inhalants, GHB, and Anabolic–Androgenic Steroids

Have you ever heard the word "resistoleros"? If you have, it was probably in reference to a Bay Area punk rock band that goes by that name. But there is another, more disturbing, use of the word. In many parts of Latin America, resistoleros are street children who are habitual glue sniffers. Their name comes from Resistol, which is a contact cement and shoemaker's glue that is widely sold in Latin American countries and favored by many young glue sniffers. According to the International Assembly of the National Council for the Social Studies (2004), millions of homeless Latin American children are sniffing glues such as Resistol. Glue sniffing gives the children a temporary "high" that helps them cope with their precarious existence, but it can also cause many long-term health problems including damage to the brain and other vital organs.

Glues belong to a broader class of abused substances known as **inhalants.** Most inhalants are perfectly legal, can easily be purchased at retail stores by people of any age, and are readily accessible in the home by anyone who can reach into a medicine cabinet or kitchen drawer, or who can walk down the stairs to the basement or open the door to the garage. Moreover, in recent years these substances have been responsible for the abrupt death of a number of children and teenagers in many countries, including the United States. Indeed, the parents of children who have died from abusing inhalants invariably say that they never knew how dangerous these substances could be.

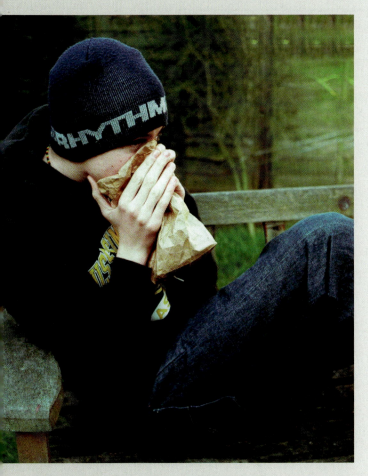

Inhalants can be taken by sniffing the fumes from a paper bag.

The first part of this chapter discusses where inhalants come from, how they affect behavioral and neural functioning, and what health risks they pose. Later sections of the chapter cover γ-hydroxybutyrate (GHB) and anabolic–androgenic steroids. Although inhalants, GHB, and steroids differ in their mechanisms of action, they share the fact that they are all newcomers to the drug abuse scene relative to many other substances such as alcohol, cannabis, tobacco, opiates, and the plant-derived hallucinogens.

Inhalants

Background

Inhalants represent a novel group of abused substances. These substances, which often come from everyday household items, have the following characteristics:

1. They are either volatile (easily vaporized) liquids or gases at room temperature.
2. They are used by either sniffing fumes from a container of the substance, inhaling the substance from a balloon, inhaling fumes from a rag saturated with the substance ("huffing"),* inhaling fumes of the substance inside of a plastic or paper bag, or spraying an aerosol of the substance directly into one's nose or mouth.
3. They do not belong to another defined class of abused substances (for example, nicotine, THC, or cocaine, all of which can be inhaled through smoking).

Most inhalants can be categorized as volatile solvents, aerosols, or gases. **Volatile solvents** are chemicals that are liquid at room temperature but give off fumes that can be inhaled. Solvents are found in numerous household and industrial products, including adhesives, correction fluids, ink used in felt-tip marking pens, paint thinners and paint removers, dry-cleaning fluids, gasoline, and industrial degreasing agents. **Aerosols** are sprays that contain various solvents and propellants. Examples are hair sprays, deodorant sprays, spray paints, vegetable oil sprays used in cooking, and sprays used for household cleaning.

---

*Although the term *huffing* has the specific meaning given here, it is also often used more generally to denote the breathing in of an inhalant.

The third category, **gases,** includes several gases found in domestic or commercial products as well as anesthetic agents used in human and veterinary medicine. Sources of gaseous inhalants include whipped cream dispensers (which contain nitrous oxide, also known as "laughing gas"), propane tanks, butane lighters, and appliances that contain refrigerants such as refrigerators, freezers, and air-conditioners. Table 15.1 lists some abused inhalants that fall within these three classes.

A fourth group of inhalants, called **nitrites,** is often placed in a separate category apart from the solvents, aerosols, and gases. Whereas most inhalants are taken in order to obtain a euphoric effect, or "high," nitrites are typi-

TABLE 15.1 Some Commonly Abused Inhalants

Compound	Principal uses
Acetone	Nail polish remover, adhesives, general solvent
Aliphatic and aromatic hydrocarbons	Gasoline, white spirits
Bromochlorodifluoromethane (BCF)	Fire extinguishers
n-Butane	Cigarette lighters, bottled fuel gas
Butanone (methyl ethyl ketone, MEK)	Adhesives, general solvent
Carbon tetrachloride	Grain fumigant, laboratory solvent
Chlorodifluoromethane (Halon 122 or Freon 22)	Aerosol propellant
Chloroform	Laboratory solvent
Dichlorodifluoromethane (Halon or Freon 12)	Aerosol propellant, refrigerant
Dichlorotetrafluoroethane (Halon 242 or Freon 114)	Aerosol propellant
Diethyl ether	Laboratory solvent
Enflurane	Anesthetic
Ethyl acetate	Adhesives
Halothane	Anesthetic
n-Hexane	General solvent
Isoflurane	Anesthetic
Methyl isobutyl ketone (MIBK)	General solvent
Nitrous oxide	Anesthetic, whipped cream dispensers
Propane	Bottled fuel gas
Tetrachloroethylene (perchloroethylene)	Dry-cleaning and degreasing agent
Toluene	Adhesives, acrylic paints, paint stripper
Trichloroethane (methylchloroform)	Dry-cleaning and degreasing agent, correction fluid
Trichloroethylene	Dry-cleaning and degreasing agent, chewing gum remover
Trichlorofluoromethane (Halon or Freon 11)	Aerosol propellant, refrigerant
Xylene	Woodwork adhesives, histology clearing agent

Source: After Dinwiddie, 1994.

cally used to heighten sexual arousal and pleasure. Furthermore, unlike other inhalants, which are thought to act directly on nerve cells, nitrites produce their subjective effects primarily by dilating blood vessels and causing muscle relaxation. Members of this group include amyl nitrite ("poppers"), butyl nitrite, and cyclohexyl nitrite. In the remainder of this section, we will focus on the first three classes of inhalants.

Behavioral and Neural Effects

Many inhalant effects are similar to alcohol intoxication

The acute effects of volatile and gaseous inhalants are often compared to those seen with alcohol intoxication. The user initially experiences euphoria, stimulation, and disinhibition, which are followed by drowsiness and lightheadedness. Heavier exposure causes stronger depressant effects, characterized by slurred speech, poor coordination, ataxia, and lethargy. Sensory distortions, even hallucinations, may occur. Very high doses can lead to anesthesia, loss of consciousness, and coma.

A British study by Evans and Raistrick (1987) surveyed groups of young people (mean ages of 15 or 16) who had abused either toluene-containing adhesives ("glue sniffing") or butane gas. Both groups reported behaving as though they were drunk while under inhalant intoxication. Euphoria was experienced in nearly all cases, but other mood changes (for example, feelings of depression or fearfulness) also occurred some of the time. Visual or auditory hallucinations were quite common. Less common but more dangerous were reports by some users of delusional ideas, including the delusion that one could fly. Users who thought they could fly actually jumped out of windows or trees, leading to at least one broken bone and various minor injuries but fortunately no fatalities.

Repeated use of inhalants can lead to tolerance, and thus a need to take higher doses in order to obtain the expected euphoric effect. Some investigators have also proposed the existence of an inhalant withdrawal syndrome with symptoms such as nausea, tremors, irritability, and sleep disturbances. However, this remains controversial at the present time.

Rewarding and reinforcing effects have been demonstrated in animals

Inhalants appear to be reinforcing, thereby linking them with most other substances of abuse. We know from subjective reports that people take inhalants to obtain pleasurable effects, but it is always valuable for researchers to have an animal model of reward or reinforcement to study. This has long been a technically challenging problem for scientists

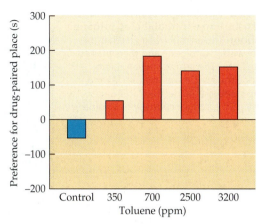

Figure 15.1   Rewarding effects of toluene in mice as shown by conditioned place preference Mice were given two training sessions per day for 5 days. Each session lasted 20 minutes and involved pairing one compartment of an airtight chamber with toluene vapor and the other compartment, which differed from the first compartment in its sensory characteristics, with air. Toluene concentrations ranged from 350 to 3200 parts per million (ppm) as shown. On the test day, no toluene was administered and the mice were allowed to move freely between the two compartments. Toluene concentrations of at least 700 ppm resulted in a significant preference for the toluene-paired side as indicated by the amount of time spent on that side. Control mice not given any toluene showed no significant preference for either side. (After Funada et al., 2002.)

working with inhalants, but progress is being made, as indicated by the recent study of Funada et al. (2002). These Japanese researchers tested the rewarding properties of toluene by means of a place-conditioning procedure using an airtight inhalation shuttlebox. As is standard for place-conditioning studies, the two compartments of the apparatus differed in the sensory cues they presented to the animals. Mice were given 10 conditioning sessions over 5 days, 1 session each day in the toluene-containing compartment, and an additional session in the compartment that just contained air. As shown in Figure 15.1, exposure to 700 parts per million (ppm) or more of toluene led to a significant preference for the toluene-associated side of the apparatus.

Inhalants reduce central nervous system (CNS) excitability by acting on specific ionotropic receptors

Because of their more recent arrival on the scene, less is known about the mechanism of action of inhalants than of other abused substances. Furthermore, all inhalants may not work the same way, due to their chemical diversity. Nevertheless, our understanding of these substances is increasing and several important findings have been made.

With respect to pharmacokinetics, inhalants are rapidly absorbed from the lungs into the bloodstream and quickly

Figure 15.2 PET images of brain uptake and distribution of radiolabeled toluene in a baboon The animal was injected intravenously with [^{11}C]toluene and then imaged 2 minutes later. The arrows show toluene being concentrated in the striatum (A) and in the deep cerebellar nuclei (B). (After Gerasimov et al., 2002; images courtesy of Madina Gerasimov.)

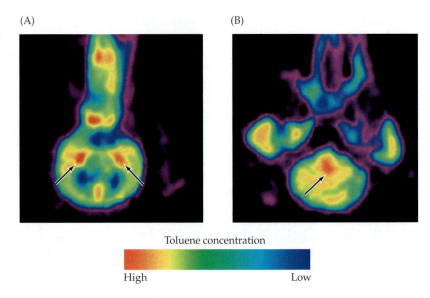

(A)   (B)

Toluene concentration

High   Low

enter the brain due to their high lipid solubility. Madina Gerasimov and her colleagues at the Brookhaven National Laboratory recently used positron emission tomography (PET) to investigate the localization of [^{11}C]toluene that had been administered to baboons (Gerasimov et al., 2002). The radiolabeled toluene reached all parts of the brain, but its distribution was not uniform (Figure 15.2A and B). Quantitative measurements of the striatum, frontal cortex, thalamus, cerebellum, and white matter showed particularly high uptake in the striatum, thalamus, and deep cerebellar nuclei. These findings indicate that localization of inhalants within the brain needs to be taken into account in trying to understand how these substances affect brain function and behavior.

The CNS-depressant actions of inhalants can best be explained by their effects on various ionotropic receptors. A number of studies have found that volatile solvents as well as anesthetics enhance the function of inhibitory GABA$_A$ and glycine receptors and inhibit the activity of excitatory NMDA glutamate receptors. A similar profile of ionotropic receptor effects has been demonstrated for other depressant drugs, particularly ethanol. Thus, it appears that inhalants reduce CNS excitability and cause behavioral impairment in much the same way as does alcohol.

Relatively little is known about the neural mechanisms underlying inhalant reinforcement. In previous chapters, we saw that dopamine (DA) plays a role in the reinforcing properties of many abused drugs. Riegel and French (2002) found that inhaled toluene activated dopaminergic neurons in the ventral tegmental area, which suggests that DA may also be involved in inhalant reinforcement. It will be important to determine whether DA receptor antagonists can block the rewarding effects of toluene in model systems such as the place-conditioning paradigm.

Significant health risks are associated with inhalant abuse

It is not uncommon for inhalants to be the first substances tried by children, even sooner than alcohol, tobacco, or mar-

ijuana. Solvents and aerosols in particular can be obtained legally and inexpensively (in fact, there are almost certainly plenty of them at home already in the kitchen, basement, or garage), and it may be difficult for parents and teachers to detect the use of inhalants if the child is careful. Government surveys indicate that about 6% of children in this country have tried inhalants at least once by the fourth grade and that inhalant use typically peaks during the seventh through the ninth grades. Indeed, inhalants were found to be the most popular substances for 12-year-olds, exceeding marijuana. This is not to say that adults don't use inhalants, because obviously some do. Nevertheless, this class of substances is unusual in its special attractiveness to children and teenagers.

The health risks of inhalant use are significant. Even a single use can lead to a fatal cardiac arrhythmia, which means a loss of normal heart rhythm. This reaction has been termed **sudden sniffing death syndrome.** Although most users obviously don't suffer heart failure, repeated inhalant use can damage the liver, kidneys, and lungs. The brain is particularly vulnerable to inhalant toxicity. Several magnetic resonance imaging (MRI) studies have shown white-matter abnormalities indicative of damage to the myelin sheaths surrounding nerve cell axons in many brain areas. One recent study compared MRI scans of chronic inhalant abusers with individuals who abused various other drugs such as cocaine, marijuana, alcohol, amphetamines, or opiates. The results indicated many more subcortical abnormalities in the inhalant-abusing group (Figure 15.3; Rosenberg et al., 2002). Moreover, the inhalant abusers also performed more poorly than the other drug abusers on several neuropsychological tests. These results suggest that chronic inhalant abuse can have damaging effects on the brain that are manifested in cognitive impairment.

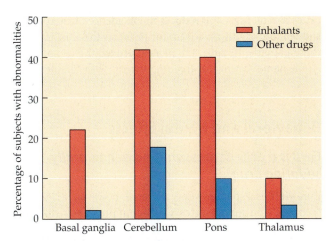

Figure 15.3 Subcortical structural abnormalities in inhalant abusers compared to abusers of other drugs Chronic abusers of either inhalants (mainly toluene-containing solvents) or other drugs were given brain scans using MRI. A much greater percentage of the inhalant abusers than the other drug abusers showed structural abnormalities in various sub-cortical areas. (After Rosenberg et al., 2002.)

Many parts of the United States have had problems with inhalant abuse, but none more than Alaska. As many as 22% of high school students surveyed in Alaska admitted to having tried inhalants, and a number of deaths have occurred. Unlike for other substances, there is little information on treatment for inhalant abuse. However, in 2001 the federal government began funding the nation's first treatment center for inhalant users, the Tundra Swan Inhalant Treatment Center, in Bethel, Alaska. Although Tundra Swan is only a small facility at this time, substance abuse workers hope that the lessons learned there will help us better understand the nature of this problem and how to treat it effectively.

Section Summary

Inhalants are abused substances that are often obtained from everyday household items. These substances are volatile liquids or gases at room temperature; are used by sniffing, inhaling, or spraying the substance; and do not belong to another defined class of abused drugs. Volatile solvents are chemicals that are liquid at room temperature but release fumes that can be inhaled. Aerosols are sprays that contain one or more solvents or propellants. There are also gaseous inhalants, which include some gases used commercially as well as anesthetic agents like nitrous oxide. Nitrites represent a fourth group of inhalants that differ from the previous types in that they are taken specifically to enhance sexual arousal.

Low doses of volatile and gaseous inhalants produce effects resembling those seen with alcohol intoxication. Users exposed to greater amounts of these substances show stronger depressant effects, including slurred speech, poor coordination, ataxia, and sleepiness. Very high doses may cause loss of consciousness and even coma. Repeated inhalant use leads to tolerance, although the existence of an inhalant withdrawal syndrome has not yet been conclusively established. Inhalants are reinforcing to humans due to their euphoric effects, and animal studies have also begun to establish the rewarding and reinforcing properties of these substances under controlled laboratory conditions.

Inhalants are rapidly absorbed from the lungs and quickly enter the brain from the bloodstream due to their high lipid solubility. Distribution within the brain does not appear to be uniform, which may influence the behavioral effects of these substances. The depressant effects of inhalants can be attributed mainly to enhancement of inhibitory GABA$_A$ and glycine receptor activity, as well as inhibition of excitatory NMDA receptors. Inhalant reinforcement may also involve release of DA due to activation of dopaminergic neurons in the ventral tegmental area.

Because of their legal status and ready availability in the home, inhalants are sometimes the first abused substances taken by children. Surveys show that inhalant use peaks during the seventh through the ninth grades. Inhalants present serious health risks involving damage to the liver, kidneys, lungs, and brain. Solvent abusers show cognitive impairment that may be related to white-matter abnormalities seen on MRI scans. There is also a rare disorder called sudden sniffing death syndrome, which is a fatal cardiac arrhythmia resulting from inhalant use. Although inhalant use and abuse is found throughout the United States, the greatest problem is found in Alaska. Little is known about the most effective treatments for inhalant abusers, but useful information will hopefully be gleaned from the treatment center that was established several years ago in Alaska.

Gamma-Hydroxybutyrate

Background

The second part of this chapter concerns **γ-hydroxybutyrate (GHB),** a simple chemical with a complicated history. As can be seen in Figure 15.4, GHB is closely related structurally to the important inhibitory neurotransmitter GABA. The pharmacologic properties of GHB were first reported in 1960 by a French team headed by Henri Laborit, the same scientist who discovered the antipsychotic drug chlorpromazine. Laborit was looking for a GABA analog that would cross the blood–brain barrier more efficiently than GABA and thus might have therapeutic potential as a CNS-depressant com-

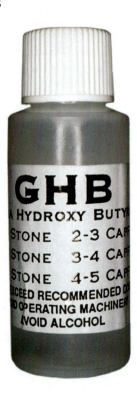

GABA   GHB   1,4-Butanediol   GBL

Figure 15.4 Chemical structures of GABA, GHB, 1,4-butanediol, and GBL

pound. Indeed, early studies showed GHB to produce sedation and even anesthesia in laboratory animals and humans, and the compound is currently available by prescription for several clinical applications (including as an anesthetic) in Europe.

In the United States, little attention was paid to GHB until the 1980s, when it began to be marketed by health food stores as a nutritional supplement for bodybuilders. Despite a lack of supporting evidence, GHB was claimed by manufacturers to reduce body fat and enhance muscle mass due to its ability to stimulate growth hormone secretion by the pituitary gland. As time went on, the Food and Drug Administration (FDA) began receiving a number of reports of GHB-related illness, and in 1990 the FDA declared the drug to be unsafe and banned over-the-counter sales.

Despite the FDA ban, GHB use continued to grow due largely to an upsurge in recreational use under various street names such as "liquid X," "liquid E," "Georgia home boy," "grievous bodily harm," "cherry meth," "organic quaalude," and "nature's quaalude." Some stores, as well as many Internet sites, sold GHB-containing formulations with commercial names like Remforce, Revivarant, Renewtrient, Blue Nitro, and SomatoPro. In addition, restrictions on GHB sales were circumvented by the introduction of kits for synthesizing the compound at home from the chemical precursors γ-butyrolactone (GBL) or 1,4-butanediol (see Figure 15.4). GHB, along with MDMA (see Chapter 11) and ketamine (see Chapter 14), is sometimes called a **club drug** because of its popularity at nightclubs and dances or "raves." Due to its intoxicating and heavily sedating effects at high doses, GHB also began to be used as a "date rape" drug (Box 15.1). Increasing concerns over the problems associated with illicit GHB use led to its designation as a Schedule I controlled substance in 2000, thus making possession of the drug illegal except for medicinal use with a prescription.

Even though GHB is not used as an anesthetic in the United States, it has found a different and surprising clinical use in this country. Specifically, in patients with the sleep dis-

order narcolepsy, GHB reduces the incidence of cataplexy, a sudden loss of muscle control or paralysis that can occur in these patients. In 2002, the FDA approved the use of GHB (trade name Xyrem) for treating patients with cataplexy.

Behavioral and Neural Effects

GHB is a CNS-depressant and behaviorally sedating drug

Pure GHB is a solid powdery material; however, it is usually sold as a solution in water. GHB-containing solutions are clear, odorless, and almost tasteless. Such solutions are often packaged in small bottles similar to those used to package shampoo in hotel rooms (Figure 15.5). Typical recreational doses range from 1 to 3 g (approximately 14 to 42 mg/kg for a 70-kg adult), although some regular users may take as much as 4 or 5 g (about 57 to 71 mg/kg) at a time.

When a GHB-containing solution is drunk, the drug is rapidly absorbed from the gastrointestinal tract, enters the bloodstream, and crosses the blood–brain barrier without difficulty. The ensuing psychological and physiological effects are strongly dose related. Low doses of GHB produce an alcohol-like experience. Users report mild euphoria, relaxation, and social disinhibition beginning approximately 15 minutes following drug ingestion. A placebo-controlled, double-blind study by Ferrara and coworkers (1999) found that oral GHB administration led to an increase in "calmness" at a dose of 12.5 mg/kg but not 25 mg/kg. Euphoria was not assessed in this study. Higher doses of GHB can cause lethargy, ataxia, slurring of speech, dizziness, nausea, and vomiting. Finally, overdosing on this compound is very dangerous, since respiration is depressed and the user may become unconscious or even comatose (Dyer, 1991). Alternatively, the individual may exhibit signs of seizure activity. Overdosing can readily occur if the user takes multiple doses over a short period of time, if there is a greater than expected concentration of GHB in the bottle, or if the drug is taken in combination with alcohol or another sedative–hypnotic drug.

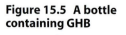

Figure 15.5 A bottle containing GHB

BOX 15.1 # Drugs and Society

"Date Rape" Drugs

Men have long used alcohol to reduce women's sexual inhibitions, thereby making them more willing sexual partners. However, in recent years a much more insidious phenomenon has emerged: the use of drugs that render a woman completely unconscious, after which she is raped by the perpetrator. Unlike the situation with alcohol, in which the woman knows she is drinking, these other substances are put clandestinely in the victim's drink so that she isn't even aware that anything is amiss until she wakes up hours later in the man's bed. Drugs are sometimes used in this way on a date, hence the term "date rape" drugs. However, there have also been instances in which a woman was raped by a total stranger after being given one of these substances.

Two compounds that are reportedly being used in this manner are GHB and a benzodiazepine called flunitrazepam (trade name Rohypnol). Rohypnol is a powerful sleep-inducing agent that is used medicinally in Europe and Mexico but is not currently approved for sale in the United States. Nevertheless, it is readily available illicitly under street names like "roofies," "rophies," or "roche" (the drug is manufactured by the Hoffmann-La Roche pharmaceutical company). Besides inducing sleep, Rohypnol may also cause anterograde amnesia, which means a lack of memory for events that occur while the recipient is under the influence of the drug. This can make it more difficult for prosecutors to prove a rape charge when Rohypnol is involved.

At the present time, government agencies do not have adequate data on the incidence of drug-facilitated sexual assaults or rapes. It appears, however, that such assaults have been on the rise in recent years. In response, Congress passed the Drug-Induced Rape Prevention and Punishment Act in 1996, which instituted tough penalties for the possession or sale of flunitrazepam. Similar legislation relating to GHB was put into place in 2000. There have also been attempts by the private sector to increase the detectability of potential date rape drugs by women. For example, Hoffmann-La Roche has replaced its old Rohypnol formulation, which was colorless when dissolved in an alcoholic beverage, with a new tablet that turns blue when dissolved. Unfortunately, some of the older tablets are still available on the street. Moreover, perpetrators may attempt to disguise the telltale blue tint emanating from the newer tablet by ordering a similarly colored tropical drink for their date.

Another commercial approach to preventing drug-facilitated rape is the marketing of coasters designed to test one's drink for possible date-rape drugs. The first such device is called the Drink Safe Coaster, which is made by Drink Safe Technologies. The Drink Safe Coaster is designed to detect both GHB and ketamine, which has also been used as a date-rape drug. The coaster does not test for flunitrazepam (Rohypnol), although Drink Safe Technologies has stated that they omitted this test because the current incidence of flunitrazepam-related date rapes is low compared to the incidence of date rapes in which the victim is drugged with GHB or ketamine. As shown in the figure, each Drink Safe Coaster contains two pairs of test circles located at the bottom corners of the card. If the coaster is being distributed by a bar or club, it may also include some type of advertisement or logo that has been selected by the proprietor of the establishment. The woman is instructed to place a drop or two of her drink on one of the pairs of test circles and wait for about one minute. A positive test is indicated by either circle turning a darker blue color, which is interpreted as a drug-contaminated drink. It is important to note that the use of the Drink Safe Coaster is not recommended for highly acidic beverages such as drinks containing large amounts of fruit juice. There are other limitations as well. The color change could be masked by the drink itself, (for example, red wine), or the bar or club could be so dark that confirming a modest color change would be difficult. Therefore, even though test coasters may help prevent some date rapes, women should remain alert for potential adulteration of their drinks even when such coasters are available and seem to indicate that everything is normal.

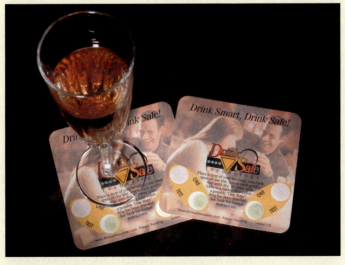

The drink-testing coaster from Drink Safe.

In laboratory animals, acute GHB administration causes sedation, reduced locomotor activity, and decreased anxiety in certain tests such as the elevated plus-maze. At higher doses, animals show signs of catalepsy. Some of these behavioral effects, particularly hypolocomotion and catalepsy, are thought to be due to GHB-induced inhibition of DA release. Electroencephalogram (EEG) recordings have also revealed the presence of a paradoxical CNS excitation at high doses of GHB that some investigators have likened to absence (petit mal) seizures in humans and that may be related to the occasional reports of seizure activity in human overdose cases. Absence seizures involve a temporary loss of consciousness and cessation of activity without the whole-body convulsions seen in a grand mal seizure.

Evidence for GHB reinforcement in animal studies has been inconsistent

As mentioned in the previous section, users report experiencing a euphoric effect when taking GHB. On the other hand, animal studies have yielded mixed results with respect to GHB as a reinforcer. Experiments with rats and mice using either self-administration or place-conditioning paradigms have generally supported the idea that GHB has rewarding and reinforcing properties (Martellotta et al., 1997, 1998; Itzhak and Ali, 2002). In contrast, two research groups that investigated intravenous self-administration of GHB in monkeys found much weaker evidence for GHB reinforcement (Beardsley et al., 1996; Woolverton et al., 1999). Interestingly, the researchers noted that in some cases the monkeys did take in enough GHB to produce noticeable sedation. Perhaps this sedative effect was either dysphoric to the animals or interfered with their lever-pressing behavior. Even in those instances where overt sedation was not observed, the subjects might have limited their GHB intake so as to avoid becoming drowsy and lethargic. Until additional experiments are performed, it will be difficult to reconcile the conflicting results obtained from the rodent and primate studies.

There are two major hypotheses concerning the mechanism of action of GHB

Currently, there are two competing hypotheses about the mechanism of action of GHB, each with some supporting evidence. The first hypothesis is that GHB's effects are mediated by activation of pre- and/or postsynaptic GABA$_B$ receptors. This hypothesis is based, in part, on research showing that some of the behavioral and physiological effects of GHB in animals can be inhibited by GABA$_B$ receptor antagonists (Madden and Johnson, 1998; Carai et al., 2001; Carter et al., 2003). For example, Carter and coworkers (2003) recently studied the ability of the antagonist CGP 35348 to alter the discriminative stimulus effects of GHB. Rats were trained to

press one lever in a Skinner box when they received GHB (200 mg/kg) and to press the other lever when they received saline vehicle. Once the task had been acquired, the animals were tested for their lever-pressing behavior in the presence of the GHB plus CGP 35348. As shown in Figure 15.6A and B, the GABA$_B$ receptor antagonist dose-dependently reduced the percentage responding on the GHB lever without altering the overall lever-pressing rate. A similar inhibition of drug-selective responding was observed in rats that had been trained to discriminate the GABA$_B$ agonist baclofen from saline. These results support the contention that the discriminative stimulus effects of GHB are mediated by activation of GABA$_B$ receptors.

Some investigators have proposed that GHB functions as a direct GABA$_B$ receptor agonist (Mathivet et al., 1997; Madden and Johnson, 1998), although it has a relatively low affinity for the receptor, which might explain why users must take rather high doses of GHB (compared to most other psychoactive compounds) to obtain the desired behavioral

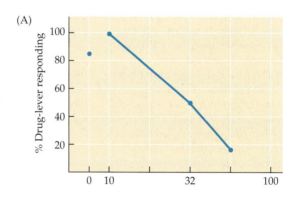

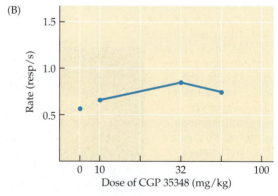

Figure 15.6 Dose-dependent blockade of the discriminative stimulus properties of GHB by the GABA$_B$ antagonist CGP 35348. Rats were trained to discriminate 200 mg/kg GHB (given intraperitoneally) from saline. In the absence of CGP 35348 (0 dose), the animals showed an average of >80% responding on the drug-appropriate lever. Pretreatment with CGP 35348 (10, 32, or 56 mg/kg) produced a dose-dependent reduction in drug-lever responding (A), while having no significant effect on lever-pressing rate (B). (After Carter et al., 2003.)

effects. An alternative explanation is that GHB is metabolized in the brain to GABA, which then stimulates $GABA_B$ receptors (Hechler et al., 1997). One problem with this notion is that the GABA formed from GHB should presumably act on both the $GABA_A$ and $GABA_B$ receptor subtypes, yet there is little evidence that GHB stimulates $GABA_A$ receptors.

The second hypothesis is that GHB's effects are mediated by a specific GHB receptor. Indeed, there are GHB binding sites in the brain that appear to be selective for this substance (Benavides et al., 1982). The structure of the proposed GHB receptor is not known, because the receptor gene has not yet been cloned. However, pharmacological studies suggest that the receptor belongs to the superfamily of G protein-coupled (metabotropic) receptors (Snead, 2000). Moreover, GHB binding sites are nonuniformly distributed in the brain, which is consistent with the idea that they represent a physiologically relevant receptor. In rats, monkeys, and humans, the highest levels of binding are generally found in the hippocampus and cerebral cortex, whereas little or no binding is observed in the cerebellum and brain stem (Hechler et al., 1987; Castelli et al., 2000). Finally, an analog of GHB called NCS-382 binds to the GHB receptor and is proposed to be a selective antagonist at this receptor (Maitre et al., 1990; Mehta et al., 2001).

Central GHB receptors are thought to be activated not only by exogenous GHB but also by GHB synthesized within the brain from GABA. GHB fulfills many of the characteristics expected of a neurotransmitter or neuromodulator substance: it is synthesized within the brain, it is released in a Ca^{2+}-dependent manner, it possesses distinct uptake systems to transport it into synaptic vesicles and to clear it from the synaptic cleft following release, and it has its own specific receptor system (Nicholson and Balster, 2001). However, there are two important reasons to question the relevance of endogenous GHB and GHB receptors for understanding the behavioral and physiological effects of exogenously administered GHB. First, naturally occurring levels of GHB in the brain are much lower than the levels produced when animals are given GHB at behaviorally effective doses. This raises the possibility that exogenous GHB could act via mechanisms different than the mechanisms underlying the actions of endogenous GHB. Second, although some effects of administered GHB are blocked by the GHB receptor antagonist NCS-382 (Maitre et al., 1990), many are not (Carai et al., 2001; Cook et al., 2002; Carter et al., 2003). Unfortunately, interpretation of these results is clouded by several findings of GHB-like effects at higher doses of NCS-382 (Carai et al., 2001; Carter et al., 2003), which may mean that this compound is a mixed agonist–antagonist rather than a pure antagonist at the GHB receptor. In conclusion, to better understand the role of GHB receptors in mediating the effects of this substance, we need new drugs that block these receptors without exerting any agonistic effects.

GHB use and abuse has been growing

Government statistics indicate that the use and abuse of GHB has increased significantly since the mid-1990s. This can be seen in the data collected by the Drug Abuse Warning Network (DAWN), a national surveillance system run by the U.S. Substance Abuse and Mental Health Service Administration. DAWN obtains information on drug-related visits to participating hospital emergency departments throughout the U.S. as well as drug-related fatalities reported by medical examiners and coroners. Figure 15.7 shows that the number of yearly emergency department visits in which GHB was mentioned as a possible contributory factor rose greatly between 1994 (56 emergency department mentions) and 2000 (4969 mentions), and then dropped somewhat in 2001. Despite this trend, it is important to recognize that GHB is still associated with far fewer adverse drug reactions than more widely used substances like alcohol (218,005 emergency department mentions in 2001), cocaine (193,034 mentions), heroin (93,064 mentions), and marijuana (110,511 mentions).

The increase in adverse reactions to GHB can also be seen in published case reports of overdose victims. One group of researchers summarized 88 cases of GHB overdose that were seen in the emergency department of San Francisco General Hospital between July 1993 and December 1996 (Chin et al., 1998). The patients had a mean age of 28 years, and about two-thirds of them were male. Well over half of the cases involved coingestion of one or more other substances, usually alcohol, amphetamine, or MDMA. About 80% of the patients suffered from a decrease in conscious awareness, including a substantial number who were comatose upon admission to the emergency department. Other symptoms displayed by significant numbers of patients were emesis (vomiting), hypothermia (reduced body temperature), bradycardia (slowed heart rate), hypotension (lowered blood pressure), and acidosis (low blood pH). All patients in this

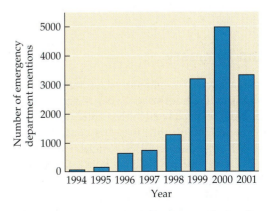

Figure 15.7 Emergency department mentions of GHB from 1994–2001. The number of emergency department mentions of GHB grew rapidly from 1994 to 2000.

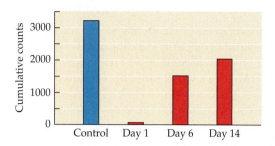

Figure 15.8 Tolerance to the locomotor-suppressant effects of GHB in mice Mice were given 200 mg/kg GHB intraperitoneally for 14 days. Locomotor activity in a photobeam apparatus was measured for 2 hours following drug administration on days 1, 6, and 14 of treatment. The figure illustrates the number of beam breaks recorded from 30 to 60 minutes post-treatment on each of these days. Compared to control mice administered saline, the GHB-treated animals showed a nearly complete cessation of locomotor activity on day 1, whereas a partial return of activity was observed on subsequent test days. (After Itzhak and Ali, 2002.)

case series regained consciousness over a period of several hours after admission, and all were discharged within 24 hours or less except for one individual who was admitted to the psychiatric ward due to suicidal ideation. Thus GHB overdose can lead to unconsciousness or coma as well as other potentially dangerous symptoms. Prompt treatment, however, usually results in an uneventful recovery.

Relatively few data are available on whether tolerance occurs following chronic GHB exposure. A recent study involving daily treatment of mice with 200 mg/kg GHB found tolerance to the activity-suppressing effects of the drug (Itzhak and Ali, 2002; Figure 15.8). GHB tolerance in humans has not been systematically investigated, but some users report an escalation in their dosing regimen that is suggestive of tolerance (Galloway et al., 1997). In extreme cases, users reach a pattern of constant dosing in which GHB is taken every 2 to 4 hours around the clock.

Information about GHB dependence is based mainly on self-report and case studies. Although such sources are not always reliable, in this case they strongly suggest that dependence and withdrawal can develop with repeated GHB use. The most common withdrawal symptoms seem to be insomnia, anxiety, and tremors (Friedman et al., 1996; Galloway et al., 1997; Craig et al., 2000). However, users of extremely high doses may experience more-severe symptoms including hallucinations, delirium, extreme agitation, and psychosis (Dyer et al., 2001; McDaniel and Miotto, 2001).

Section Summary

GHB is an analog of the inhibitory neurotransmitter GABA. The drug is used clinically as a sedative and anesthetic in Europe, and it was marketed in the United States as a bodybuilding supplement until over-the-counter sales were banned in 1990. However, GHB is available in prescription form for treating patients who suffer from cataplexy. Illicit use of GHB often occurs at nightclubs and dances, and unfortunately it has been used occasionally as a "date rape" drug.

GHB is usually taken orally in the form of an aqueous solution. Low doses produce alcohol-like effects including mild euphoria, relaxation, and social disinhibition. Higher

doses are associated with stronger sedating effects as well as dizziness, nausea, and vomiting. Severe overdosing with GHB causes severe respiratory depression, unconsciousness, and even coma.

Animals treated with GHB exhibit sedation, reduced locomotor activity, decreased anxiety behavior, and catalepsy at high doses. Some of these effects may be related to a drug-induced reduction in DA release. High doses of GHB can also lead to EEG excitation resembling absence (petit mal) seizures in humans. Rodent studies suggest that GHB has reinforcing properties; however, relatively little self-administration of GHB was observed when monkeys were given access to this compound.

There are two competing hypotheses concerning the mechanism of action of GHB. One hypothesis is that its effects are mediated by activation of pre- and/or postsynaptic $GABA_B$ receptors. Such activation might occur through the direct stimulation of these receptors by GHB. Alternatively, GHB could be metabolized to GABA within the brain, after which the excess GABA is released and stimulates $GABA_B$ receptors. The second hypothesis is that the effects of GHB are mediated by a specific receptor for this substance. Although no one has yet cloned a GHB receptor gene, there are binding sites for GHB that are present at relatively high levels in the hippocampus and cerebral cortex. Moreover, there is evidence that GHB may itself be a neurotransmitter or neuromodulator within the brain: it is synthesized enzymatically from GABA, it is released in a Ca^{2+}-dependent manner, it possess vesicular and plasma membrane uptake systems, and it appears to have its own receptor. Nevertheless, the relationship between the endogenous GHB system and the behavioral effects of exogenously administered GHB is not yet clear.

Use and abuse of GHB has increased significantly since the mid-1990s. This is reflected in the incidence of adverse reactions to GHB overdose, including many that require visits to hospital emergency departments. There is some evidence for tolerance, dependence, and withdrawal with repeated GHB use, although more research needs to be done in this area. Typical withdrawal symptoms include insomnia, anxiety, and tremors, although use of extremely high doses can apparently cause a psychotic reaction involving hallucinations, delirium, and extreme agitation.

Anabolic–Androgenic Steroids

Every few years, it seems, newspaper headlines blurt out the sad fact that yet another one of our sports heroes has been found guilty of taking some kind of banned performance-enhancing substance. Although there are many such substances available now, especially to a world-class athlete, one important category of performance enhancers is the **anabolic–androgenic steroids.** These are defined as steroid hormones that increase muscle mass (the anabolic part) and also have masculinizing, or testosterone-like, properties (the androgenic part). On the street, these substances are usually just called anabolic steroids, but there are no members of the group that aren't also androgenic. Nevertheless, it is more convenient to use the shorthand term *anabolic steroids,* and that is the term that we will use in the remainder of this chapter.

Why are anabolic steroids being brought up in a chapter on substances of abuse? There is significant evidence that these hormones are abused by some users, and some researchers have theorized that anabolic steroids can produce an addiction-like dependence. Before we discuss these ideas, however, we will present basic information on these substances and how they entered the realm of bodybuilding and athletic competition.

Background and History

Anabolic steroids are structurally related to testosterone

The chemical and trade names of some common anabolic steroids are presented in Table 15.2. Some of these compounds are taken orally, while others are injected intramuscularly. The latter are formulated for depot injection and maintain their potency for periods ranging from several days to 3 weeks, depending on the steroid. As shown in Figure 15.9, these compounds are all structurally related to testosterone, the principal androgen synthesized by the testes. However, because it is the anabolic rather than androgenic effects that are desired by most users, the chemical modifications that differentiate various synthetic steroids from

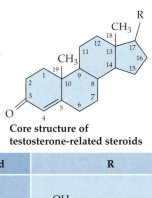

Core structure of testosterone-related steroids

Compound	R
Testosterone	— OH
Testosterone enanthate	— O — CO(CH$_2$)$_5$CH$_3$
Testosterone undecanoate	— O — CO(CH$_2$)$_9$CH$_3$
Testosterone cypionate	— O — COCH$_2$CH$_2$ ⬠
Nandrolone decanoate	— O — CO(CH$_2$)$_8$CH$_3$ (no methyl group at position 19)
Nandrolone phenproprionate	— O — CO(CH$_2$)$_2$ ⬡ (no methyl group at position 19)

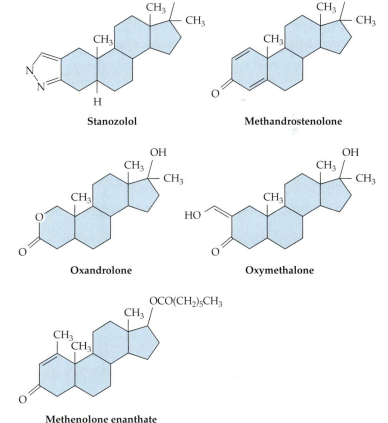

Stanozolol

Methandrostenolone

Oxandrolone

Oxymethalone

Methenolone enanthate

Figure 15.9 Chemical structures of some commonly abused anabolic steroids

TABLE 15.2 Some Common Anabolic Steroids

Generic name	Trade name	Route of administration
Methandrostenolone	Dianabol	Oral
Testosterone undecanoate	Andriol	Oral
Oxandrolone	Oxandrin	Oral
Oxymetholone	Anadrol	Oral
Stanozolol	Winstrol	Oral or injection
Testosterone cypionate	Depot-Testosterone	Injection
Testosterone enanthate	Primotetson	Injection
Nandrolone phenylpropionate	Durabolin	Injection
Nandrolone decanoate	Deca-Durabolin	Injection
Methenolone enanthate	Primobolan Depot	Injection

testosterone are aimed at selectively enhancing their anabolic potency. Because the oral steroids are potentially vulnerable to first-pass metabolism in the liver, these compounds are chemically designed to minimize this problem and thus retain adequate bioavailability.

Anabolic steroids were developed to help build muscle mass and enhance athletic performance

American athletes knew little about these compounds before the 1954 World Weightlifting Championships held in Vienna, Austria. Until 1953, American weightlifters had routinely beaten the Soviet team, but the Soviets outscored the Americans in that year and again in 1954. During the Vienna competition, the U.S. and Soviet Union team physicians reportedly went out in the evening for entertainment, and after a few drinks, the physician for the Soviet Union squad confided that some of his men were using testosterone. Dr. John Ziegler, who was the American physician, went back home and began to experiment with testosterone, but he didn't like the strong androgenic side effects. Ziegler expressed the need for a more anabolic, less androgenic compound to the giant pharmaceutical company Ciba. Within a few years, Ciba introduced Dianabol, an orally active compound with enhanced anabolic properties. When Dianabol was administered to elite weightlifters at the famous York Barbell Club in Pennsylvania, the drug produced spectacular results. Once the news got out, many similar compounds quickly followed and strength athletes began to view steroids as the only way to reach the highest level of achievement. According to a 1969 article in the magazine *Track and Field News* entitled "Steroids: Breakfast of Champions," these substances were readily available to athletes either from physicians who were willing to write the necessary prescription or even from some pharmacists who dispensed steroids without requiring a prescription (Hendershott, 1969).

However, as we will see later, there is a dark side to anabolic steroids in terms of their potential for serious side effects and possible dependence. Ziegler later recognized the monster that he had helped create, and by the time of his death in 1984 he profoundly regretted that part of his life.

Besides the Soviet Union, the German Democratic Republic (GDR, or East Germany) began secretly giving anabolic steroids to its elite athletes in the 1960s (Franke and Beredonk, 1997). The most commonly used compound in the GDR was chlordehydromethyltestosterone, known as Oral-Turinabol. The East Germans had especially great success with their female athletes, who won many Olympic and world championships with the aid of anabolic steroids. Figure 15.10 illustrates the increased performance of a female shot-putter over an 11-week period of Oral-Turinabol treatment. Unfortunately, as we will see later, these competitors paid a high price for their achievements due to the powerful side effects of anabolic steroids in women.

By the mid-1980s, there were increasing reports of rampant anabolic steroid use not only in professional sports but also reaching down into colleges and even high schools. In response, the U.S. Congress held a series of hearings between 1988 and 1990 that culminated in the Anabolic Control Act

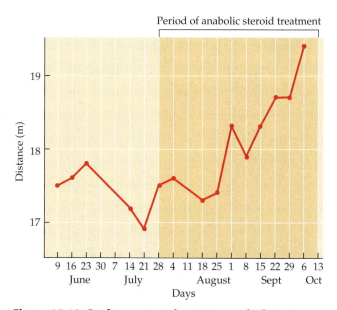

Figure 15.10 Performance enhancement of a former East German female shot-putter as a result of anabolic steroid treatment. Shot-put distance increased markedly over the 11-week period during which the athlete was being given anabolic steroids. (After Franke and Beredonk, 1997.)

of 1991. This legislation classified 27 specific anabolic steroid preparations as Schedule III controlled substances, thus making their use illegal without a medical prescription. In addition, these substances are banned by many amateur and professional sports organizations, including the National Collegiate Athletic Association, the International Olympic Committee, the National Football League, the National Basketball Association, and most recently Major League Baseball.

Although users had long touted the beneficial effects of anabolic steroids on muscle mass and strength, many researchers remained unconvinced by these anecdotal reports because properly controlled scientific studies were lacking and arguments could be made that placebo effects, increased training motivation, or other confounding factors might be responsible for the enhanced performance of anabolic steroid users. However, a series of recent studies by Shalender Bhasin and his colleagues at the Charles R. Drew University of Medicine and Science have shown that giving high doses of testosterone to healthy young men leads to muscle fiber hypertrophy (increased size), increased muscle mass, and enhanced strength (Bhasin et al., 1996, 2001; Sinha-Hikim et al., 2002). Some of the results from one of these studies are presented in Figure 15.11 (Bhasin et al., 2001). The subjects were given weekly injections of testosterone enanthate at different doses for a period of 20 weeks. They also received another drug at the same time to suppress endogenous testosterone secretion so that their testosterone levels would depend solely on the exogenous treatment. The lowest doses (25 and 50 mg per week) produced subnormal circulating testosterone concentrations, the 125 mg-dose produced concentrations in the normal range, and the 600-mg dose produced testosterone levels that were at least 4 times the average pretreatment concentration. As shown in Figure 15.11A–C, anabolic steroid administration caused dose-dependent increases in muscle volume and strength. In contrast, sexual function was unchanged (Figure 15.11D), indicating that this aspect of androgen action is not influenced by testosterone level within the dose range used and

Figure 15.11 Increased muscle strength and volume following chronic testosterone administration to men The subjects were healthy men, 18 to 35 years of age, who had prior weightlifting experience but who had not previously taken anabolic steroids. All subjects were given monthly treatments with a long-acting drug to suppress their endogenous testosterone synthesis. Matched groups were also administered weekly intramuscular injections of testosterone enanthate for 20 weeks at doses ranging from 25 to 600 mg per injection. A comparison of circulating testosterone levels at the beginning of the study (baseline) with levels present at the 16-week time point showed that the 25- and 50-mg doses produced testosterone concentrations significantly below baseline, the 125-mg dose produced concentrations similar to baseline, and the 300- and 600-mg doses produced testosterone levels that were approximately 2 to 4 times baseline, respectively (data not shown). Leg press strength (A), thigh muscle volume (B), quadriceps muscle volume (C), and sexual function as determined by sexual activity and desire (D) were assessed at baseline and at the end of the 20-week dosing period. Muscle strength and volume were enhanced by increasing doses of testosterone, whereas sexual function remained relatively constant regardless of dose. (After Bhasin et al., 2001.)

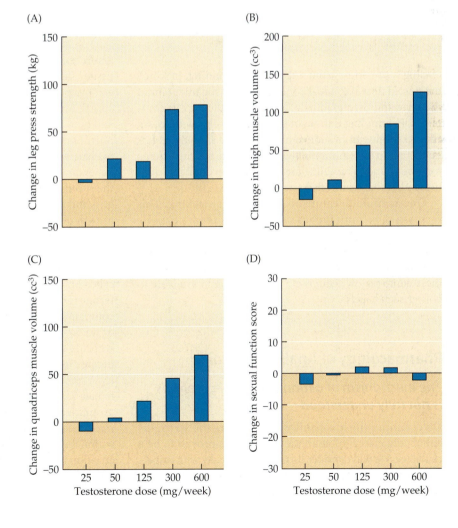

over the time period of testing. The findings of Bhasin's group are very important because they were obtained under carefully controlled conditions. However, it is worth noting that even greater effects may be obtained by users taking still higher doses of steroids and combining the treatment with intensive strength training.

Anabolic steroids are taken in specific patterns and combinations

Anabolic steroids are taken in a variety of different doses, patterns, and combinations (Mottram and George, 2000). Endurance athletes (for example, marathon runners) and sprinters tend to take relatively low doses of steroids, whereas bodybuilders and strength athletes like weightlifters may take up to 100 times the therapeutic doses of these hormones. Anabolic steroids are often used in patterns called **cycling.** Cycles are typically 6 to 12 weeks in duration, with periods of abstinence between successive cycles. Athletes use cycling for the following reasons:

1. To minimize the development of tolerance to the drug
2. To reduce the occurrence of adverse side effects
3. To maximize performance at an athletic competition; and
4. To avoid detection of a banned substance

Cycling is sometimes combined with **pyramiding,** in which the steroid dose is gradually increased until the midpoint of the cycle and then gradually decreased as the cycle is completed. Pyramiding is thought to reduce possible withdrawal effects resulting from sudden termination of steroid use. It is important to note, however, that many of the reasons offered for cycling and pyramiding are based on anecdotal information rather than controlled scientific studies.

One additional feature of steroid use is **stacking.** This refers to the simultaneous use of two or more anabolic steroids. Stacking is often done by combining a short-acting oral steroid with a long-acting injectable preparation. While users may believe that stacking enhances the effectiveness of these compounds, again there is little research available to bolster such beliefs.

Pharmacology of Anabolic Steroids

The mechanism of action of anabolic steroids is not fully understood

Determining the mechanisms underlying the strength-enhancing effects of anabolic steroids has proven to be a challenge. We will consider this issue specifically with respect to testosterone, as all anabolic steroid preparations either contain testosterone itself or are testosterone derivatives. Testosterone and other androgens are agonists at the **andro-**

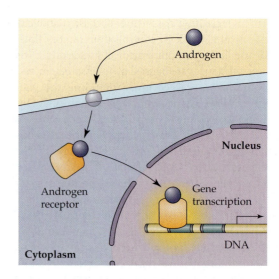

Figure 15.12 Mechanism of action of androgens on gene transcription Androgens enter target cells by diffusing across the cell membrane. After the hormone binds to androgen receptors in the cell cytoplasm, the hormone–receptor complex translocates to the cell nucleus, where it alters the transcription of specific genes.

gen receptor. These receptors are present in many different tissues, including skeletal muscle. In the inactive state, androgen receptors are located in the cytoplasm of the cell (Figure 15.12). Androgen molecules diffuse across the cell membrane and bind to the receptor, thereby activating it. The activated hormone–receptor complex then translocates into the cell nucleus, where it regulates the transcription of specific genes, depending on the cell type. Researchers haven't yet identified the specific muscle cell genes that are "turned on" by androgens, but the overall effect is to increase protein synthesis and growth of the muscle.

The actions of testosterone are complicated by the fact that this substance is converted enzymatically to two other bioactive hormones within the body. In some tissues, an enzyme called **5α-reductase** converts testosterone to **dihydrotestosterone (DHT),** which also has potent androgenic effects. This conversion does not occur in skeletal muscle, which has little or no 5α-reductase activity. In fact, some synthetic anabolic steroids were designed to avoid this metabolic reaction because it decreases the ratio of anabolic to androgenic activity. A second enzyme, **aromatase,** converts testosterone to the female sex hormone **estradiol** in a chemical reaction called **aromatization.** Aromatization is a normal process, even in males, and it plays a vital role in some of testosterone's actions within the CNS. In the present circumstance, however, aromatization is extremely undesirable because it leads to the feminizing side effects of steroid use. Again, some of the synthetic anabolic steroids were created to resist aromatization and thus minimize these particular side effects.

As suggested in the preceding discussion, the muscle-building effects of anabolic steroids are believed to be mediated at least partly by activation of androgen receptors. However, at least for men, this hypothesis has been questioned based on the idea that these receptors may be saturated (that is, completely filled) at normal physiological levels of testosterone. If this is true and the androgen receptors are already maximally activated, then how can raising the amount of circulating steroids produce a change in the muscle? We don't yet know the answer to this question, but there is recent evidence that anabolic steroid treatment can induce androgen receptor expression in muscle (Sheffield-Moore et al., 1999). Increasing the number of androgen receptors in the tissue would allow steroids to produce greater anabolic effects than they would in the presence of normal receptor expression. Another possibility stems from the fact that at high levels, androgens act as antagonists to glucocorticoid hormones (see Chapter 3). In muscle, glucocorticoids are **catabolic,** which means that they tend to produce an overall decrease in protein synthesis and an increase in protein breakdown. Hence, a second mechanism of action for anabolic steroids could be their anticatabolic effects via glucocorticoid antagonism. Further studies are needed to investigate these and other hypotheses of anabolic steroid action.

Many adverse side effects are associated with anabolic steroid use

Table 15.3 presents some of the potential adverse side effects of anabolic steroid use. Some of these effects are relatively common (for example, acne; Figure 15.13A), whereas others are rare (peliosis hepatis). Many side effects, such as those involving the cardiovascular system, are reversible if the person stops using steroids. Others, however, can be irreversible, like the masculinizing effects that occur in women (Figure 15.13B). Which side effects occur depends on a number of factors, including the age and sex of the user, the type of steroid used (especially oral vs. injectable), the dose, and the pattern and duration of use. As mentioned in the table, liver toxicity is mainly associated with oral steroids, but other side effects can occur with either oral or injectable forms. The documented decrease in high-density lipoprotein (HDL) cholesterol is noteworthy because it puts the user at increased risk for heart disease. Young people who are still growing also need to be concerned about the possible stunting effects of anabolic steroids produced by premature closure of the epiphyses.*

The behavioral effects of anabolic steroids have been a matter of considerable debate over the years. This debate has focused mainly on two issues: (1) whether anabolic steroids cause increased irritability and aggressive behavior; and (2) whether users develop dependence on these compounds. We will focus on the first question here and take up the issue of dependence in the next section.

A variety of different approaches have been used to investigate the effects of anabolic steroids on mood and aggressiveness (Bahrke et al., 1996). Many surveys and retrospective studies seem to indicate an association between anabolic steroid use and increased irritability and aggressive behavior. Numerous case studies have also been reported in which men who were not previously aggressive or violent began to show such characteristics while on steroids. This phenomenon, which is called "'roid rage" on the street, is discussed in Box 15.2.

Controlled studies of anger or aggressive behavior in response to anabolic steroids have yielded less consistent results, with some studies finding that steroids have signifi-

*These are the end regions of long bones that retain the capacity to further lengthen the bone. Once the epiphyses are "closed," the individual stops growing.

Figure 15.13 Facial acne and facial hair growth in anabolic steroid users Anabolic steroids can cause severe acne in users (A) and can also stimulate the growth of facial hair in women (B). (Photographs courtesy of Dr. Michael Scott.)

(A)

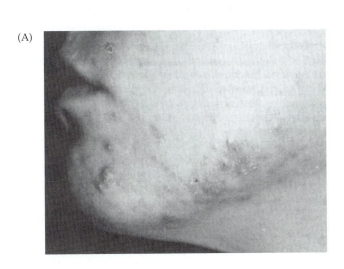

(B)

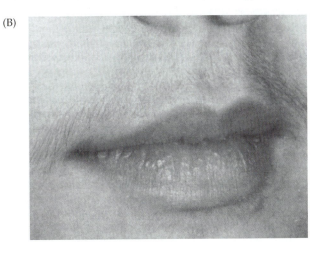

cant effects on mood or aggressive behavior but other studies reporting no such effects (Bahrke et al., 1996). Some of this inconsistency may be due to differing treatment regimens or methods for assessing aggressiveness. However, another important factor emerged from the recent double-blind, placebo-controlled study of Pope et al. (2000). Despite the fact that testosterone administration led to significant overall increases in manic symptoms and aggressive behavior, these effects were highly variable across subjects. Thus, 84% of the subjects exhibited little mood change in response to the treatment, 12% developed mild symptoms of mania, and just 4% showed strong manic symptoms. These findings suggest that some people are more susceptible than others to developing mood shifts and behavioral changes in response to anabolic steroid use. Such differential susceptibility could also explain why 'roid rage only occurs in a small subset of steroid users.

Do anabolic steroids cause dependence?

By the late 1980s and early 1990s, reports began to appear suggesting that some anabolic steroid users meet *DSM (Diagnostic and Statistical Manual of Mental Disorders)* criteria for dependence on these substances. A recent review of this literature, which includes individual case reports, case series, and surveys, found a total of 165 published instances of presumed steroid dependence (Brower, 2002). According to survey studies (Brower et al., 1991; Midgley et al., 1999), some of the commonly reported signs of dependence using the standard *DSM* criteria are:

1. Withdrawal symptoms when use of the substance (steroid) is stopped

2. Taking more of the substance than originally intended

3. Inability to cut down or control usage despite a desire to do so

4. Spending a large amount of time on activities related to obtaining and using the substance

5. Continued substance use despite problems caused by such use

6. Replacement of other activities with substance use

TABLE 15.3 Possible Health Consequences of Anabolic Steroid Use

Category	Effects
Cardiovascular effects	Hypertension (high blood pressure)
	Increased blood clotting
	Increased red blood cells
	Decreased HDL cholesterol (the "good" kind of cholesterol)
Effects on the liver (particularly from oral steroid use)	Jaundice
	Peliosis hepatis (blood-filled cysts in the liver)
	Tumors
Effects on the skin and hair	Oily skin and scalp
	Severe acne
	Male pattern baldness
Growth effects	Growth stunting in adolescents due to premature epiphyseal closure
Behavioral effects	Increased libido (sex drive)
	Increased irritability and aggressiveness
	Dependence
Specific effects on men	Testicular shrinkage
	Reduced sperm counts and possible infertility
	Prostate enlargement
	Gynecomastia (breast development)
Specific effects on women	Menstrual abnormalities
	Deepening of the voice
	Excessive hair growth, especially on the face
	Enlargement of the clitoris
	Decreased breast size

Withdrawal symptoms can include fatigue, depressed mood, insomnia, restlessness, anorexia, decreased libido, dissatisfaction with body image, and a desire for more steroids (Brower et al., 1990, 1991). Evaluation of anabolic steroid dependence is hampered by an absence of large-scale controlled studies that would enable us to gauge the prevalence of the problem. There is no indication in the literature that a lot of steroid users are presenting themselves for psychiatric treatment. This could mean that severe dependence on anabolic steroids is a relatively rare phenomenon, but it is also possible that dependent steroid users are reluctant to seek treatment for various reasons.

Information on the potential abuse liability of testosterone has also been obtained from studies in laboratory animals. To our knowledge, there are no published reports of self-administration by animals of testosterone or any other anabolic steroid. On the other hand, systemic injections of testosterone or one of its biologically active metabolites have been shown to produce a conditioned place preference in male rats

BOX 15.2 Drugs and Society

Anabolic Steroids and "'Roid Rage"

You may have heard the term "'roid rage" to describe a sudden eruption of intense anger or violent behavior by someone taking anabolic steroids. Case reports have documented instances in which violent outbursts appear to be linked to heavy steroid use. One extreme case is described in Katz and Pope (1990). Mr. X, as he is referred to, was a 23-year-old male who had been bodybuilding for 5 years. While in high school and prior to beginning his use of steroids, Mr. X drank alcohol socially and occasionally snorted cocaine with friends. He had no history of psychiatric illness, nor was he known to have ever committed a violent act. Indeed, his father was a minister, and Mr. X himself had been an active member of the church's youth ministry. He was described by friends as a considerate, religious person.

At the age of 21, Mr. X began the first of two cycles of anabolic steroid use in order to improve his competitive standing as a bodybuilder. During this time, he started to experience severe mood swings, including noticeable increases in irritability and argumentativeness. Quoting Katz and Pope,

On more than one occasion he tore chunks of aluminum out of cans with his teeth to intimidate bystanders. He also ripped telephones out of the wall on impulse. At this time, he met *DSM-III-R* criteria for a manic episode with decreased desire and need for sleep, explosive temper, extremely reckless behaviors with a high potential for dangerous and undesirable consequences, continued irritability, and grandiosity that reached delusional proportions. While out one weekend evening with some friends during the second course of anabolic steroids, the group stopped at a small market. While in the parking lot, Mr. X, without known or observed provocation, suddenly wrapped his arms around the telephone booth, tore it from its base, and threw it across the lot. The group left immediately and soon thereafter saw a hitchhiker on the road. Mr. X told the driver to stop. After the hitchhiker, a stranger to all present, entered the vehicle, Mr. X instructed the driver to drive to a remote spot in the woods. Once there, without instigation, Mr. X beat the victim repeatedly, tied him between two poles, smashed a wooden board over his back, and kicked him. The hitchhiker was found dead the next morning. (p. 220)

Mr. X was arrested, convicted, and incarcerated for his crime. Once off steroids, however, he reverted to his previous personality traits. In prison he was described as quiet, modest, and accommodating. Indeed, he was astonished at the acts he had committed that fateful evening.

While case reports such as this do not prove an association between anabolic steroids and violent behavior, they suggest that such an association may occasionally occur. Nevertheless, such extreme 'roid rage is a rare event even among heavy users. Controlled studies of steroid administration indicate that some individuals appear to be particularly susceptible to steroid-induced aggressiveness (see text), and we might speculate that steroid users who engage in violent acts (such as Mr. X) are among the susceptible group.

(Alexander et al., 1994; Frye et al., 2001). Because the cellular events triggered by steroid hormone receptors occur much more slowly than the rapid events triggered by neurotransmitter receptors (that is, altered gene transcription vs. ion channel opening or second-messenger synthesis), it is possible that place-conditioning procedures are better suited than self-administration methods for demonstrating the rewarding effects of anabolic steroids.

Further investigation demonstrated that place conditioning could be established with injections of testosterone or its metabolites directly into the nucleus accumbens, a brain area strongly associated with drug (particularly psychostimulant) reward (Packard et al., 1997; Frye et al., 2002). Moreover, the conditioned place preference produced by peripheral testosterone injections was completely blocked by either peripher-

al or intra-accumbens administration of the mixed D_1/D_2 dopamine receptor antagonist α-flupenthixol (Packard et al., 1998; Figure 15.14). Taken together, the place-conditioning studies argue that testosterone can be rewarding under the appropriate conditions, and they additionally provide a neuroanatomical and neurochemical link with other abused substances that have been shown to activate the accumbens dopamine system.

Even though anabolic steroids can apparently produce rewarding effects, dependence on these substances does not seem to have the same features as dependence on more typical drugs of abuse such as alcohol, nicotine, cocaine, and heroin. Under controlled laboratory conditions, administration of varying doses of testosterone to subjects who were not steroid users failed to produce any feelings of euphoria

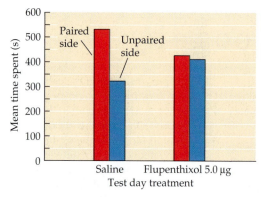

Figure 15.14 Blockade of a testosterone conditioned place preference by microinjection of the dopamine receptor antagonist α-flupenthixol into the nucleus accumbens Rats were given 8 days of training during which testosterone (0.8 mg/kg intraperitoneally) or vehicle was administered once daily while the animal was confined to one or the other compartment of a place-conditioning apparatus for 30 minutes. Preference for the testosterone-paired side was tested on day 9. Some rats received 5.0 μg of α-flupenthixol into the nucleus accumbens on the test day, while others received an intra-accumbens injection of saline instead. The animals given saline on the test day showed a conditioned preference for the chamber previously paired with testosterone, whereas this preference was not observed in the animals given α-flupenthixol on the test day. (After Packard et al., 1998.)

(Fingerhood et al., 1997). Indeed, the hormone wasn't even reliably detected compared to placebo treatment in a drug discrimination paradigm. Moreover, users don't typically report strong cravings when withdrawing from steroids, which differs from the intense cravings usually experienced by cocaine-, heroin-, alcohol-, or nicotine-dependent individuals undergoing forced abstinence. In humans at least, it seems likely that the reinforcement obtained from taking anabolic steroids stems principally from their performance-boosting and body image-enhancing effects. As Brower (2002) points out, anabolic steroid dependence occurs in weightlifters who are highly motivated to increase their strength and who participate in a culture that places a premium on physical attractiveness, fitness, and competitiveness. He proposes that the development of steroid dependence is due to the "muscle-active" effects of these compounds rather than any specific psychoactive effects. However, based in part on the animal literature summarized in the preceding paragraphs, Brower goes on to speculate that with repeated high-dose usage, a second stage of steroid dependence may develop that is mediated by brain reward mechanisms. This interesting theory remains to be tested experimentally.

Section Summary

Anabolic–androgenic steroids are hormones that increase muscle mass and strength and also produce masculinizing effects in the user. These substances either contain the naturally occurring male sex hormone testosterone or are similar to testosterone in their chemical structure. Some anabolic steroids are taken orally, others by intramuscular injection.

Anabolic steroids were developed for their muscle-building and performance-enhancing effects. The Soviet Union was the first country in which steroids were administered to athletic competitors; however, the practice quickly spread to other countries. When the use and abuse of these substances became more widespread and numerous adverse side effects began to emerge, steroids were classified as Schedule III controlled substances in the United States. They were also banned by a variety of national and international athletic organizations.

Despite anecdotal reports and case studies of performance enhancement by anabolic steroids, researchers were skeptical about these claims for many years due to an absence of appropriate double-blind, placebo-controlled studies. However, controlled experimental studies published over the past 10 years have demonstrated the dose-dependent effects of testosterone on muscle fiber size, muscle mass, and strength. Thus at the present time there is no longer any doubt about the effectiveness of anabolic steroids.

Anabolic steroids are usually taken in specific patterns and combinations. In the case of cycling, the steroid is taken in alternating on and off periods. Cycling can be combined with pyramiding, in which the dose is increased during the early part of the cycle and then gradually decreased after the peak dose is reached at the midpoint of the cycle. Some users also combine two or more steroids, often one that is injected and another that is taken orally. This practice is known as stacking.

Testosterone and other androgens are agonists at androgen receptors. When activated by binding an androgen, these receptors translocate to the cell nucleus, where they modulate gene transcription. Muscle cells possess androgen receptors, but it is thought that these receptors may already be maximally occupied by normal circulating levels of testosterone. This would make it difficult to explain how supraphysiological androgen levels could produce their anabolic effects. One possibility is that high androgen concentrations increase receptor expression by the muscles, thereby permitting enhanced hormone action. It is also possible that high doses of anabolic steroids exert an anticatabolic effect through an antagonistic action against glucocorticoids.

There are a number of adverse side effects of anabolic steroids that affect the cardiovascular and reproductive systems. These substances can produce masculinizing effects in female users and growth stunting in adolescents. Oral steroids pose the additional risk of causing liver damage. Behavioral side effects include heightened irritability and aggressiveness that reaches extreme proportions in a small number of cases.

Anabolic steroid dependence and withdrawal have been reported in some users. Although androgen self-administration has not been demonstrated in experimental animals, there are several studies showing rewarding effects through place conditioning. There is also evidence that the nucleus accumbens dopamine system may be involved in androgen reward. Nevertheless, anabolic steroid dependence does not show the same intensity as dependence on many other drugs of abuse. Brower has proposed a two-stage hypothesis of anabolic steroid dependence in which these substances are initially taken for their muscle-active effects but may eventually engender direct reinforcing effects with prolonged high-dose use.

Recommended Readings

Brower, K. J. (2002). Anabolic steroid abuse and dependence. *Curr. Psychiatry Rep.*, 4, 377–387.

Dinwiddie, S. H. (1994). Abuse of inhalants: A review. *Addiction*, 89, 925–939.

Nicholson, K. L., and Balster, R. L. (2001). GHB: A new and novel drug of abuse. *Drug Alcohol Depend.*, 63, 1–22.

Voy, R. (1991). *Drugs, Sports, and Politics.* Leisure Press, Champaign, Illinois.

Characteristics of Affective Disorders

The *Diagnostic and Statistical Manual of Mental Disorders* (*DSM-IV*) describes two principal types of affective disorder: **major depression** and **bipolar disorder.** Both of these are characterized by extreme and inappropriate exaggeration of mood (or affect). Major depression, also called unipolar depression, is characterized by recurring episodes of dysphoria and negative thinking that is also reflected in behavior. Bipolar disorder (also called bipolar depression), is also cyclic, but moods swing from depression to mania over time. The thinking and behavior of individuals with affective disorders are consistent with the exaggerated mood, but the mood does not reflect a realistic appraisal of the environment. Mood disorders are among the most common form of mental illness today and were described as early as 400 B.C. by Hippocrates. The Greeks called depression *melancholia,* meaning "black bile," and recognized that it was associated with anxiety and heavy alcohol use. However, only in the last 150 years has it been recognized as a disorder of brain function.

Major depression damages the quality of life

We are all familiar with the essential feelings associated with depression: feeling down and blue, feeling listless, and lacking energy to do even the fun things we normally enjoy. The state of sadness that occurs in response to situations such as the loss of a loved one, failure to achieve goals, or disappointment in love is called **reactive depression** and does not constitute mental illness unless symptoms are disproportionate to the event or significantly prolonged. The fact that we all have experienced depression does not make the clinical condition any easier to understand. In clinical depression, the mood disorder is so severe that the individual withdraws from life and all social interactions. The intense pain and loneliness may make suicide seem like the only option. Pathological depression resembles the emotional state that we have all experienced but differs significantly both in intensity and duration.

The dysphoric mood is characterized by a loss of interest in almost everything and an inability to experience pleasure in anything (anhedonia). Most depressed patients express feelings of hopelessness, worthlessness, sadness, guilt, and desperation. Frequently, patients exhibit loss of appetite, insomnia, crying, diminished sexual desire, loss of ambition, fatigue, and either motor retardation or agitation. Self-devaluation and loss of self-esteem are very common and are combined with a complete sense of hopelessness about the future. Individuals may stop eating or caring for themselves physically, sometimes remaining in bed for prolonged periods. Other physical symptoms may include localized pain, severe digestive disturbances, and difficulty breathing.

Thoughts of suicide are common; one estimate of suicide rates suggests that 7 to 15% of depressed individuals commit suicide, in contrast to a rate of 1 to 1.5% in the overall population. Table 16.1 summarizes the *DSM-IV* criteria for major depression and manic episodes. Although there are some common features of clinical depression, symptom clusters do vary with the individual. Furthermore, particular patterns of symptoms suggest that there are depression subtypes that may or may not be associated with distinct pathophysiologies.

If left untreated, most episodes of unipolar depression improve in about 6 to 9 months. However, the episodes usually recur throughout life, often increasing in frequency and intensity in later years. Although stress often precedes the first episodes of depression, later episodes are more likely to occur without the influence of psychosocial stress. Estimates of the incidence of depression vary significantly, but it is generally believed that 15 to 20% of the population experience depressive symptoms at any given time. The lifetime risk for a first episode of unipolar depression is between 3 and 4% for men and from 5 to 9% for women. The gender difference in the risk for depression is a topic of considerable interest and debate. The mean age of onset for depression is 27 years. This figure has decreased in recent years: Figure 16.1 shows that among Americans born before 1905, only 1% developed depression by age 75, whereas among those born since 1955, 6% had become depressed by age 24.

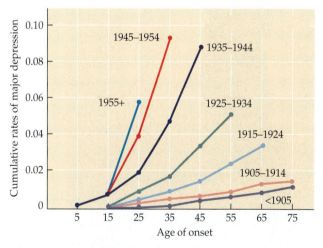

Figure 16.1 Age of onset of major depression Americans are developing major depression at higher rates and younger ages than previously, according to this analysis of data. The study evaluated 18,244 subjects at five sites, grouped in cohorts based on year of birth. Cross-cultural surveys indicate a similar phenomenon worldwide. (After Barlow and Durand, 1995.)

16

Affective Disorders

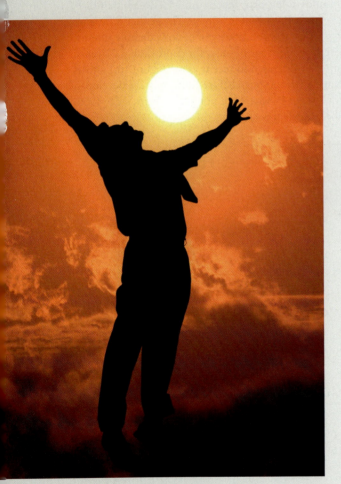

Barbara, a 39 year-old woman who had studied operatic singing, suffered from manic episodes. During one of them she started keeping her family up all night with prayer and loud singing. She was often not tired for days, scarcely sleeping at all. During one manic period she slept only two and a half hours a day. When interviewed by the psychiatrist at the hospital, she was wearing a flamboyant long red skirt with a peasant blouse and was heavily ornamented with huge earrings and numerous necklaces, bracelets, and medals pinned to her shirt. She talked fast, too loudly, and too much, frequently breaking into song. She could not be interrupted to answer the doctor's questions. Her talking and singing emphasized her intimate relationship with God, and she said that her beautiful singing voice was God's gift, which she had to share with those less fortunate. She drove to New York City to inform the Metropolitan Opera that she might have time for several performances in between her other vocal activities. Although Barbara has a beautiful voice and grandiose plans, she has not managed to create a career in singing due to the intrusion of mental illness and multiple hospitalizations, often for suicide attempts (Lickey and Gordon, 1991).

Excessive energy and unlimited confidence may lead the manic individual to impulsive and dangerous behavior.

TABLE 16.1 Symptoms of Manic Episodes and Major Depression

Diagnosis	Symptom
Manic episode	Inflated self-esteem or grandiosity
	Decreased need for sleep (e.g., feeling rested after only 3 hours of sleep)
	Greater talkativeness than usual or pressure to keep talking
	Flight of ideas or feeling that thoughts are racing
	Distractibility (i.e., attention too easily drawn to unimportant external stimuli)
	Increase in goal-directed activity (either socially, at work, or sexually); agitation
	Excess involvement in pleasurable activities that have a high potential for painful consequences (e.g., unrestrained buying sprees, sexual indiscretions, or foolish investments)
Major depressive episode	Depressed mood (or irritable mood in children and adolescents) most of the day, nearly every day
	Diminished interest or pleasure in most activities most of the day, every day
	Significant changes in body weight or appetite (gain or loss)
	Insomnia or hypersomnia nearly every day
	Psychomotor agitation (increased activity) or retardation (decreased activity)
	Fatigue or loss of energy
	Feelings of worthlessness or excessive or inappropriate guilt
	Diminished ability to think or concentrate; indecisiveness
	Recurrent thoughts of death, recurrent suicidal ideation without a specific plan, or a suicide attempt or specific plan for committing suicide

Source: American Psychiatric Association, 1994.

In bipolar disorder moods alternate from mania to depression

The second type of exaggerated mood is mania. Mania rarely occurs alone but rather alternates with periods of depression to form bipolar disorder. The primary symptom of mania is elation. Manic individuals feel faultless, full of fun, and bursting with energy. Their need for sleep is significantly reduced. They tend to be more talkative than usual and experience racing thoughts and ideas. In some individuals the predominant mood is irritability, belligerence, and impatience because the rest of us are just too slow. They tend to make impulsive decisions of the grandiose sort and have unlimited confidence in themselves. The manic individual becomes involved in activities that have a high potential for negative consequences that often go unrecognized by the individual, such as foolish business investments, reckless driving, buying sprees, or sexual indiscretions. However, some individuals during a manic phase are capable of highly productive efforts when channeled appropriately. A high proportion of creative individuals in the arts and sciences have experienced bipolar disorder and find that during the manic periods their thought processes quicken and they feel both creative and productive. Is creativity linked to mental illness? Box 16.1 considers that possibility.

The incidence of bipolar disorder is the same in men and women: it occurs in approximately 1% of the population. The time of onset for bipolar illness is typically between 20 and 30 years of age, and episodes continue throughout the life span.

Risk factors for mood disorders are biological and environmental

Most scientists agree that psychiatric disorders develop in a given individual because of the interaction of genes and environmental events. Individuals with particular clusters of genes inherit the tendency to express certain traits or behaviors that increase their vulnerability to specific disorders. Having those genes does not mean you will develop the disorder, but exposure to particular environmental events is more likely to trigger the disorder in the vulnerable individual. Heredity, environmental stress, and altered biological rhythms are risk factors for affective disorders.

Role of heredity   Evidence for a genetic contribution to affective disorders comes from several sources. **Adoption studies** help to clarify the role of genetics and family environment. In these studies, individuals with a firm diagnosis

Drugs and Society

Mood Disorders and Creativity

The old belief that genius is allied to madness may have its origins in the behaviors of mystics and soothsayers who frequently experienced unusual states of consciousness while revealing their prophesies. Edgar Allan Poe may have been one of the first contemporary authors to suggest that his creative talent might in fact "spring from disease of thought— from moods of mind." Several questions pose themselves. Is the occurrence of mental illness higher in populations of creative people than in average individuals? If so, then is mental disorder responsible for the special talent we call creativity or are there common factors that may contribute to both creative endeavors and vulnerability to mental disorders? Many influential poets, artists, and composers either wrote about their intense mood changes or have been diagnosed with either mania or depression. However, it is certainly true that the majority of creative individuals do not suffer from mood disorders or mental illness.

To begin to answer some of our questions, we need reliable statistical evidence rather than merely anecdotal reports. To evaluate the hypothesis that a relationship exists between mood disorders and creative behavior, we need to have systematic data collection, which may include structured interviews, along with control groups that are matched on significant variables such as education, socioeconomic level, etc. Also, we cannot rely on "madness" as our defining criterion for mental illness. Instead, strict diagnostic criteria such as the *DSM-IV* definition of mood disorders must be used. As an expert in the field, Kay Jamison (1985) has compiled data from a number of statistical studies that show extremely high

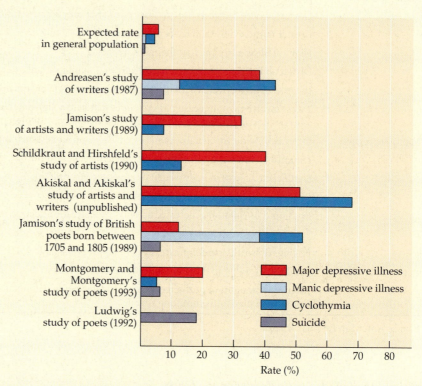

rates of depression, mania, cyclothymia (a less severe form of manic–depressive illness), and suicide among creative people compared to controls. Overall, these investigations show a suicide rate 18 times higher in individuals who have significantly contributed to the arts and literature compared to the general population, as well as an incidence of depression 8 to 10 times higher and an incidence of manic–depressive illness 10 to 20 times higher.

Although there is no way to be sure, Jamison argues that some of the classic symptoms of mood disorders may promote some unique talents. For example, individuals with mania or a less severe condition called hypomania experience expansive thinking and grandiose moods. Hypomanic speech uses more rhyme, alliteration, and unique vocabulary. Tests have also shown that word associations are more rapid during a hypomanic state. Depression produces subdued behav-

ior, inward-directed thoughts, and questioning. Perhaps some individuals who experience manic–depressive episodes use the altered states to view the world as a place of opposing forces and ambiguities and, as a result, develop insights into the constantly changing nature of life.

Does this mean mood disorders should go untreated? Certainly not, because these are serious and dangerous conditions that should not be trivialized. Left untreated, a mood disorder often worsens to the point that the individual cannot work at all. Furthermore, treatment becomes less effective later in the course of the disorder. Some may abuse alcohol or illicit drugs seeking relief. Unfortunately, the side effects of the mood-stabilizing drugs may cause a loss in cognitive skills. The ultimate goal of therapeutics for bipolar disorder should be to control the extremes but not impair the normal range of human emotional experience.

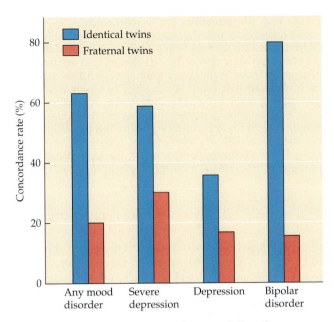

Figure 16.2 Concordance rate for mood disorders among identical and fraternal twins Identical twins are far more likely to share mood disorders than are fraternal twins, especially in the case of bipolar disorder. Concordance for clinical depression depends to some extent on severity. In this case, severe depression is defined as three or more episodes of depression. Data derived from 110 pairs of twins. (After Bertelsen et al., 1977.)

who were adopted at an early age are the focus of the research. If a heritable component exists, one would expect to see that, compared with controls, the individual with affective disorder has more biological relatives with the same disorder, despite being raised in a different environment. Although adoption studies suggest a role for genetics, the results have not always been consistent.

The best evidence for a heritable component to affective illness comes from **twin studies,** which show a significant difference between monozygotic (identical) and dizygotic (fraternal) twins in the rate of concordance for the disorders. The data in Figure 16.2 show that if one twin has a mood disorder, the concordance rate (i.e., the likelihood of the other twin sharing the trait) for a monozygotic twin is approximately 65%. This means that if one of the pair of identical twins (having the same genes) experiences affective illness, the probability that the other twin will also experience some affective disorder is 65%. In contrast, the concordance rate for dizygotic twins (who are genetically no more similar than other siblings) is 20%. The difference in these two rates suggests the extent to which genetics contributes to the disorder. Keep in mind that if genetics were the only determining factor, the concordance rate in identical twins would be 100%. The genetics of an individual can certainly make him more vulnerable, but whether or not he actually develops the disorder must also depend on other psychosocial or pathophysiological factors.

If you look again at Figure 16.2 you will see that the concordance rate is also dependent on the severity of clinical depression: more severe mood disorders may have a stronger genetic contribution than less severe disorders. The figure also shows that the genetic contribution to bipolar disorder is significantly greater than that to major depression. Eighty percent concordance in monozygotic twins compared to 16% in dizygotic twins indicates a very strong role for heredity in bipolar disorder.

Despite **linkage studies,** which look for similarities in gene location on chromosomes in families with affected members, and other more sophisticated methods of molecular biology that examine DNA fragments, no single dominant gene for affective disorders is known. We may well find that the genes involved confer a general vulnerability to a host of mood and anxiety disorders. The particular disorder that is expressed in an individual may ultimately be determined by developmental or psychosocial factors.

Role of stress Both neurobiological studies and family studies indicate that anxiety and depression are closely related. First, anxiety along with its associated physiological symptoms is a frequent accompaniment to depression. Second, intense environmental stress and anxiety often precede episodes of depression, particularly early on in the course of the disorder. Further, altered patterns of stress hormone levels are frequently found in depressed patients. Chapter 17 will further develop the realtionship between anxiety and depresssion. Despite the importance of environmental stress, keep in mind that identical life stresses may be perceived very differently by individuals. Many people seem resilient and capable of coping despite extraordinary stresses, while others seem to succumb to relatively minor problems. It is likely that genetics plays a role in determining how one responds physically and behaviorally to daily traumas and stress. The dual importance of nature (genetics) and nurture (environment) can never be ignored.

The importance of stress to the etiology of depression and its mediation by the hypothalamic–pituitary–adrenal (HPA) axis is a significant focus in neuroscience. In response to stress, multiple neurotransmitters (including norepinephrine, acetylcholine, and γ-aminobutyric acid [GABA]) regulate the secretion of corticotropin-releasing factor (CRF) from hypothalamic cells. CRF controls the release of adrenocorticotropic hormone (ACTH) from the pituitary into the blood. ACTH in turn acts on the adrenal gland to increase secretion of cortisol and other glucocorticoids, which all play a role in the mobilization of energy to deal with stress (Figure 16.3). Normally, cortisol feeds back to shut down HPA activation, resulting in transient activity of the system and brief surges in cortisol.

Among the most consistent neuroendocrine abnormalities in depressed individuals is abnormal secretion of corti-

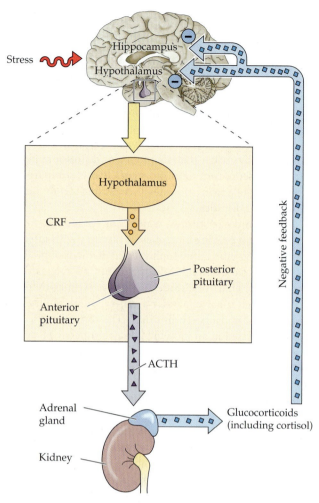

Figure 16.3 The HPA axis Our normal response to stress includes activation of the hypothalamus, which initiates a cascade of events beginning with the release of CRF. CRF acts at the anterior pituitary to induce ACTH release. ACTH in turn causes the adrenal cortex to release cortisol and other glucocorticoids into the general circulation to enhance energy production to deal with stress. Notice the dual negative-feedback loop initiated by high levels of glucocorticoids in the blood that directly reduces hypothalamic release of CRF while at the same time acting on the hippocampus, which also inhibits HPA function.

Figure 16.4 Abnormalities in glucocorticoids (A) Many (but not all) depressed patients have elevated cortisol levels, compared with controls. Each dot represents a single individual. (B) Differences exist between the circadian changes in blood cortisol levels of depressed patients and healthy control subjects. The measures were made each hour over a 1-day period. The decline in cortisol that normally occurs in the early morning and evening occurs to a lesser extent in depressed patients. (C) Depressed individuals fail to respond with reduced cortisol levels after injection with 1 mg dexamethasone (DEX). The injected glucocorticoid also normally reduces both CRF release from the hypothalamus and pituitary release of ACTH. (B after Kandel, 1991; C after Klein, 2000.)

Second, the high level of cortisol found in depressed patients is characterized by an abnormal circadian rhythm in cortisol secretion. The elevated and relatively flat pattern (depicted in Figure 16.4B) may reflect a more general abnormality in the biological clock, since altered rhythmicity also occurs for body temperature changes and sleep patterns (see below). Third, since many depressed individuals have elevated cortisol, it is not surprising that some fail to respond to dexamethasone challenge. Dexamethasone is a synthetic glucocorticoid that should act as a negative-feedback stimulus to suppress hypothalamic release of CRF and pituitary release of ACTH, resulting in decreased cortisol levels (Figure 16.4C). Several studies have suggested that patients who remain nonresponders to dexamethasone (i.e., fail to have cortisol release suppressed) after successful antidepressant treatment have a higher probability of relapse than those who show normal response.

Although usually adrenal glucocorticoids (including cortisol) are helpful in preparing an organism for stress, when the levels are persistently elevated, several systems begin to show pathological changes. Besides having damaging effects on immune-system and organ function, glucocorticoids are also associated with neuronal atrophy in the hippocampus, leading to cognitive impairment, imbalances in the serotonin (5-HT) system correlated with anxiety, and hormonal changes associated with depression (McEwen et al., 1994). The section on the neurobiological models of depression later in the chapter will provide more detail on the role of glucocorticoids in depression.

Altered biological rhythms   Cortisol secretion is not the only biological rhythm that is disturbed in major depression. Altered sleep rhythms are among the most common and persistent symptoms of depression. Circadian rhythm controls the onset, pattern, and termination of sleep. The normal sleep cycle is quite regular, having four stages of non-REM sleep (stages 1 to 4) lasting a total of 70 to 100 minutes followed by a 10- to 15-minute period of rapid eye movement (REM) sleep, during which time dreaming occurs. This cycle is repeated four or five times a night. Depressed individuals show several distinct abnormalities in their sleep rhythm (Figure 16.5A). First, there is a long period before sleep

sol, which is demonstrated in several ways. First, many depressed patients have elevated levels of cortisol (Figure 16.4A) in response to a greater-than-normal release of ACTH. Although both the pituitary and adrenal glands are enlarged due to hypersecretion, evidence from several sources suggests that the abnormality is not in the glands but is in the brain. The hypersecretion is most likely due to abnormal regulation of CRF by the hypothalamus. Numerous studies have found higher-than-normal levels of CRF in the cerebrospinal fluid (CSF) of depressed patients and increased numbers of CRF-producing cells in the hypothalamus in postmortem brain tissue. It is important to note that antidepressant drug treatment and electroconvulsive therapy reduce CRF levels in depressed patients.

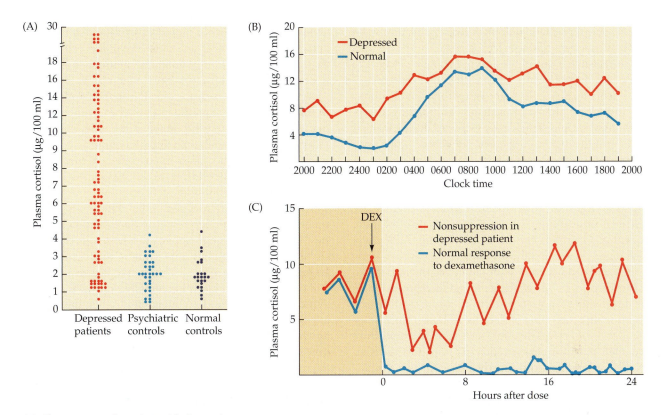

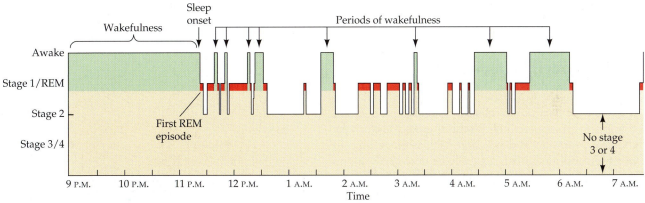

(A) Sleep pattern of a patient with depression

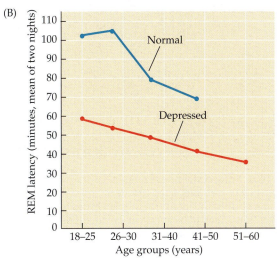

Figure 16.5 Altered sleep architecture in depression (A) In depressed patients, the onset of sleep is delayed and REM periods (colored red) get shorter as the night goes on rather than longer, which is typical in healthy adults. Also, notice the many awakenings that occur during the night due to the failure to reach deep sleep (stages 3 and 4). (B) REM episodes begin sooner after the onset of sleep in depressed than in nondepressed individuals.

onset. Second, there is a significant decrease in the time spent in slow-wave sleep, or deep sleep (stages 3 and 4), which leads to repeated awakenings during the night. Third, the onset of REM sleep occurs much earlier after the onset of sleep (Figure 16.5B). In extreme cases, the individual may enter REM sleep almost immediately after falling asleep. Fourth, REM sleep is significantly increased during the first one third of the night in depressed individuals, while non-depressed individuals have proportionately more REM sleep in the final one third of sleep. Also, while normal REM periods tend to increase in duration during the night, depressed patients do not show such a pattern. Finally, when ocular movement is measured, depressed individuals show more frequent and vigorous eye movements during REM sleep, which suggests more-intense dreaming.

Although we don't know what the altered rhythms mean, the irregularities in sleep patterns found in depressed individuals resemble the sleep patterns of normal individuals who must alter their time of sleep by 12 hours. Since other indicators of biological rhythms, such as body temperature fluctuation and hormonal secretion (e.g., cortisol), are often also altered, one might consider the possibility that the biological clocks of people with depression are "phase-shifted." In some individuals, the three rhythms are out of harmony (called desynchronization) or are mismatched. The implications of these irregularities have led to several novel treatment strategies, described in Box 16.2.

Animal Models of Depression

Animal models are used to study the neurobiology of depression and to evaluate the mechanism of antidepressant drugs, as well as to screen new drugs for effectiveness. Although the affective symptoms of depression, such as the feelings of worthlessness and guilt, can really be described only in human terms, several animal models have provided important tools to evaluate drugs and neurochemistry. There is no available model that mimics all the symptoms of depression; instead they consider specific aspects of the disorder such as reductions in psychomotor activity, neuroendocrine responses, cognitive changes, or such functions as eating and sleeping. Therefore, their usefulness in evaluating the complex etiology of depression is limited.

One of the oldest methods used to identify clinically useful antidepressants is the antagonism or reversal of **reserpine-induced sedation.** In terms of face validity, psychomotor slowing seems to be most similar to human depression, although other reserpine-induced effects can be used as readily. For example, reserpine-induced ptosis (drooping eyelids) and hypersecretion of tears and saliva also provide ready measures and are frequently used in animal research. The validity of the model has been further demonstrated by the

almost universal ability of clinically useful antidepressants to antagonize the effects of reserpine. The model is limited in that it is dependent on monoamine neurochemistry and does not identify novel approaches to therapeutics.

A more complex measure, called the **behavioral despair,** or **forced swim test,** requires rats or mice to swim in a cylinder from which there is no escape. After early attempts to escape are unsuccessful, the animals assume an immobile posture except for the minimal movements needed to keep their heads above water (Figure 16.6). The model is based on the idea that the immobility reflects a lowered mood in which the animals are resigned to their fate and have given up hope. Effective antidepressants reduce the time spent in this "freezing" phase of immobility relative to untreated control animals. This test has similarities to the **learned helplessness** test described in Chapter 4 (see Figure 4.25). You will recall that the subjects are initially exposed to aversive events over which they have no control. When the subjects are placed in a new situation in which a response could alter an aversive event, they fail to make the appropriate response. The animal behavior resembles clinical depression in that depressed humans frequently fail to respond to environmental changes and express feelings of hopelessness and the belief that nothing they do has an effect.

In order to evaluate the importance of stress as a vulnerability factor in the development of depression, **maternal separation** can be used. Stress is induced by separating young

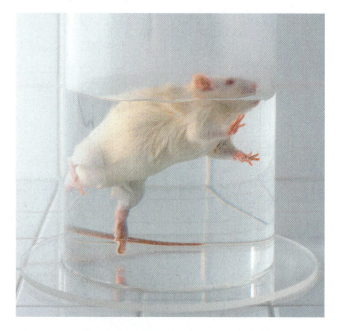

Figure 16.6 Forced swim test After initial attempts to escape, the rat in the water-filled cylinder is shown in a posture reflecting a sense of futility. Antidepressant drugs reduce the amount of time spent in the immobile posture. (Courtesy of Porsolt and Partners Pharmacology.)

BOX 16.2 Clinical Applications

Sleep Deprivation Therapy

For those of us who chronically seem to work and play too hard and deprive ourselves of sleep, it may be difficult to believe that sleep deprivation can have benefits. But according to a summary of results compiled from 61 studies completed over 20 years, involving more than 1700 individuals with depression, total sleep deprivation significantly reduced depressive symptoms in 59% of the patients (Wu and Bunney, 1990). Figure A shows a typical profile of symptoms before and after total sleep deprivation. It may be worth noting that the patients who responded to sleep deprivation were those who did *not* show the normal hormonal response to dexamethasone. Perhaps this finding indicates that a subset of depressed individuals have an underlying neurohormonal dysfunction. Unfortunately, the depressive symptoms returned following a single night of sleep (Figure B).

A more practical approach uses partial sleep deprivation, especially effective during the second half of the night, or sleep phase shifting. Experimental data suggest that changing the sleep–waking cycle (e.g., sleep onset at 5 P.M. and waking at 2 A.M.) reduces depressive symptoms, perhaps by resetting the normal phase relationship between the sleep–waking cycle and the other rhythms. An additional benefit is that when classic antidepressant medication is used along with partial sleep deprivation, depressed patients respond more quickly than they do using the antidepressant drugs alone or using partial sleep deprivation alone.

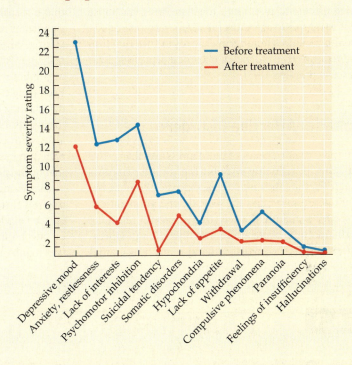

(A) Therapeutic effect of sleep deprivation The effect of sleep deprivation on a profile of symptoms in patients with unipolar depression. The difference between the two curves represents changes in symptom severity before (the upper profile line) and after (the lower profile line) 24 hours of sleep deprivation. (After Pflug, 1988.)

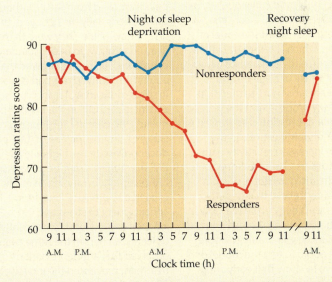

(B) Effects of sleep deprivation on mood rating for two groups of patients Notice that individuals who respond to sleep deprivation with reduced depression rating scores (responders) return to their previous condition after one night of sleep. (After Wu and Bunney, 1990.)

animals (usually rats) from their mothers for brief periods daily during the first few weeks of life. Early stress provides the opportunity to evaluate long-term behavioral and neuroendocrine abnormalties in the animals as adults. Nemeroff (1998) used this model to evaluate the hypothesis that abuse or neglect early in life activates the stress response at the time, but also produces long-term changes in CRF function that may predispose the individual to clinical depression later in life (discussed in Box 16.3).

Therapies for Affective Disorders

There are three major classes of antidepressants that prove highly effective in reducing symptoms of mood disorders (Table 16.2). They are the monoamine oxidase inhibitors, the tricyclic antidepressants, and the second-generation antidepressants, which include the selective serotonin reuptake blockers. In addition, there are several atypical antidepressants as well as electroconvulsive therapy and transcranial magnetic stimulation. Lithium therapy will be considered separately because of its primary importance in treating bipolar disorder.

Having a variety of antidepressant drugs available means that a majority of clinically depressed individuals can find significant relief. However, double-blind, placebo-controlled trials of antidepressants show that no one specific drug or drug type is more effective than any other, and there is no way to predict which patient will respond to a particular drug. Each drug is effective in about two thirds of cases of clinical depression. The different pharmacological characteristics of the agents mean that they will reduce different symptoms and also produce distinct but characteristic side effects. Each patient must usually undergo trials to find an antidepressant that optimally balances effectiveness and side effects.

Every one of the treatment methods currently available requires chronic administration, suggesting that although we understand how each works acutely at the synapse, the clinical effect must depend on compensatory changes in function that require time to develop. Although significant changes in

---

BOX 16.3 Pharmacology in Action

Stress–Diathesis Model of Depression

Nemeroff (1998) and colleagues developed a model of mood disorders called the stress–diathesis model of depression, which refers to the interaction between early experience (stresses such as abuse or neglect) and genetic predisposition (diathesis). In essence they propose that the genetic character of depression is expressed in lowered monoamine levels in the brain or in increased reactivity of the HPA axis to stress. These factors create a lower threshold for depression. In addition, they believe that negative, stressful events early in life may lower the threshold even further, leaving the individual more vulnerable to depression as an adult. To test the model one would have to show that early stress not only produces immediate activity of the HPA axis but also causes a persistent activation of CRF-containing neurons. If such were the case, then these individuals would respond more strongly to stress as adults than control subjects.

The design to test the model used newborn rats that were stressed by being removed from their mothers for brief periods daily for 10 days of their first 21 days of life. They were then allowed to grow up under standard conditions. The results showed that as adults the deprived rats had elevations in stress-induced ACTH and cortisol and increased CRF in the brain. A permanent increase in CRF gene expression explains the increase in CRF production. Despite the higher levels of CRF, the studies also found increased CRF receptor density, which might be expected to produce long-term enhancement of stress and CRF-induced depression. More recently, other researchers in the same group observed that antidepressant drug treatment prevented the increase in CRF and reduced the fearful behaviors (for example, freezing in novel situations) normally exhibited by the rats. When treatment was terminated, all the abnormalities returned. How the blocking of 5-HT reuptake modifies the CRF axis is not immediately evident but is certainly the focus of future research.

The implications of this type of research are very clear. Several million children are abused or neglected in the United States each year. Based on the animal evidence, we would expect these children to be exposed to events that permanently modify their developing brains, leaving them more vulnerable to stress and depression as adults.

The research also suggests a new direction for antidepressant drug development and therapeutic regimens. The reemergence of biological abnormalities after termination of drug treatment suggests that treatment may need to be continued indefinitely to prevent the recurrence of depressive episodes. Also, the potential to develop a new class of antidepressants that block CRF receptors could lead to a new therapeutic approach to the treatment of at least some cases of depression.

TABLE 16.2 Major Classes of Antidepressants and Their Most Notable Side Effects

Class	Antidepressants	Side effects
Monoamine oxidase inhibitors	Phenelzine (Nardil) Tranylcypromine (Parnate) Isocarboxazid (Marplan)	Insomnia, weight gain, hypertension, drug interactions, tyramine effect
Classic tricyclics	Imipramine (Tofranil) Amitriptyline (Elavil) Desipramine (Norpramine)	Sedation, anticholinergic effects, cardiovascular toxicity
Second-generation:		
Selective serotonin reuptake inhibitors	Fluoxetine (Prozac) Sertraline (Zoloft) Paroxetine (Paxil)	Insomnia, gastrointestinal disturbances, sexual dysfunction, serotonin syndrome
Atypical antidepressants	Maprotiline (Ludiomil) Bupropion (Wellbutrin) Mirtazapine (Remeron)	Varies with individual mechanism of action
Electroconvulsive shock and transcranial magnetic stimulation		Memory impairment, confusion, amnesia

symptoms can occur during the first 1 to 3 weeks of drug treatment, maximum effectiveness may not be achieved until after 4 to 6 weeks of therapy. This time lag is especially worrisome in patients who are severely depressed and suicidal. Some symptoms, including irregularities in sleep and appetite, are the first signs that show improvement, followed over the next few weeks by mood enhancement. Several long-term studies from the National Institute of Mental Health suggest a period of maintenance drug treatment for at least 6 to 8 months after symptoms are reduced. Because maintenance therapy significantly reduces the probability of relapse, treatment is extended indefinitely for some individuals.

Although we are treating antidepressant drugs and drugs used for anxiety (Chapter 17) as separate entities, we would like to make it clear that the distinction is often more semantic than real. As we noted earlier, stress and anxiety are components of affective disorders, and the trend in drug treatment further blurs the distinction. Antidepressant drugs reduce the anxiety that accompanies depression, and they are increasingly being used to treat anxiety disorders unrelated to depression.

Monoamine oxidase inhibitors are the oldest antidepressant drugs

The first true antidepressant action was discovered quite by accident due to a lucky clinical observation. The drug iproniazid was used in the early 1950s to treat tuberculosis but had significant mood-elevating effects unrelated to its effects on the disease. Following that observation, iproniazid was found to inhibit monoamine oxidase (MAO). Although met with enthusiasm following their early introduction as antidepressants, the **MAO inhibitors (MAO-Is)** fell into disfavor

because of their reputation for having severe and dangerous side effects (see below). However, over the years it has become apparent that, with appropriate dietary restrictions, MAO-Is can be used safely and often work well for patients who are treatment-resistant (those who do not respond to other drugs) and who reject the idea of electroconvulsive therapy. In addition to their use in affective disorders, MAO-Is are also used in the treatment of several anxiety states and have positive effects on the eating behavior and mood of patients with bulimia and anorexia nervosa. The currently available MAO-Is include phenelzine (Nardil), tranylcypromine (Parnate), and isocarboxazid (Marplan).

Mechanism of action You will recall from Chapter 5 that MAO is an enzyme found inside the cells of many tissues, including neurons. The normal function of the enzyme is to metabolize the monoamine neurotransmitters in the presynaptic terminals that are not contained in protective synaptic vesicles. The inhibition of MAO increases the amount of neurotransmitter available for release. A single dose of a MAO-I increases norepinephrine (NE), dopamine (DA), and 5-HT and thus increases the action of the transmitters at their receptors. It was initially assumed that the enhanced neurotransmitter function was responsible for the antidepressant action; however, those biochemical changes occur within hours, while the antidepressant effects require weeks of chronic treatment. It is now apparent that neuron adaptation involving change in receptor density or second-messenger function must play an important part in these drug effects (Figure 16.7A–C).

Side effects The more common side effects of MAO-Is include changes in blood pressure, sleep disturbances

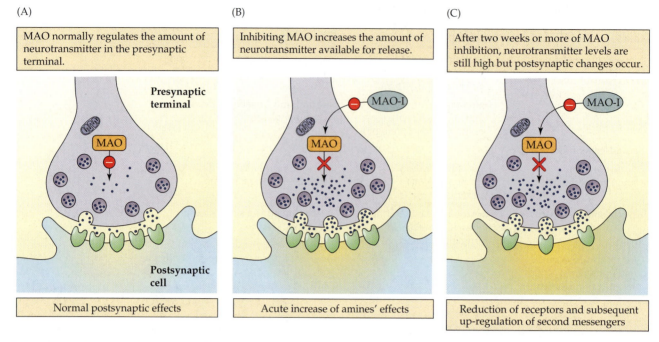

(A) MAO normally regulates the amount of neurotransmitter in the presynaptic terminal.

Presynaptic terminal

MAO

Postsynaptic cell

Normal postsynaptic effects

(B) Inhibiting MAO increases the amount of neurotransmitter available for release.

MAO-I

MAO

Acute increase of amines' effects

(C) After two weeks or more of MAO inhibition, neurotransmitter levels are still high but postsynaptic changes occur.

MAO-I

MAO

Reduction of receptors and subsequent up-regulation of second messengers

Figure 16.7 Acute and long-term effects of MAO-Is on synaptic function (A) Presynaptic MAO degrades neurotransmitter molecules that are not in vesicles to keep amines at "normal" levels. (B) MAO-Is inhibit the enzyme, causing an elevation in available neurotransmitter for release, resulting in increased action at receptors. (C) After 10 days to 2 weeks of antidepressant treatment, the amount of neurotransmitter in the synapse is still elevated over control conditions, but neural adaptation has occurred: down-regulation of amine receptors and up-regulation of the cyclic adenosine monophosphate (cAMP) second-messenger system. Other antidepressant drugs produce similar adaptive changes in neurons.

including insomnia, and overeating, especially of carbohydrates, which may lead to excessive weight gain. In addition to these side effects, there are three other types of side effects that are significantly more dangerous. First, because inhibition of MAO elevates NE levels in peripheral nerves of the sympathetic branch of the autonomic nervous system as well as in the CNS, any prescription or over-the-counter drug that enhances NE function will have a much greater effect than normal. For example, nasal sprays, cold medications, antiasthma drugs, amphetamine, and cocaine will all have greater-than-expected effects and produce elevated blood pressure, sweating, and increased body temperature. Second, some serious side effects are due to the inhibition of MAO in the liver as well as in the brain. The MAO in the liver is responsible for deaminating tyramine, which is a naturally occurring

amine formed as a by-product of fermentation in many foods, including cheeses, certain meats, pickled products, and other food. These foods must be avoided by individu-

TABLE 16.3 Dietary Restrictions for Patients Taking MAO-Is

Food group	Examples
Dairy	Unpasteurized milk and yogurt; aged cheese; other cheeses including blue, Boursault, brick, Brie, Camembert, cheddar, Colby, Emmenthaler, Gouda, Gruyere, mozzarella, Parmesan, provolone, Romano, Roquefort, and Stilton
Meat and meat alternatives	Aged game; liver; canned meats; yeast extracts; salami; dry sausage; salted, dried, smoked, or pickled fish such as herring, cod, and caviar; peanuts
Breads, cereals, and grains	Homemade yeast breads with substantial quantities of yeast; bread or crackers containing cheese
Vegetables and fruits	Italian broad beans, sauerkraut, bananas, red plums, avocados, raspberries
Miscellaneous	Alcoholic beverages including red and white table wines, ale, beer, champagne, sherry, and vermouth; yeast concentrates, soup cubes, commercial gravies, or meat extracts; soups containing items that must be avoided; soy sauce; soy bean curd (hoison)

als using MAO-Is (Table 16.3). Elevated tyramine levels release the higher-than-normal stores of NE at nerve endings, causing a dramatic increase in blood pressure. Blood pressure may reach critical levels and is accompanied by headache, sweating, nausea, vomiting, and sometimes stroke. Third, MAO-Is also inhibit other liver enzymes such as the cytochrome P450 enzymes (see Chapter 1), which normally degrade such drugs as barbiturates, alcohol, opiates, aspirin, and many others. The effects of these drugs are prolonged and intensified in the presence of MAO-Is.

Tricyclic antidepressants are highly effective

This class of antidepressant is named for its characteristic three-ring structure (Figure 16.8), which is closely related to that of the antipsychotic drugs in the phenothiazine class (see Chapter 17). Although the prototypical **tricyclic antidepressant (TCA)** imipramine

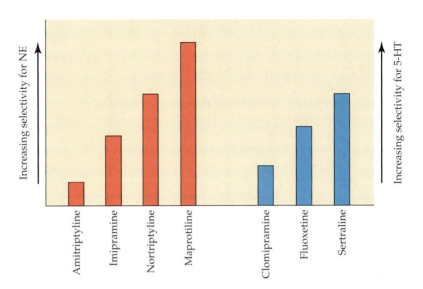

Figure 16.9 Relative specificity of several antidepressant drugs that depend on reuptake blockade to enhance monoamine action Those in blue are relatively specific for blocking 5-HT reuptake and belong to the class called selective serotonin reuptake inhibitors. Those in red, such as maprotiline, are rather specific norepinephrine reuptake blockers. Drugs such as imipramine, amitriptyline, and clomipramine block reuptake of both monoamines but show a slight preference for one or the other.

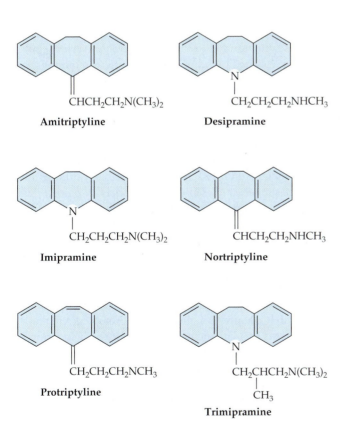

Amitriptyline

Desipramine

Imipramine

Nortriptyline

Protriptyline

Trimipramine

Figure 16.8 Tricyclic antidepressants are named for their characteristic three-ring structure.

(Tofranil) failed its original test for antipsychotic effects, it did appear to have mood-elevating actions. Many other tricyclics were subsequently developed.

Mechanism of action The drugs in this class act by binding to the presynaptic transporter proteins and inhibiting reuptake of neurotransmitters into the presynaptic terminal. Inhibition of reuptake prolongs the duration of transmitter action at the synapse, ultimately producing changes in both pre- and postsynaptic receptors. Although many of the drugs in this class are equally effective in inhibiting the reuptake of NE and 5-HT, some are more effective on one transmitter than the other. Although this difference does not change their antidepressant action, it does determine the drugs' side effects. Figure 16.9 provides a visual representation of the relative NE and 5-HT reuptake-blocking potencies of several TCAs and some second-generation antidepressants as well. As was true for the MAOIs, the immediate increase in NE and 5-HT function is not correlated to clinical effectiveness, which takes several weeks. Clearly, an acute increase in synaptic activity is only the first step in antidepressant action; neuronal adaptation, occurring over a period of time, also plays an important role (see Figure 16.7). In addition to reuptake blockade, most of the TCAs also block acetylcholine, histamine, and α-adrenergic receptors, which contribute to their side effects.

Side effects Although we assume that TCA action is due to enhancement of monoamine activity followed by compensatory changes in the transmitter systems, the receptor-blocking activity contributes to side effects. Histamine receptor blockade is responsible for the sedation and fatigue that are frequent side effects that limit the drugs' usefulness in individuals who must remain alert. On the other hand, for patients who experience agitation, the sedative effects may be welcome. Anticholinergic side effects are troublesome for others and include dry mouth, constipation, urinary retention, dizziness, confusion, impaired memory, and blurred vision. The α_1-blockade in combination with the NE reuptake-blocking effects lead to several potentially dangerous cardiovascular side effects, including orthostatic hypotension, tachycardia, and arrhythmias. This particular set of side effects makes it especially difficult to treat depression in elderly patients with known cardiac disorders.

In addition, toxicity following overdose causes cardiovascular depression, delirium, convulsions, respiratory depression, and coma. Heart arrhythmias may produce cardiac arrest and fatalities. Since the fatalities associated with TCA treatment occur at approximately 10 times the normal dose, these drugs have a relatively low therapeutic index (TD_{50}/ED_{50}), particularly when used by patients demonstrating suicidal tendencies.

Second-generation antidepressants have different side effects

In an attempt to offer drugs with fewer side effects and more rapid onset of action, a host of new antidepressants have been developed. In general, they are designed to be more selective in their action with the hopes of eliminating the anticholinergic and cardiovascular effects produced by the older drugs while still elevating levels of NE and/or 5-HT to provide antidepressant action. None are more effective, however, nor do they have a more rapid onset. The most significant difference is in the nature of their side effects, which are related to their neurochemical mechanisms of action. Many are considered safer than the older drugs if taken as an overdose.

The **selective serotonin reuptake inhibitors (SSRIs)** deserve special mention because they are often the first choice among antidepressants because of their greater relative safety. In addition to major depression, the drugs are also used to treat several distinct disorders: panic and anxiety disorders, obsessive–compulsive disorder, obesity, and alcoholism.

Mechanism of action Drugs in this class, which include fluoxetine (Prozac), sertraline (Zoloft), and paroxetine (Paxil), are more selective than TCAs in enhancing serotonin function because they block the presynaptic reuptake transporter for 5-HT to a greater extent than the noradrenergic transporter. As is true for all of the antidepressants discussed, we assume that the antidepressant action requires compensatory changes in neurons that occur over several weeks.

Side effects The side effects of the SSRIs are different from the TCAs because the drugs do not alter NE, histamine, or acetylcholine. Hence, the frequent TCA-induced side effects of sedation, cardiovascular toxicity, and anticholinergic effects are absent. Nevertheless, SSRIs produce a different pattern of side effects because they enhance 5-HT function at all serotonergic receptors. While the antidepressant action may be related to increased 5-HT function at serotonergic receptors, increased 5-HT activity at other receptors causes side effects: anxiety, restlessness, movement disorders, muscle rigidity, nausea, headache, insomnia, and sexual dysfunction. The sexual dysfunction, which occurs in 40 to 70% of patients, is a frequent reason for terminating therapy, particularly among young, male patients.

Although the SSRIs are generally safer than the older drugs, they have potentially life-threatening effects when combined with other serotonergic agonists or with drugs that interfere with the normal metabolism of the SSRIs. These effects, referred to as the **serotonin syndrome,** are characterized by severe agitation, disorientation and confusion, ataxia, muscle spasms, and exaggerated autonomic nervous system functions including fever, shivering, chills, diarrhea, elevated blood pressure, and increased heart rate (Lane and Baldwin, 1997).

One other distinctive characteristic of the SSRIs compared with the older antidepressants is their ability to cause physical dependence. As many as 60% of patients suffer withdrawal effects following drug termination (Zajecka et al., 1997). The withdrawal symptoms, which can last for several weeks, include dizziness and ataxia, nausea, vomiting and diarrhea, fatigue, chills, sensory disturbances, insomnia, vivid dreams and increased anxiety, agitation, and irritability. Although the SSRIs avoid many of the dangerous side effects of the older drugs, caution in their use is still warranted.

Although the SSRIs are second generation antidepressants, some of the newest antidepressants are once again **dual NE/5-HT modulators.** Mirtazapine (Remeron), a drug approved by the U.S. Food and Drug Administration in 1997, was developed with two concepts in mind. First, the most current thinking suggests that enhancing both NE and 5-HT function is more beneficial than acting on a single monoamine. Second, in order to reduce side effects, the drug specifically blocks selected receptors. Early trials showed clear clinical benefits in a broad range of patients when compared with placebo and equal effectiveness compared with the TCA amitriptyline, but with fewer (65%) adverse side effects compared with placebo (70%) or amitriptyline (87%). As a representative of the newest dual-action drugs, mirtazapine offers the promise of clinical efficacy with limited side effects (Pinder, 1997).

Third-generation antidepressants have distinctive mechanisms of action

Third-generation antidepressants are currently in the development and testing stage. The goals for the newest drugs will be to continue to minimize side effects and toxicity as well as speed up the onset of effectiveness. Despite our best attempts, it is evident that neuropharmacology is still unsure about the cellular changes that produce effective antidepressant action, but it is clear that a series of molecular changes underlie the therapies. The two newest approaches, CRF receptor antagonism and enhancement of the cyclic adenosine monophosphate (cAMP) intracellular second-messenger system, will be discussed later in the chapter, in the section on neurobiological models of depression.

Electroconvulsive therapy is safe and highly effective

In the early 1900s, a Hungarian psychiatrist noted that several of his patients showed improvement in their moods after having spontaneous seizures. This observation encouraged others to induce convulsions in psychiatric patients by administering camphor and oil or insulin. Such treatment was the predecessor of electroconvulsive therapy (ECT), which was introduced in 1938 and is used today to treat affective disorders, both clinical depression and bipolar disorder. Generally, ECT is used on the depressed patient who is unresponsive to pharmacotherapy. The effectiveness of ECT (80 to 90%) is higher than that of more conventional treatments, but because its administration is technically more difficult and expensive, its use is limited to the most resistant cases. In addition, although it produces no pain or awareness of the seizure and has a low incidence of side effects, public concern has limited its use (Fink, 1987).

Although there are a variety of methods to produce seizures, using either electricity or drugs, ECT is used most often because it is more reliable and does not cause the fear reaction of some drugs. Furthermore, ECT is easier and safer to administer and produces the least discomfort and side effects because of the routine use of anesthesia, muscle relaxation (to prevent the convulsion), and oxygenation (to maintain respiration). As is true for antidepressant drugs, ECT treatment must be administered several times a week for several weeks to be fully effective (e.g., three times a week for 3 weeks).

Mechanism of action   ECT enhances the function of several neurotransmitter systems, including NE, 5-HT, DA, and GABA, and these changes are probably responsible for its antidepressant action. As is true for many of the pharma-cotherapies, the repeated treatment leads to down-regulation of β_2- and α_2-adrenergic receptors.

Side effects   ECT has a low incidence of side effects, which makes this treatment most appropriate for those with cardiovascular disorders, the elderly, the medically ill, or pregnant women. The most significant side effect is cognitive impairment, taking the form of confusion and memory loss. ECT may disrupt the ability to retain new information (anterograde amnesia) for several days or weeks after treatment. In addition, significant retrograde amnesia for events preceding the treatment may also occur. Patients may have difficulty remembering events that occurred during the series of ECT treatments and several months prior to the treatment.

Transcranial magnetic stimulation is easy to administer

Transcranial magnetic stimulation (TMS) is a new brain-stimulation technique that has been recently tested for antidepressant effects. The treatment involves placing a small coil of wires on the scalp and applying a brief but powerful electric current that induces a strong, localized magnetic field. The magnetic field moves unimpeded through the skull and induces a weaker, localized electric current in the brain. Depending on the stimulation frequency, TMS may either excite the brain or inhibit neural activity.

Several recent clinical trials (Berman et al., 2000; George et al., 2000; Grunhaus et al., 2000) evaluated the effects of TMS, applied for approximately 20 days to the left dorsolateral prefrontal cortex, on symptoms of depression. Overall results showed that active TMS significantly reduced depressive symptoms compared with sham TMS treatment. TMS was very similar to ECT in its ability to reduce Hamilton Depression Rating Scale scores; however, it was only modestly effective for delusional depression and may not work with patients who are treatment-resistant. Nevertheless, more-intense evaluation of the parameters of administration may yield further improvements in TMS's efficacy while maintaining its mild side effect profile. Additionally, the method is non-invasive and almost painless, and it does not produce convulsions or require anesthesia, so it can be performed on an outpatient basis, unlike ECT.

Drugs for treating bipolar disorder stabilize the highs and the lows

For the majority of patients with bipolar disorder, **lithium carbonate** (Carbolith, Eskalith) is the most effective medication and is the usual drug of choice. Although lithium has no effect on mood or behavior in healthy individuals, J. Cade in 1949 discovered that it had powerful effects on patients with mania. One to two weeks of lithium use eliminates or

(A)

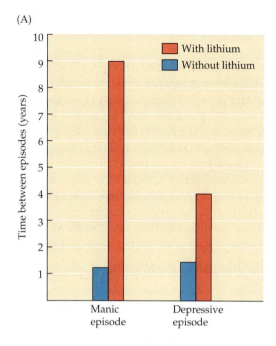

(B)

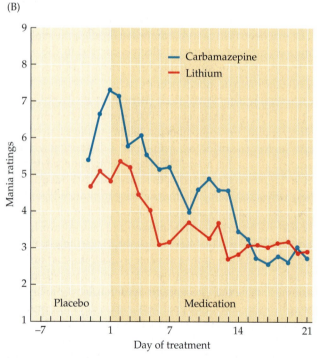

Figure 16.10 Lithium's effectiveness for bipolar disorder
(A) Maintenance therapy with lithium significantly reduces the occurrence of manic episodes so that on the average, the time between manic periods is 9 years, compared with 14 months without treatment. Depressive episodes also occur less often, averaging 4 years between episodes with lithium treatment and 17 months without. (B) The time course and extent of effectiveness of the newer drug carbamazepine is virtually identical to that of lithium in reducing manic symptoms in patients with bipolar disorder. (A after Lickey and Gordon, 1991; B after Post et al., 1984.)

reduces symptoms in approximately 60 to 80% of manic episodes without causing depression or producing sedation. The drug is somewhat less effective in terminating episodes of depression, so it is often administered along with a TCA or other antidepressant drug. Most important is that it is useful for reducing the occurrence of future episodes of mania and depression. Patients who continue with lithium treatment have an average hospital stay of less than 2 weeks per year, while without lithium therapy they spend an average of 8 to 13 weeks per year in the hospital. Figure 16.10A graphically demonstrates that without lithium maintenance the typical bipolar patient has an episode of mania every 14 months and a period of depression every 17 months on average. Lithium maintenance reduces the recurrence of mania to once in 9 years and depressive episodes to about every 4 years (Lickey and Gordon, 1991).

Treatment of bipolar disorder with a mood stabilizer is a lifelong necessity for most patients. Either abrupt termination or gradual withdrawal of lithium results in recurring periods of mania and heightened suicide risk. Despite the risks, many patients stop taking the drug. In some cases, side effects are a significant problem for the patient, especially if they involve impaired memory and confusion. In other cases, patients stop taking the drug because they fail to experience normal mood changes, which diminishes the richness of life. Finally, others object to the loss of the manic phase of bipolar disorder because that time is perceived as a period of heightened creativity and productiveness.

Mechanism of action It is probably not surprising to find that lithium enhances 5-HT actions: it elevates brain tryptophan, 5-HT, and 5-HIAA (the principal 5-HT metabolite) as well as increasing 5-HT release, which ultimately alters receptor response in several brain areas. Lithium reduces catecholamine activity by enhancing reuptake and reducing release. Despite these neurochemical changes, it is unlikely that lithium acts on individual neurotransmitters to normalize mood swings of both mania and depression. Given that the drug flattens the extremes of emotion in both directions, it is more likely that it modifies synaptic transmission at points beyond the neurotransmitter receptors, for instance on second-messenger function. Lithium has pronounced effects on adenylyl cyclase, phosphoinositide cycling, G protein coupling, and brain neurotrophic factors. Its ability to alter intracellular actions regardless of the triggering neurotransmitter may explain its effects in both mania and depression.

Side effects Lithium is not metabolized but is excreted by the kidney in its intact form at a rate inversely related to sodium levels. Sodium depletion due to extreme sweating, diarrhea, vomiting, dehydration, use of diuretic medication, or adherence to severely salt-restricted diets may lead to potentially toxic levels of lithium. The effective therapeutic range of lithium concentration in the blood is 0.7 to 1.2 mM. Since toxic effects begin to occur at blood levels of 2.0 mM, the therapeutic index is very low, and a patient's blood level of lithium must be monitored on a regular basis. Side effects are generally quite mild at therapeutic doses but may include increased thirst and urination, impaired concentration and memory, fatigue, tremor, and weight gain. Toxic effects are more severe and include cramps, vomiting, diarrhea, kidney dysfunction, coarse tremor, confusion, and irritability. Levels of lithium above 3.0 mM may lead to seizures, coma, and death (Calabrese et al., 1995).

Other therapies for bipolar disorder   Because of lithium's potential for toxicity, alternative therapies have been developed. Of the alternatives, the anticonvulsant drugs carbamazepine (Tegretol) (Figure 16.10B) and valproate (Depakene) are the most common; however, several newer drugs such as topiramate (Topamax) and tiagabine (Gabitril) are similarly effective when compared with lithium but have a different toxicity profile. Further discussion of these drugs is beyond the scope of this text and is left to others (Calabrese et al., 1995; Guay, 1995).

Section Summary

Affective disorders constitute clinical depression and bipolar disorder, also called manic–depressive disorder. In both cases the symptoms occur in discrete episodes that recur throughout life. Family studies, adoption studies, and twin studies demonstrate the importance of genetics to both disorders but particularly to manic–depressive disorder. Nevertheless, environmental factors such as stress contribute to the onset and course of the psychopathology.

Significant abnormalities in biological rhythms are associated with clinical depression. The most consistent neuroendocrine abnormality is elevated cortisol. Higher cortisol levels are reported in response to elevated ACTH, which is under the control of hypothalamic CRF-secreting neurons. Depressed individuals also fail to show the normal rise and fall of cortisol secretion that occurs during the day in healthy individuals. Some depressed patients are also unresponsive to the negative feedback normally produced by high levels of cortisol or by administration of dexamethasone.

Depressed individuals also show distinct circadian irregularities in the sleep cycle. Altering the total amount of sleep with sleep deprivation or by changing the timing of the sleep–waking cycle has significant antidepressant effects for some individuals.

Animal models of depression are useful for screening new drug treatments and also for studying the neurochemistry of the disorder. The three major classes of antidepressant drugs are monoamine oxidase inhibitors, tricyclic antidepressants, and second-generation antidepressants, including selective serotonin reuptake inhibitors and several atypical agents. Electroconvulsive therapy is a safe and effective procedure that is used primarily when other antidepressant treatments are ineffective. Transcranial magnetic stimulation is another, newer method of stimulating the CNS that is currently being tested.

Each antidepressant drug is effective in about two thirds of cases and has a unique combination of side effects based on its neurochemical effects. Although neuropharmacologists know the mechanisms of action of the drugs, it is still not clear which of their neurochemical actions is responsible for their effectiveness in treating depression. What we are sure about is that regardless of the acute effects on neurotransmitters, it requires several weeks of repeated administration for the therapeutic effects to set in. The time course strongly suggests that the CNS must make compensatory modifications before a drug's effectiveness can be realized. Current research is investigating second-messenger changes after chronic treatment and on neuroendocrine response.

Bipolar disorder is most often treated with lithium, which reduces mania and depression and also prevents the recurrence of mood swings. Lithium's potential for toxicity has led to the testing of other types of drugs, including several that are used as antiseizure medications.

Neurochemical Basis of Mood Disorders

The earliest attempt to develop a cohesive theory of the neurochemical basis of affective disorders was the **monoamine hypothesis.** The monoamine hypothesis originated with the observation that reserpine, a drug effective in reducing high blood pressure, induces depression as a side effect in a significant number of patients. The drug prevents the packaging of neurotransmitters into vesicles, leaving the molecules in the cytoplasm, where MAO degrades them. In this way, reserpine treatment produces empty vesicles and reduces the levels of dopamine, norepinephrine, and serotonin (all monoamines). Could it be that the reduced level of monoamines in the CNS is responsible for the depressed mood? This possibility seemed increasingly likely when the mechanism of action of two types of antidepressants (MAO-Is and TCAs) was considered. Despite their varied synaptic action, the antidepressant drugs acutely increase the function of NE or 5-HT or both. In addition, drugs in both classes reverse reserpine-induced reduction in motor activity, a classic animal model for testing antidepressant agents that was described earlier (Figure 16.11). The drug studies were combined with the early data showing reduced levels of the NE metabolite MHPG (suggesting lowered NE synaptic activity) and reduced 5-HIAA in the CSF, plasma, or urine of depressed patients. These measures suggest low utilization of the monoamines. In addition, the

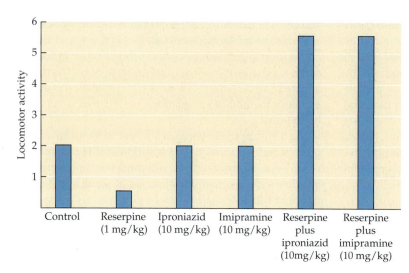

Figure 16.11 Effects of reserpine, the MAO-I iproniazid, and the TCA imipramine on rat locomotor activity Reserpine clearly reduces motor activity of rats compared to control treatment, while neither of the antidepressants has any effect on motor activity when given alone. However, a dramatic increase in motor behavior occurs when reserpine is given in combination with either of the antidepressants. The reversal of reserpine-induced depression parallels the changes in brain amines and contributes to the monoamine hypothesis of affective disorders. (From Snyder, 1996.)

manic-like activity produced by amphetamine and cocaine is correlated with the increase in catecholamines in the synapse following enhanced release or blocked reuptake. Prolonged use of the drugs causes depletion of the amines, resulting in depression, lethargy, and craving. All of these pieces of evidence formed the basis of the monoamine hypothesis of affective disorders (Schildkraut, 1965).

Although many new questions have challenged the original hypothesis, when it was first proposed the best evidence supported the idea that depression is associated with low levels of monoamines, whereas mania coincides with excess monoamine activity. Because reserpine acts on all monoamines and the early antidepressants also were nonselective in increasing NE and 5-HT, it really was not clear which of the neurotransmitters was most important in the etiology of depression. Unfortunately, we have not yet resolved this issue, and more and more researchers are coming to the conclusion that both of these amines are likely to play a role in clinical depression and that other neurotransmitters may also contribute to the complex pattern of symptoms. There is increasing evidence that there is anatomical and functional interaction between the noradrenergic neurons in the locus coeruleus and the serotonergic neurons originating in the midbrain raphe. Each of the two transmitter systems seems to be capable of modulating the other. In the meantime, it is important to remember that neurotransmitter systems should be considered not in isolation but

instead as a part of a complex network of interacting neurons.

Although we now know that the monoamine hypothesis is overly simple, it provided an important theoretical model that was the focus of enormous amounts of research over many years. It provided the basis for new drug development, the creation and testing of new animal models, and the formulation of new questions that could not be answered within the old theory. As is always the case in good science, new and often conflicting evidence must be accounted for and old theories modified.

The monoamine hypothesis as originally stated was based heavily on acute antidepressant drug effects. It is too simplistic to account for the complex syndrome of affective disorders, and it fails to resolve several discrepancies. The most important of these is the discrepancy in time between the rapid neurochemical actions of antidepressants and the slow onset of clinical effects over several weeks. This disparity in time course clearly demonstrates that the acute enhancement of monoamine function is not the neurochemical basis for therapeutic activity. Newer testable models of the neurobiological basis of affective disorders still use three basic approaches: (1) developing animal models; (2) evaluating the mechanism of action of effective drug treatment; and (3) examining neurobiological differences in patient populations. The most common ways of evaluating groups of patients are by measuring neurochemical differences in biological fluids or brain tissue postmortem, evaluating response to drug challenge, and visualizing the brain with positron emission tomography (PET) or magnetic resonance imaging. Using patients is most problematic in that results are frequently inconsistent due to variability among patients in symptoms, history of drug use, lifestyle issues, and so forth.

Serotonin dysfunction contributes to mood disorders

Serotonin continues to be a focus of research because it has a significant influence on sensitivity to pain, emotionality, and response to negative consequences as well as to reward. The effects of 5-HT on sleep, eating, and thermoregulation are likewise well documented and intuitively seem to contribute to depressive symptoms. Rats with depleted stores of 5-HT are irritable and aggressive, appear overly sensitive to pain, and show altered patterns of eating and satiety. Parallels in humans suffering from major affective disorders can be easily seen.

Measuring 5-HT in humans Although there is no solid evidence for abnormal 5-HT function in depressed patients, several measures can provide a clue to CNS function. First, the most common way to determine the level of 5-HT function (called **turnover**) is by measuring the principal metabolite of serotonin 5-hydroxyindole acetic acid (5-HIAA). It is generally assumed that high 5-HIAA reflects increased function of serotonergic neurons and low 5-HIAA the converse. Lower 5-HIAA levels have been found in postmortem brains of depressed individuals, most consistently in the brains of suicide victims. Several studies have also reported lower 5-HIAA levels in the CSF of depressed individuals. Measuring monoamine metabolites in other body fluids such as blood or urine is much easier, but the results may or may not indicate CNS function.

Second, blood level of **tryptophan,** the 5-HT precursor, is another measure of serotonergic function that frequently appears low in depressed patients compared to controls. Further, in one double-blind, placebo-controlled study, Delgado and coworkers (1990) rapidly depleted tryptophan in patients who had shown a good response to antidepressant treatment. Depression scores showed that 14 out of 21 patients had a recurrence of symptoms despite continued antidepressant medication. The depression scores were negatively correlated with free plasma tryptophan levels.

Third, **receptor binding studies** in postmortem brain samples from unmedicated individuals with mood disorders have found *increased* density of postsynaptic 5-HT$_2$ receptors, which may be considered a compensatory response to low serotonergic activity. In accord with this finding, animal studies show that chronic antidepressant treatment leads to a fairly consistent decrease (down-regulation) in 5-HT$_2$ receptors. Table 16.4 gives you some idea of the variety of antidepressant treatments that produce this down-regulation. Only the clinically effective use of chronic ECT fails to reduce these receptors.

Challenge studies provide one additional way to evaluate receptor function indirectly in vivo by measuring the magnitude of a biological response to administered agonists or antagonists (Brown et al., 1994). For the serotonergic system, the biological response measured is most often hormonal, including changes in cortisol, prolactin, or growth hormone, although other physiological measures may also be used, such as body temperature. The magnitude of the response is considered an indicator of the sensitivity or function of the receptor. Overall, the agonist-induced increase in prolactin

TABLE 16.4 **Effects of Chronic Antidepressant Treatment on Serotonin Neurons**

Antidepressant treatment	Effect on 5-HT$_2$ receptor binding[a]	Electrophysiological response to 5-HT
Tricyclics		
Amitriptyline	↓ or =	↑
Chlorimipramine	↓	↑
Desmethylimipramine	most ↓	↑
Imipramine	↓ or =	↑
Second-generation		
Fluoxetine	↓ or =	=
Iprindole	↓	↑
Mianserin	↓	↑
Trazodone	↓	↑
MAO-Is		
Tranylcypromine	↓	↓
Clorgyline	↓	↓
ECT	= or ↑	↑

Source: After Willner, 1995.

[a] ↑ enhancement; = no change; ↓ reduction.

suggests that 5-HT receptors are less sensitive in depressed patients. Sensitivity to 5-HT is restored by chronic administration of certain antidepressants.

Finally, we can utilize some of the newest imaging techniques to visualize changes in brain function and receptors in human subjects. PET imaging (Figure 16.12) provides the first look at blood flow changes in the brains of patients with

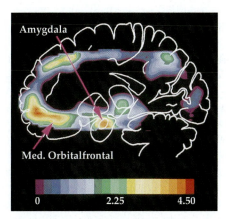

Amygdala

Med. Orbitalfrontal

| 0 | 2.25 | 4.50 |

Figure 16.12 **PET scan of blood flow in the brain in a patient with unipolar depression** Increased metabolic activity occurs in the amygdala and medial orbitofrontal cortex. Activation is shown in red and orange. (Courtesy of Wayne C. Drevets.)

depression compared to normal blood flow in control subjects. Increased activity in part of the medial orbitofrontal cortex and the amygdala support their role in the regulation of emotion. The increase in metabolic activity in the amygdala is correlated with the severity of depression and returns to normal after antidepressant drug treatment. Increased activity of the orbitofrontal cortex may reflect the individual's effort to control unpleasant thoughts and emotions (Drevets, 2001).

Antidepressant effects on 5-HT in animals   In addition to evaluating depressed patients, we can look at the long-term effects of antidepressant drugs on 5-HT by using animals. Animal studies have shown that most antidepressants increase 5-HT by blocking reuptake or inhibiting MAO. The increased synaptic 5-HT has postsynaptic action but also acts on 5-HT autoreceptors to slow the firing rate of cells and reduce 5-HT synthesis as well as release. Therefore, the two effects tend to cancel one another out. Overall, lower neuronal activity reduces metabolism of 5-HT to 5-HIAA, indicating reduced turnover (Figure 16.13). However, chronic treatment results in tolerance and reduces the action of the autoreceptor (down-regulation) and in that way gradually increases the amount of 5-HT in the synapse. The reuptake transporter blockade is still effective, so at this point the two actions both produce an increase in 5-HT. Since the therapeutic effects of antidepressants take several weeks to develop, the delay in autoreceptor desensitization and subsequent enhanced 5-HT activity may be in part responsible for the delayed therapeutic onset (Blier et al., 1990).

Animal studies also show that electrophysiological response to the application of 5-HT agonists is *enhanced* by long-term antidepressant treatment. De Montigny (1981) examined responses of single cells in rat forebrain to the application of 5-HT. Results showed that 2 days of antidepressant pretreatment produced no change in the sensitivity

(A) Acute effects of antidepressants

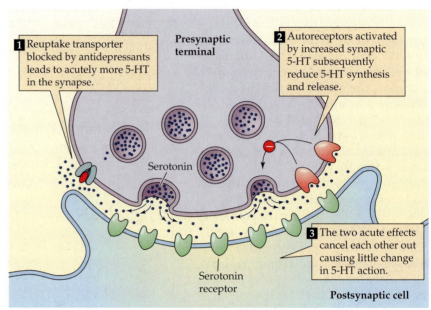

1 Reuptake transporter blocked by antidepressants leads to acutely more 5-HT in the synapse.

Presynaptic terminal

2 Autoreceptors activated by increased synaptic 5-HT subsequently reduce 5-HT synthesis and release.

Serotonin

3 The two acute effects cancel each other out causing little change in 5-HT action.

Serotonin receptor

Postsynaptic cell

(B) Chronic effects of antidepressants

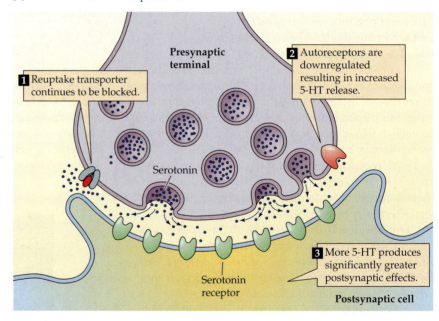

1 Reuptake transporter continues to be blocked.

Presynaptic terminal

2 Autoreceptors are downregulated resulting in increased 5-HT release.

Serotonin

3 More 5-HT produces significantly greater postsynaptic effects.

Serotonin receptor

Postsynaptic cell

Figure 16.13 Effects of antidepressants on serotonergic cells (A) The initial effects of reuptake blockade include increased 5-HT in the synapse and activity at both postsynaptic receptors and autoreceptors. Autoreceptor activation reduces the rate of firing of the cell as well as the rate of synthesis and release of 5-HT and subsequently also reduces the rate of formation of 5-HIAA. (B) With repeated administration, the autoreceptors become less sensitive and their inhibition of serotonergic neurons decreases, which leads to an increase in 5-HT function and 5-HIAA. The desensitization of the autoreceptors coincides with the onset of clinical effectiveness.

of the neurons to 5-HT but that after 4 to 7 days of pretreatment the response was moderately increased. Following 15 days of antidepressant administration, there was a large increase in sensitivity to 5-HT. The time course of this physiological change is related to the onset of clinical antidepressant effects. Although the argument for enhanced sensitivity of serotonergic neurons is among the most consistent (see Table 16.4), the fact that the enhanced physiological response occurs in brain areas where 5-HT$_2$ receptors are reduced is difficult to reconcile (Caldecott-Hazard et al., 1991). Differences in pre- and postsynaptic receptors may be one explanation.

Norepinephrine activity is altered by antidepressants

Norepinephrine also continues to be a focus of research because it has a known role in neuroendocrine function, reward mechanisms, attention and arousal, and response to stress, each of which may contribute to the symptoms of the affective disorders. In animal studies, electrical stimulation of the locus coeruleus, the cluster of noradrenergic cell bodies in the pons, produces vigilance, anxiety, and inhibition of exploratory behavior. Electrical recording in animals shows that locus coeruleus firing increases during threatening situations and decreases during usual functions such as sleeping, grooming, and feeding. Other studies with animals have shown that antidepressant drugs tend to reduce the firing rate of the locus coeruleus and subsequently reduce NE metabolites in the brain.

Unfortunately, results of studies with depressed patients are difficult to interpret. Levels of the principal noradrenergic metabolite MHPG in the body fluids of depressed patients have been found to be higher, lower, and no different from those of controls. In general, MHPG is usually found to be elevated in patients undergoing treatment, suggesting an increase in turnover with antidepressant use. Although no consistent differences have been found in noradrenergic receptor binding in untreated depressed or bipolar patients, chronic antidepressant treatment leads to down-regulation of both β-receptors and α$_2$-autoreceptors. Unfortunately, when both α$_2$- and β-receptors are down-regulated, they have opposite effects on adrenergic synapses. Since α$_2$-autoreceptors acutely reduce noradrenergic cell function by decreasing the rate of firing and reducing NE release, α$_2$-autoreceptor down-regulation increases both of these cell functions. Using α$_2$-challenge measures, the majority of experiments show that chronic, but not acute, antidepressant treatment produces a reduction in autoreceptor responsiveness that coincides with the increase in turnover described earlier.

One of the most consistent findings regarding catecholamine response to chronic antidepressant treatment is the down-regulation of β-receptors, which requires 7 to 21 days of treatment, a lag that parallels that seen in the onset of therapeutic response in depressed patients. Similar results occur with the vast majority of antidepressant drugs tested, including the TCAs, MAO-Is, SSRIs, and second-generation antidepressants. ECT, lithium under some conditions, and even REM sleep deprivation seem to reduce β-receptors.

Norepinephrine and serotonin modulate one another

Because the most consistent chronic effects of antidepressants are down-regulation of β-receptors and 5-HT$_2$ receptors and an enhanced physiological response to 5-HT, Sulser (1989) proposed a "serotonin–norepinephrine" hypothesis of depression. Both anatomical and functional interactions exist between the noradrenergic neurons originating in the locus coeruleus and the serotonergic neurons in the raphe nuclei (Figure 16.14), and each system is capable of modulating the other. Destroying 5-HT terminals with the neurotoxin 5,6-dihydroxytryptamine prevents the down-regulation of β-receptors that follows chronic antidepressant treatment. Others have shown that 5-HT agonists can indirectly stimulate the noradrenergic system, causing β-receptor down-regulation, and that increased noradrenergic function may also increase electrophysiological activity in the raphe nuclei. Sulser suggests that norepinephrine function involves multiple feedback loops that use a variety of neurotransmitters, including 5-HT, acetylcholine, DA, GABA, and opioid peptides. For more information on the contribution of these neurotransmitters to the symptoms of depression, refer to several excellent reviews (Caldecott-Hazard and colleagues, 1991; Brown et al., 1994; Willner, 1995).

Section Summary

The monoamine hypothesis of affective disorders states that depression is due to hypofunctioning of noradrenergic and/or serotonergic neurons in the brain, while mania is caused by excess monoamines. Unfortunately, the measures used to evaluate monoamine function in depressed patients do not consistently support the hypothesis and suggest an interactive role of multiple neurotransmitter systems. Also, although acute antidepressant drug treatment fits the model, we know that effectiveness does not occur with the acute elevation of amines but requires biological changes that occur over a period of weeks.

Results from the many animal and human studies summarized here are frequently inconsistent, which suggests that we still do not have a complete understanding of serotonergic function in depression and treatment. However, what we do know is worth summarizing briefly. Serotonin turnover and plasma tryptophan levels are frequently reduced in non-

(A) **Norepinephrine**

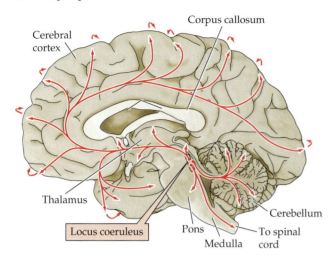

(B) **Serotonin**

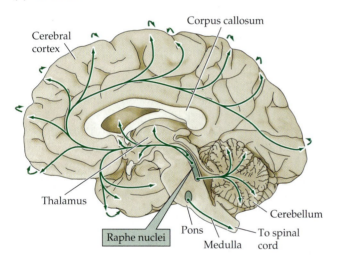

Figure 16.14 Two monoamine pathways in the human brain This schematic diagram shows noradrenergic pathways originating in the locus coeruleus (A) and serotonergic pathways originating in the raphe nuclei (B). The overlapping nature and interaction of the two neurotransmitter systems is very apparent.

reduced 5-HT turnover. However, chronic treatment causes downregulation of autoreceptors so serotonergic turnover is ultimately increased. Electrophysiological response to applied 5-HT agonists, like the human challenge studies, shows increased sensitivity of receptors with chronic drug treatment.

One of the most consistent changes after chronic antidepressants is down-regulation of β-receptors. This decrease occurs after several weeks of treatment with a majority of antidepressant drugs. Beta-receptor down-regulation also follows chronic ECT, lithium administration, and some types of sleep deprivation treatment. Ample evidence exists to demonstrate anatomical and functional interactions between serotonergic and noradrenergic neurons, indicating that each system is capable of modulating the other. It is apparent that both of these monoamines, as well as other neurotransmitters including dopamine, acetylcholine, GABA, and opioids, likely interact to form the complex combination of symptoms of affective disorder.

Neurobiological Models of Depression

In addition to the consideration of neurotransmitter function in depression, other hypotheses pose alternative neurobiological models that are now being tested. One such hypothesis, the **glucocorticoid hypothesis,** focuses on the stress-related neuroendocrine abnormalities that are frequently found in depressed individuals (see the section on biological rhythms earlier in the chapter; see also Aborelius et al., 1999 for an excellent review). The abnormal secretion of CRF from the hypothalamus is apparently responsible for the hypersecretion of ACTH from the pituitary and cortisol from the adrenal cortex. The hypothalamic CRF neurons are normally controlled by other areas of the CNS: the amygdala, which is central to emotional responses, normally stimulates the CRF circuit, while the hippocampus has inhibitory control (see Figure 16.3). The hippocampus has receptors that when activated by high levels of glucocorticoids (such as cortisol) help to inhibit CRF release from the hypothalamus, subsequently returning glucocorticoid levels to normal. However, when stress is intense and/or prolonged, glucocorticoid levels remain high and, as shown in animal studies, hippocampal neurons are damaged and no longer respond. The principal damage includes decreases in dendritic branches and loss of dendritic spines, as well as a reduction in the formation of new hippocampal cells (neurogenesis). Cell loss means reduced response to circulating cortisol and loss of inhibition of the HPA axis, inducing further glucocorticoid-mediated hippocampal cell loss.

One might speculate that the elevated cortisol levels found in depressed individuals contribute to cell death and some of the cognitive symptoms of depression. Small reductions in hippocampal volume are found in magnetic reso-

medicated depressed patients while postsynaptic serotonergic receptors are increased in number perhaps to compensate for the low 5-HT utilization. Chronic antidepressant treatment tends to reverse each of these. Challenge studies indicate reduced receptor sensitivity in depression that is restored by treatment.

Data from animal studies generally support the evidence gathered from depressed patients. Although antidepressant treatment acutely increases 5-HT in the synapse, the autoreceptor activation more than compensates so that there is nance imaging scans of depressed patients. Further, antidepressant drugs and ECT reduce CRF levels in depressed patients. In animals, several types of antidepressant drugs also reverse the loss of dendrites and increase neurogenesis in the hippocampus and other brain areas. Finally, intracerebroventricular administration of CRF elicits stress-related behavioral and physiological responses in animals, including the expected enhancement of cortisol levels and sympathetic nervous system activity. CRF also elicits behaviors in animals that are closely correlated with symptoms of clinical depression in humans: arousal, insomnia, decreased eating, reduced sexual activity, and anxiety.

The glucocorticoid hypothesis of affective disorder is the basis for the clinical tests of CRF receptor antagonists, which show early promise as antidepressants. Preliminary clinical studies (Zobel et al., 2000) found significant improvement in both depression and anxiety scores using the CRF receptor antagonist R121919. Minimal side effects were found in this preliminary study, and even at the higher doses tested only minor elevations in liver enzyme values were noted.

A second closely related neurobiological model looks at potential mechanisms underlying the hippocampal cell loss following stress: deficits in neurotrophic factors such as **BDNF (brain-derived neurotrophic factor).** Neurotrophic factors are important proteins that are needed during brain development but also regulate changes in cells and their survival in adult brains. The **neurotrophic hypothesis** suggests that low BDNF may be responsible for the loss in dendritic branches and spines and that antidepressants may protect vulnerable cells by preventing the decrease in BDNF. Evidence in support can be briefly summarized: (1) chronic stress reduces BDNF in the hippocampus in rats; (2) chronic but not acute antidepressant treatment increases BDNF in both animals and humans; and (3) antidepressants prevent stress-induced reductions in BDNF (Figure 16.15). A direct connection between BDNF and depression is more difficult to determine. However, Shirayama and coworkers (2002) injected BDNF intracerebrally into regions of the hippocampus in rats and found antidepressant effects in the forced swim test and learned helplessness test.

Since the production of BDNF is dependent on the cAMP second-messenger system, it is significant that *chronic* antidepressant drug treatment up-regulates several components of the system in the hippocampus and frontal cortex. This up-regulation occurs despite the down-regulation of the β-receptors (βARs) and 5-HT receptors that are coupled to the cAMP cascade (Figure 16.16). Up-regulation occurs in several stages of the cascade, including enhanced coupling between stimulatory G protein and adenylyl cyclase, increase in cAMP-dependent protein kinase (PKA), and increase in cAMP response element binding protein (CREB), which is a transduction factor that induces protein synthesis of BDNF and other proteins.

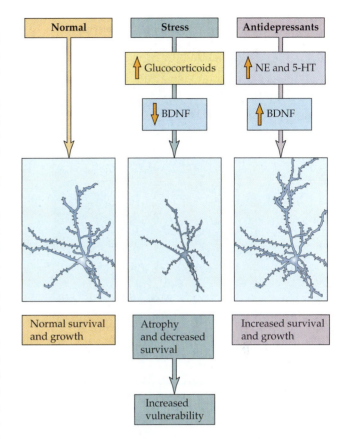

Figure 16.15 Effect of stress and antidepressant treatment on BDNF in hippocampal cells The box on the left shows a typical hippocampal cell in the CA3 area. Chronic stress (center) elevates glucocorticoids and decreases BDNF, which may be responsible for the loss of dendritic trees and make the cells more vulnerable to a variety of detrimental factors. Chronic antidepressant treatment (right) not only alters monoamine transmission but also increases BDNF. BDNF may protect the cells from further damage and help repair those already damaged. (After Duman et al., 1999.)

Although at present there is no way to directly inject BDNF into humans as a test for antidepressant activity, elevating CREB in the hippocampus of laboratory animals produced antidepressant effects in the forced swim and learned helplessness tests (Chen et al., 2001). One might consider that enhancing any portion of the cAMP cascade could ultimately enhance BDNF production and relieve depression. One approach involves inhibiting **phosphodiesterase**, the enzyme that normally degrades cAMP to 5′-AMP. One phosphodiesterase inhibitor, rolipram, reduced symptoms in a small trial of depressed patients, but side effects prohibit its regular use. More selective inhibitors may prove effective with reduced side effects. A second approach involves activating the transcription factor CREB, which in turn induces the production of BDNF to promote cell survival and relieve depression.

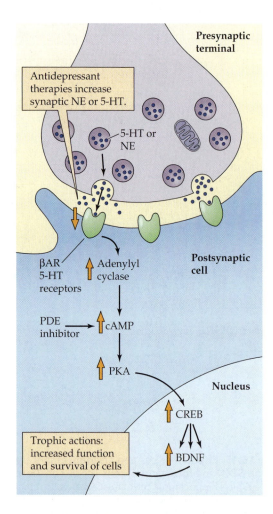

Figure 16.16 Up-regulation of second-messenger pathway by chronic antidepressant treatment The increase in NE and 5-HT caused by acute antidepressant treatment produces down-regulation of their receptors when treatment is chronic. In response to the reduction in receptors the cAMP pathway is up-regulated, producing increases in adenylyl cyclase activity, cAMP, PKA, and the transcription factor within the nucleus, CREB. CREB increases the synthesis of several proteins, including BDNF. (After Duman et al., 1997.)

Brain levels of CREB are low in depressed patients and are increased by most antidepressant drugs after several weeks. It is tempting to try to develop therapeutic methods that might rapidly enhance CREB and the neurotrophic factors.

Although the possibilities are exciting, application to human therapeutics is clearly a long way off.

These two neurobiological hypotheses, along with a third, which considers the impairment of brain reward pathways, are discussed in detail in an excellent review by Nestler and colleagues (2002). They provide both an overview and supporting evidence as well as a discussion of future directions for research.

Section Summary

Several new neurobiological models of depression focus on the role of stress and the HPA axis because stress-induced elevation of CRF initiates the release of ACTH from the pituitary and subsequently of glucocorticoids (e,g., cortisol) from the adrenal cortex. Prolonged elevation of glucocorticoids during chronic stress damages hippocampal cells, which prevents the normal hippocampal inhibition of the HPA axis, causing further glucocorticoid-induced brain damage. Chronic antidepressant treatment in depressed patients seems to reduce CRF levels, and animal studies show that chronic treatment reverses hippocampal cell damage.

Chronic antidepressant treatment also up-regulates the cAMP cascade, despite the fact that the drugs down-regulate the receptors coupled to the system. The enhanced coupling between G protein and adenylyl cyclase and the increase in cAMP, PKA, and CREB induce the synthesis of BDNF, a trophic factor that protects neurons. Future research will determine whether there is a direct connection between the symptoms of depression, BDNF levels, and brain cell loss that can be reversed by antidepressants.

Recommended Readings

Jamison, K. R. (1993). *Touched with Fire: Manic-Depressive Illness and the Artistic Temperament.* Free Press/Macmillan, New York.

Nemeroff, C. B. (1998). The neurobiology of depression. *Sci. Am.,* June, 42–49.

Nestler, E. J., Barrot, M., KiLeone, R. J., Eisch, A. J., Gold, S. J., and Monteggia, L. M. (2002). Neurobiology of depression. *Neuron,* 34, 13–25.

17 *Anxiety Disorders*

*R*ichard was a 19-year-old college freshman majoring in philosophy when he withdrew from school because of incapacitating ritualistic behavior. These rituals included excessive hand washing and showering; ceremonial rituals for dressing and studying; compulsive placement of any objects he handled; grotesque hissing, coughing, and head tossing while he was eating; and shuffling and wiping his feet while walking. Over the prior 2 years Richard's behavior had steadily deteriorated, and finally he had isolated himself from his family and friends, refusing meals and neglecting his personal appearance. He had not cut his hair in 5 years, nor had he shaved or trimmed his beard. Any time he walked anywhere he would take very small steps on his toes while continually looking back, checking and rechecking.

Richard was clearly in a good deal of pain and his life was totally disordered. He had lost the desire to be with family and friends because his behavior was so embarrassing to him. He recognized that his thoughts and behaviors were not rational but had no control over their occurrence (Barlow and Durand, 1995). After reading the section on clinical anxiety disorders, see if you can make the diagnosis for Richard and recommend treatment strategies.

Feelings of fear, helplessness, and horror may lead to anxiety disorders.

Characteristics of Anxiety Disorders

Having just completed Chapter 16, which describes major disorders of affect or mood—notably clinical depression and bipolar disorder—we turn now to yet another class of mood disorders. These maladaptive reactions have *anxiety* as a major component. As a group, they produce an enormous amount of suffering, contribute to low productivity, and generate a poor quality of life for a large number of individuals. Although the incidence of each syndrome varies, it has been estimated that 10 to 30% of Americans will suffer from a significant anxiety disorder at some point in their lives. The ways in which that anxiety is expressed vary greatly and include episodes of panic, phobic avoidance of anxiety-eliciting stimuli, intrusive thoughts or compulsive behaviors, and damaging negative thinking patterns. In addition, anxiety is a factor commonly associated with other psychopathology, particularly clinical depression. The link between anxiety and depression is well documented: According to the National Comorbid Survey, 58% of patients with major depression also show signs of anxiety disorder (Ninan, 1999). Furthermore, both neurobiological and pharmacological evidence support the idea of a common link between the two. Before describing some of the psychiatric disorders in which anxiety is a major characteristic, let's look a little closer at anxiety itself.

Anxiety is important for survival

Most anxiety presents itself as a subjectively unsettling feeling of concern or worry that is displayed by behaviors including a worried facial expression as well as bodily responses such as increased muscle tension, restlessness, impaired concentration, sleep disturbances, and irritability. In addition, activation of the sympathetic branch of the autonomic nervous system (ANS) produces increased heart rate, sweating, shortness of breath, and other signs of the "fight-or-flight" response (see Chapter 2). Anxiety can vary in intensity from feelings of vague discomfort to intense sensations of terror.

Evolutionarily, anxiety is important to survival since it warns us of danger and activates the fight-or-flight response, enabling us to cope with impending emergency. Unfortunately, many of the dangers we face in the modern world do not involve fighting off or running from predators like the saber-toothed tiger, when increased heart rate and blood pressure, elevated blood glucose, and surges of adrenaline would be beneficial. Most of the anxiety-provoking situations that we face demand instead that we restrain our aggressive impulses (wanting to attack our hostile boss), think clearly (during a difficult exam), and remain in the anxiety-producing situation (giving a speech to a large group) until a resolution occurs. In these circumstances, the fight-or-flight response is not helpful and may impair our ability to perform at our best.

Nevertheless, despite its unpleasantness, anxiety in small doses is clearly a necessary stimulus for optimum performance in many everyday situations. Anxiety before an exam encourages more study; anxiety before public speaking forces us to practice our presentation one more time; anxiety before a first date prompts us to recheck our plans for the evening. Regardless of whether we are students, factory workers, or businesspeople, it is anxiety that boosts our energy level and pushes us to work harder and longer. But sometimes we experience too much of a good thing. When anxiety increases beyond a certain level, performance deteriorates noticeably, particularly on complex tasks. What begins as increasing alertness and focus becomes preoccupation with our own agitation that distracts us from our task. The ANS prepares our bodies for emergency; our muscles are tense; and we may suffer from digestive problems, sleep disturbances leading to fatigue, and psychosomatic illness. The overanxious student often cannot focus on an important exam because he is too preoccupied with thoughts of how awful it would be to fail. Worst of all, because high anxiety has damaged our performance, our failures provide more reason to be anxious, creating an escalating circular pattern (Figure 17.1). Once we begin to have negative feelings about ourselves and our lack of productivity, depression may develop.

Anxiety disorders are different from everyday worry

Among the disorders that are recognized as anxiety syndromes by the American Psychiatric Association, this chapter will consider the five principal categories: generalized anxiety disorder, panic disorder, several types of phobias, post-traumatic stress disorder, and obsessive–compulsive disorder.

Brief episodes of anxiety, even when rather intense, are not likely to be harmful and may be quite rational in many situations. **Acute anxiety** occurs in response to real-life stressors, and symptoms occur only in response to these events. Pharmacological treatment is very effective in providing relief from the anxiety associated with major life changes such as death of a loved one, divorce or permanent disability, or sudden stressors like major surgery that trigger intense anxiety. The anxiolytics (drugs that reduce anxiety) in the benzodiazepine class are extremely effective for relieving this type of anxiety.

Generalized anxiety disorder   Although acute anxiety may at times need to be treated, it is generally not long-lasting and is not considered a clinical disorder. In contrast, for some people the symptoms of anxiety have no real focus, and

Figure 17.1 Three-component model of anxiety shows that stress induces the cyclic interaction of bodily response, ineffective behavior, and upsetting thoughts. Potential stressors may be perceived as a threat, which initiates portions of the anxiety responses. Each of the three components influence the others, potentially escalating the overall damaging effect of anxiety. For other individuals, the stressor may be perceived as a challenge, which engages more constructive behavior. Individual differences based on genetic traits and early experience may make some people more or less vulnerable to stressors. (After Rosenthal and Rosenthal, 1980.)

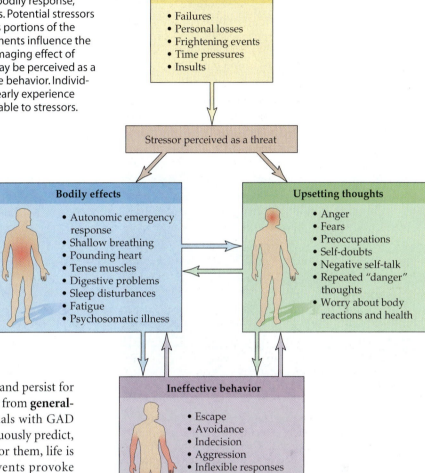

they can be present for much of the day, and persist for months or years. These individuals suffer from **generalized anxiety disorder (GAD).** Individuals with GAD show signs of constant worry and continuously predict, anticipate, or imagine dreadful events. For them, life is generally stressful, and even minor events provoke worry. Being late for an appointment, not completing a task, or making a minor mistake are all causes of worry. The most common physical symptoms include muscle tension and agitation that lead to fatigue, poor concentration, irritability, and sleep difficulties. As you might expect, the chronic anxiety reduces the individual's performance on many tasks and decreases the pleasure derived from his or her efforts. GAD is one of the more common anxiety disorders, afflicting an estimated 5% of the general population between the ages of 15 and 45 (Wittchen et al., 1994). Most cases begin gradually, usually in the teens or early adulthood, and persist throughout life. Although some genetic contribution is suggested by the fact that GAD tends to run in families, twin studies are not consistent in supporting the role of heritability.

Panic attacks and panic disorder   In contrast to anxiety, which is the anticipation of potential danger, fear is the physiological reaction to immediate danger that prepares us to fight or run away. When an individual experiences all the effects of a fear reaction without a threatening stimulus, he

is having a **panic attack.** The sudden intense fearfulness is accompanied by strong arousal of the sympathetic ANS. The symptoms associated with panic include heart pounding or chest pain, sweating, shortness of breath, faintness, choking, and the fear of losing control or dying (Figure 17.2). These symptoms, which last minutes to even hours, may occur (1) in response to a particular environmental cue (producing a phobia); (2) totally without warning in unexpected fashion; or (3) in a situation where an attack occurred previously, thus making it more likely to occur again. The latter two cases are the basis for **panic disorder.** Panic disorder usually begins in the late twenties and may last for many years, with attacks occurring at different frequencies and intensities over that time. In panic disorder, the individual experiences both panic (in the form of individual attacks) and anxiety (called **anticipatory anxiety**) over the possibility that she may have

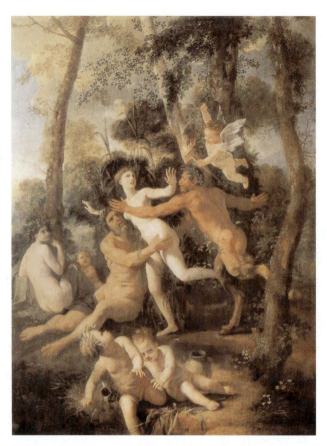

Figure 17.2 The word panic comes from Pan, the Greek god of pastures and shepherds, who is represented as having the legs, horns, and ears of a goat. It was believed that if he were awakened from his nap by travelers, he would let out a blood-curdling scream that would often scare them to death.

TABLE 17.1 Typical Situations Avoided by a Person with Agoraphobia

Shopping malls

Cars (as driver or passenger)

Buses

Trains

Subways

Wide streets

Tunnels

Restaurants

Theaters

Being far from home

Staying at home alone

Waiting in line

Supermarkets

Stores

Crowds

Planes

Elevators

Escalators

Source: Barlow and Durand, 1995.

an attack in a place that is not safe, for example, in the middle of a movie theater or during a church service, where it would be embarrassing or perhaps impossible to escape. The anxiety associated with being in an "unsafe" place leads to **agoraphobia,** a fear of public places and subsequent avoidance of many common situations (Table 17.1). Individuals with agoraphobia often lead very limited lives because they never leave the safety of their own homes.

Unlike some of the other anxiety disorders, a genetic predisposition for panic is well documented. The concordance rate is significantly higher in monozygotic than in dizygotic twins. Furthermore, a significant number of patients with panic disorder have parents with the same diagnosis.

It is not entirely clear whether people with panic disorder have a more reactive ANS, but panic attacks can be triggered in individuals with the disorder by a variety of stimuli that activate the ANS. These include injection with lactic acid (a product of muscle exertion), caffeine, or yohimbine (an α_2-adrenergic receptor antagonist), or breathing air with increased amounts of carbon dioxide. Because these same techniques do not elicit panic in normal individuals, they have been useful in studying panic disorder in the laboratory (see Nutt et al., 1998).

Phobias   **Phobias** involve fears that the individual recognizes as irrational. Fears may focus on specific objects or situations such as high places, closed-in spaces, water, mice, or snakes, or they may relate to social or interpersonal situations such as speaking in public. Phobias can affect the individual's daily existence and reduce his quality of life. Although many of us have irrational fears of things like spiders, usually we can avoid those things with little modification of lifestyle (Figure 17.3). However, for some people an irrational fear significantly alters their daily activities. One example of such an individual is John Madden, the well-known American sports announcer and former football coach. He suffers from claustrophobia and is overwhelmed with anxiety when traveling within the confined space of an airplane. Although he maintains a busy schedule of cross-country appearances for television, he travels only by train or on a bus designed for his use.

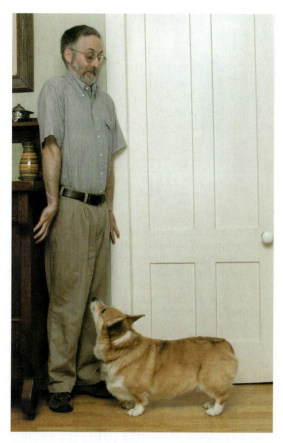

Figure 17.3 Cynophobia causes individuals to suffer signs of anxiety in the presence of dogs or even in response to items closely associated with the animals. Other animals like snakes, mice, or cats are also frequent bases for phobias and phobic avoidance.

to the heart of danger, for there you will find safety." Medication for phobias is rarely needed.

Social phobia involves fear of being around others because the individual is concerned that he might do something embarrassing. Social phobia is far more than extreme shyness and restricts such activities as public speaking, attending parties, taking exams, and even eating in public places. Evidence suggests cognitive therapy that modifies negative thoughts such as the likelihood of looking foolish, plus social-skills training, is frequently highly beneficial.

Post-traumatic stress disorder   Severe and chronic emotional disorders can occur after traumatic events such as war, natural disasters like hurricanes or earthquakes, terrorist attacks such as 9/11, physical assault, or auto accidents. In each case the individual involved feels not only fear but also a sense of helplessness and horror. Many of the individuals who witnessed the terrorist attack on the World Trade Center in New York City have developed **post-traumatic stress disorder (PTSD),** and the soldiers returning from the war in Iraq show a particularly high rate of PTSD. Individuals with PTSD frequently experience nightmares and memories that may occur as sudden flashbacks of the traumatic event. In addition, they show increased physiological reactivity to reminders of the trauma, sleep disturbances, avoidance of stimuli associated with the trauma, and a numbing of emotional responses for many years after the original stress. Many exhibit sudden outbursts of irritability that can emotionally injure family and friends who are making an effort to be supportive. The individuals often feel detached from others and fail to experience the full range of emotions, which leads to diminished interest in life activities. In addition, the probability of attempting suicide is significantly

While there is an almost infinite list of items that can elicit phobic anxiety (Table 17.2), what people fear is at least partially determined by culture. For instance, in the Chinese culture *pa-leng* is a morbid fear of the cold and loss of body heat. This fear is based on the Chinese belief that yin represents the cold, dark, and energy-draining parts of life that optimally should be balanced with yang, the warm, light, and sustaining elements. People with *pa-leng* often wear several layers of clothing even on extremely hot days. Fortunately, phobias can usually be effectively treated with behavior therapy that involves presenting the fear-inducing stimulus in gradual increments, allowing the individual to maintain a relaxed state while confronting the source of her fear. This technique, called **behavioral desensitization,** is a common modern treatment method but may reflect an ancient Chinese proverb: "Go straight

TABLE 17.2 Some Common (*) and Less Common Phobias

Phobia	Fear of
Acrophobia*	Heights
Aichmophobia	Sharp, pointed objects; knives
Ailurophobia	Cats
Algophobia	Pain
Astraphobia*	Storms, thunder, lightning
Claustrophobia*	Tight enclosures
Hematophobia*	Blood
Monophobia*	Being alone
Nyctophobia	Darkness, night
Ochlophobia	Crowds
Pyrophobia	Fire
Thanatophobia*	Death
Xenophobia*	Strangers

greater in these individuals, as is the incidence of substance abuse, marital problems, depression, and feelings of guilt and anger. Children also develop PTSD following trauma, although their symptoms are somewhat different.

Although statistics tell us that lifetime prevalence of PTSD varies from 1 to 10% in the United States, the occurrence varies widely depending on the trauma. For example, approximately 3% of people who have experienced a personal attack, 4 to 16% surviving a natural disaster, 30% of war veterans, as many as 50% of those who have experienced rape, and 50 to 75% of prisoners of war who were torture victims develop PTSD (Yehuda et al., 1998). Given the frequent occurrence of war, starvation, forced immigration, terrorist activities, and ethnic and religious conflict that has occurred globally in the recent past, it is painful to think of the number of cases of PTSD around the world.

Although PTSD is clearly related to the intensity of the traumatic event, some individuals seem far more susceptible than others. Clearly, not all war veterans in active combat develop PTSD, nor do all women who experience rape. Family studies of individuals who develop PTSD after trauma show that as many as 74% had a family history of psychopathology (PTSD, anxiety, depression, or antisocial behavior). The significantly higher concordance among monozygotic twins than dizygotic twins further supports the genetic vulnerability model. The interaction of family history and the magnitude of trauma is suggested by the fact that under conditions of high stress, people with a family history of PTSD may be only slightly more vulnerable to PTSD. However, when the magnitude of trauma is less intense, biologically vulnerable individuals are significantly more likely to show signs of the disorder. One possibility is that vulnerable individuals may perceive events as more traumatic than other individuals.

Children who have parents with PTSD have an increased risk for PTSD and also tend to have lower-than-normal blood cortisol (a stress hormone). The hormonal difference may be a marker that predicts vulnerability. Although on the surface it seems odd to have low stress hormones associated with an anxiety disorder, it is possible that the normal feedback mechanism that turns off cortisol secretion is hypersensitive in PTSD. Yehuda and colleagues (2000) show that in the high-risk population of Holocaust survivor offspring, those who both developed PTSD themselves and had a parent with PTSD had the lowest levels of cortisol (shown in Figure 17.4). Those whose parents had PTSD but did not themselves show PTSD had intermediate levels, and those who neither had a family history of PTSD nor had symptoms themselves had cortisol levels equal to controls. While there is almost certainly a genetic contribution to this susceptibility, the extent of social support after the trauma may also be a significant factor. An additional factor that increases the risk of not only PTSD but also other anxiety disorders

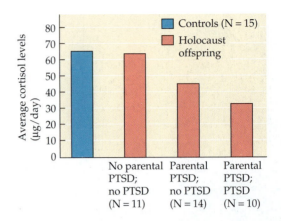

Figure 17.4 Average blood cortisol levels in several groups of offspring of Holocaust survivors and control subjects Subjects with no parental history of PTSD and no PTSD themselves had similar cortisol levels to controls. A family history of PTSD was associated with reduced cortisol in the absence of symptoms. The lowest cortisol levels occurred in subjects with PTSD who also had a family history of the disorder. (After Yehuda et al., 2000.)

and associated depression is a history of chronic stress, abuse, or trauma.

Obsessive–compulsive disorder   Have you ever made an attempt to forget some peculiar, sexual, or aggressive thought and found the thought recurring over and over? Have you ever checked your alarm clock before you got ready for bed and then felt compelled to check it again and again before you climbed into the sack even though you know you set it correctly? Having experienced those normal events will help you begin to understand **obsessive–compulsive disorder (OCD)**. However, while these examples are trivial ones, OCD is anything but trivial. It is a severe, chronic psychiatric problem that may require hospitalization, or in the most extreme cases psychosurgery, to control the symptoms. The disorder is characterized by recurring, persistent, intrusive, and troublesome thoughts of contamination, violence, sex, or religion (**obsessions**) that the individual tries to resist but which cause a great deal of anxiety, guilt, and shame. **Compulsions** are repetitive rituals considered attempts to relieve the tremendous anxiety generated by the obsessive thoughts, although they may be directly related or totally unrelated to the obsessive ideas. In the first instance, an individual may wash his hands hundreds of times a day until the skin is raw and bleeding because of an obsession about contracting a fatal disease. Other compulsions are unrelated to obsessions; they may involve meaningless repetitive acts like counting each crack in the sidewalk, jumping through doorways, or chewing each bite of food 100 times because of the belief that a family member may otherwise become fatally ill. Figure 17.5 shows the incidence of particular

(A) **Obsessions**

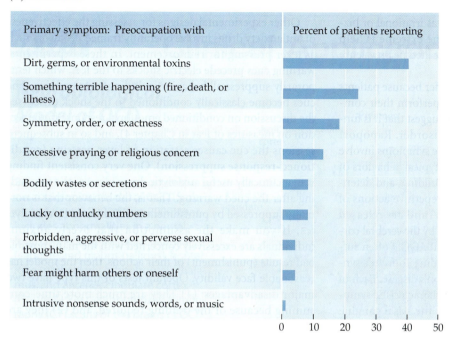

Primary symptom: Preoccupation with	Percent of patients reporting
Dirt, germs, or environmental toxins	
Something terrible happening (fire, death, or illness)	
Symmetry, order, or exactness	
Excessive praying or religious concern	
Bodily wastes or secretions	
Lucky or unlucky numbers	
Forbidden, aggressive, or perverse sexual thoughts	
Fear might harm others or oneself	
Intrusive nonsense sounds, words, or music	

(B) **Compulsions**

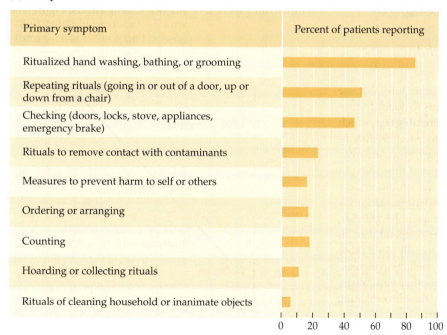

Primary symptom	Percent of patients reporting
Ritualized hand washing, bathing, or grooming	
Repeating rituals (going in or out of a door, up or down from a chair)	
Checking (doors, locks, stove, appliances, emergency brake)	
Rituals to remove contact with contaminants	
Measures to prevent harm to self or others	
Ordering or arranging	
Counting	
Hoarding or collecting rituals	
Rituals of cleaning household or inanimate objects	

Figure 17.5 Occurrence of OCD symptoms Percentage of child and adolescent patients reporting particular obsessions and compulsions as their chief symptom. (After Rapoport, 1989.)

obsessions and compulsions in a population of young patients with OCD. Regardless of the compulsion, the individual is convinced that unless the compulsive ritual is completed, disastrous consequences will occur. These activities are recognized by sufferers as inappropriate or irrational and consume most of their waking hours, yet they feel forced to do them against their will. The disorder causes intense emotional distress but is often left untreated because the individual is so

BOX 17.1 (continued)

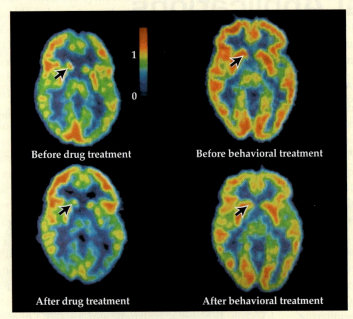

Before drug treatment

Before behavioral treatment

After drug treatment

After behavioral treatment

(B) PET scans of the brains of patients with OCD show hyperactivity in the head of the caudate. Both SSRI treatment (bottom left) and cognitive therapy (bottom right) reduce the hyperactivity in the caudate compared to pretreatment levels (top left and right). (From Baxter et al., 1992.)

Horizontal view

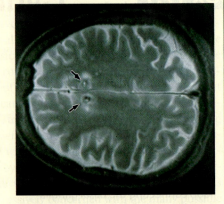

Sagittal view

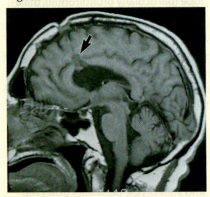

(C) Magnetic resonance image (MRI) of the brain of a patient with OCD The patient had neurosurgery to disrupt the neural connections of the cingulate cortex (see arrows) from the frontal cortex, basal ganglia, and thalamus. (From Martuza et al., 1990; courtesy of Robert L. Martuza.)

basal ganglia and the thalamus, is successful in relieving symptoms in 50 to 70% of cases (Mindus et al., 1994). It appears that interrupting the circuitry at any one of several points may relieve symptoms of OCD. These results demonstrate the importance of considering the functional interaction of multiple brain areas when looking for the biological basis of any psychiatric disorder. Understanding the neural network associated with behavior also means that psychopharmacology can be used to target the symptoms at multiple sites by modulating the synaptic connections.

shows the strong correlation between the effectiveness of anxiolytic drugs from several classes in a conflict procedure and the potency of these drugs in clinical trials with human patients.

Drugs for Treating Anxiety

Drugs that are used to relieve anxiety are called **anxiolytics.** Many belong to the class of **sedative–hypnotics,** which is part of a still larger category, the **CNS depressants.** CNS depressants include the barbiturates, the benzodiazepines, and alcohol. All of these drugs reduce neuron excitability by enhancing the inhibitory effects of the amino acid neurotransmitter GABA (γ-aminobutyric acid). As you may know,

the oldest known anxiety-reducing drug is alcohol, and it is still popular as an over-the-counter remedy for stress (see Chapter 9). However, because it is difficult to administer in accurate doses and has a very poor therapeutic index, it has no medical use.

To be considered an anxiolytic, a drug should relieve the feelings of tension and worry and signs of stress that are typical of the anxious individual. As we saw in animal models, drugs in this class increase behaviors that are normally suppressed by anxiety or punishment. Drugs that relieve anxiety often also produce a calm and relaxed state, with drowsiness and mental clouding, incoordination, and prolonged reaction time. At higher doses these drugs also induce sleep, and they are therefore sometimes called hypnotics (Figure 17.7). At the highest doses CNS depressants induce coma and

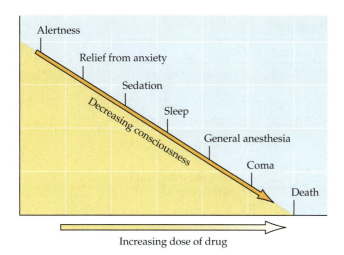

Figure 17.7 Dose-dependent effects of CNS depressants on levels of consciousness With increasing doses, the level of awareness and arousability gradually decreases along a continuum until death occurs.

the barbiturates have essentially been replaced by the benzodiazepines in the treatment of anxiety disorders, our discussion of these drugs will be brief.

Pharmacokinetics   All of the barbiturates have a similar basic ring structure (Figure 17.8) but vary in the length and complexity of the side chain attached to the ring. These molecular differences are responsible for their differences in lipid solubility. The **ultrashort-acting** barbiturates such as thiopental (Pentothal) and hexobarbital (Evipal) are highly lipid soluble and readily penetrate into the brain to put an individual to sleep within 10 to 20 seconds when intravenously administered. Consciousness returns in about 20 to 30 minutes because of the redistribution of drug to inactive drug depots in muscle and fat.

The **short/intermediate-acting** barbiturates are moderately lipid soluble and take longer to reach significant brain levels. They are likely to produce relaxation and sleep in about 20 to 40 minutes and last about 5 to 8 hours. Their moderate lipid solubility is also responsible for their longer duration of action because termination depends more on liver metabolism than on redistribution, which is characteristic of very lipid-soluble drugs. This group (including amobarbital [Amytal] and secobarbital [Seconal]) is most likely to be prescribed for insomnia but also includes those drugs most likely to be abused.

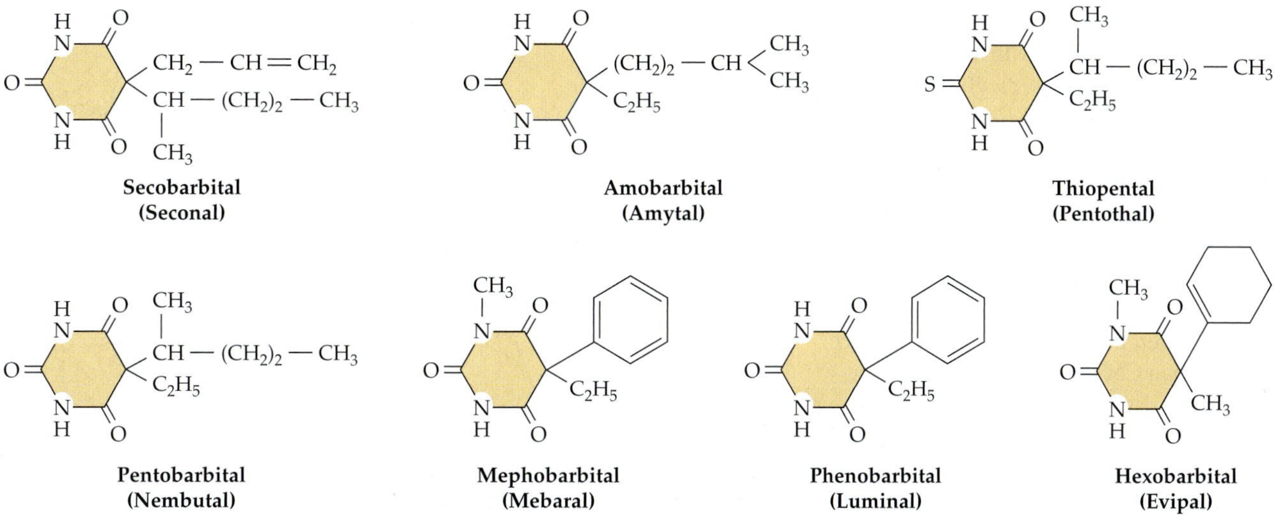

death, although even at therapeutic doses they can be fatal if combined with other drugs. Selected sedative–hypnotics also reduce seizures and may be used to treat epilepsy. Others produce muscle relaxation as needed to treat muscle spasms, for example, following an auto accident.

Barbiturates are the oldest sedative hypnotics

Sodium amytal was the first barbiturate, but as many as 50 others with different profiles of bioavailability were developed. The pharmacokinetic factors of absorption, distribution, and metabolism described in Chapter 1 determine each drug's onset of effect and duration of action, and it is on this basis that the drugs are classified into three groups. Because

Secobarbital (Seconal)

Amobarbital (Amytal)

Thiopental (Pentothal)

Pentobarbital (Nembutal)

Mephobarbital (Mebaral)

Phenobarbital (Luminal)

Hexobarbital (Evipal)

Figure 17.8 Chemical structure of the barbiturates The barbiturates all have a similar molecular ring structure (highlighted in orange) with distinct side chains that affect their lipid solubility. Each drug's lipid solubility determines how quickly it enters the brain, binds to drug depots, and is metabolized.

TABLE 17.3 Duration of Action and Uses of Major Barbiturates

Duration of action	Lipid solubility	Onset	Duration	Use
Ultrashort Thiopental (Pentothal) Methohexital (Brevital)	High	10–20 s	20–30 min	Intravenous anesthesia
Short/intermediate Amobarbital (Amytal) Secobarbital (Seconal) Pentobarbital (Nembutal)	Moderate	20–40 min	5–8 h	Surgical anesthesia and sleep induction
Long Phenobarbital (Luminal) Mephobarbital (Mebaral)	Low	Over 1 h	10–12 h	Prolonged sedation and seizure control

Finally, the **long-acting** drugs have poor lipid penetration, so their onset takes an hour or more, but their slow metabolism produces prolonged action for 10 to 12 hours. These characteristics are optimal for treating seizure disorders because a stable blood level can be maintained. Phenobarbital (Luminal) is commonly used in this way. Table 17.3 summarizes these characteristics and provides examples.

Side effects Although barbiturates readily induce sleep, it is not a normal, restful sleep. The drugs alter sleep architecture by reducing the amount of REM (rapid eye movement) sleep and causing a rebound in REM after withdrawal.

Second, the anxiolytic effects of these drugs are accompanied by pronounced cognitive side effects including mental clouding, loss of judgment, and slowed reflexes, making driving particularly dangerous. High doses also lead to gross intoxication, staggering, jumbled speech, and impaired thinking. Coma and death due to respiratory depression occur at 10 to 20 times the normal therapeutic dose. These drugs are extremely dangerous when combined with alcohol.

Third, when used repeatedly barbiturates increase the number of liver microsomal enzymes. This increase enhances drug metabolism, producing lower blood levels (metabolic tolerance) and reduced effectiveness. Since the same liver enzymes metabolize many other drugs, cross-tolerance diminishes the effectiveness of other drugs as well. Further, pharmacodynamic tolerance occurs when CNS neurons adapt to the presence of the drug and become less responsive with chronic drug use. Mood changes and sedation seem to show the greatest and most rapid tolerance, while the lethal respiratory-depressant action of the drug does not show tolerance at all. Therefore, as one gradually increases the dose of drug needed to achieve a desired effect, the margin of safety (therapeutic index) becomes less (Figure 17.9).

Fourth, barbiturates produce significant physical dependence and potential for abuse. Terminating drug use after extended treatment produces a potentially fatal rebound hyperexcitability withdrawal syndrome similar to that for alcohol. Although gradual reduction in the dose of the drug will decrease the intensity of withdrawal, because receptors are not suddenly deprived of the drug molecule, the withdrawal syndrome will be longer in duration.

Illicit use Despite their high cost, the short/intermediate-acting barbiturates like Seconal, Nembutal, and Amytal have been popular with drug abusers, who refer to them as red devils, yellow jackets, and blue angels, respectively, based on the color of the capsules. Table 17.4 provides some of the more common street names. The potent reinforcing effect of these drugs is demonstrated by the high rate of self-administration found in rats and monkeys tested in an operant

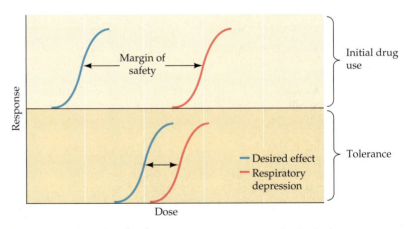

Figure 17.9 Margin of safety Dose–response curves for the barbiturate-induced desired effect (mood change or sedation) and lethal respiratory depression. The top panel shows that with early drug use (nontolerant) the individual experiences mood effects without significant respiratory depression. However, as tolerance develops with repeated use (bottom panel), larger amounts of drug are needed to experience the mood change (the curve shifts to the right) but no change in the dose causing depression of respiration occurs. The margin of safety shrinks dramatically in the tolerant individual.

TABLE 17.4 Street Names for Various Barbiturates

Type of barbiturate[a]	Street name
Pentobarbital (Nembutal)	Abbotts, blockbusters, nebbies, nembies, yellow bullets, yellow dolls, yellow jackets, yellows
Amobarbital (Amytal)	Blue angels, bluebirds, blue bullets, blue devils, blue dolls, blue heavens, blues
Secobarbital (Seconal)	F-40s, Mexican reds, R.D.s, redbirds, red bullets, red devils, red dolls, reds, seggies, pinks
Secobarbital and amobarbital (Tuinal)	Christmas trees, double trouble, gorilla pills, rainbows, tootsies, trees
Barbiturates in general	Downers, goofballs, G.B.s, idiot pills, King Kong pills, peanuts, pink ladies, sleepers, softballs, stumblers

[a]Illicit "barbiturate" capsules often contain a combination of several other substances such as strychnine, arsenic, laxatives, or sugar.

chamber. Street use in humans frequently involves oral ingestion of high doses in a binge fashion that may be a substitute for alcohol or in combination with alcohol (a particularly dangerous practice) to enhance the effect. Other users inject the barbiturate intravenously to produce a "high" similar to that achieved with heroin. Injected barbiturates may then replace heroin if the preferred drug is unavailable, or the two drugs may be taken in combination. However, there is no cross dependence between barbiturates and heroin or other opiates, so opiate withdrawal is not specifically reduced by barbiturate use. Simultaneous use of a CNS stimulant like amphetamine and a barbiturate apparently produces an unusual mood elevation that is "smoother" than with the stimulant alone. Other users take "uppers" in the day and, to compensate for the stimulant-induced insomnia, a barbiturate at night. Clearly these drug combinations create particularly hazardous situations: acute drug interactions as well as significant potential for chronic dependence.

The high incidence of side effects and lethality, rapid tolerance, and great abuse potential of barbiturates prompted the search for a novel anxiolytic drug without these undesirable characteristics. The benzodiazepines were introduced in 1960 and in general have replaced the prescription of barbiturates. The decline in prescriptions for barbiturates over the years has made these drugs less available and caused a parallel decline in abuse.

Benzodiazepines are highly effective for anxiety reduction

The first benzodiazepine (BDZ) to be introduced was chlordiazepoxide (Librium). It represented the first true anxiolytic that targeted anxiety without producing excessive seda-

tion. It has a low incidence of tolerance, a less severe withdrawal syndrome than barbiturates, and a very safe therapeutic index. Within a few years diazepam (Valium), oxazepam (Serax), flurazepam (Dalmane), and at least a dozen other chemically related drugs were developed.

Pharmacokinetics All BDZs have a common molecular structure (Figure 17.10) and similar mechanism of action. As was true for the barbiturates, the choice of a particular benzodiazepine for a given therapeutic situation depends primarily on the speed of onset and duration of drug action. Their duration of action is determined by (1) differences in their

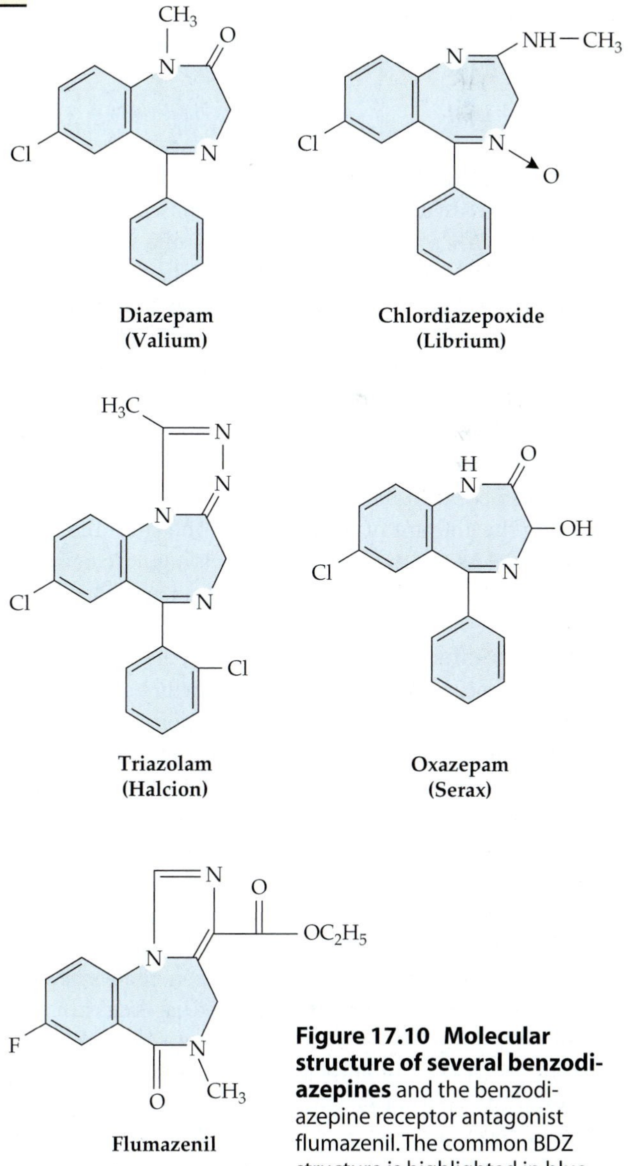

Figure 17.10 Molecular structure of several benzodiazepines and the benzodiazepine receptor antagonist flumazenil. The common BDZ structure is highlighted in blue.

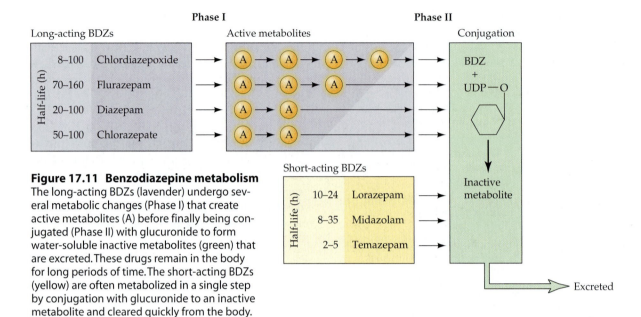

Figure 17.11 Benzodiazepine metabolism
The long-acting BDZs (lavender) undergo several metabolic changes (Phase I) that create active metabolites (A) before finally being conjugated (Phase II) with glucuronide to form water-soluble inactive metabolites (green) that are excreted. These drugs remain in the body for long periods of time. The short-acting BDZs (yellow) are often metabolized in a single step by conjugation with glucuronide to an inactive metabolite and cleared quickly from the body.

method of biotransformation and (2) the extent of redistribution to inactive depots such as skeletal muscle and fat. The long-acting BDZs undergo several metabolic steps to produce multiple active metabolites that may have half-lives of 60 hours or more (Figure 17.11). These can be problematic for elderly individuals, who may rapidly accumulate drug in the body because of their reduced metabolic capacity. The short-acting BDZs, such as midazolam (Versed) and lorazepam (Ativan), are metabolized in one step into inactive metabolites by conjugation with glucuronide. Redistribution also contributes to the short duration of action by reducing the amount of drug available to act on the CNS. The slow release from inert depots back into circulation is responsible for any drug hangover effects that might occur.

Therapeutic effects   Unlike barbiturates, the BDZs cannot be used for deep anesthesia, but they are useful for presurgical anesthesia during which the patient is conscious but less aware of his surroundings and quite relaxed. They are also commonly used before major dental work as well as for a wide range of stressful diagnostic procedures. One of the newer benzodiazepines is midazolam (Versed), used for rapid onset of relaxation and deep sleep during brief surgical procedures done with local anesthetics. Because it has a short half-life, recovery takes only a few hours without hangover. It also induces an anterograde amnesia that creates an illusion of anesthesia in some patients, which is considered a beneficial drug effect.

In other cases, however, the drug-induced amnesia is highly undesirable. Recently a benzodiazepine that is marketed outside the United States as a sleep aid has been illegally imported and used as a "date rape" drug. Flunitrazepam

(Rohypnol) is quite potent and, when combined with alcohol, impairs judgment and causes amnesia along with significant sedation. There have been a limited number of reports of women who have been sexually assaulted and found themselves in unfamiliar locations with no memory of the events surrounding the attack. Although such situations produced serious concern on college campuses and at social establishments serving alcohol, the number of documented cases is quite small and the risk is low. However, because of the illicit use, the U.S. Drug Enforcement Administration has classified flunitrazepam as a Schedule I drug, (i.e., a drug with high potential for abuse and no medical use). (See Chapter 15 for more on other "date rape" drugs.)

The most popular use for BDZs is anxiety relief. Benzodiazepines relieve the sense of worry and fearfulness as well as the physical symptoms associated with anxiety with less mental clouding, loss of judgment, and motor incoordination than is typical of other sedative–hypnotics. The mild sedation that accompanies use of some of the BDZs decreases with repeated use over a week to 10 days, but little or no tolerance occurs for the antianxiety effects. Nevertheless, in older individuals with slower drug metabolism excessive confusion and reduced cognitive function may be quite serious and resemble senile dementia.

Several of the longer-acting benzodiazepines are useful **hypnotics.** BDZs shorten the time needed to fall asleep and increase the duration of sleep time, as well as reduce the number of nighttime awakenings. Despite their relative safety, all sleep medications pose potential problems (Box 17.2). Some BDZs are useful **muscle relaxants** and others are **anticonvulsants** for the management of particular forms of epilepsy. Intravenous diazepam is the treatment of choice for status epilepticus, a period of severe and persistent seizures

BOX 17.2   Clinical Applications

Treating Insomnia

Sleep is an altered state of consciousness that fascinates laymen and scientists alike. Although all mammals and birds engage in sleep, we do not really understand why sleep is important, although recovery from brain metabolic fatigue and memory consolidation are two possibilities. What is apparent is that the need for sleep is an extraordinarily powerful motivation. Although human beings are quite capable of starving themselves to death by overcoming the need to eat, the need to sleep cannot be ignored.

Sleep is not a unidimensional state but consists of several well-defined stages of consciousness characterized by distinct brain electrical activity patterns (Figure A), proceeding from dozing and light sleep in stages 1 and 2 to deep and restful sleep in stages 3 and 4 (slow-wave sleep). In addition, another type of sleep occurs, known as rapid eye movement (REM) sleep.

REM sleep is characterized by increased heart rate and respiration, loss of muscle tone, rapid darting eye movements, and brain waves that look like wakefulness. If the individual is wakened during REM sleep, she usually reports experiencing a narrative-like dream. This sleep cycle repeats four or five times a night, with an elongation of REM periods toward morning and a corresponding decrease in slow-wave sleep (see Figure A). The sleep architecture is quite similar in all normal, healthy adults, but there are large interindividual differences in sleep latency (the time to fall asleep) that vary from several minutes to a half hour or more. Total sleep duration is also highly variable: Some adults need 8 to 10 hours of sleep per night to feel rested, whereas others need only 5 or 6, and in rare instances only 2 to 3 hours. When you fail to sleep the optimum number of hours in a night, you become sleep-deprived. As students, you surely know the symptoms of sleep deprivation: daytime fatigue and drowsiness,

impaired performance, irritability, and feelings of depression. After too many nights of inadequate sleep, the stresses of the day seem more troublesome and the joys diminish. Although your sleep deprivation is often self-imposed, for others insomnia can be a chronic problem.

Insomnia is defined as a failure to fall asleep, an inability to maintain sleep, or a dissatisfaction with the quality of sleep that leads to sleep deprivation. Occasional insomnia occurs at some time for almost everyone because of jet lag, time changes in work schedules, pain or illness, hormonal changes, everyday stresses, or drug-induced stimulation (e.g., from cold medications). Although occasional sleep deprivation is harmless, the deprived individual may contribute to accidents, lose productivity, and show impaired judgment. As much as 15% of the population have serious and chronic insomnia.

Generally, treating insomnia involves little more than eliminating disruptive stimuli in the bedroom,

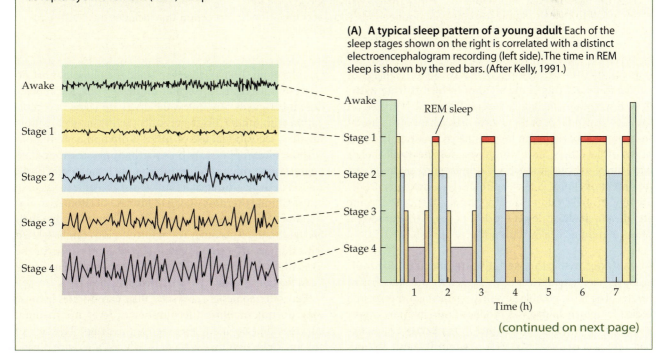

(A) A typical sleep pattern of a young adult Each of the sleep stages shown on the right is correlated with a distinct electroencephalogram recording (left side). The time in REM sleep is shown by the red bars. (After Kelly, 1991.)

Awake

Stage 1

Stage 2

Stage 3

Stage 4

REM sleep

Time (h)

(continued on next page)

BOX 17.2 (continued)

reducing aches and pains, and avoiding such drugs as caffeine, alcohol, tobacco, nasal decongestants, and so forth. Regular physical exercise during the day and a warm bath several hours before bedtime may help. Several over-the-counter sleep aids (e.g., Sominex and Unisom) containing antihistamines (H_1 receptor blockers) such as diphenhydramine or doxylamine are available. These drugs are normally used to treat allergies but have drowsiness as a side effect. Although some people consider them to be effective, laboratory sleep studies show that they do not have a significant effect on inducing or sustaining sleep. Furthermore, rapid tolerance and potential side effects make them minimally useful at best.

In cases when self-help techniques do not improve the quality of sleep, prescription drugs can be very effective, but at a cost. Compare the sleep patterns for an individual using barbiturate sleeping pills initially and then after chronic use (Figure B). Initially, the barbiturates readily induce sleep and decrease spontaneous awakenings, although grogginess and "hangover" the next day may impair functioning. With chronic nightly use and

increased doses, however, drug tolerance is apparent by the longer sleep latency (1 hour) and the 12 awakenings during the night. Also, both REM sleep and the most restful sleep (stages 3 and 4) are suppressed. When the drug is stopped, the amount of REM sleep becomes greater than normal and the character of the dreams may be more intense, producing vivid dreams and nightmares along with insomnia. Occasionally, waking "daymares" occur that cause the individual to panic. Chronic use and increased doses also increase the probability of physical dependence.

Benzodiazepines are the most-prescribed hypnotics because those with rapid onset and short action are effective in helping individuals fall asleep and are eliminated from the body during a normal night's sleep. The slower-onset and longer-acting benzodiazepines are used for people who fall asleep readily but suffer from nighttime or early-morning waking. Unfortunately, the longer-acting drugs are also more likely to cause reduced alertness the next day since they remain in active form for longer periods. Drug accumulation is

common in the elderly, who metabolize BDZs more slowly, leading to incoordination and confusion that resembles dementia. In addition, although benzodiazepines are considered to produce a more "natural" sleep because they have minimal effects on REM episodes, they do apparently increase stage 2 sleep at the expense of the more restful stage 4. Although tolerance and physical dependence are less than with barbiturates, rebound withdrawal insomnia often occurs after chronic use. More importantly, people who learn to rely on drugs to induce sleep lie awake at night worrying that they will not sleep when they have not taken a pill.

Recently, TV advertising has promoted zolpidem (Ambien) as the newest sleep-inducing drug. Zolpidem is a short-acting nonbenzodiazepine hypnotic that nevertheless binds to BDZ receptors on the GABA complex. It effectively induces sedation and sleep, but has no specific anxiolytic, anticonvulsant, or muscle-relaxing effects. Its distinctive activity may be explained by its selective action at one subtype of $GABA_A$ receptor that includes the BDZ1

---

that can be life-threatening. BDZs are also the drugs of choice in preventing acute **alcohol** or **barbiturate withdrawal** symptoms, including seizures. This action is based on the cross dependence of these three drugs; hence withdrawal from any one of them can be terminated by administration of any of the others. Since withdrawal from heavy alcohol or barbiturate use can produce a life-threatening situation, the treatment of choice is to substitute a long-acting benzodiazepine (usually Valium) to stop the abstinence syndrome and then to gradually lower the dose of the BDZ over several weeks to minimize the withdrawal.

Advantages over other sedative–hypnotics
Benzodiazepines have several clear advantages over the older barbiturates. The most notable advantage is the high therapeutic index. Extremely high doses produce disorientation, cognitive impairments, and amnesia and in some cases a paradoxical increase in aggressiveness, irritability, and anxiety

(Hobbs et al., 1996). However, since they have almost no effect on the respiratory center in the medulla, lethal overdose is extremely rare unless the drugs are taken in combination with other CNS depressants such as alcohol. Unfortunately, recreational use of BDZs is often in combination with alcohol, opiates such as methadone, or other CNS depressants, which can produce highly toxic interactions. Although there is no specific antagonist available for alcohol or barbiturate overdose, the BDZ flumazenil (Romazicon) is a competitive antagonist for the BDZ receptor. Individuals brought to the emergency room unconscious can be treated with flumazenil, which quickly reverses the effects of the BDZ while the non-BDZ depressant is gradually eliminated from the body through normal metabolic processes.

Benzodiazepines are also safer than barbiturates because they do not increase the number of liver microsomal enzymes that normally metabolize the drugs. The lack of enzyme induction means there is reduced tolerance during

BOX 17.2 (continued)

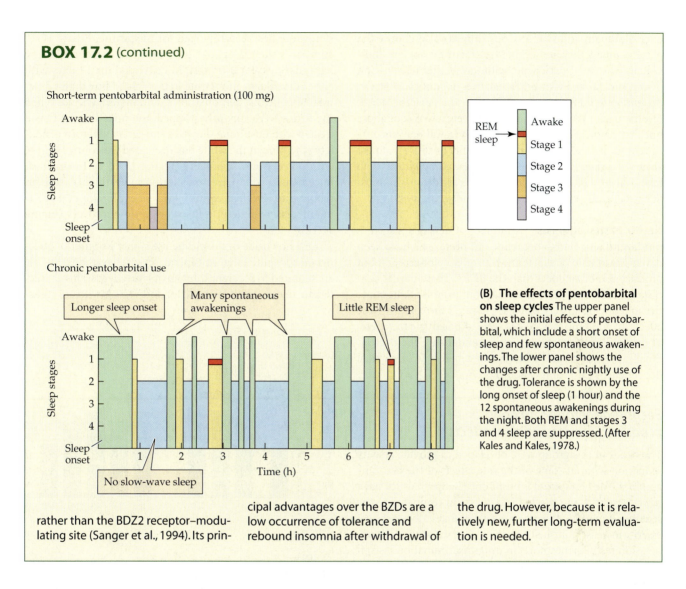

Short-term pentobarbital administration (100 mg)

Chronic pentobarbital use

Longer sleep onset

Many spontaneous awakenings

Little REM sleep

No slow-wave sleep

(B) The effects of pentobarbital on sleep cycles The upper panel shows the initial effects of pentobarbital, which include a short onset of sleep and few spontaneous awakenings. The lower panel shows the changes after chronic nightly use of the drug. Tolerance is shown by the long onset of sleep (1 hour) and the 12 spontaneous awakenings during the night. Both REM and stages 3 and 4 sleep are suppressed. (After Kales and Kales, 1978.)

rather than the BDZ2 receptor–modulating site (Sanger et al., 1994). Its principal advantages over the BZDs are a low occurrence of tolerance and rebound insomnia after withdrawal of the drug. However, because it is relatively new, further long-term evaluation is needed.

repeated drug administration and also fewer drug interactions.

Benzodiazepines have a reputation for lower probability of physical dependence and abuse. Nevertheless, chronic use and physical dependence do occur. The abstinence syndrome, which is milder than that of the barbiturates and not life-threatening, develops gradually over several weeks, especially for those drugs with a very long half-life. The symptoms may include insomnia, restlessness, headache, anxiety, mild depression, subtle perceptual distortions, muscle pain, and muscle twitches (Carvey, 1998). The most severe symptoms, which resemble those of other CNS depressants, include panic, delirium, and seizures. These occur in individuals who are abusing the drugs at high doses for prolonged periods, often in combination with other drugs.

In initial research, laboratory animals did not readily self-administer benzodiazepines in an operant chamber, suggesting that the drugs have little reinforcement value and low abuse potential in humans. However, BDZs with more rapid onset are more likely to be self-administered by animals. Furthermore, in animals that are first trained to self-administer a barbiturate, the reinforcing effects of BDZs are more apparent. In drug-discrimination tests (see Chapter 4) in which rats are taught to discriminate between barbiturates and saline by pressing a lever for reinforcement, BDZs will substitute for barbiturates. However, rats can also be trained to discriminate chlordiazepoxide from barbiturates and alcohol. These results indicate that the subjective drug-induced states of the 3 drugs must be similar if they substitute for each other in the discrimination test yet have some qualitative differences that can be distinguished. Overall, animal studies suggest that the reinforcement value of BDZs is much less than that of barbiturates (Griffiths et al., 1991).

Over the years, concern about the abuse potential of these drugs has led to fewer prescriptions. However, studies with humans show that normal volunteers prefer to take a placebo over diazepam and that anxious subjects also choose the placebo unless they are seeking treatment for anxiety. Individuals who are experiencing withdrawal after termination of chronic diazepam or other sedative–hypnotics, however, do tend to self-administer a BDZ rather than placebo. These results suggest that BDZs have a relatively low risk of abuse but that physical dependence and withdrawal may encourage continued use. Overall, the probability of abuse is almost always associated with polydrug use; that is, individuals who have a history of drug or alcohol abuse are those who most likely will abuse benzodiazepines (Woods et al., 1995).

Newer partial agonists   A number of new drugs such as imidazenil, etizolam, abecarnil, and bretazenil have been developed to bind readily to the benzodiazepine receptor but produce less of an effect than the BDZs. These partial agonists are still in experimental stages but promise to be effective in reducing anxiety with even fewer of the cognitive side effects. In addition, they do not seem to potentiate the effects of other CNS depressants, further enhancing their safety. Finally, they are associated with a low incidence of physical dependence (Costa and Guidotti, 1996).

Second-generation anxiolytics produce distinctive clinical effects

The drugs in this group were developed to provide anxiety reduction without some of the side effects of the benzodiazepines. The best known is buspirone (BuSpar), which has a novel structure and mechanism of action compared to the sedative–hypnotics. It is also unusual in that it does not necessarily increase punished behaviors as in the water-lick suppression test. Furthermore, in drug-discrimination tests, it does not substitute for either barbiturates or BDZs. Clearly, buspirone has distinctive subjective effects as well as a distinctive mechanism of action.

In clinical tests, buspirone has significant anxiolytic actions, although it is much less effective in reducing the physical symptoms of anxiety than the cognitive aspects of worry and poor concentration. Some suggest that it may be best used in combination with other pharmacotherapies or along with cognitive behavior therapy (Harvey and Balon, 1995).

Buspirone has several advantages over the benzodiazepines, including its usefulness in treating depression that often accompanies anxiety. In addition, its anxiety reduction is not accompanied by sedation, confusion, or mental clouding. Buspirone does not enhance the CNS-depressant effects of alcohol or other CNS depressants, so it is still safer than the BDZs. It also has a minimum of severe side effects, and fatalities have not been reported. Further, it has little or no potential for recreational use or dependence. In fact, some patients report a dysphoric effect, described as a feeling of restlessness and malaise. Finally, no rebound withdrawal

syndrome has been reported for buspirone. Figure 17.12 compares the effects of buspirone and diazepam in the light–dark exploration test. Mice treated for 14 days with either drug spent more time in the lighted box than saline-treated controls, demonstrating antianxiety effects. When the drugs were abruptly stopped, the mice that had been treated with buspirone showed a slow gradual return of anxiety (the time in the white box decreased) to control values, with no rebound in anxiety (Figure 17.12A). In contrast, mice treated with diazepam showed an abstinence-induced rebound to less than control levels of exploration (suggesting increased anxiety) followed by a slow recovery (Figure 17.12B).

One downside of buspirone use is that its onset of effectiveness is quite long. In general, several weeks of daily use are required to see significant anxiolytic effects. This characteristic makes it less desirable for individuals who are accus-

(A) Buspirone

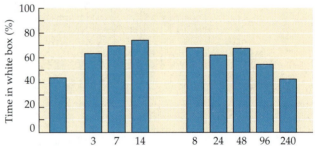

(B) Diazepam

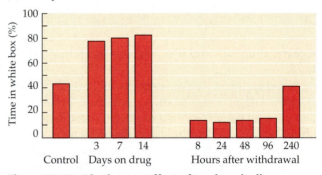

Figure 17.12 Abstinence effect after chronic diazepam but not buspirone Mice treated with buspirone (A) or diazepam (B) for 14 consecutive days and placed in the light–dark test on day 3, 7, and 14 showed reduced anxiety by exploring the bright box for more time than control mice. Neither drug produced tolerance over the 14 days. When the test was repeated at various times after drug withdrawal, the buspirone-treated mice showed a gradual return of anxiety. In contrast, mice treated with diazepam showed an abstinence-induced rebound in anxiety. This effect is shown by levels of exploration significantly less than control levels, followed by a slow recovery. (After Costall and Naylor, 1991.)

tomed to the immediate relief induced by BDZs. Also, its delayed action makes it less useful for patients who take the drug only when needed for situational anxiety. Second, buspirone, as well as other structurally related drugs (gepirone and ipsapirone), does not show cross-tolerance or cross dependence with BDZs or sedative–hypnotics. This feature makes it inappropriate for use as a substitution in cases of alcohol or barbiturate withdrawal. Third, it lacks the hypnotic effects necessary to treat insomnia, has no muscle-relaxant effects, and does not control seizures.

Buspirone has unusual characteristics because, unlike the sedative–hypnotics, it does not enhance GABA function but instead acts as a partial agonist at serotonergic 5-HT$_{1A}$ receptors. These receptors are found in heavy concentration in the limbic system, including the amygdala and the frontal and entorhinal cortices. Although some of these receptors are thought to be located postsynaptically, autoradiographic and immunohistochemical studies also show 5-HT$_{1A}$ somatodendritic autoreceptors in the nucleus of the raphe. The neurochemical basis of the anxiolytic action is not fully explained, but Charney and colleagues (1990) suggest that down-regulation of the 5-HT receptors may be responsible for the delayed onset of action.

Antidepressants relieve anxiety and depression

Several of the anxiety disorders described in earlier sections are effectively treated with antidepressant drugs. These drugs are important because anxiety and depression very often occur in the same individual and a single drug can be used to treat both conditions. However, several antidepressants have beneficial effects in treating anxiety apart from their antidepressant action. For example, in OCD the selective serotonin reuptake inhibitors (SSRIs) clomipramine (Anafranil), fluoxetine (Prozac), fluvoxamine (Luvox), and sertraline (Zoloft) have been found effective in reducing symptoms, possibly because they each enhance serotonin (5-HT) function by blocking reuptake of the monoamine. The benefits are apparently unrelated to the SSRIs' antidepressant action, as shown in the results of an experiment by Leonard et al. (1989). In this double-blind crossover experiment, investigators compared the effects of two antidepressants: desipramine (DMI), which blocks norepinephrine reuptake and has minimal effects on 5-HT, and clomipramine (CMI), which selectively blocks 5-HT reuptake. After 3 weeks of placebo treatment to establish a baseline of symptom severity, one group received DMI and the other CMI for a 5-week period. After 5 weeks the drugs were switched for the two groups. Figure 17.13 shows that the 5-HT agonist CMI was consistently more effective in relieving symptoms of OCD. Further, when patients on CMI switched to DMI, their symptoms reappeared, which shows the selective effect of the serotonergic antidepressant.

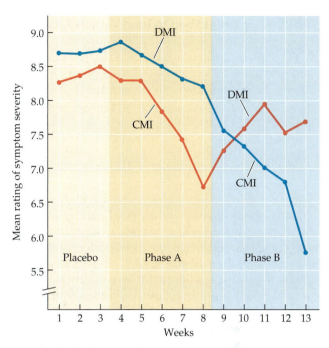

Figure 17.13 Mean rating of symptoms in patients with OCD when treated with desipramine (DMI) or clomipramine (CMI) In this crossover study, during drug treatment in phase A, the CMI group had fewer symptoms. In phase B, when the treatments were reversed for the two groups, the CMI-treated group again showed greater improvement. Patients who were treated with DMI during phase B showed a return of symptoms. (After Leonard et al, 1989.)

Tricyclic antidepressants such as imipramine (Tofranil) and monoamine oxidase inhibitors (e.g., phenelzine [Nardil] and tranylcypromine [Parnate]) are also often effective in treating some anxiety disorders, including panic, phobic disorders, and GAD, although side effects are often troublesome (see Chapter 16). Since the side effects of SSRIs are sometimes less disturbing to patients and they have a more favorable therapeutic index, the serotonergic drugs are more often prescribed as a first choice. In addition, because abuse potential of the SSRIs is low, they may be used on occasions when benzodiazepine dependence is a concern. Table 17.5 provides a summary of a variety of treatment options. Keep in mind that behavioral therapy is the principal way of treating simple phobias and, along with cognitive therapy, is a significant approach in treating GAD, social phobia, OCD, and PTSD.

Section Summary

Anxiety disorders are the most common psychiatric diagnoses, affecting between 10 and 30% of the population. Despite the utility of anxiety in providing motivation and drive, excess anxiety can be debilitating and damage the quality of life. Five

TABLE 17.5 Drugs Used to Treat Various Anxiety Disorders

Drug class	Trade name	Anxiety disorders
Benzodiazepines	Valium, Xanax	GAD, PTSD, panic disorder
Tricyclic antidepressants	Tofranil, Aventil	Panic disorder, GAD, OCD, PTSD
Monoamine oxidase inhibitors	Nardil, Parnate	Social phobia, panic disorder
Selective serotonin reuptake inhibitors	Prozac, Zoloft, Paxil	Social phobia, panic disorder, OCD, PTSD
Buspirone	BuSpar	GAD, panic disorder, OCD

common anxiety disorders include general anxiety disorder (GAD), panic disorder with or without agoraphobia, several types of phobias, post-traumatic stress disorder (PTSD), and obsessive–compulsive disorder (OCD). Although all are classified as psychiatric conditions that have anxiety as a major component, each has unique, clearly definable symptoms and apparently distinct biological contributions.

Animal models of anxiety depend on either naturalistic avoidance of situations such as brightly lit areas or conditioned approach–avoidance situations (conflict procedures). Although the models are good predictors of anxiety reduction in general, they are not specific for the multiple disorder subtypes. Nevertheless, each of the disorders described can be effectively treated with pharmacotherapy and/or cognitive behavior therapy.

Barbiturates reduce anxiety and induce sedation and sleep and are categorized primarily by their duration of action. Some of the longest acting, such as phenobarbital, remain useful in treating seizure disorders. However, their significant cognitive side effects, great potential for dangerous overdose, rapid development of tolerance, and high abuse potential make them less popular than the newer benzodiazepines (BDZs).

The long-acting benzodiazepines are effective anxiolytics that can be used to relieve acute anxiety as well as that associated with GAD and panic disorder. Overall, they are safer, have fewer side effects, produce less tolerance and physical dependence, and have lower abuse potential than barbiturates and other sedative–hypnotic drugs. Several BDZs effectively reduce insomnia, produce muscle relaxation, and have anticonvulsant effects. Because BDZs show cross dependence with both alcohol and barbiturates, they are administered to prevent the dangerous withdrawal syndrome of sedative–hypnotics before being gradually withdrawn. Several agents are being developed to further minimize side effects. Partial agonists that act at the BDZ receptor are one class that may increase safety. In addition, anxiety-reducing drugs such as buspirone that work by distinct neurochemical mechanisms provide a novel approach to the treatment of anxiety disorders. Finally, several antidepressant drugs are also useful in treating selected anxiety disorders.

Neurochemical Basis of Anxiety and Anxiolytics

Although the classic sedative–hypnotic drugs affect the functioning of many types of neurons in the CNS, their primary mechanism of action involves enhancing GABA transmission. Since GABA is the major inhibitory neurotransmitter in the nervous system, it has receptors on most cells in the CNS to exert widespread inhibitory effects. You may recall that the $GABA_A$ receptor complex regulates a chloride (Cl^-) channel that increases chloride current into the cell to move the membrane potential farther away from the threshold for firing. Therefore, GABA agonists produce a local hyperpolarization, or inhibitory postsynaptic potential, and inhibit cell firing. Both barbiturates and benzodiazepines have binding sites as part of the $GABA_A$ receptor complex and enhance the inhibitory effects of GABA. Figure 17.14A shows the hyperpolarization caused by GABA and its enhancement by diazepam.

When BDZs bind to their receptor on the $GABA_A$ complex, they enhance the effect of GABA by increasing the number of times the channel opens. However, in the absence of GABA the benzodiazepines have no effect on Cl^- channel opening. Apparently the presence of a BDZ alters the physical state of the receptors so that GABA opens the channels more easily. As you would expect, the addition of the competitive antagonist flumazenil prevents the BDZ-induced enhancement of GABA action but does not affect GABA-induced hyperpolarization (Figure 17.14B). In contrast, the addition of a GABA antagonist prevents GABA from opening the channel, and the presence of a benzodiazepine has no further effect.

Competition experiments that measured the effectiveness of various BDZs in displacing [^{3}H]diazepam showed a positive correlation between the ability to displace the radioligand and the clinically effective dose for relieving anxiety (Figure 17.15). This means that the drugs that bind most readily to the BDZ receptor (i.e., require low concentrations to displace [^{3}H]diazepam) are also clinically effective at low doses. Likewise, BDZs that bind less easily need higher doses to be effective.

Barbiturates also increase the affinity of the $GABA_A$ receptor for GABA; however, they increase the duration of the opening of GABA-activated chloride channels rather than the number of openings. In addition to enhancing GABA's action at the receptor, barbiturates also directly open the Cl^- channel without GABA. This additional action may explain why barbiturates can be lethal while benzodiazepines are not.

(A)

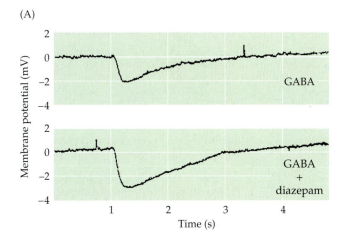

(B)

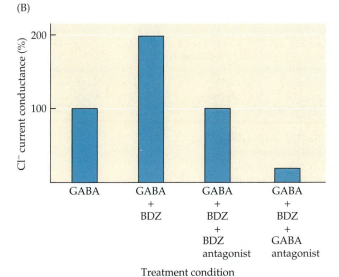

Figure 17.14 Effects of GABA and diazepam on membrane potentials and chloride flux (A) Electrical recording of the hyperpolarizing effect of GABA and the enhanced hyperpolarization caused by the addition of diazepam to a mouse spinal cord neuron. Diazepam alone would produce little or no hyperpolarization. (B) GABA alone increases the conductance of Cl⁻ through its channel. Adding a BDZ enhances the amount of Cl⁻ movement into the cell. Blocking the BDZ receptor prevents the drug's enhancement of GABA but not the effect of GABA itself. A GABA antagonist prevents GABA from opening the Cl⁻ channel, and the presence of BDZ has no effect. (After Kandel, 2000.)

Multiple neurotransmitters mediate anxiety

A wide variety of lesion and drug studies in psychobiology suggest that the central nucleus of the amygdala orchestrates the components of anxiety: autonomic activation, defensive behavior, enhanced reflexes, activation of the hypothalamic–pituitary adrenal (HPA) axis, and other responses

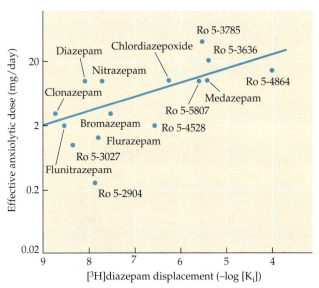

Figure 17.15 Correlation of benzodiazepine binding and antianxiety effect The ability of the benzodiazepines (including several experimental compounds having the "Ro" designation) to displace [³H]diazepam from the BDZ receptor is correlated with the doses required for anxiolytic action. The negative log scale on the x-axis reflects increasing concentrations from left to right. Therefore, the benzodiazepines that displace labeled diazepam at low concentrations (e.g., clonazepam and flunitrazepam) also tend to be those that require lower doses to reduce anxiety. Those that are less effective at binding (needing higher concentrations) to the diazepam site (e.g., Ro 5-4864) also need higher doses for antianxiety effects. (After Braestrup and Squires, 1978.)

(LeDoux, 1996). Stimulation of the amygdala has widespread effects because of its multiple connections with brain areas that are responsible for how emotion is expressed (refer to Figure 17.16 for details). In addition, it identifies the emotional significance of events and aids in the formation of emotional memories. For example, lesioning the amygdala prevents the development of conditioned emotional responses and also blocks innate fear. Also, intracerebral injection of various drugs into the amygdala produces anxiolytic effects in a number of animal tests of anxiety. Furthermore, lesioning selected brain areas that receive projection neurons from the amygdala can eliminate specific components of the anxiety response. For example, lesioning the periaqueductal gray prevents the freezing response. The anatomical complexity of emotion and its importance to survival makes it highly likely that many neurotransmitters modulate the anxiety response.

While activation of the amygdala elicits emotional responses, the prefrontal cortex (particularly the orbitofrontal and medial frontal) exerts inhibitory control over the

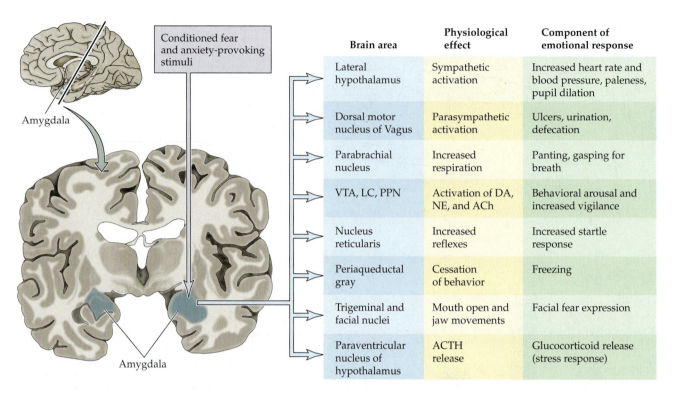

Brain area	Physiological effect	Component of emotional response
Lateral hypothalamus	Sympathetic activation	Increased heart rate and blood pressure, paleness, pupil dilation
Dorsal motor nucleus of Vagus	Parasympathetic activation	Ulcers, urination, defecation
Parabrachial nucleus	Increased respiration	Panting, gasping for breath
VTA, LC, PPN	Activation of DA, NE, and ACh	Behavioral arousal and increased vigilance
Nucleus reticularis	Increased reflexes	Increased startle response
Periaqueductal gray	Cessation of behavior	Freezing
Trigeminal and facial nuclei	Mouth open and jaw movements	Facial fear expression
Paraventricular nucleus of hypothalamus	ACTH release	Glucocorticoid release (stress response)

Figure 17.16 The amygdala coordinates components of emotion. The amygdala has neuronal connections with all of these brain areas that produce individual pieces of emotional expression. VTA, ventral tegmental area; LC, locus coeruleus; PPN, pedunculopontine nucleus; DA, dopamine; NE, norepinephrine; ACh, acetylcholine; ACTH, adrenocorticotropic hormone.

more primitive responses of the limbic system. Without the "cognitive" control of the prefrontal cortex, the anxiety response produces more limited patterns of behavior that may not be suitable for coping with modern stressors that are not resolved by fighting or running away.

Role of GABA in anxiety   The ability of BDZs to modulate GABA clearly implicates the neurotransmitter in anxiety. The importance of GABA is directly shown by the reduction in anxiety produced by local administration of GABA or the GABA agonist musimol into the amygdala. Intracranial administration of BDZs into the amygdala also has anxiolytic effects in several animal tests, including the light–dark crossing test, freezing response, elevated plus-maze, and operant conflict tests. The anticonflict effects can be reversed by flumazenil and also by coadministration of the GABA antagonist bicuculline into the amygdala. Furthermore, Sanders and Shekhar (1995) found that intra-amygdaloid injection of flumazenil or bicuculline also blocks *systemic* antianxiety effects of chlordiazepoxide in the social interaction test. The bicuculline effect demonstrates the necessity for GABA activity in the anxiolytic effects of BDZs. The amygdala, particularly the basolateral nucleus, is clearly an important site mediating the antianxiety effects of BDZs.

However, since BDZs can still have anxiety-reducing effects following destruction of the amygdala, multiple redundant brain areas must be involved in the response to anxiety (see Davis, 1997, for an excellent summary).

Role of natural ligands for BDZ receptors in anxiety   We certainly might wonder about the function of BDZ receptors under normal circumstances when we are not taking anxiolytic drugs. The receptors were identified in 1977, and their location was mapped in the rat brain using autoradiography. Their high concentration in the amygdala and other parts of the limbic system, which regulate the fear/anxiety response, and in the cerebral cortex (particularly the frontal lobe), which exerts control over limbic structures, provides the first clue to their function. A PET scan of BDZ receptors in the human brain also shows their wide distribution (Figure 17.17).

In Chapter 7 you read about the existence of endogenous substances called inverse agonists that bind to the BDZ site and produce the opposite actions of the drugs, namely increased anxiety, arousal, and seizures. One class of inverse agonists is the β-carbolines, which when administered to humans produce extreme anxiety and an overwhelming sense of panic. These inverse agonists are presumed to

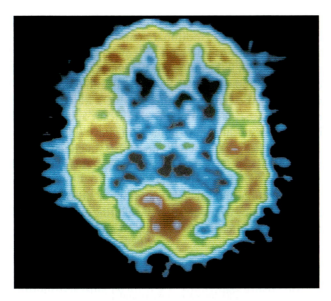

Figure 17.17 PET scan of benzodiazepine receptors in the human brain The highest concentrations are shown in orange and red. (Courtesy of Goran Sedvall.)

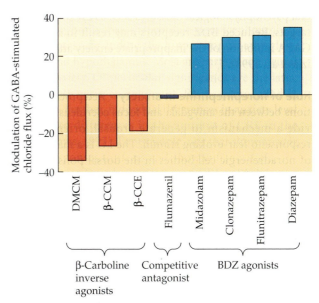

Figure 17.18 The anxiety-producing β-carbolines are inverse agonists at the BDZ receptor. They not only prevent the effect of GABA on chloride flux but produce the opposite effect, which leads to cell excitation. The anxiolytic BDZs are agonists and enhance GABA's effects. The competitive antagonist flumazenil binds to the BDZ receptor but has no action of its own. However, it prevents either the BDZs or the inverse agonists from acting. DMCM, methyl-6,7-dimethoxy-4-ethyl-β-carboline-3-carboxylate; β-CCM, methyl-β-carboline-3-carboxylate;. β-CCE, β-carboline-3-carboxylic acid ethylester. (After Richards et al., 1991.)

uncouple the GABA receptors from the Cl⁻ channels so that GABA is less effective in causing entry of Cl⁻ into the cell (Figure 17.18), leading to increased membrane excitability. A second family of inverse agonists are peptides related to the large peptide called diazepam binding inhibitor. The anxiety-inducing effects of diazepam binding inhibitor are described in Box 7.2 in Chapter 7.

Other ligands called endozepines may represent natural anxiety-*reducing* agents that act at the benzodiazepine site. Drugan and coworkers (1994) propose that when an individual learns how to cope with her stress, anxiety may be reduced by the increase of natural BDZs. The effects of the natural ligands and those of the BDZ drugs suggest these receptors are important in regulating normal anxiety and may contribute to abnormal anxiety as well.

Other evidence suggesting that BDZ receptors mediate anxiety comes from studies that look at natural differences in animal anxiety in conflict situations such as the water-lick suppression test. In any group of animals, some (the "laid-back" type) become adapted to the tongue shock with repeated exposure and drink despite the shock, while their "uptight" littermates dramatically avoid drinking. The more emotional animals have fewer BDZ receptors in several brain areas (Sepinwall and Cook, 1980). Other studies find a correlation between anxiety in the elevated plus-maze and decreased number of GABA and BDZ receptors in mouse cerebral cortex (Rago et al., 1988). In patients with panic disorder, PET scans show less benzodiazepine binding in the CNS, particularly in portions of the frontal lobes (Figure 17.19). These patients are also less sensitive to BDZs on sev-

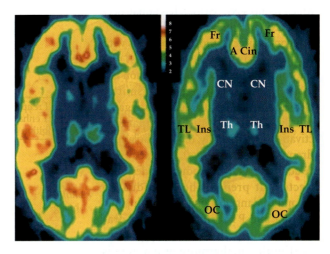

Figure 17.19 PET scans of a control subject (left panel) and a patient with panic disorder (right panel) The scans made in the horizontal plane with the frontal cortex at the top show decreased density of BDZ receptors in the patient with panic disorder, particularly in the frontal cortex (Fr) and insula (Ins), areas important in anxiety modulation. Other brain areas also show reduced numbers of BDZ receptors. Warm colors indicate the most receptors; cool colors indicate fewer. Receptors were labeled with [¹¹C] flumazenil. A Cin, anterior cingulate; TL, temporal lobe; CN, caudate nucleus; Th, Thalamus; OC, occipital cortex. (From Malizia et al., 1998.)

Section Summary

The classic sedative–hypnotic drugs, which include alcohol as well as the benzodiazepines and barbiturates, potentiate the effects of GABA by binding to modulatory sites on the GABA receptor to enhance chloride conductance and produce an inhibitory effect. This enhanced inhibitory action potentially modifies all the neurotransmitters normally regulated by GABA. BDZs increase the number of channel openings caused by GABA binding, but the drugs alone have no effect on chloride conductance. Barbiturates increase the duration of opening time of GABA-activated chloride channels and also have a direct effect on chloride conductance in the absence of GABA. The latter action may explain why barbiturates, unlike BDZs, can cause severe side effects and have the potential for fatalities. Some endogenous ligands for BDZ receptors act as inverse agonists (β-carbolines) to increase anxiety, while others (endozepines) may be natural anxiety-reducing chemicals that compete for the same site.

The neural basis of anxiety focuses on limbic structures, particularly the amygdala, which controls the components of emotional responding, and the frontal cortex, which exerts control over the amygdala. Both animal and human studies support the idea that GABA and its modification by natural BDZs and inverse agonists regulate anxiety. Since GABA is a major inhibitory neurotransmitter throughout the nervous system, changes in GABA function modify several other neurotransmitters, all of which may contribute to the evolutionarily vital anxiety response. Interactions among NE, 5-HT, CRF, and DA, particularly in the amygdala and locus coeruleus, probably modulate appropriate levels of anxiety for given conditions but also may contribute to the damaging effects of the anxiety disorders.

Recommended Readings

LeDoux, J. E. (1996). *The Emotional Brain.* Simon and Schuster, New York.

Ninan, P. T. (1999). The functional anatomy, neurochemistry, and pharmacology of anxiety. *J. Clin. Psychiatry,* 60(Suppl. 22), 12–17.

Rapoport, J. L. (1989). The biology of obsessions and compulsions. *Sci. Am.,* March, 83–89.

Shader, R. I., and Greenblatt, D. J. (1995). The pharmacotherapy of acute anxiety. In *Psychopharmacology: The Fourth Generation of Progress* (F. E. Bloom and D. J. Kupfer, eds.), pp. 1341–1348. Raven Press, New York.

18 *Schizophrenia*

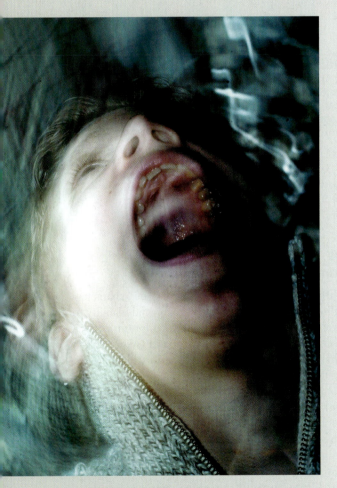

The symptoms of schizophrenia frequently lead to personal isolation and failure to achieve a meaningful and productive lifestyle.

When Jill, a 23-year-old secretary, quit her job, she knew something was happening to her, but didn't know what it was. She had suddenly become withdrawn and preoccupied with her own thoughts, considering the meaning of existence and religious issues. She was so absorbed that she stopped taking care of herself and failed to shower, wash her hair, or clean her clothes. One morning at dawn, she was called to her mission as she looked out her window and saw an especially bright planet followed by the sudden burst of sun rays. When a dog barked she knew she had been chosen for the task of saving the United States from cataclysmic destruction. Although she didn't know how the disaster would occur, many signs were revealed, such as when a fly landed on the television and cleaned its wings during satellite pictures of the planet Neptune. That clearly meant the time was near. Unfortunately, her enemies were aware of her role because they could read her mind, and each time she developed a plan, they stole it from her brain and prevented it. So Jill started wearing a black hat to keep her thoughts in her own mind. But the enemy voices talked about her constantly, swore at her, and plotted to stop her. They put snakes in her stomach and poisoned the medication that she was given during her first of many stays in the hospital (Lickey and Gordon, 1991).

Characteristics of Schizophrenia

Chapter 18 describes the characteristics of the devastating mental disorder known as schizophrenia and the drug therapies that are currently available to treat it. It also describes several models that attempt to explain the neuropathology that leads to its hallmark abnormal behavior and multiple symptoms.

Major mental disorders called psychoses are characterized by severe distortions of reality and disturbances in perception, intellectual functioning, affect (emotional expression), motivation, social relationships, and motor behavior. Schizophrenia is one relatively common form of psychosis and manic–depressive psychosis (discussed in Chapter 16) is another. Individuals with schizophrenia demonstrate many different symptoms, including hearing voices that are not there, holding unrealistic ideas and beliefs, and communicating in a way that is difficult to understand. They are frequently so incapacitated that voluntary or involuntary hospitalization is required.

Although drug use or environmental toxins may cause brief episodes of psychosis, schizophrenia is generally a chronic condition. While its symptoms can usually be controlled to some extent, schizophrenia cannot at this time be cured or prevented. Despite therapy, approximately 30% of people with schizophrenia spend a significant portion of their lives in mental hospitals, accounting for a majority of the total hospital beds in these facilities. Approximately 1 to 1.5% of the world's population will suffer from schizophrenia during their lifetimes. Another 2 to 3% will suffer from less severe schizophrenic symptoms but not meet the diagnostic criteria.

Symptoms of schizophrenia most often begin during the late teenage years and early twenties, although the disorder may first occur in childhood. The early onset of the disorder means that the episodes recurring throughout life disrupt the individual's most productive years. Although epidemiological studies have indicated that schizophrenia affects men and women equally, a clear gender difference in the age of onset and course of this disorder exists. Figure 18.1 shows that the onset of schizophrenia among 470 patients is highest in early adulthood for both sexes. However, for men the onset decreases rapidly with age. The onset for women is lower than for men until age 36. At that time more women than men demonstrate a first episode, and that difference continues into old age (Howard et al., 1993). The implication of the gender difference in onset is not clear, but it may suggest the existence of two qualitatively distinct subtypes of the disorder. Schizophrenia can destroy lives and also cause a great deal of pain and suffering, not only to afflicted individuals but also to their families as they attempt to cope emotionally and financially with the disorder. On that basis, the direct (e.g., hospitalization and medication costs) and indirect (loss of productive employment, participation in society, and fam-

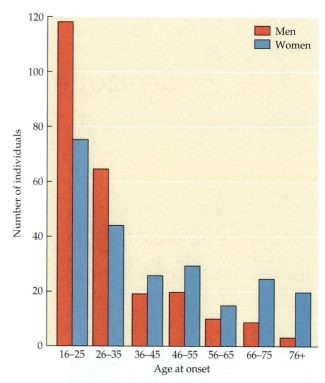

Figure 18.1 Gender differences in age at onset of schizophrenia Although both sexes show peak onset of symptoms between 16 and 25 years of age, this sample of 470 patients shows that more women than men experience their first episode after age 36, a difference that continues in every age bracket through old age. (After Howard et al., 1993.)

ily stress) costs of schizophrenia have been estimated to be between $30 billion and $50 billion a year in the United States.

There is no defining cluster of schizophrenic symptoms

Schizophrenia is very clearly a thought disorder, characterized by illogical thinking, lack of reasoning, and inability to recognize reality; however, the specific symptoms show a great deal of individual variation. Disturbances in perception (hallucinations) are a frequent occurrence in schizophrenia. These hallucinations are most often auditory and generally consist of voices that are insulting or commanding. For a closer look at auditory hallucinations, turn to Box 18.1. Tactile hallucinations are often electrical, tingling, or burning sensations. Bizarre delusions (beliefs not based on reality) are also common. Particularly prevalent are delusions of persecution involving the individual's belief that others are spying on or planning to harm him. Also quite common is the delusion that one's thoughts are broadcast from one's head to the world or that thoughts and feelings are not one's own but are imposed by an outside source, such as from outer space. Because the form of thought is disturbed, communication is confused and illogical and often does not even follow the rules of semantics. Speech may be vague or repetitive or shift from one subject to another, totally unrelated subject.

In many individuals with schizophrenia, emotions are either absent or totally inappropriate to the situation. Inappropriate emotion is demonstrated, for example, by the individual who smiles or laughs while describing electrical tortures. Individuals who lack emotion show no expression, speak in a monotone, and report a lack of feeling. Sudden and unpredictable changes of emotion are also common.

People with schizophrenia are frequently withdrawn, preoccupied with their own thoughts and delusions. Extreme apathy and an inability to initiate activities (avolition) frequently mean that the individual has no interest in performing everyday activities, including maintaining personal hygiene, which further isolates the individual from the main-

stream. Motor activity is generally reduced and characterized by inappropriate and bizarre postures, rigidity that resists efforts to be moved, or purposeless and sterotyped movements, for example, rocking or pacing. At times people with schizophrenia, particularly the paranoid type, can be agitated and violent (Krakowski and Menahem, 1997).

Diagnosis   Although the symptoms described above seem to be easily recognizable, the diagnosis of schizophrenia is not so simple. One reason is that no two individuals show the identical pattern of symptoms, nor is there a single symptom that occurs in every patient with schizophrenia. Furthermore, symptoms increase and decrease over time, and the predominant symptoms or symptom clusters often change over the years in the same individual, which may lead to a change in diagnosis. The question of whether schizophrenia is a single disorder or a collection of disorders has never been fully resolved.

BOX 18.1   Clinical Applications

The Functional Neuroanatomy of Hallucinations

One prominent core characteristic of schizophrenia is the occurrence of hallucinations, which are perceptions in the absence of external stimuli. Almost everyone has on occasion experienced things that are not there, but for many patients with schizophrenia the perceptions are frequent and seem to be very real. Although the most common hallucinations are auditory, the experience varies from individual to individual. The voices may be familiar ones such as a parent or spouse, or unrecognized voices that may be interpreted as "foreign agents," such as a radio transmitter implanted in the individual's head, or as the voices of angels. In many cases words and/or their meanings are not intelligible, but the message is clearly understood by the individual. Unfortunately, although the message may be harmless, such as a suggestion to

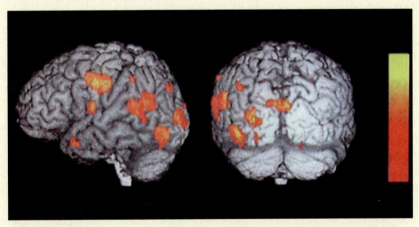

Left lateral and posterior surface views of the brain showing areas of increased cerebral blood flow during visual and auditory hallucinations. (From Silbersweig et al., 1991.)

mow the lawn, often the voices are harsh, critical, or demanding. The voices may accuse the individual of inappropriate actions, such as having raped a woman when in fact he just passed her on the street. In other instances, the voices direct the individual to perform certain behaviors that can lead to violent and destructive ends. Finally, although in many cases the hallucinations persist over

long periods, in other cases the voices occur primarily when the individual is not engaged in a task or has limited sensory input.

Among the more exciting research into the etiology of hallucinations is the use of PET or SPECT imaging to scan the brain during an ongoing hallucination. Several laboratories have

(continued on next page)

BOX 18.1 (continued)

produced intriguing results, although the functional neuroanatomy of the hallucinations is not identical in each individual. When the scans (refer to the figure) of several individuals were compared, some consistent results became apparent. First, in the vast majority of cases, the areas activated were located in the left cerebral hemisphere, which reflects the characteristic auditory–linguistic nature of the hallucinations and the fact that the left hemisphere specializes in language function in the majority of people. The most active brain areas are within the auditory–linguistic association cortex rather than the primary cortex, which is consistent with the internally generated nature of the experience. Psychological theories have suggested that auditory hallucinations represent "inner speech," that is, the individual is listening to his or her own thoughts and cannot tell the difference from listening to an outside source. However, Broca's area in the frontal lobe, which is responsible

for generating fluent speech, is not consistently activated, so inner speech may be involved but may not be the central pathological process. Left temporal lobe sites (including Wernicke's area and the middle temporal gyrus) are usually active during the hallucination, and electrical stimulation of these areas can produce auditory hallucinations in a healthy individual. Further, temporal lobe activity during epileptic seizures is often associated with auditory hallucinations.

Other neocortical areas that are active reflect the content of the individual hallucination. Activation in the visual association cortex (specialized for higher-order visual perception) accompanies visual components of a hallucination. We might add that the classic hypofrontality (reduced activity in prefrontal regions) associated with schizophrenia may also contribute to the phenomenon. Hypofrontality and the resulting lack of inhibition and internal monitoring

may lead the individual to falsely attribute internally generated perceptions to the external environment.

Somewhat surprising is that it is not only cortical areas that are active. There is also a common pattern of deep brain activity: subcortical regions including the thalamus and limbic (e.g., hippocampus, cingulate cortex) and parahippocampal areas show increased activity and are probably responsible for attention and the emotional component of the experience. These areas are highly interconnected with one another and with the activated association cortices. Cellular abnormalities in these brain regions are commonly reported in schizophrenia, and abnormal dopamine and glutamate activity are believed to be involved in disrupting these cortical–subcortical circuits, producing symptoms (see text). Further details on the functional neuroanatomy of hallucinations can be found in a variety of sources (McGuire et al., 1993; Silbersweig et al., 1995).

Historically, schizophrenia has been organized into subtypes, classified as **catatonic** (alternating periods of immobility and excited agitation), **paranoid** (characteristic delusions of grandeur or persecution), **hebephrenic** (silly and immature emotionality with disorganized behavior), and **undifferentiated** (cases not meeting the criteria of the other subtypes). These categories are based on the observations of Emil Kraepelin, a German psychiatrist who viewed these symptom patterns as manifestations of a single disorder in the early 1900s. Similar categories are used in the *Diagnostic and Statistical Manual of Mental Disorders* prepared by the American Psychiatric Association, now in its fourth revision (*DSM-IV*, 1994).

A second useful classification scheme, stemming from the work of Crow (1980) and modified more recently by Andreasen (1990), is that of **positive** and **negative symptoms.** The positive symptoms of schizophrenia include the more dramatic symptoms of the disorder, such as the delusions and hallucinations, disorganized speech, and bizarre behavior. Patients who demonstrate predominately positive symptoms tend to be older when they experienced a sudden onset of symptoms and appeared relatively normal in their

younger years before the symptoms occurred. These patients respond well to conventional antipsychotic medications that block dopamine receptors (D_2), while their symptoms are made worse by drugs that enhance dopamine function. Current thinking suggests that neurochemical abnormalities are significant to this disorder (see the section on abnormal dopamine function).

Negative symptoms are characterized by a decline of normal functions and include reduced speech (alogia), deficits in emotional responsiveness (flattened affect), loss of initiative and motivation (avolition), social withdrawal, loss of ability to derive pleasure from normally pleasurable activities (anhedonia), and intellectual impairment. These symptoms are among the most resistant to classic antipsychotic drugs but are reduced by the newer "atypical" antipsychotics (see the section on neuroleptics and atypical antipsychotics). Unlike patients with prominent positive symptoms, patients with negative symptoms tend to show early onset of some symptoms and a long course of progressive deterioration, perhaps reflecting long-term neurodegeneration or developmental errors.

Long-term outcome depends on pharmacological treatment

Before the advent of drug therapy, the history of treatment for schizophrenia was rather dismal (Figure 18.2A). The mentally ill were maintained in huge mental hospitals where treatment was limited to isolation or restraint, "shock" therapy using insulin-induced seizures or electric current, or surgery such as prefrontal lobotomy. Figure 18.2B shows a steady increase in the number of hospitalized psychiatric patients in the United States from 1900 to 1956 because such patients were usually permanently hospitalized. In 1956, the number of hospitalized patients began a sudden and steady decline despite a continued increase in initial admissions. This reduction coincided with the introduction of drug therapy, in particular the use of chlorpromazine (Thorazine). Chlorpromazine, a drug in the phenothiazine class, was initially used to enhance surgical anesthesia because it produces a sense of calmness and reduced awareness of environmental stimuli when administered before surgery. When tried with schizophrenic patients, chlorpromazine was especially effective because it calmed the excited patient and activated the patient who was profoundly withdrawn. Many modifications of the chlorpromazine molecule have already been made, and the development of new compounds to reduce symptoms with fewer side effects continues today.

Figure 18.2 Treatment of the mentally ill (A) Drawing depicting one of the available methods of "treatment" of the mentally ill during the early 1800s. (B) Patient populations in public mental institutions in the United States increased from 1900 to 1956. At that point a dramatic decline occurred in the number of institutionalized patients following the introduction of antipsychotic drugs. (After Bassuk and Gerson, 1978.)

Preclinical Models of Schizophrenia

Animal models of schizophrenia are important for identifying the neurochemical and genetic basis for the disorder. They are also vital for screening new antipsychotic drugs. Developing such models is difficult, however, because the primary symptom is profound thought disorder, a cortical process not found in lower animals.

The toxic reaction to high doses of central nervous system (CNS) stimulants is a model that is still considered among the best. It was found quite accidentally when clinicians realized that people who abuse CNS stimulants (amphetamine and cocaine) frequently show signs of thought disorder. Addicts hospitalized with stimulant toxicity often have well-formed paranoid delusions; various stereotyped, compulsive behaviors; and either visual or auditory hallucinations. Even trained clinicians find the symptoms to be indistinguishable from those of paranoid schizophrenia. Also, when amphetamine is administered to patients with schizophrenia, the patients report that their existing symptoms get worse, not that new symptoms are produced. Finally, amphetamine-induced psychosis can be treated with the same drugs that are most effective in treating schizophrenia.

In animals, high doses of amphetamine produce a characteristic stereotyped sniffing, licking, and gnawing. Because stereotyped behavior also occurs in response to high doses of amphetamine in humans and is similar to the compulsive repetitions of meaningless behavior seen in schizophrenia, the **amphetamine-induced stereotypy** is used in the laboratory as an animal model for schizophrenia. For many years it has been a classic screening device to identify effective antipsychotic drugs. Because high doses of amphetamine release dopamine, the abnormal behaviors produced by the

(A)

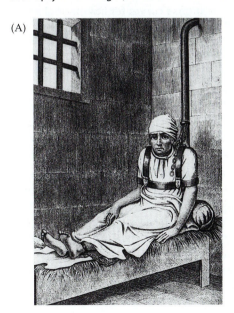

(B)

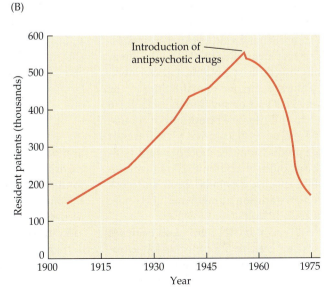

drug support the dopamine hypothesis of schizophrenia (see the section on this hypothesis later in the chapter).

A second screening procedure compares the dose–response curve for the antipsychotic drug's inhibition of motor activity induced by apomorphine (a dopamine agonist) with the curve for the drug's effectiveness in producing catalepsy (maintenance of abnormal postures). Although the animal models for measuring drug-induced running and the peculiar posturing of catalepsy may not seem to reflect psychotic behavior and extrapyramidal symptoms, respectively, they have provided consistent preclinical results. Drugs that are effective in reducing psychotic symptoms in humans quite consistently also reduce apomorphine-induced running as well as amphetamine-induced stereotyped behaviors. Likewise, neuroleptics that do not produce catalepsy in rats have low incidences of motor side effects. Figure 18.3 shows that for the classic antipsychotic haloperidol, the dose–response curves for inhibiting apomorphine-induced locomotion and producing catalepsy are very similar, suggesting that doses that are effective in reducing the locomotion are almost identical to those that induce catalepsy. In contrast, the dose–response curves for the atypical antipsychotic remoxipride show a much larger difference in doses required to inhibit hyperactivity and induce catalepsy. This type of preclinical screening predicts a lower incidence of motor side effects with the atypical drugs, and clinical evaluation with patients supports that conclusion.

Another drug-induced syndrome produced in humans by high doses of phencyclidine (PCP; "angel dust") forms the basis for the dopamine–glutamate hypothesis of schizophrenia (see the section on this hypothesis later in the chapter). At low doses, PCP produces symptoms of drunkenness and mild stimulation, which progress to loss of body boundaries and withdrawal from social interaction. The symptoms of severe PCP intoxication include disorientation, muteness, profound cognitive impairments, various motor symptoms (e.g., agitation, grimacing, rigidity, catalepsy, tremors), and occasionally paranoid delusions (see Chapter 14). **PCP-induced psychosis** in normal individuals closely resembles an acute episode of schizophrenia. Repeated use of PCP may produce long-lasting psychotic symptoms. Furthermore, PCP intensifies the primary symptoms of schizophrenia. The usefulness of studying PCP's action stems from its ability to produce both positive and negative symptoms of schizophrenia (Javitt and Zukin, 1991), unlike toxic doses of amphetamine, which produce only the more dramatic positive symptoms of paranoid schizophrenia. Note that both amphetamine and PCP enhance dopamine release and block reuptake, while PCP in addition antagonizes glutamate transmission (Lahti et al., 1995).

One very different type of model is based on evidence that schizophrenics fail to "gate," or filter, most of the sensory stimuli they receive. Such a defect may lead to sensory

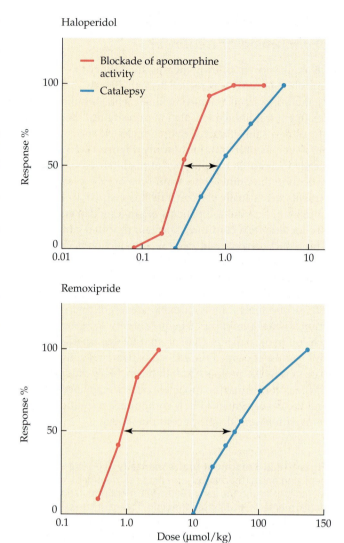

Figure 18.3 Dose–response curves for haloperidol and remoxipride for blocking apomorphine-induced hyperactivity and producing catalepsy in rats The horizontal distance between the curves on each graph represents the difference in potency of the drug required to produce both of the effects. The wider the separation of the curves, the lower the likelihood that the effective antipsychotic dose will produce motor side effects in humans.

overload and fragmented thinking, because schizophrenics are overwhelmed by sights and sounds and odors in the environment that they cannot filter out. The acoustic startle response is one of the most reliable and generalizable models used to study sensory-filtering deficits, and it can be utilized easily in both animals and human subjects. Box 18.2 describes the technique called **prepulse inhibition of startle (PPI)** and demonstrates the elegance of this model.

Classic Neuroleptics and Atypical Antipsychotics

Drugs useful in treating schizophrenia are called antipsychotic drugs or **neuroleptics,** a term that refers to their ability to selectively reduce emotionality and psychomotor activity. A large number of drugs are included in this category, and they are commonly divided into two classes: traditional neuroleptics and the newer second-generation (often called "atypical") antipsychotics. Although none of the drugs is consistently more effective than the others, a particular individual may respond better to one drug than to another. Therefore, treatment may require testing several antipsychotic drugs to find the one most effective for a given patient. The classic antipsychotic drugs are the phenothiazines, such as chlorpromazine (Thorazine), and the butyrophenones, such as haloperidol (Haldol). Since the phenothiazines are still the largest and most commonly used class of antipsychotic drug, much of our discussion will focus on them. The second-generation antipsychotics, such as clozapine (Clozaril), risperidone (Risperdal), and aripiprazole (Abilitat) are noteworthy because they appear to relieve negative symptoms more effectively than conventional antipsychotics and they produce fewer side effects involving abnormal movements (e.g., tremors, rigidity). These drugs are discussed later in the chapter.

Phenothiazines and butyrophenones are traditional neuroleptics

Chlorpromazine was the first phenothiazine used in psychiatry, but many small changes in the shape of the drug molecule produced a family of related compounds that differ in potency, clinical effectiveness, and side effects. Figure 18.4 shows the three-ring phenothiazine nucleus and the structural relationships of several other drugs in this class. By changing the chemical groups at the R_1 and R_2 positions, many new compounds can be created that vary in their effects. For example, chlorpromazine (which has a chlorine at R_2) is much more potent than promazine

(which has hydrogen at the R_2 position). By substituting at R_1, an antipsychotic (thioridazine [Melleril]) with fewer motor side effects is created. Further changes at R_1 and R_2 produce drugs (trifluoperazine [Stelazine], fluphenazine [Prolixene]) that further vary in potency and side effects. This structure–activity relationship provides clear evidence that molecular modifications alter the ability of the drugs to bind to specific receptor-recognition sites in the cell membranes.

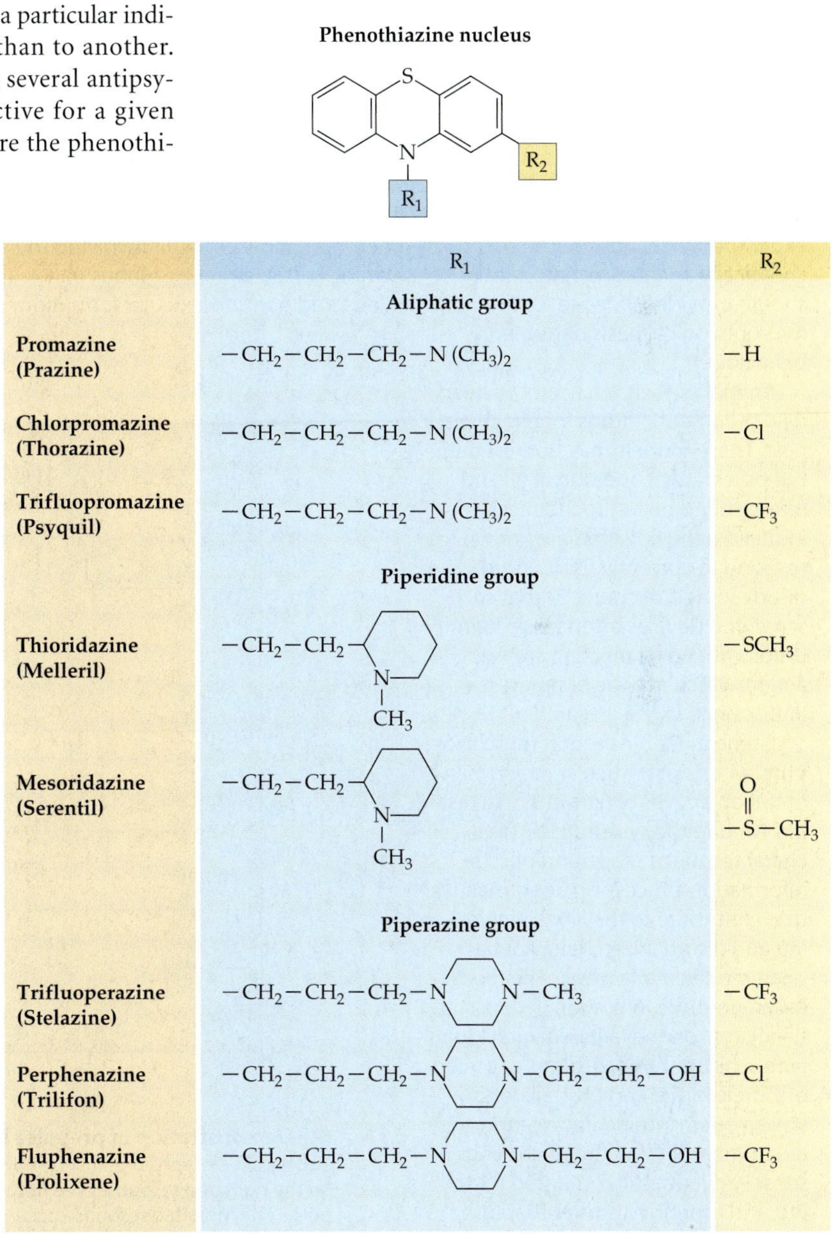

Phenothiazine nucleus

	R_1			R_2
	Aliphatic group			
Promazine (Prazine)	$-CH_2-CH_2-CH_2-N(CH_3)_2$			$-H$
Chlorpromazine (Thorazine)	$-CH_2-CH_2-CH_2-N(CH_3)_2$			$-Cl$
Trifluopromazine (Psyquil)	$-CH_2-CH_2-CH_2-N(CH_3)_2$			$-CF_3$
	Piperidine group			
Thioridazine (Melleril)	$-CH_2-CH_2$ (piperidine, N–CH₃)			$-SCH_3$
Mesoridazine (Serentil)	$-CH_2-CH_2$ (piperidine, N–CH₃)			$-S(=O)-CH_3$
	Piperazine group			
Trifluoperazine (Stelazine)	$-CH_2-CH_2-CH_2-N$ (piperazine) $N-CH_3$			$-CF_3$
Perphenazine (Trilifon)	$-CH_2-CH_2-CH_2-N$ (piperazine) $N-CH_2-CH_2-OH$			$-Cl$
Fluphenazine (Prolixene)	$-CH_2-CH_2-CH_2-N$ (piperazine) $N-CH_2-CH_2-OH$			$-CF_3$

Figure 18.4 Phenothiazine nucleus and related compounds Minor molecular modifications determine the three major subgroups of phenothiazines and change drug potency, pharmacological activity, and side effects.

BOX 18.2

Pharmacology in Action

Animal Model—Prepulse Inhibition of Startle

No single animal model can mimic the complex symptomatology of schizophrenia, so each one tends to focus on one aspect of the disorder and experimentally induce homologous (similar) changes in animal behavior. It is assumed that subsequent attempts to manipulate the experimental response both neurochemically and neuroanatomically should provide evidence for the neurobiological basis of human behavior.

Animal models are used to screen new therapeutic drugs for effectiveness. These models may not resemble the psychiatric condition at all and may depend on neurochemically induced behaviors that are known to respond to currently useful drugs. The disadvantage, of course, is that such screening devices often fail to identify drugs with novel mechanisms of action, which may be of greatest importance to the researcher.

Of the available models for schizophrenia, one in particular meets many of the objectives of conventional testing. Among the symptom clusters characteristic of schizophrenia, the information-processing abnormalities that contribute to the illogical thinking and disorganized behavior has been modeled effectively. The model called prepulse inhibition (PPI) of startle focuses on the failure of individuals with schizophrenia to "gate," or screen out, irrelevant stimuli. By failing to screen out incoming information, they are bombarded by stimuli, causing sensory overload, fragmented thinking, and thought disorder. Prepulse inhibition refers to a reduction in the reflex startle response to a strong, rapid-onset stimulus (either a sudden loud tone or sudden bright light) when it is preceded by a prepulse (occurring 30 to 500 milliseconds before) that is too weak to elicit a startle response itself. The experimental design is shown in Figure A. Apparently, under normal conditions the prepulse activates a neural circuit that inhibits the reflex to the second stimulus. Although the startle response itself is a relatively simple reflex, the inhibition of the reflex is exerted by a neuroanatomical circuit involving the limbic cortex, striatum, globus pallidus, and pontine reticular formation.

Abnormalities in each of these brain areas have been implicated in the etiology of schizophrenia; therefore, failure of the prepulse to inhibit the startle response would be anticipated. Many studies have shown that PPI is diminished in schizophrenia, which means that patients do not inhibit the startle as effectively as normal subjects, as shown in Figure B. Deficits in PPI occur in other clinical conditions that involve some part of the cortical–striatal–pallidal–pontine circuit, such as obsessive–compulsive disorder, attention deficit disorder, Huntington's disease, and others. Thus, PPI deficiency is associated not with a

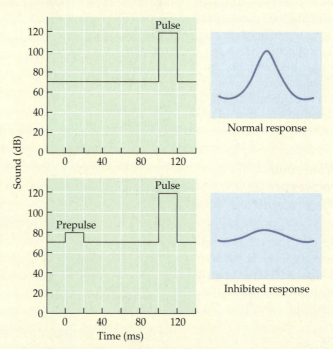

(A) Demonstration of prepulse inhibition of startle for a normal subject The graphs on the left show the stimulus presentation; the graphs on the right, the response. The normal startle response follows the single pulse. The inhibited response occurs in a normal subject when a prepulse occurs shortly before the major pulse.

BOX 18.2 (continued)

specific psychopathology but with deficits in gating resulting from abnormalities in a particular brain circuit.

PPI has several advantages that make it an appealing animal model. First, the reflex is simple to measure and produces reliable results. PPI is exhibited in virtually all mammals, including primates, and requires no training. In human studies the eye-blink reflex is measured, while in rats the whole-body flinch is evaluated.

Support for the dopamine hypothesis comes from findings that PPI is disrupted by systemic administration of dopamine agonists and reinstated by dopamine receptor–blocking antipsychotic drugs. That is, treatment with apomorphine or other dopaminergic drugs interferes with the normal gating function. The ability of antipsychotics, including the atypical antipsychotic clozapine, to restore PPI in apomorphine-treated rats at doses that

strongly correlate with clinical potency further validates this model (Figure C). However, PPI is also disrupted by systemic administration of serotonin agonists and glutamate antagonists and by a variety of surgical or neurochemical manipulations of the cortical–striatal–pallidal–pontine circuit. Since structural or functional abnormalities in schizophrenic patients have been reported at every level of the gating circuit as well as in glutamate and serotonin function, the PPI model may provide unique information on the pathology underlying schizophrenia.

This chapter describes the interaction of factors that contribute to the occurrence of schizophrenia: genetic, anatomical, and environmental. The PPI model is especially appealing because it also responds to each of these factors. First, genetically distinct rat strains differ significantly in the dopaminergic modulation of PPI. Also,

rats that have been bred for apomorphine sensitivity or lack of sensitivity show parallel differences in PPI. Thus, if genes control susceptibility to apomorphine-induced gating disruption, such a model may provide information about genetic-mediated susceptibility to schizophrenia. Second, some evidence exists to suggest that early brain lesioning may have an impact on apomorphine-induced disruption of PPI in the adult animal. Third, developmental influences such as isolation stress early in life significantly reduce PPI (impaired gating), and this effect is reversed by both typical and atypical antipsychotic drugs (Varty and Higgins, 1995). Such parallels make PPI modeling of schizophrenia a particularly appealing design and one that may provide a good deal of new information. A more detailed description of these experiments and the PPI model can be found in Swerdlow and Geyer (1998).

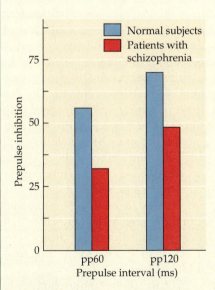

(B) Failure of prepulse inhibition in schizophrenia at two different prepulse intervals

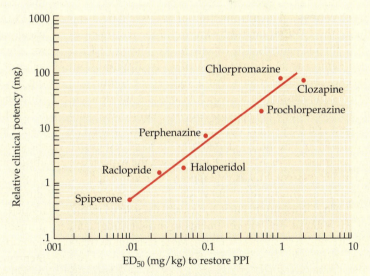

(C) Antipsychotic drugs that are clinically effective at low doses also restore the prepulse inhibition at low doses. High-dose antipsychotics also require higher doses to restore the prepulse inhibition.

Pharmacokinetics   Antipsychotics are only slowly and incompletely absorbed from the gastrointestinal tract. Nevertheless, they are still most often administered orally because they are used over extended periods of time. Intramuscular preparations of some of these drugs are also available for patients who are unable or unwilling to take an oral dose. For individuals who fail to take the drug reliably, a depot injection administered either intramuscularly or subcutaneously may be used. The slowly dissolving preparation releases drug into the system so gradually that administration is needed only every 4 to 6 weeks. The drugs are distributed throughout the body, with the highest concentrations in the liver and lungs. Binding to inactive sites such as blood proteins and fat is significant and release from these sites is quite gradual, resulting in a slow rate of elimination. In addition, metabolism is also quite slow, so that metabolites can be found in the urine many months after treatment has been terminated. Because of the binding to inactive sites and the slow metabolism, the half-life of these drugs ranges from 11 to 58 hours, so only a single dose is needed each day. The long half-life also explains why symptoms reappear gradually after drug termination.

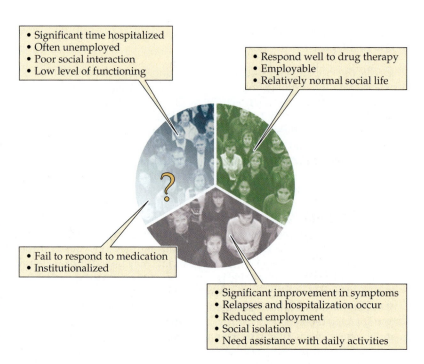

- Significant time hospitalized
- Often unemployed
- Poor social interaction
- Low level of functioning

- Respond well to drug therapy
- Employable
- Relatively normal social life

- Fail to respond to medication
- Institutionalized

- Significant improvement in symptoms
- Relapses and hospitalization occur
- Reduced employment
- Social isolation
- Need assistance with daily activities

Figure 18.5 The law of thirds approximates the effectiveness of antipsychotic drug treatment. Overall, approximately two-thirds of patients treated with antipsychotic drugs show significant improvement. The question mark indicates that some unspecified fraction of the least responsive third fails to respond to treatment at all.

Effectiveness   The introduction of antipsychotic drugs during the 1950s dramatically improved the treatment of schizophrenic patients. The effectiveness of these drugs has been demonstrated hundreds of times in double-blind, placebo-controlled trials. For a significant number of patients, the antipsychotics reduce symptoms and decrease the average length of hospitalization. Not only do they calm agitated and excited patients, but they also make socially withdrawn and inwardly focused patients more responsive and communicative. After only a few doses, the hyperactive and manic symptoms usually disappear, whereas the positive symptoms of schizophrenia may gradually improve over several weeks. Delusions, hallucinations, and disordered thinking are reduced, and improvements in insight, judgment, self-care, and seclusiveness are seen. More resistant to treatment are the negative symptoms of schizophrenia.

Although estimates of effectiveness vary, psychiatrists often refer to the **law of thirds** (Figure 18.5). One third of the patients treated with antipsychotics show excellent symptom reduction in response to the drugs and may not experience subsequent hospitalizations even when they discontinue medication. These individuals show few residual signs of the disorder. They are employed outside the institution, may marry, and maintain a relatively normal social life. The second third show significant improvement of symptoms but

may experience relapses that require hospitalization from time to time. These individuals may be employed, although usually at a reduced occupational level, and they may remain socially isolated. Some require significant help in day-to-day living, for example, in maintaining personal hygiene, preparing meals, or keeping scheduled appointments. The final third show a lesser degree of recovery and may spend a significant amount of time each year in a psychiatric institution. These patients need much more help in dealing with the stresses of everyday living. Since many of the behavioral abnormalities remain, these individuals are often unemployed, have few social relationships, and exist on the margins of society. Estimates suggest that over 30% of the adult homeless population in the United States may suffer from unmedicated or inadequately medicated psychosis. Some portion of this final third fail to respond to any drug treatment and remain institutionalized.

Following a patient's initial recovery, antipsychotic drugs are prescribed as maintenance therapy to prevent relapse. Recovered patients maintained on antipsychotics have about a 55% chance of remaining in the community for 2 years after leaving the hospital, compared with a 20% chance for those on placebo. Thus drug maintenance more than doubles an individual's chances of avoiding significant relapse. Unfortunately, because the side effects of these drugs (discussed later in this chapter) are often debilitating and extremely unpleasant, many patients fail to continue treatment, which leads to a high relapse rate.

Although psychotherapy and group therapy are not considered substitutes for pharmacotherapy, social-skills training and family therapy are important additions to drug treatment. Psychoeducation involves enhancing social competence and family problem solving, teaching vocational skills, minimizing stress, and enhancing cooperation with medication schedules (Goldstein, 1995).

Dopamine receptor antagonism is responsible for antipsychotic action

Neuroleptic drugs modify several neurotransmitter systems; however, their clinical effectiveness is best correlated to their ability to antagonize dopamine (DA) transmission by competitively blocking DA receptors or by inhibiting DA release. Evidence comes from several sources, including the drugs' three-dimensional structures, their side effects, receptor binding studies, changes in DA turnover, second-messenger function, and neuroendocrine effects.

First, the three-dimensional shape of the phenothiazines, as determined by X-ray crystallography, can be superimposed on the three-dimensional structure of DA. Changing small molecular groups, such as removing a molecule at R_2 (see Figure 18.4), alters the ability of the phenothiazine to look like DA and in this way reduces its pharmacological activity. Second, the common occurrence of parkinsonian side effects indirectly suggests that neuroleptics reduce the normal dopamine-mediated inhibition of cholinergic cells in the striatum, which is responsible for Parkinson's Disease (see the section on parkinsonism).

Receptor binding   A strong positive correlation exists between the ability of antipsychotic drugs to displace a labeled ligand on dopamine receptors and average clinical daily dose (Figure 18.6A). Drugs that readily bind to the DA receptor at low concentration because of their high affinity also reduce symptoms at low doses. Likewise, antipsychotics that require higher concentrations to bind to DA receptors require higher doses to be clinically effective. Although

antipsychotic drugs bind to other neurotransmitter receptors in addition to dopamine, there is no clear relationship between clinical effectiveness and the binding to serotonin (Figure 18.6B), α-adrenergic, or histamine receptors. Therefore, the correlation with DA receptor binding establishes quite clearly the mechanism of antipsychotic drug action.

Now that it is clear that there are subtle differences among DA receptors, neuropharmacologists have been concerned

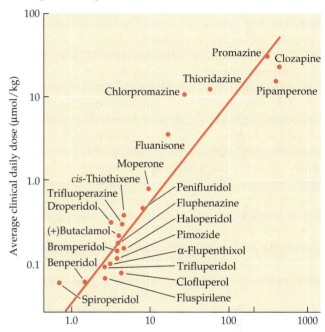

(A) Dopamine receptors

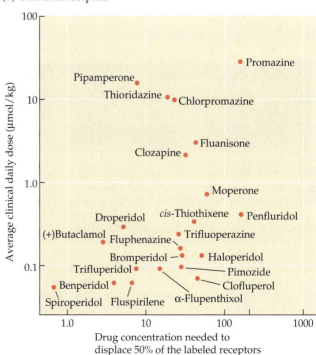

(B) Serotonin receptors

Figure 18.6 Correlation between antipsychotic drug binding to neurotransmitter receptors and clinical effectiveness The receptor binding studies were accomplished by first labeling the receptors with an appropriate radioactive ligand for each neurotransmitter. The antipsychotic drug was added in increasing concentrations until it competed successfully for half of the labeled sites. That value (K_i) is plotted along the x-axis, and the corresponding average clinical daily dose for that drug is plotted on the y-axis. A clear positive correlation is found for dopamine receptor binding (A), while serotonin receptor binding shows no apparent correlation with effectiveness (B). Further experiments found no correlation between clinical effects and binding to either α-adrenergic or histamine receptors. (After Snyder, 1996.)

with finding which receptor subtype is responsible for specific effects of the neuroleptics. Researchers hope that new drugs can be designed to act at a particular receptor subtype to reduce psychotic symptoms without acting on other subtypes that produce serious side effects. Attention has been focused on the D_1, D_2, D_3, and D_4 receptor subtypes. Neuroleptics have a particularly high affinity for D_2 receptors, which serve as both normal postsynaptic receptors and autoreceptors and are located in the basal ganglia, nucleus accumbens, amygdala, hippocampus, and cerebral cortex. Figure 18.7 shows a series of positron emission tomography (PET) images in which D_2 receptors in the basal ganglia were labeled with [^{11}C]raclopride. The bright areas show the binding of the labeled drug to D_2 receptors. The control is a scan of a healthy man injected only with the [^{11}C]raclopride to show maximum binding. The remaining scans are from schizophrenic patients given [^{11}C]raclopride in addition to one of the antipsychotic drugs. Reduction of radioactive ligand binding indicates competition for the sites. Striatal D_2 receptors were almost completely blocked by haloperidol and risperidone, but clozapine had less affinity. Although a drug's ability to bind to the D_2 receptor is closely correlated to its effectiveness in reducing psychotic symptoms, some of the atypical antipsychotics, such as clozapine, may produce their unique effects by acting on a combination of receptor types.

In addition to reducing dopaminergic transmission by blocking postsynaptic D_2 receptors, the antipsychotics also readily block D_2 autoreceptors. The inhibitory autoreceptors are responsible for controlling the rate of firing of the cell as well as the rate of synthesis and release of neurotransmitter. Applying a DA agonist, such as apomorphine, to the DA cell bodies in the substantia nigra (origin of nigrostriatal cells) or ventral tegmentum (origin of mesolimbic and mesocor-

tical neurons) stimulates the autoreceptors and decreases the rate of firing of the dopaminergic neurons. This inhibition is antagonized by administration of an effective neuroleptic drug such as chlorpromazine, but not by an inactive phenothiazine. The increase in firing rate after antipsychotic administration is accompanied by increased turnover (synthesis, release, and metabolism) of DA.

DA turnover   Clinical response to antipsychotic treatment is associated with an initial increase in dopamine metabolism, which is determined by measuring the concentration of the principal DA metabolite, homovanillic acid (HVA). An increase in metabolism is assumed to reflect an increase in neurotransmitter release. The initial increase in HVA is followed by a gradual decrease with chronic treatment. Patients who are good responders to treatment have higher initial levels of plasma HVA than do nonresponders. They also show greater drug-induced reductions of the metabolite over time (Siever et al., 1993). Patients with negative symptoms do not show the initial increase in HVA, nor do they show the decline in HVA with continued neuroleptic treatment. The changes in DA metabolism can be explained by neuroleptic action at D_2 autoreceptors. The increase in DA utilization follows the acute blockade of autoreceptors on dopaminergic cells. However, chronic blockade with neuroleptics leads to supersensitivity (up-regulation) of the autoreceptors, allowing them to respond appropriately to DA by reducing DA synthesis, release, and metabolism. An alternative explanation for the gradual decrease in turnover, posed by Grace (1992), suggests that after the initial neuroleptic-induced increase in DA turnover, dopaminergic cells have the ability to temporarily inactivate themselves. This temporary inactivation, called depolarization block, would reduce the release of DA and its subsequent metabolism. The time-dependent change in receptors and depolarization block help to explain the gradual onset of effectiveness of antipsychotic drugs.

Prolactin release   Further evidence for DA receptor blockade comes from neuroendocrine measures of prolactin. Under normal conditions, DA inhibits prolactin release. By blocking D_2 receptors in the pituitary gland, neuroleptics stimulate the secretion of prolactin, which leads to lactation, a disturbing side effect of antipsychotic drug use. Measuring serum prolactin in patients provides an easy measure of D_2 receptor function in the CNS.

Slow homeostatic changes   Although the clinical effectiveness of antipsychotics is closely correlated with dopamine receptor blockade, the time courses of the two events are significantly different. While the receptor blockade is almost immediate, several weeks of treatment are necessary before symptoms begin to subside. This disparity in time course suggests that the drugs are not directly targeting the locus of the disorder but are gradually inducing the nervous system

| Control | Haloperidol | Clozapine | Risperidone |

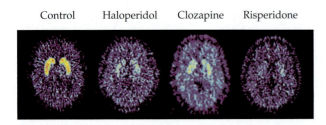

Figure 18.7 D$_2$ receptor occupancy by antipsychotic drugs PET scans of a healthy, untreated male (control) and three patients with schizophrenia treated with the traditional neuroleptic haloperidol or with an atypical antipsychotic drug, clozapine or risperidone. In all subjects, striatal D$_2$ receptors were labeled with [^{11}C]raclopride. The scans show that the radioactive label of striatal D$_2$ receptors was almost completely displaced by haloperidol and risperidone binding but less effectively by clozapine. These and other differences in receptor antagonism are thought to be responsible for the ability of the atypical neuroleptics to reduce symptoms without producing serious motor side effects. (Courtesy of Svante Nyberg and Anna-Lena Nordstöm, Karolinska Institute.)

to make adaptive changes that lead to clinical improvement. Some of the slow homeostatic changes that occur over time are depolarization block, change in receptor number, and altered dopamine turnover.

Side effects are directly related to neurochemical action

Unfortunately, the classic antipsychotic drugs frequently produce a large number of side effects, some of which are so disturbing that nonhospitalized patients stop taking the drug and suffer a relapse of psychiatric symptoms. Because patient compliance (cooperation in following the treatment schedule) is a large problem, clinicians most often choose the neuroleptic to prescribe based on minimizing the side effects for a given patient.

Neuroleptic-induced DA receptor antagonism occurs in each of the DA pathways described in Chapter 5 and is responsible not only for the clinical effectiveness of antipsychotics but also for many of their side effects. There are four dopamine pathways in the brain that are important for understanding antipsychotic drug action, three of which are illustrated in Figure 5.7.

1. The mesolimbic pathway projects from the ventral tegmental area to the nucleus accumbens and other limbic areas. It is involved in many behaviors, as well as the pleasure derived from drugs of abuse and the delusions and hallucinations of schizophrenia. It is reasonable to consider the mesolimbic pathway as the site for the drug-induced reduction of positive symptoms.

2. The mesocortical pathway also projects from the ventral tegmental area but sends axons to the limbic cortex, where it may have a role in the cognitive effects and negative symptoms of schizophrenia.

3. The nigrostriatal pathway begins in the substantia nigra and projects to the striatum, where it contributes to the modulation of movement. Parkinsonian symptoms are caused by DA receptor blockade in the striatum. Therefore, neuroleptic effects on nigrostriatal DA are likely to be responsible for parkinsonian tremors and other motor side effects.

4. Projecting from the hypothalamus to the pituitary gland are the short neurons that constitute the tuberohypophyseal pathway, which regulates pituitary hormone

secretion. Blockade of DA receptors in this pathway is the likely source of the neuroendocrine side effects.

Parkinsonism   The most serious and troublesome side effects of classic antipsychotics are the movement disorders that resemble the symptoms of Parkinson's disease (see Chapter 5) and involve the extrapyramidal motor system. **Parkinsonian symptoms** include tremors, akinesia (a slowing or loss of voluntary movements), muscle rigidity, akathesia (a strong feeling of discomfort in the legs and an inability to sit still, which compels the patient to get up and walk about), and loss of facial expression. We know that Parkinson's disease is caused by a lack of dopamine function in the striatum (a subcortical brain area that modulates movement) and subsequent excess cholinergic neural activity (Figure 18.8).

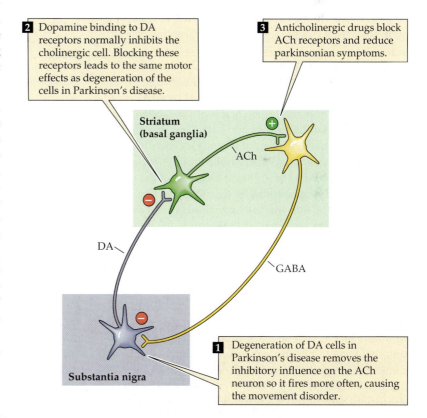

2 Dopamine binding to DA receptors normally inhibits the cholinergic cell. Blocking these receptors leads to the same motor effects as degeneration of the cells in Parkinson's disease.

3 Anticholinergic drugs block ACh receptors and reduce parkinsonian symptoms.

Striatum (basal ganglia)

ACh

DA

GABA

Substantia nigra

1 Degeneration of DA cells in Parkinson's disease removes the inhibitory influence on the ACh neuron so it fires more often, causing the movement disorder.

Figure 18.8 Schematic diagram showing the neurotransmitters involved in parkinsonian symptoms Parkinson's disease is caused by degeneration of the nigrostriatal dopaminergic neurons, which begin in the substantia nigra. The reduced dopaminergic cell function causes a loss of inhibitory control of the cholinergic cells in the striatum, so the cholinergic cells fire at higher rates. Drug-induced parkinsonian symptoms follow DA receptor blockade in the striatum and subsequent excess acetylcholine activity, which is functionally similar to the loss of dopaminergic cells in Parkinson's disease. Anticholinergic drugs reduce the symptoms of Parkinson's disease and the side effects of antipsychotic drug treatment.

Knowing that the classic antipsychotic drugs block dopamine receptors, we assume that drug-induced parkinsonism is due to dopamine blockade in that area of the brain. To verify this hypothesis, experiments using PET showed that neuroleptic-treated patients with parkinsonian symptoms had *more* dopamine receptors of the D_2 type in the striatum than did those without those side effects (Farde et al., 1992). Such compensatory receptor up-regulation is likely to occur after *reduced* dopamine transmission. Therefore, it is assumed that the antipsychotic-induced tremors are due to the blockade of dopamine receptors in the striatum, the projection region of the nigrostriatal dopaminergic neurons. Since one way to treat the symptoms of Parkinson's disease is to reduce excess acetylcholine activity, neuroleptic drugs that have anticholinergic action have been developed to minimize the parkinsonian side effects. One such example is thioridazine. Alternatively, combining antipsychotic drug treatment with an anticholinergic drug such as benztropine (Cogentin) is also a common treatment approach. In addition, several of the atypical antipsychotics, such as clozapine and risperidone, produce a lower-than-normal incidence of extrapyramidal side effects (see the section on atypical antipsychotics).

Tardive dyskinesia   A second type of motor side effect associated with prolonged use of antipsychotic drugs is **tardive dyskinesia (TD).** TD is characterized by stereotyped involuntary movements, particularly of the face and jaw, such as sucking and lip smacking, lateral jaw movements, and "fly-catching" movements of the tongue. There may also be purposeless, quick, and uncontrolled movements of the arms and legs or slow squirming movements of the trunk, limbs, and neck. Estimates suggest that TD appears in about 10 to 20% of patients treated with neuroleptics overall. Although TD may appear in any age group, the incidence increases to 50% in patients over 60 years of age and may exceed 70% in geriatric patients. It is generally assumed that the dose of neuroleptic and duration of treatment are related to the occurrence of TD. To demonstrate the importance of treatment duration, Figure 18.9 shows the cumulative incidence of TD in a group of 362 chronic psychiatric patients who were maintained on antipsychotic drugs. The conclusion that two out of three patients maintained on antipsychotics for a period of 25 years will develop TD is a sobering one that should encourage further research into treatment strategies that minimize such side effects. Although the symptoms are considered to be irreversible in some patients, for many individuals improvement does gradually occur. However, in many cases the symptoms are much worse when the drug is first terminated and persist for long periods after the withdrawal of neuroleptics. Reversal of TD occurs most readily in younger patients.

Despite a good deal of research with both animal and human models, the underlying neuropathology responsible

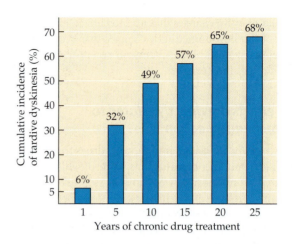

Figure 18.9   Cumulative incidence of tardive dyskinesia in a group of psychiatric patients maintained on antipsychotic medication. Evaluation of the patients showed an average incidence of approximately 6% for each of the first 5 years, with a cumulative incidence of 30% at the end of 5 years of chronic medication. By combining data, the investigators estimated the 10-year and 25-year risks. Clearly, long-term treatment increases the probability of developing tardive dyskynesia.

for TD is not known. A hypersensitivity of some DA receptors and a D_1–D_2 receptor imbalance are possibilities, but neurotoxic effects of free-radical by-products from catecholamine metabolism has also received some support. However, GABA (γ-aminobutyric acid) insufficiency, cholinergic hypofunction, or a serotonin–dopamine interaction may contribute to TD (Casey, 1995).

Neuroendocrine effects   Blockade of receptors in the dopamine pathway that regulates pituitary function produces a variety of neuroendocrine effects. These effects include breast enlargement and tenderness, decreased sex drive, lack of menstruation, increased release of prolactin (frequently producing lactation), and inhibition of growth hormone release. Reduced growth hormone release represents a significant therapeutic issue when medicating children and adolescents. In addition, significant weight gain and the inability to regulate body temperature can be disturbing side effects, particularly for young people who are concerned with body image.

Neuroleptic malignant syndrome   Of the possible side effects, **neuroleptic malignant syndrome (NMS)** is the most serious and life-threatening. NMS is characterized by fever, rigidity, altered consciousness, and autonomic nervous system instability (including rapid heart rate and fluctuations in blood pressure). NMS is potentially lethal, but rapid diagnosis and immediate action have significantly reduced the mortality risk.

Additional side effects Antipsychotic drugs have not only dopamine-blocking effects but also anticholinergic and antiadrenergic actions. These complex interactions produce widespread effects on the autonomic nervous system. For example, blocking cholinergic synapses produces effects such as dry mouth, blurred vision, constipation, difficulty in urination, and decreased gastric secretion and motility. Orthostatic hypotension (low blood pressure when an individual stands upright) from the antiadrenergic action of antipsychotics leads to dizziness, faintness, or blacking out. Many of these drugs produce significant sedation, which may be very troublesome for some patients but useful for those who suffer from agitation and restlessness.

In general, the particular phenothiazine chosen for a patient depends on its side effects. For example, chlorpromazine or thioridazine may be used because they tend to minimize the extrapyramidal side effects, although their sedative effects may be undesirable and the probability of autonomic side effects is relatively high. Haloperidol, in contrast, tends to produce less sedation and fewer autonomic side effects but is associated with a greater probability of movement disorders. Many of the newest antipsychotic drugs have been developed to provide professionals with more options for matching a particular patient and the side effects he or she can tolerate. For example, clozapine, the best-known atypical antipsychotic, causes a low incidence of extrapyramidal side effects and TD; however, it may produce cardiovascular irregularities, cause hypersalivation and weight gain, and increase the risk of seizures. In addition, the risk of bone marrow toxicity posed with this drug necessitates regular and careful monitoring of blood cell count. (Clozapine is discussed further in subsequent sections.) Table 18.1 lists a number of traditional and atypical antipsychotic drugs and rates the incidence of specific side effects for each drug.

Tolerance and dependence Clinically, the antipsychotic drugs cause little or no tolerance, physical dependence, or abuse potential (psychological dependence). Patients can take the same dose of these drugs for years without seeing a reduction in the effectiveness in reducing psychotic symptoms. However, some tolerance to the sedative, hypotensive, and anticholinergic effects develops gradually over a period

TABLE 18.1 Partial List of Commonly Used Traditional and Atypical Antipsychotic Drugs and Their Side Effects

Generic name (trade name)	Sedation	Autonomic side effects[a]	Hypotension[b]	Motor disorders
Typical antipsychotics				
Chlorpromazine (Thorazine)	High	High	High	Moderate
Prochlorperazine (Compazine)	Moderate	Low	Low	High
Triflupromazine (Vesprin)	High	Moderate	Moderate	Moderate
Thioridazine (Mellaril)	Moderate–high	Moderate–high	Moderate–high	Low
Trifluoperazine (Stelazine)	Low–moderate	Low–moderate	Low	High
Fluphenazine (Prolixin)	Low	Low	Low	High
Perphenazine (Trilafon)	Low–moderate	Low	Low	High
Mesoridazine (Serentil)	High	Moderate	Moderate	Low
Thiothixene (Navane)	Low	Low–moderate	Low	Moderate–high
Haloperidol (Haldol)	Low	Very low	Low	High–very high
Loxapine (Loxitane)	Moderate	Low	Low	Moderate
Molindone (Moban)	Moderate	Low	Very low	Low–moderate
Atypical antipsychotics				
Clozapine (Clozaril)	Moderate–high	Moderate	Moderate–high	Low
Olanzapine (Zyprexa)	Moderate	Low	Moderate	Very low
Risperidone (Risperdal)	Low–moderate	Very low–low	Moderate	Low
Quetiapine (Seroquel)	Moderate	Moderate	Moderate	Very low
Ziprasidone (Zeldox)	Low	Low	Moderate	Very low

Source: After Grilly, 2002; Julien, 2002; Jibson and Tandon, 1998.

[a]Includes blurred vision, dry mouth, reduced gastric secretion and motility, urinary retention, and constipation.

[b]Drop in blood pressure upon standing upright (orthostatic), dizziness, faintness, or blacking out.

of weeks. The lack of physical dependence is demonstrated by the absence of withdrawal symptoms following abrupt cessation of these drugs even after years of administration. The lack of abstinence syndrome may be due to the long half-life of the drugs and the prolonged presence of the drugs and their active metabolites in the body before excretion. However, abrupt termination of the drugs may unmask signs of TD.

Since the neuroleptics do not produce euphoria and have subjectively unpleasant effects, these drugs are rarely abused. Animal studies also demonstrate a low incidence of self-administration and a tendency to avoid these drugs. Despite the drugs' unpleasant nature and disagreeable side effects, the antipsychotics are not lethal and have a high therapeutic index, which makes them unlikely candidates for drug overdose.

Atypical antipsychotics are distinctive in several ways

The principal difference between the second-generation, or atypical, neuroleptics and the traditional neuroleptics is that the newer agents generally reduce symptoms of schizophrenia without causing significant extrapyramidal side effects. Second, many do not produce the predicted results in behavioral screening tests. Third, some atypical antipsychotics can reduce negative as well as positive symptoms and are effective in treatment-resistant patients. Unfortunately, there seems to be no single neurochemical characteristic that identifies neuroleptics that produce atypical effects. The best current explanation is that the drugs either block D_2 receptors incompletely or block other receptors to restore an imbalance that exists among neurotransmitters (Seeman, 1990).

Selective D_2 receptor antagonists Since effective antipsychotic drugs block D_2 receptors, the first attempts to develop new drugs with fewer side effects evaluated **selective D_2 receptor antagonists.** Examples of such drugs include sulpiride, raclopride, and remoxipride. All three bind specifically to D_2 receptors along with a slight affinity for D_3 receptors, which may explain why their behavioral effects differ from those of traditional neuroleptics. Their selectivity for DA receptors also means that effects on the autonomic nervous system and cardiovascular system are minimal and sedation is mild. However, hormonal side effects tend to be common, and the risk of fatal blood disorders (especially with remoxipride) reduces the utility of the drugs.

Broad-spectrum antipsychotics A second trend in neuropharmacology is to evaluate **broad-spectrum antipsychotics** that block other receptor types in addition to D_2 receptors. The rationale for this work is the clinical effectiveness of clozapine, a drug that has relatively weak affinities for D_1 and D_2 and substantial serotonergic, muscarinic, and histaminergic affinities, as well a high affinity for the D_4 receptor. While there is general agreement that D_2 receptors are important for antipsychotic effects, some laboratories hypothesize that typical and atypical neuroleptics can be differentiated by their ratio of antagonism for various receptors. For instance, a high degree of binding to D_4 receptors, found in high concentration in the mesolimbic system and frontal cortex, may enhance the therapeutic effect but minimize the nigrostriatal motor symptoms associated with D_2 occupation. Other evidence suggests the importance of antagonism of the 5-HT_2 receptor in combination with D_2 blockade (Meltzer, 1999). Figure 18.10 shows that the atypical neuroleptics clozapine and risperidone readily bind to 5-HT_2 receptors, while haloperidol does not. In contrast, haloperidol almost completely blocks D_2 receptors (see Figure 18.7), while the atypical drugs show a partial effect on D_2. Whether this difference in receptor antagonism is responsible for selectively reducing negative symptoms or for minimizing extrapyramidal effects is not known. However, Csernansky and coworkers (1990) found a positive correlation between 5-HIAA (a 5-HT metabolite) in cerebrospinal fluid (CSF) and negative-symptom rates, which would suggest that increased 5-HT function is associated with the symptoms. Muscarinic receptor antagonism and the ratio of D_1 to D_2 receptor occupation are also considered possible factors in defining atypical neuroleptic action (Richelson, 1995).

Clozapine is the best-known atypical antipsychotic. Preclinical animal testing shows that it blocks apomorphine-

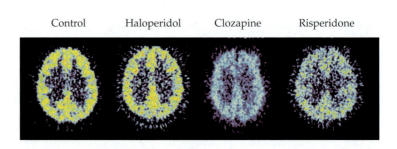

| Control | Haloperidol | Clozapine | Risperidone |

Figure 18.10 5-HT_2 receptor binding by atypical antipsychotics
PET scans of a healthy, untreated male (control) and three patients with schizophrenia treated with the traditional neuroleptic haloperidol or with an atypical antipsychotic drug, clozapine or risperidone. In all subjects, neocortical 5-HT_2 receptors were labeled with [^{11}C]N-methylspiperone ([^{11}C]NMSP). The scans show that both atypical antipsychotics but not haloperidol reduced 5-HT_2 binding. These and other differences in receptor antagonism are thought to be responsible for the ability of atypical neuroleptics to reduce schizophrenic symptoms (negative as well as positive) with a minimum of motor side effects. (Courtesy of Svante Nyberg and Anna-Lena Nordstöm, Karolinska Institute.)

induced hyperactivity but does not produce catalepsy except at high doses, which predicts a low incidence of motor side effects. Although clozapine is no more effective than standard neuroleptics in treating the positive symptoms of schizophrenia, it is often effective in patients who do not respond to classic antipsychotic treatment. Clozapine produces significant improvement in 60% of patients who do not respond to typical neuroleptics. However, response to clozapine may not be evident until after 5 months of treatment (Meltzer, 1995). Why there is such a long delay in effectiveness is not known. Clozapine is also the first antipsychotic that can reduce negative symptoms as well as reduce anxiety and tension. Unfortunately, the drug has a wide variety of side effects because of its action on multiple receptors. Clozapine reduces the seizure threshold, making seizures more likely in the vulnerable individual. It also produces hypersalivation, weight gain, and cardiovascular problems. A more serious side effect is the occurrence of agranulocytosis, a serious blood abnormality that can be detected only with frequent blood screening tests. The increased expense of testing and seriousness of side effects restrict the use of clozapine to selected patients.

The development of the multireceptor antipsychotic risperidone (Risperdal) is particularly exciting because the drug seems to have many of the benefits of clozapine without the risk of blood disorders. Risperidone is chemically unrelated to any other antipsychotic and is a potent $5-HT_{2A}$, $5-HT_7$, α_1- and α_2-adrenergic, and histamine H_1 receptor antagonist. It is also a D_2 receptor antagonist comparable to haloperidol, although it is a relatively weak antagonist at D_1 and D_4 receptors. Preclinical testing shows that risperidone blocks apomorphine-induced hyperactivity at a dose that produces only mild catalepsy, so its profile suggests antipsychotic effectiveness with minimal extrapyramidal symptoms. Data compiled from four well-designed, double-blind studies comparing the effectiveness of risperidone, haloperidol, and placebo are shown in Figure 18.11 (Lindenmayer, 1994). Clearly, administration of placebo produced only minimal changes in the scores for the three categories: (1) positive symptoms; (2) negative symptoms; and (3) general psychopathology. Haloperidol dramatically improved the positive symptoms but had little effect on the other two measures. Risperidone improved all 7 items on the positive scale, all 7 on the negative scale, and 13 out of 16 items on the psychopathology scale. Furthermore, risperidone did not produce any more extrapyramidal symptoms than did placebo. However, the most common side effects with risperidone are insomnia, anxiety, agitation, sedation, dizziness, hypotension, weight gain, and menstrual disturbances. Risperidone has great potential because of its unique combination of clinical effects and lack of the most serious usual side effects. Unfortunately, risperidone may increase a user's probability of developing diabetes, which is a serious problem that will require further investigation.

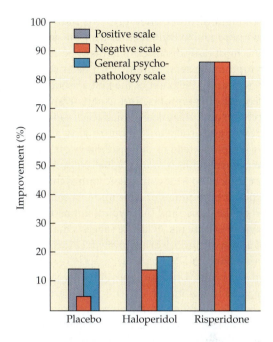

Figure 18.11 Improvement in positive symptoms, negative symptoms, and general psychopathology in patients with schizophrenia treated with placebo, haloperidol, and risperidone. While haloperidol improved the positive symptoms, it was no more effective than placebo for alleviating negative symptoms and general psychopathology. In contrast, risperidone significantly improved all three measures of the disorder. (After Lindenmayer, 1994.)

Dopamine system stabilizers Among the newest of the atypical antipsychotics are the **dopamine system stabilizers.** The prototypic drug aripiprazole (Abilitat) is a dopamine agonist–antagonist, which means that the drug readily binds to DA receptors but produces less of an effect than DA itself. Hence aripiprazole competes with DA for DA receptors in overactive synapses, reducing the effect of DA for as long as the drug is bound. By reducing excessive DA activity, the positive symptoms are reduced. In contrast, the same drug stimulates DA receptors in brain areas where there may be too little DA, thus reducing negative symptoms. In clinical trials the drug had a low incidence of side effects. There was little evidence of cardiotoxicity or motor side effects. The reported adverse effects such as headache, agitation, insomnia, and nervousness were minor. Aripiprazole may represent a new class of antipsychotics that is more readily accepted because of fewer unpleasant side effects.

Section Summary

Schizophrenia is a chronic, debilitating psychiatric disorder that occurs in about 1% of the world's population. This severe thought disorder often prevents individuals from engaging in productive interaction with the world around them. It is most easily discussed in terms of positive and negative symptom clusters. Patients with positive symptoms tend to be older at the onset of the first episode, experience abrupt onset of symptoms, and usually respond well to antipsychotic drug treatment, which leads some to suggest an underlying neurochemical abnormality. Patients with negative symptoms tend to show pathology earlier in life, so the onset of symptoms is more gradual. Negative symptoms are more difficult to treat with classic antipsychotic drugs.

The positive symptoms of schizophrenia are significantly reduced by the classic and the atypical antipsychotic drugs in a majority of patients. Evidence suggests that the mechanism of action of effective drugs involves DA receptor blockade (particularly of D_2 receptors), especially in the limbic areas of the brain. Unfortunately, effectiveness is often accompanied by significant side effects that are unpleasant and sometimes disabling. Among the most troublesome are the motor side effects: parkinsonian symptoms and tardive dyskinesia. Further chemical refinements that improve the drugs' specificities for receptor subtypes may enhance safety, selectivity, and effectiveness. Atypical antipsychotics are distinct in that they reduce negative symptoms as well as positive symptoms while also reducing the potential for serious motor side effects. These differences may be due to their action at 5-HT receptors or at dopamine D_1 or D_4 receptors in addition to D_2 receptors.

Etiology of Schizophrenia

Scientists from several disciplines use a variety of strategies to uncover the causes of schizophrenia. The goal is to develop an integrated approach to psychopathology considering anatomical, neurochemical, and functional factors. Schizophrenia is best understood as a disorder having a genetic component that makes the individual more vulnerable to particular environmental factors than the average person.

Abnormalities of brain structure and function occur in individuals with schizophrenia

Until recently, differences in the brains of individuals with schizophrenia compared with controls could not be detected. However, with the development of new techniques in neuroscience, differences of several kinds have been found, including structural differences, functional abnormalities, and irregularities in psychophysiological measures.

Structural abnormalities   Brain imaging techniques such as computerized tomography and magnetic resonance imaging continue to produce evidence of structural abnormali-

28-year-old male identical twins

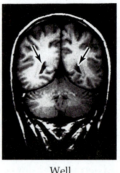 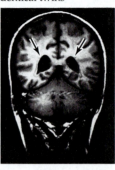

Well   Affected

Figure 18.12 Brain images of twins not concordant for schizophrenia The arrows in the figure point to the ventricles filled with cerebrospinal fluid. The healthy twin has normal-sized ventricles, while his schizophrenic twin has ventricles that are much enlarged. (Courtesy of Drs. E. Fuller Torrey and Daniel Weinberger.)

ties in the brains of people with schizophrenia. Many studies show cerebral atrophy (shrinking or wasting away) and enlargement of fluid-filled ventricles following cell loss (Figure 18.12). Among the brain areas showing reduced volume are the basal ganglia, temporal lobe, and several limbic regions, such as the hippocampus. The temporal lobe and hippocampal changes in people with chronic schizophrenia compared with controls are some of the most consistent magnetic resonance imaging findings (DeLisi et al., 1991). Structural differences in these areas also occur between monozygotic twins when only one has the disorder. Numerous studies show that hippocampal cells of patients with schizophrenia are more disorganized (Figure 18.13A) than those of healthy subjects (Figure 18.13B) and that selected cortical layers in the brains of patients with schizophrenia are atrophied. Involvement of the hippocampus and dopamine-rich basal ganglia may be related to the memory impairment and poor cognitive function found in most individuals with schizophrenia.

Investigators are always concerned that some brain changes may be due to progressive deterioration during the course of illness rather than cause the illness or may be due to the effects of antipsychotic medication used chronically over many years. However, most brain changes, such as enlarged ventricles, are not correlated with either the duration of time since the onset of symptoms or the duration of time since the first hospitalization. In contrast, a significant correlation does exist between ventricle size and age of the individual when symptoms were first diagnosed. Based on these results, researchers conclude that ventricular enlargement is not due to a progressive loss of brain cells, but may represent abnormalities of brain growth and development preceding the onset of symptoms. Additional evidence for this idea is the discovery that the more subtle abnormalities

Figure 18.13 Disorganization of cells in the hippocampus Histological cross sections of hippocampus showing the disorganized cells in the brain of a patient with schizophrenia (A) compared to the brain of a normal control (B). Corresponding schematic diagrams showing the haphazard arrangement of pyramidal cells in the hippocampus of the patient with schizophrenia and the normal parallel organization in normal controls. (From Kovelman and Scheibel, 1984.)

(A) Patient with schizophrenia   (B) Normal control

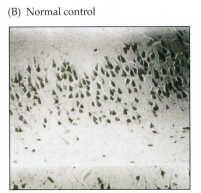

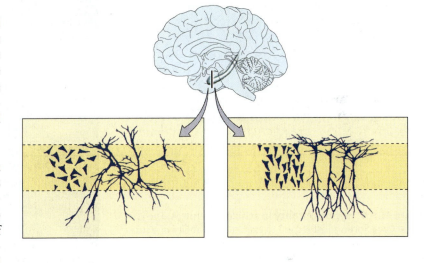

in cell structure are rarely accompanied by gliosis (multiplication of astrocytes and microglia). Since gliosis is a response to neuronal damage that occurs in the mature brain, but not in the immature brain, it is likely that the cell abnormalities occurred during the developmental process (Weinberger, 1995).

Functional abnormalities   In addition to structural abnormalities in the brains of individuals with schizophrenia, regional brain function in these individuals also differs from that in controls. Measures of brain function include rate of cell metabolism, blood flow, electrical activity, and chemical changes. The most consistent difference is reduced function of the prefrontal cortex, called hypofrontality (Buchsbaum, 1990). PET and single-photon emission computerized tomography (SPECT) studies show less increase in cerebral blood flow in the frontal cortex of patients with schizophrenia than normal subjects while they perform cognitive tasks requiring planning and strategy, such as the Wisconsin Card Sorting Test (Figure 18.14A). Reduced blood flow is associated with less glucose use, which in turn is a good indicator of how active the brain cells are. Figure 18.14B shows that the frontal cortex is less active in patients with schizophrenia compared to their nonschizophrenic twins both at rest and during the Wisconsin Card Sorting Test. Hypofrontality in schizophrenia is especially interesting because the negative symptoms of schizophrenia resemble the deficits seen following surgical disconnection of the frontal lobes (prefrontal lobotomy). Included in these deficits are poor social functioning, loss of motivation, defective attention, emotional blunting, and inability to shift strategies during problem solving (Gur, 1995).

Psychophysiological irregularities   Several potential markers for schizophrenia have been evaluated and may be useful in diagnosis. A majority of patients with schizophrenia demonstrate eye-movement dysfunctions such as the inability to visually track an object. With their heads held still, they are unable to follow a moving pendulum with their eyes. This deficit is not related to drug treatment or institutionalization (Lieberman et al., 1993). Since failure to track is also found in many of the relatives of patients with schizophrenia, genetic research suggests that the defective eye-tracking gene may be inherited along with the genes for schizophrenia.

A second neurophysiological abnormality involves brain electrical activity measured by electroencephalography (EEG). The EEG records neural activity associated with the perception of an event and related cognitive processes. Normal individuals show localized stimulus-induced electrical activity in a specific area of the brain depending on the nature of the stimulus. In contrast, individuals with schizophrenia respond to specific stimuli with widespread electrical activity in the brain. The differences in eye movement and EEG patterns suggest a defect in stimulus perception and psychological processing of the information (Baribeau and Laurent, 1991).

(A)

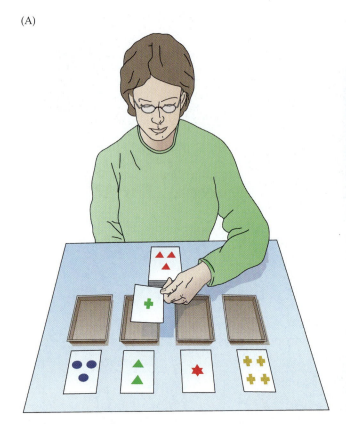

(B)

At rest

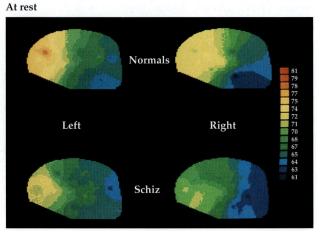

During card-sorting task

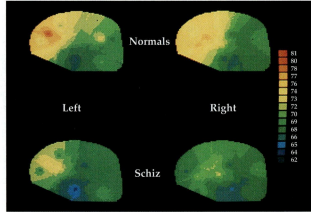

Figure 18.14 Hypofrontality in schizophrenia (A) The Wisconsin Card Sorting Test is used to evaluate the ability of a subject to shift response strategies based on feedback from the tester. The subject is presented with stimulus cards having simple designs that differ in color, shape, and number of elements. The subject is asked to sort the remaining cards into piles. With each attempt, the subject is told whether the choice is correct or incorrect. Over the test period, the sorting principle may first be color and then shift to form or number. Patients with schizophrenia and those with frontal lobe lesions fail to shift strategies and may continue to sort based on the original stimulus (e.g., color) despite being told that color sorting is no longer correct. (B) PET scans comparing frontal lobe activity of a patient with schizophrenia and nonschizophrenic twin. The sibling with schizophrenia has less frontal lobe activity at rest (top) as well as during a frontal lobe challenge with the Wisconsin Card Sorting Test (bottom). (B courtesy of Karen Berman.)

Genetic, environmental, and developmental factors interact

Although schizophrenia is an ancient disorder described as early as 1000 B.C., its causes remain unknown. Schizophrenia is increasingly regarded as a neurodevelopmental disorder with a strong genetic component; however, psychological, biological, and sociological factors combine in a unique manner to contribute to the psychopathology, its course, and its outcome.

Heredity The importance of heredity has been demonstrated by numerous family, twin, and adoption studies conducted by investigators who have taken advantage of the excellent record-keeping system of Denmark to show that relatives of individuals with schizophrenia are afflicted with the disorder much more frequently than members of the general population. In fact, the closer the genetic relationship, the greater the probability of schizophrenia in the relative. Gottesman (1991) summarized a large number of family and twin studies of individuals with schizophrenia completed between 1920 and 1987 (Figure 18.15). These data demonstrate that the risk of having schizophrenia varies according to how many genes one shares with someone who has the disorder. Compared with the lifetime risk in the general population of about 1%, first-degree relatives such as parents, children, and siblings have an average lifetime risk 12 times greater (ranging from 6 to 17%), while more distant (second-degree) relatives, including uncles and aunts, nephews and nieces, grandchildren, and half siblings, have

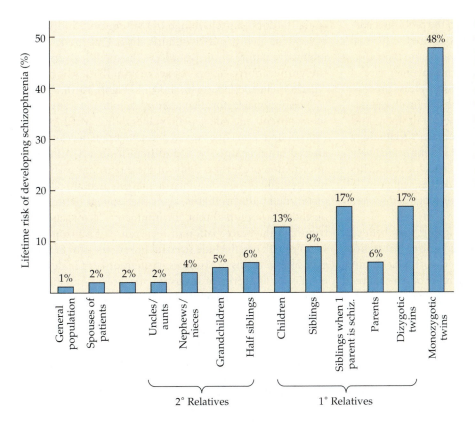

Figure 18.15 Lifetime risks of developing schizophrenia among relatives of an affected individual. Data are summarized from about 40 family and twin studies conducted between 1920 and 1987. Compared to a 1% risk of developing schizophrenia in the general population, second-degree relatives have an average risk of 4%, first-degree relatives have a 6 to 17% risk, and monozygotic twins have a 48% risk. (After Gottesman, 1991.)

an average risk of 4% (ranging from 2 to 6%). Dizygotic twins, who have the genetic similarity of siblings but who share the prenatal environment, show a concordance of 17%, which means that if one twin of the pair develops schizophrenia, the probability of the second twin developing the disorder is 17%. In comparison, monozygotic (identical) twins, who have identical genes, have a concordance of 48%. This concordance exists even when the twins are reared apart in different environments. While the concordance is striking, it is important to point out that other factors must be involved in the occurrence of the disorder, because if genetic abnormalities were totally responsible, concordance for identical twins would be 100%.

Current molecular genetic research is trying to identify the specific genes that predict vulnerability to schizophrenia (Tsuang, 2000). The task is difficult because multiple genes located at different **loci** (sites on our chromosomes) are involved. Multiple gene abnormalities would explain why the risk of having schizophrenia increases with the number of affected relatives in the family. It also might explain why the symptom clusters vary in intensity from individual to individual.

Despite the difficulties, loci on a dozen chromosomes have been identified as likely sites for "schizophrenia genes," with the most promising being on chromosomes 13, 8, 22, and 6. Some have been identified by **linkage studies,** which look for similarities at the loci in families with affected

members. A second approach considers **candidate genes,** genes that on prior physiological or theoretical grounds are suspected to be involved in disease development, progression, or clinical manifestation. In the case of schizophrenia, identification of candidate genes falls into three possible areas. First, genetic correlates of neurophysiological characteristics typical of the schizophrenic individual are evaluated, such as the defective filtering of auditory stimuli, eye-tracking dysfunction, ventricular enlargement, and so forth. Second, neurochemical models or studies of pharmacological response may provide an additional focus in the search for candidate genes. A productive line of research evaluates differences in alleles associated with neurotransmitters and receptors, including dopamine, glutamate, and GABA, and with second-messenger systems, including G proteins, adenylyl cyclase, and protein kinases. Third, because schizophrenia is considered a neurodevelopmental disorder, gene mutations that affect proteins needed for key events during brain development, such as growth factors, are significant. Early gene-induced errors could produce the major permanent modifications of brain structure seen in schizophrenia.

New developments in technology like **DNA microarray** provide the means for rapid screening of large amounts of genomic data. The method, described in Chapter 4, can identify complex gene expression patterns. For example, Mirnics et al. (2000) reported multiple defects in the gene groups related to presynaptic function in the prefrontal cortex of individuals with schizophrenia compared to normal controls. In particular, they found the greatest and most consistent defects in proteins needed for normal maintenance of synaptic vesicles and in those needed for the release process. However, other differences in gene expression involve glutamate and GABA transmission, energy metabolism, and growth factors. Although the use of microarray technology to study the complexity of the nervous system is relatively new and requires verification by other techniques, this method, along with other genomic approaches, will provide future advances in clarifying complex neurological diseases.

Developmental errors   Many investigators now believe that genetic vulnerability increases the probability that errors during perinatal (including prenatal and postnatal) brain development will contribute to the occurrence of schizophrenia (Lewis and Levitt, 2002). The abnormal pattern of cortical connections and other brain structure irregularities that exist in the brains of individuals with schizophrenia are likely to be due to disruptions in the normal processes of cell multiplication and cell loss that continue into adolescence. Keshavan et al. (1994) found significant abnormalities in the elimination of cells (pruning) that normally occurs during puberty. Excessive pruning in the prefrontal cortex (associated with negative symptoms) and failure of pruning in certain subcortical structures (associated with positive symptoms) occur more often in the brains of individuals with schizophrenia than in healthy individuals. Alterations in these normal processes could be caused by genetic programming errors, early brain insults, and environmental factors. The nature and extent of interaction of these factors remains unclear.

Evidence from several sources shows a higher occurrence of perinatal complications among individuals with schizophrenia than in the general population. Brain insult during pregnancy and delivery caused by oxygen deprivation, drug use, infections, endocrine disorders, or other factors occurs with higher frequency in individuals with schizophrenia. Exposure to viral infection (e.g., pneumonia, influenza, measles, or polio) during the second trimester of pregnancy significantly increases the risk of schizophrenia in the child (Tsuang, 2000). Severe malnutrition, as demonstrated in Holland during World War II, also represents an assault on the fetus that increases the probability of schizophrenia. While none of these stresses alone may explain the occurrence of the illness, in the individual who is genetically at risk, the assault may increase its probability.

Biopsychosocial interaction   It is easy to imagine an interactive basis for schizophrenia that depends on genetic predisposition, structural brain-wiring errors, and subsequent biochemical abnormalities, plus environmental or social factors that challenge the susceptible individual beyond his ability to deal with the stress. One model of the interactive nature of the disorder is the modified version of the vulnerability–stress model originally developed by Nuechterlein and Liberman, shown in Figure 18.16.

The personal factors that identify an individual at risk for schizophrenia include genetic vulnerability, which may be expressed in terms of errors in perinatal brain development, altered brain chemistry, and difficulties in attention and information processing. Some of these personal risk factors may actually be neuropsychiatric markers that are part of a prodromal pattern, that is, signs that appear before clear diagnostic symptoms occur. Environmental factors also contribute to the exacerbation or recurrence of schizophrenic symptoms. These include stressful life events—for example, exposure to toxins or stressors in utero or later in development, such as a series of adversities that are beyond the individual's control. The family climate may also contribute to stress when it is dysfunctional, critical, and emotionally turbulent and when communication patterns are distorted. Excessive social stimulation or pressure to perform may also represent environmental stressors that precipitate illness.

Other factors, both personal and environmental, reduce one's probability of developing schizophrenia. The protectors include the ability of the individual to use coping techniques that provide her with a feeling of competence in dealing with her problems, as well as the use of antipsychotic medication once she has been diagnosed with schizophrenia. Environmental protectors include learning effective problem-solving strategies to deal with stresses within the family and community, and psychosocial therapies that help family members to modify the stress-producing, negative emotional climate. The stressors and protectors change and interact throughout the individual's life, contributing to the nature and onset of symptoms as well as the recurrence of episodes over the life span. For a vivid example of the complex interaction of genetics and environment in the disorder, refer to Box 18.3, that describes a set of quadruplets who share the same genes and who all developed schizophrenia, which, however, varied in its onset and symptoms.

The benefit of such a model is that being able to identify the high-risk individual means that intervention strategies can be applied before the onset of the symptoms. In addition to heredity, several behavioral characteristics of early infancy may signal potential problems, particularly if the infant has other risk factors. The infant behaviors identified were passivity and apathy, less responsiveness to verbal commands, more difficult temperament, and poor sensorimotor performance. In later childhood, deficits on attentional and information-processing tasks, along with impairments in fine motor coordination, were the best predictors of psychiatric disorders in adolescence.

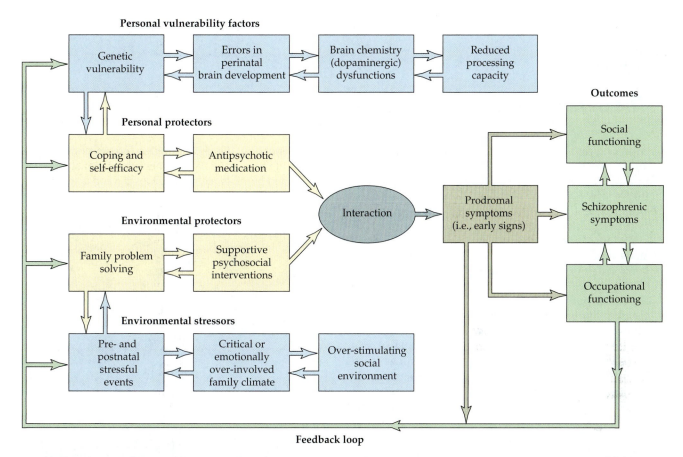

Figure 18.16 A modified representation of the vulnerability–stress model originally developed by Nuechterlein and Liberman. The blue boxes represent factors that contribute to the original onset or the reappearance of schizophrenic symptoms. The yellow boxes represent factors that reduce the probability of the occurrence of symptoms. An interaction among all the factors determines whether an individual will develop the early signs (prodromal symptoms) of illness. These symptoms further alter social functioning and occupational functioning, which contributes to the occurrence of schizophrenic symptoms. Note that each of the final outcome boxes on the right provide feedback to and interact with each of the vulnerability factors and protectors. (After Goldstein, 1987.)

Neurochemical Models of Schizophrenia

To identify the neurochemical basis for any mental disorder, three general approaches can be taken. First, neurochemical correlates of animal and human models of the disorder can be studied. Second, the neuronal mechanisms of effective drug treatment are considered, keeping in mind that it is dangerous to assume that because the neurochemical effects of a drug reverse the symptoms, the drug is acting at the specific site of the disorder. Third, the functioning of neurotransmitter systems in patient populations is assessed by measuring biological amines in blood, CSF, urine, or in postmortem brain tissue. Brain imaging techniques provide the newest way of evaluating CNS function in patient populations. Based on these three approaches, evidence strongly suggests that although several neurotransmitters probably play a role in schizophrenic symptoms, malfunction of dopaminergic transmission is almost certainly involved.

Abnormal dopamine function contributes to schizophrenic symptoms

The finding that amphetamine can produce a psychotic reaction in healthy individuals that can be reversed by DA antagonists initially suggested the **dopamine hypothesis** of schizophrenia. Also, patients with schizophrenia who have been given amphetamine and cocaine say that the drugs make their symptoms worse but do not produce different symptoms. In addition, stereotyped behavior in rats can be elicited by intracerebral injection of amphetamine into forebrain DA areas and can be blocked by administration of DA receptor blockers, such as haloperidol.

Clinical Applications

The Genain Quadruplets

A startling case history documented and compiled over a number of years by David Rosenthal and colleagues at the National Institute of Mental Health (Rosenthal, 1963) has provided fascinating insights into the interaction of genetics and environment. The study involved a set of identical female quadruplets all of whom have schizophrenia. They were nicknamed the Genain quadruplets to protect their identity; *genain* is Greek for "dreadful gene." The in-depth case study was warranted because the probability of the birth of quadruplets developing a relatively rare disorder is quite low. This "experiment of nature" provided a rare and valuable database. The data collected came from years of interviews with all family members by case workers; interviews with members of the community who knew the family personally; records from schools, physicians, clinics, and hospitals; newspaper accounts of the family; an elaborate family scrapbook begun by the siblings' mother at the time of birth; and a variety of psychological test results. A synthesis of this work can be found in a text edited by David Rosenthal and colleagues, *The Genain Quadruplets: A Case Study and Theoretical Analysis of Heredity and Environment in Schizophrenia.*

The monozygotic (coming from a single fertilized egg) quadruplets shared the same genetic predisposition to schizophrenia and they were raised in the same dysfunctional family. Yet it is clear that they exhibited the disorder in different ways. Although we tend to think of children raised in the same family as experiencing similar good and bad parenting, both prenatal and family experiences can and do differ

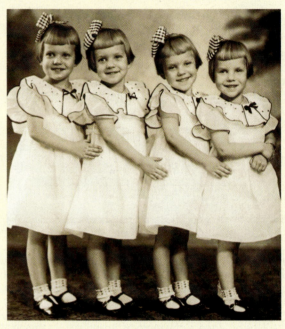

The Genain quadruplets at five years old

The correlation between D_2 receptor blockade and effectiveness in reducing schizophrenic symptoms has already been discussed. The time-dependent development of depolarization blockade following chronic neuroleptic treatment also argues for the importance of dopaminergic function in the disorder. Finally, the finding that antipsychotic treatment induces changes in DA turnover, as determined by plasma HVA levels, further supports the DA hypothesis of schizophrenia, which suggests that excess DA function is related to the manifestation of the positive symptoms.

Of the approaches used to understand the neurochemistry of schizophrenia, the evaluation of dopamine functioning in patient populations has been the least consistent. To substantiate the DA hypothesis, we would expect to see an increase in DA activity either through increased turnover (synthesis, release, metabolism) or by altered receptor number. Although the change in the dopamine metabolite HVA in response to antipsychotic treatment (i.e., an initial increase followed by a significant decrease over several weeks) predicts treatment outcome, under baseline (nondrug) conditions neither plasma nor CSF HVA levels are consistently different in patients with schizophrenia compared to control subjects. Nor are HVA levels correlated with symptom type or severity (Friedhoff and Silva, 1995). These data might be interpreted to mean that DA functioning is not increased in the brains of individuals with schizophrenia.

However, Laruelle and colleagues (1999) found that in patients with schizophrenia, a challenge dose of amphetamine elicited a significantly greater release of DA than in control subjects. This effect was found at the onset of illness and in patients who had never taken neuroleptic drugs. Hence the hyperdopaminergic state is not due to prolonged illness, hos-

BOX 18.3 (continued)

between siblings. Apparently, even identical quadruplets can experience very different social and emotional environments within the same household. For instance, an individual child's behaviors evoke reactions from those around her, which in turn influence the child's responses. Hester, the least-favorite daughter, cried more than the others after coming home from the hospital, contributing to stress and anxiety in the family. Her "bad" image persisted through childhood, and she was described by her parents as a habitual masturbator at age 3 (which was more likely a problem for the parents than for the child). Her response to the correction and criticism was to display temper tantrums and damage property. She continued to have social problems as she grew up, and at the time of her hospitalization at age 24, she was living in a world dominated by fear, anxiety, and anger.

Not only did the four sisters display different symptoms over the years, but their ages at the first hospitalization varied (ages 22, 23, 24, and the last more than 10 years later). The actual age of onset of schizophrenia is more difficult to determine, since psychopathological behaviors frequently show gradual appearance. An example taken from Rosenthal describes Nora, who had a background of "nervousness." At age 19, Nora developed phobias and compulsions about telephones and getting tuberculosis. At age 20, she developed crying spells, nausea, increased tiredness, and bodily concerns and symptoms. She regularly "visualized" her father in a casket. At age 21, she could no longer cope with the stresses of work and quit her job. During this time she walked and talked in her sleep, was dysphoric, and would stand on her elbows and knees until her elbows bled. However, a coworker to whom she wrote said that her letters were perfectly rational. Soon after she had suicidal urges and thought she was mentally ill. At age 22, she felt people were talking about her and walking on her and that she was losing her eyesight. She experienced panic, had severe "head pains," and stayed in bed day and night. At this point she was hospitalized for the first time. From this example you can see that distinguishing between prodromal pattern (symptoms occurring before diagnosis) and time of onset of schizophrenia is not a simple task.

The quadruplets differed not only in the variety of symptoms they displayed and age of first hospitalization but also in the ultimate outcome of their disease. The four of them represent the full range of possible outcomes. After the initial episode, Myra was never hospitalized again, and at the time of writing she seemed contentedly married. Nora was hospitalized repeatedly but had a marginal adjustment while outside the hospital. Iris experienced more-chronic hospitalization, and her clinical condition fluctuated from periods of severe catatonic withdrawal and hebephrenic symptoms to times of marginal adjustment when she was able to leave the hospital. Hester further deteriorated and remained hospitalized.

These four individuals with identical genes shared a vulnerability to schizophrenia but differed significantly in their expression of symptoms and the course and outcome of the disorder. The interpretation of the data leads to the conclusion that both pre- and postnatal environmental stressors clearly interact with genetics to determine the ultimate outcome.

---

pitalization, or chronic drug treatment. Further, a correlation was found between the exaggerated DA response and the worsening of the positive symptoms. Other evidence for DA involvement comes from several studies that found increased D_2 receptors in the basal ganglia, nucleus accumbens, and substantia nigra of postmortem schizophrenic brains. PET scan quantification of DA receptors also suggests increased D_2 receptors in drug-free patients with schizophrenia, particularly in patients with positive symptoms as well as those who are more acutely ill (Kahn and Davis, 1995).

Much of the evidence has been synthesized into a **DA imbalance hypothesis** described by Davis and colleagues (Davis et al., 1991). They suggest that schizophrenic symptoms are due to reduced DA function in mesocortical neurons along with excess DA function in mesolimbic dopaminergic neurons. The negative symptoms and impaired thinking may be explained by impaired prefrontal cortex function (low mesocortical activity). In contrast, positive symptoms seem to respond to reducing DA function in mesolimbic neurons.

The neurodevelopmental model integrates anatomical and neurochemical evidence

Weinberger (1995) has developed a **neurodevelopmental model** that combines evidence of altered dopaminergic function with the loss of specific nerve cells (as described earlier in the section on etiology) and symptom clusters. For instance, several pieces of evidence associate negative symptoms (flat affect, social withdrawal, lack of motivation, poor insight, and intellectual impairment) with reduced frontal lobe function. First, the negative symptoms of schizophrenia resemble the characteristics of patients with lesions of the frontal lobe (e.g., following frontal lobotomy). Also, the severity of the negative symptoms is correlated with reduced prefrontal cell metabolism when evaluated by PET scan. In addition, neuropsychological testing in humans shows a relationship between poor test performance on tasks requiring frontal lobe function, reduced cerebral blood flow in the prefrontal cortex during mentally challenging tasks, and decreased DA function as determined by lowered CSF HVA. Further, in animal experiments, prefrontal lesions produce deficits in behaviors that require insight and strategy. Animal studies also implicate mesocortical cells in normal response to stress. Mesocortical cells respond with increased DA turnover not only to acute stress but also to learned stress, for instance, when an animal is returned to a previously stressful environment. In sum, these results suggest that the onset of negative symptoms of schizophrenia is due to the occurrence of early mesocortical damage (Figure 18.17). However, although the cell loss occurs relatively early in life, the abnormal behavior may not appear until the system would normally reach functional maturity (i.e., after puberty, when development and myelination are complete). Thus complex cognitive functions, including insightful behavior and the ability to respond to the social stresses commonly occurring at adolescence, would be expected to be compromised.

The second part of the model attempts to explain positive symptoms of schizophrenia with evidence of hyperactive sub-

cortical cells. In animal studies, lesioning of prefrontal dopaminergic neurons produces chronic subcortical DA hyperactivity, manifested by increased DA turnover (Kahn and Davis, 1995). In addition, when DA agonists such as apomorphine are injected into the prefrontal cortex, DA metabolites are reduced in the striatum. Thus when the inhibitory cortical feedback is lost, mesolimbic cells increase their activity. Furthermore, studies of epileptic patients suggest that psychotic experiences, hallucinations, perceptual distortions, and irrational fears are associated with electrical discharge in limbic regions. Thus Weinberger (1995) suggests that excessive mesolimbic DA activity following mesocortical cell loss could explain the more dramatic positive symptoms of schizophrenia. Those are the same symptoms that are most readily reversed by neuroleptic-induced DA receptor blockade.

The neurodevelopmental model (see Figure 18.17) makes no attempt to identify the cause of the proposed early mesocortical cell loss. The defect could be due to one of many factors, including genetically programmed errors, inadequate maternal nutrition, obstetrical complications, viral infection, and other possibilities discussed earlier in the chapter. Weinberger argues that such a lesion produces few symptoms early in life, but reveals itself later at a time when social stresses demand maximum prefrontal cognitive function. Loss of the DA input prevents the individual from making appropriate responses and instead leads to confused thinking, perseveration of inappropriate behavior, and social with-

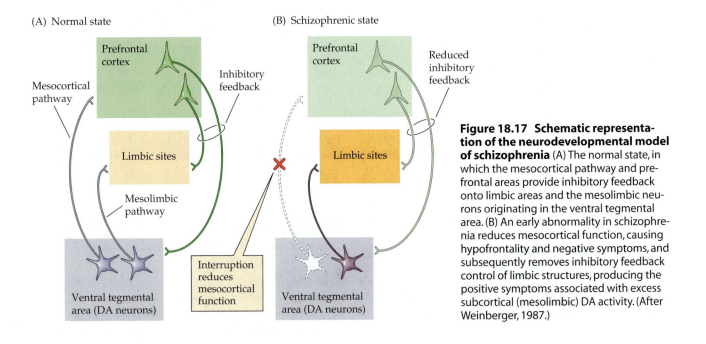

(A) Normal state

(B) Schizophrenic state

Figure 18.17 Schematic representation of the neurodevelopmental model of schizophrenia (A) The normal state, in which the mesocortical pathway and prefrontal areas provide inhibitory feedback onto limbic areas and the mesolimbic neurons originating in the ventral tegmental area. (B) An early abnormality in schizophrenia reduces mesocortical function, causing hypofrontality and negative symptoms, and subsequently removes inhibitory feedback control of limbic structures, producing the positive symptoms associated with excess subcortical (mesolimbic) DA activity. (After Weinberger, 1987.)

drawal. The loss of inhibitory cortical feedback onto subcortical neurons plus the stress-induced increase in mesolimbic cell function lead to agitation, fearfulness, and hallucinations. The appeal of this model of schizophrenia is in its ability to incorporate many distinct pieces of the puzzle (neurochemical, anatomical, developmental, and social stress). It also provides several testable hypotheses on which to design future research.

Glutamate and other neurotransmitters contribute to symptoms

Since many of the cortical cells that project to subcortical centers use glutamate as a neurotransmitter, the loss of prefrontal cells may be reflected in low glutamate function in patients with schizophrenia. Grace (1992) proposes a **glutamate–dopamine model** that emphasizes the importance of presynaptic modulation of dopaminergic cells by glutamate. Although the neurochemical interaction is too complex to include in this chapter, the conclusion is that cortical glutamate activity should normally indirectly reduce DA cell firing, producing less DA release. Therefore, loss of glutamate input to subcortical DA centers would lead to excess DA activity and the positive symptoms of schizophrenia, which could be modulated by DA receptor-blocking antipsychotic drugs. Some direct evidence for low CSF glutamate levels in patients with schizophrenia has been found. In addition, in synaptosomes prepared from postmortem brains of patients with schizophrenia, depolarization-induced release of glutamate is reduced. Also, changes in glutamate receptors in several brain areas of individuals with schizophrenia have been described (Ulas and Cotman, 1993). Of particular interest is that clozapine interacts with the glutamate receptor and increases glutamate levels in the prefrontal cortex of rats. Classic neuroleptics, like haloperidol, also modify glutamate function to some extent; this suggests a new target for the development of antipsychotic drugs. For a detailed discussion of the interaction of glutamate and DA in the production of schizophrenic symptoms, as well as an analysis of the neuronal circuitry and receptor types involved, see Bunney et al. (1995).

Because the circuitry of the limbic structures and the frontal cortex are complex, it is not surprising that many other neurotransmitters modulate or interact with DA transmission. Acetylcholine, GABA, norepinephrine, serotonin, and endorphins may each play a part in the presentation of individual symptoms of schizophrenia.

Section Summary

Compared with healthy individuals, individuals with schizophrenia have significant differences in brain structure and function. Brain shrinkage and cell disorganization occur in the basal ganglia, temporal lobe, prefrontal cortex, and several limbic areas, including the hippocampus. Ventricles are significantly enlarged. The correlation between ventricular size and age at diagnosis plus the lack of gliosis suggest that the cell loss is not degenerative but more likely an error of neurodevelopment. PET measures of cell activity consistently show diminished activity of the frontal lobe. The failure of the prefrontal cortex is reflected in many symptoms: poor social functioning, lack of motivation, poor attention, and problem-solving deficits.

The etiology of schizophrenia has clear genetic components, which are being investigated using techniques of molecular biology including linkage studies, candidate genes, and DNA microarray. Neurodevelopmental deficits that may be induced by prenatal events may also be significant risk factors for developing the disorder. In addition, both personal and environmental factors may trigger the disorder in vulnerable individuals, while others with similar physiology are protected by certain life events.

A significant amount of evidence also points to a role for DA in the etiology of schizophrenia. However, abnormalities in DA transmission do not account for all aspects of the disorder, nor is the DA hypothesis free from contradictions. It is important to remember that the clinical effects of antipsychotic drugs take several weeks to develop, which suggests that the drugs are not acting at the site of the disorder but are causing an adaptive change in the nervous system that reduces symptoms. There is evidence that DA interacts with other neurotransmitters, for example, glutamate, and it is likely that schizophrenia involves the complex interaction of multiple neuronal pathways.

Recommended Readings

Lewis, D. A., and Levitt, P. (2002). Schizophrenia as a disorder of neurodevelopment. *Annu. Rev. Neurosci.*, 25, 409–432.

Rosenthal, D. (ed.). (1963). *The Genain Quadruplets: A Case Study and Theoretical Analysis of Heredity and Environment in Schizophrenia.* Basic Books, Inc., New York.

Tsuang, M. (2000). Schizophrenia: Genes and environment. *Biol. Psychiatry*, 47, 210–220.

Glossary

A

absolute refractory period   Short period of time after an action potential characterized by the inability to open Na^+ channels and the inability to respond to subsequent stimuli.

absorption   Movement of a drug from the site of administration to the circulatory system.

abstinence syndrome   Condition characterized by unpleasant symptoms when an individual tries to cease drug use.

acetaldehyde dehydrogenase (ALDH)   Enzyme in the liver that metabolizes the acetaldehyde intermediate formed by alcohol oxidation into acetic acid.

acetylcholine (ACh)   Neurotransmitter involved with the central and peripheral nervous system and synthesized by the cholinergic neurons. It is the target of many of the deadliest neurotoxins.

acetylcholinesterase (AChE)   Enzyme that controls levels of ACh by breaking it down into choline and acetic acid.

acetyl coenzyme A (acetyl CoA)   Precursor necessary for ACh synthesis.

action potential   Rapid change in electrical signal that is transmitted down the axon.

active zone   Area along the axon terminal, near the postsynaptic cell, that is specialized for neurotransmitter release.

acute anxiety   Response to a stressful event, and only to a stressful event, that results in extreme apprehension.

acute tolerance   Rapid tolerance formed after a single administration of a drug, as is the case with alcohol.

additive effects   Drug interactions characterized by the collective sum of the two individual drug effects.

adenosine   Blockade of receptors for this substance is responsible for caffeine's stimulant effects.

adoption study   Study used to understand how heredity contributes to a disorder by comparing the incidence of the disorder in the biological and adoptive parents of people adopted at an early age who have the disorder. A higher incidence of the disorder among biological parents than adoptive parents suggests a hereditary influence.

adrenal cortex   Outer portion of the adrenal gland that secretes glucocorticoids.

adrenal gland   An endocrine gland that is located above the kidney and secretes EPI, NE, and glucocorticoids. It is composed of the adrenal medulla and the adrenal cortex.

adrenal medulla   Inner portion of the adrenal gland that secretes the catecholamines EPI and NE.

adrenergic   Adjectival form of adrenaline, also called epinephrine (EPI). May be used broadly to include both NE- and EPI-related features.

adrenoceptor   Receptor to which NE and EPI bind; part of the metabotropic receptor family. Also known as an adrenergic receptor.

adrenocorticotropic hormone (ACTH)   Hormone secreted by the anterior pituitary that stimulates glucocorticoid synthesis and release from the adrenal cortex.

aerosols   Class of inhalants characterized by sprays, such as hair or deodorant sprays, containing various chemicals used as solvents and propellants.

affinity   Attraction between a molecule and a receptor.

agonist   Substance that binds to a receptor causing stimulation.

agoraphobia   Fear of public places.

albuterol   Drug that selectively stimulates the β-adrenoceptor. It is used in asthma treatments.

alcohol abuse   Less severe form of alcoholism, characterized by consumption of alcohol in excess.

alcohol dehydrogenase   Enzyme in the liver and stomach that oxidizes alcohol into acetaldehyde.

alcohol dependence   More severe form of alcoholism, characterized by a physical reliance on alcohol.

alcoholic cirrhosis   Condition seen in chronic alcohol abusers caused by accumulation of acetaldehyde in the liver that kills cells, stimulates scar tissue formation, and promotes cell death as scar tissue cuts off blood supplies.

alcoholic hepatitis   Condition seen in chronic alcohol abusers caused by accumulation of acetaldehyde in the liver and characterized by inflammation of the liver, fever, jaundice, and pain.

alcoholism   A form of substance abuse characterized by compulsive alcohol seeking and use despite damaging social and health effects.

alcohol or barbiturate withdrawal   Symptoms associated with the termination of alcohol, barbiturate, or benzodiazepine use. The three drugs are cross dependent; administration of one alleviates withdrawal symptoms of the other.

alcohol poisoning   Toxic effects associated with the ingestion of excess alcohol, characterized by unconsciousness, vomiting, irregular breathing, and cold, clammy skin.

alkaloid   A nitrogenous organic compound often found in plants.

all-or-none   Term used to describe the observation that the size of an action potential is independent of the amount of stimulation; all that is required to generate an action potential is to reach the threshold.

allylglycine   Drug that blocks GABA synthesis, inducing convulsions.

α-methyl-para-tyrosine (AMPT)   Drug that inhibits TH activity, thereby reducing catecholamine synthesis.

5α-reductase   Enzyme that converts testosterone into DHT.

amino acids   Essential building blocks of proteins, some of which also act as neurotransmitters.

amotivational syndrome   Symptoms of cannabis use that relate to poor educational achievement and motivation.

AMPA receptor   An ionotropic glutamate receptor selective for the synthetic amino acid agonist AMPA.

amphetamine   Psychostimulant that acts by increasing catecholamine release in nerve cells.

amphetamine-induced stereotypy   Model for schizophrenia induced by giving animals high doses of amphetamine.

amygdala   Part of the limbic system that helps to modulate emotional behavior.

amyotrophic lateral sclerosis (ALS)   Neurological disorder characterized by degeneration of the motor neurons of the spinal cord and cortex. Also known as Lou Gehrig's disease.

anabolic–androgenic steroids   Group of performance enhancers characterized by their ability to increase muscle mass and produce masculine qualities. The name may be shortened to anabolic steroids.

analeptics   Drugs that act as circulatory, respiratory, or general CNS stimulants.

anandamide   Common chemical name of the arachidonic acid derivative that functions as an endogenous ligand for cannabinoid receptors in the brain.

androgen receptor   Target site of testosterone and other androgens, located within the cytoplasm of the cell and present in many tissues.

androgens   Male sex hormones secreted by the testes.

anesthetic   Substance that depresses the CNS, decreasing all sensations in the body and causing unconsciousness.

antagonist   Substance that reduces the effect of an agonist by binding to the receptor and inhibiting the subsequent binding of active ligands.

anterior   Located near the front or head of an animal.

anterior pituitary   Portion of the pituitary gland that secretes the hormones TSH, ACTH, FSH, LH, GH, and PRL.

antibody   Protein produced by the immune system for the purpose of recognizing, attacking, and destroying a specific foreign substance (i.e., an antigen).

anticipatory anxiety   Feeling of extreme worry over the possibility that a certain unpleasant event will occur in a particular, often public, situation.

anticonvulsants   Drugs, such as benzodiazepines, that prevent or control seizures. They are used to treat epilepsy.

antisense nucleotide   A nucleotide that binds to a particular mRNA sequence, delaying translation and increasing mRNA degradation. Antisense nucleotides are used to create reversible suppression of gene expression.

antitussives   Drugs that suppress the coughing reflex.

anxiolytics   Drugs that alleviate feelings of anxiety in humans and that reduce anxiety-related behaviors in animals.

apomorphine   Drug that is a D_1 and D_2 receptor agonist and causes behavioral activation. It may also be used to treat erectile dysfunction by acting through DA receptors in the brain to increase penile blood flow.

apoptosis   Cell death resulting from a programmed series of biochemical events designed to eliminate unnecessary cells. It may also be called programmed cell death.

arachidonoyl ethanolamide   Formal chemical name of anandamide.

2-arachidonoylglycerol (2-AG)   An arachidonic acid derivative that functions as an endogenous ligand for brain cannabinoid receptors.

arachnoid   Membrane consisting of a weblike sublayer that covers the brain and spinal cord.

area postrema   Area in the medulla of the brain stem that is not isolated from chemicals in the blood. It is responsible for inducing a vomiting response when a toxic substance is present in the blood.

arecoline   Chemical from the seeds of the betel nut palm *Areca catechu* that stimulates muscarinic receptors.

aromatase   Enzyme that converts testosterone into estradiol.

aromatic amino acid decarboxylase (AADC)   An enzyme that catalyzes the removal of a carboxyl group from certain amino acids. It is responsible for the conversion of DOPA to DA in catecholaminergic neurons and the conversion of 5-HTP to 5-HT in serotonergic neurons.

aromatization   Chemical reaction that creates a compound with an aromatic ring structure such as that involving the conversion of testosterone to estradiol.

aspartate   The ionized form of aspartic acid. It is an excitatory amino acid neurotransmitter of the CNS.

association cortex   Portion of the cerebral cortex associated with multisensory integration and advanced processing of information.

astrocytes   Star-shaped cells of the nerve tissue that have numerous extensions and that modulate the chemical environment around neurons.

atropine Drug found in nightshade, *Atropa belladonna*, and henbane, *Hyoscyamus niger*, that blocks muscarinic receptors.

autoimmune disorder Condition in which the immune system attacks part of one's own body.

autonomic nervous system (ANS) The set of nerves that regulate nonvoluntary movement of smooth muscles and glands, controlling digestive processes, blood pressure, body temperature, and other aspects of the internal environment.

autoradiography Process used to detect the amount and location of bound radioligand by using a specialized film to create an image of where the radioligand is located within a tissue slice.

autoreceptors Neuronal receptors in a cell that are specific for the same neurotransmitter released by that cell. They typically inhibit further neurotransmitter release.

axoaxonic synapse Junction used for communication between the axon terminals of two neurons, permitting the presynaptic cell to control neurotransmitter release from the postsynaptic cell at the terminals.

axodendritic synapse Junction used for communication between the axon terminal of a presynaptic neuron and a dendrite of a postsynaptic neuron.

axon Long fiber extending from the soma of the nerve cell that conducts electrical signals away from the cell body.

axon collaterals Branches formed when an axon splits, giving the neuron the ability to signal more cells.

axon hillock Location at the head of an axon where the electrical signal is generated.

axon terminal End of the axon where the signal may be passed to the dendrites of the next nerve cell.

axoplasmic transport Method of transporting proteins along structures of the cytoskeleton to designations throughout a neuron.

axosomatic synapse Junction used for communication between a nerve terminal and a nerve cell body.

B

baclofen (Lioresal) Drug that is a selective agonist for the $GABA_B$ receptors. It is used as a muscle relaxant and an antispastic agent.

barbiturates Drugs that act as a CNS depressant, in part by enhancing $GABA_A$ receptor activity.

basal forebrain cholinergic system (BFCS) Collection of cholinergic nerve cells that innervates the cerebral cortex and limbic system structures. Damage to this system contributes to the symptoms of Alzheimer's disease.

basal ganglia Mass of gray matter located near the base of the cerebral hemisphere. It includes the caudate, putamen, and globus pallidus. The structures help regulate motor control.

behavioral desensitization Technique used to treat phobias by introducing the fear-inducing stimulus in increments, allowing the patient to maintain a relaxed feeling in its presence.

behavioral despair Technique used to measure depression in animals by placing them in a cylinder of water from which they cannot escape and recording the time it takes for them to abandon attempts to escape.

behavioral supersensitivity An increased response to a drug treatment as a direct result of previous drug history or drug intake.

behavioral tolerance Isolated tolerance formed for a drug in a particular environmental setting that does not carry over to a new environment or situation.

benzodiazepines (BDZs) Drugs that act as CNS depressants in part by enhancing $GABA_A$ receptor activity.

benzoylecgonine Major metabolite of cocaine breakdown. It can be detected in the urine of a user days following the last dose.

benztropine mesylate (Cogentin) Anticholinergic drug used to treat early symptoms of Parkinson's disease.

bicuculline Drug that blocks the binding of GABA to the $GABA_A$ receptor and acts as a convulsant.

binge drinking Consumption of five or more alcoholic drinks in a row.

bioavailability Concentration of drug present in the blood that is free to bind to specific target sites.

biogenic amine A transmitter that is made by a living organism and contains at least one amine group.

biopsychosocial model Model of addiction that attempts to give a full account of addiction by incorporating biological, psychological, and sociological factors.

biotransformation Inactivation of a drug through a chemical change, usually by metabolic processes in the liver.

bipolar disorder Type of affective disorder characterized by extreme mood swings between depression and mania.

blackout Amnesia directly associated with heavy alcohol consumption.

blood alcohol concentration The amount of alcohol in a given unit of blood, usually given as a percent representing milligrams of alcohol per 100 milliliters of blood.

brain-derived neurotrophic factor (BDNF) Protein of the CNS that stimulates early neuron survival and growth as well as some neuronal signaling. It is also implicated in the neurotrophic hypothesis of depression.

brain stem Portion of the brain, consisting of the medulla, pons, and midbrain, that connects it to the spinal cord.

breaking point The point at which an animal will no longer expend the effort required to receive the reward (e.g., in a drug self-administration paradigm).

broad-spectrum antipsychotics Class of drugs used to treat schizophrenia by blocking a wide range of receptors in addition to the D_2 receptor.

buprenorphine (Buprenex) An opioid agonist-antagonist that may be substituted for methadone and yields similar treatment results.

buspirone (Buspar) Drug that stimulates $5\text{-}HT_{1A}$ receptors. Symptoms include increased appetite, reduced anxiety, reduced alcohol cravings, and a lower body temperature. It is prescribed as an antianxiety medication.

C

caffeinism   Syndrome caused by taking excessive amounts of caffeine and characterized by restlessness, insomnia, anxiety, and physiological disturbances.

calcium/calmodulin kinase (CaMK)   Enzyme stimulated by calcium and calmodulin that phosphorylates specific proteins in a signaling pathway.

candidate gene   A gene that is suspected of involvement in the development, progression, or manifestation of a disease.

cannabinoid receptor   Receptor for cannabinoids, including THC and anandamide. In the CNS, they are concentrated in the basal ganglia, cerebellum, hippocampus, and cerebral cortex.

cannabinoids   Collection of over 60 compounds found uniquely in cannabis plants.

carbon monoxide (CO)   Gas that acts as a signaling molecule in the brain and is deadly in high concentrations.

case-control method   Technique used to identify genes associated with a disorder by comparing the genes of unrelated affected and unaffected people to determine if those who are affected are more likely to possess a particular allele.

catabolic   Chemicals, such as glucocorticoids, that decrease protein synthesis and increase protein breakdown.

catalepsy   State characterized by a lack of spontaneous movement. It is usually associated with D_2 receptor blockers (a DA receptor subtype), but can also be induced with a D_1 blocker.

catatonic schizophrenia   Subtype characterized by alternating periods of activity and inactivity.

catecholamines   Group of neurotransmitters and hormones characterized by two chemical similarities: a core structure of catechol and a nitrogen-containing amine. They belong to a wider group of transmitters called monoamines or biogenic amines.

catechol-O-methyltransferase (COMT)   One of the enzymes responsible for metabolic breakdown of catecholamines.

caudal   Located near the back or rear of an animal.

CB1   Cannabinoid receptor of the metabotropic receptor family located in the CNS.

CB2   Cannabinoid receptor located primarily in the immune system.

central canal   Channel within the center of the spinal cord. It is filled with CSF.

cerebellar peduncles   Large bundles of axons that connect the cerebellum to the pons, midbrain, or medulla oblongata.

cerebellum   Large structure of the metencephalon that is located on the dorsal surface of the brain and that is connected to the pons by the cerebellar peduncles. It is an important sensorimotor control center of the brain.

cerebral cortex   Tissue that forms the outside of the cerebral hemispheres and is important for higher order cognitive functions.

cerebral hemispheres   The largest regions of the brain. They include the external cerebral cortex, the underlying white matter, and some subcortical structures.

cerebral ventricles   Cavities within the brain filled with CSF.

cerebrospinal fluid (CSF)   Fluid that surrounds the brain and spinal cord, providing cushioning that protects against trauma.

cGMP phosphodiesterase   Enzyme that catalyzes the breakdown of cGMP.

challenge study   Method to indirectly measure receptor function by recording the magnitude of a biological response to an agonist or antagonist.

chippers   Individuals who are long-term smokers, but are not dependent on nicotine and can maintain a smoking rate of only a few cigarettes per day.

choline   Precursor necessary for ACh synthesis.

choline acetyltransferase (ChAT)   Enzyme that catalyzes the synthesis of ACh from acetyl CoA and choline.

cholinergic   Adjectival form of ACh.

choline transporter   Protein in the membrane of the cholinergic nerve terminal involved with the uptake of choline from the synaptic cleft.

choroid plexus   Gland that produces the CSF. Located in the lateral ventricle of each hemisphere.

chromaffin cells   The cells of the adrenal medulla.

chromosomes   Linear strands of DNA that carry genes.

cingulate   Major portion of the limbic cortex. Its anterior component is responsible for modulating the emotional component of pain.

classical conditioning   Repeated pairing of a conditioned with an unconditioned stimulus, eventually causing the conditioned stimulus to elicit a (conditioned) response that is similar to the original unconditioned response.

clonidine   An α_2-adrenergic agonist that stimulates autoreceptors and inhibits noradrenergic cell firing. It is used to reduce symptoms of opioid withdrawal.

cloning   Method used to produce large numbers of genetically identical cells. The term can also describe the isolation and characterization of an individual gene.

clozapine (Clozaril)   Drug that inhibits $5\text{-}HT_{2A}$ and D_2 dopamine receptors. It is used to treat schizophrenia.

club drug   Street name for GHB, as well as MDMA and ketamine, coined as a result of their popularity at nightclubs.

CNS depressants   Large category of drugs that inhibit nerve cell firing within the central nervous system. They include sedative–hypnotics and are used to induce sleep and to treat symptoms of anxiety.

co-agonists   Substances needed simultaneously to activate a specific receptor.

cocaethylene   Metabolite formed from the interaction of cocaine and alcohol. It produces biological effects similar to those of cocaine.

cocaine   Stimulant drug that blocks reuptake of DA, NE, and 5-HT by neurons, thereby increasing their concentration in the synaptic cleft.

cocaine binges   Periods of cocaine use lasting hours or days with little or no sleep.

coding region   Portion of the gene that codes for the amino acid sequence of a protein.

comorbidity   Diagnosis of simultaneous but distinct disease processes in an individual, such as the propensity for drug abusers to be diagnosed with other psychiatric problems.

competitive antagonist   Drug that competes with an agonist for receptor sites, reducing the effect of the agonist. The drug may be displaced by adding excess agonist.

compulsions   Repetitive tasks that an individual feels obligated to complete in an effort to quell the anxiety caused by obsessive thoughts.

computerized tomography (CT)   Technique used to form a three-dimensional map of the brain by using an X-ray to take systematic readings of two-dimensional brain "slices."

concentration gradient   Difference in the amount or concentration of a substance on each side of a biological barrier, such as the cell membrane.

conditioned emotional response   Learned response to a neutral stimulus given just prior to a negative stimulus (e.g., an electric shock) in an effort to create a fear association to the neutral stimulus.

conditioned place preference   Method used to determine the rewarding effects of a drug by allowing an animal to associate the drug with a specific environment and measuring its subsequent preference for that environment.

conditioned-response suppression   Learned response to a neutral stimulus given just prior to a negative stimulus in an effort to cue an animal to stop (suppress) its behavior.

conflict procedure   Method that creates a dilemma for an animal by giving it the choice of selecting a reward that is followed by a negative stimulus.

conflict test   Method used to evaluate the level of anxiety felt by an animal by associating a behavior with both a positive and a negative stimulus and observing its propensity to perform the behavior.

construct validity   Term used to describe the relationship between a testing procedure done on animals and its ability to predict clinical effects on humans, regardless of the similarity between their test responses.

continuum of drug use   Progression of drug use relating to the amount and pattern of drug-taking behavior and the consequences that ultimately affect a user's health and behavior.

convergence   Process by which neurons receive and integrate the numerous signals from other cells.

coronal   Sections cut parallel to the face.

corpus callosum   Large pathway connecting corresponding areas of the two brain hemispheres, allowing communication between each half of the brain.

correlational relationship   Connection between an event and a result that appears directly related, but cannot be assumed to be directly related due to other events that potentially explain both.

corticosterone   A glucocorticoid secreted by the adrenal cortex of rats and mice.

corticotropin-releasing hormone (CRH)   Hormone synthesized by neurons of the hypothalamus that stimulates ACTH release. Also known as corticotrophin-releasing factor (CRF).

cortisol   Specific glucocorticoid secreted by the adrenal cortex of primates.

cotinine   Principal product of nicotine metabolism by the liver.

counteradaptation   Process whereby repeated drug use results in changes that weaken the effect of the drug on the individual.

crack   Form of cocaine made by adding baking soda to a solution of cocaine HCl, heating the mixture, and drying the solid.

cranial nerves   The 12 pairs of nerves originating at the brain and leading primarily to regions of the head and neck.

craving   Strong urge addicts feel, compelling them to take a drug.

cross dependence   Developed need for a specific drug that can be substituted with other drugs in the same or similar class, eliminating or reducing signs of withdrawal.

cross-tolerance   Developed tolerance to a specific drug that also reduces the effectiveness of a different drug.

cyclic adenosine monophosphate (cAMP)   Second messenger that activates PKA and is controlled by DA, NE, 5-HT, and endorphins.

cyclic guanosine monophosphate (cGMP)   Second messenger that activates PKG and is controlled in part by NO.

cycling   Pattern of steroid use characterized by 6 to 12 weeks of drug use, followed by a period of abstinence before repeating the drug use pattern.

cytochrome P450   Class of liver enzymes, in the microsomal enzyme group, responsible for oxidizing the majority of psychoactive drugs, including alcohol.

cytochrome P450 2A6 (CYP2A6)   Specific type of cytochrome P450 that metabolizes nicotine into cotinine.

cytoplasm   Salty gelatinous fluid of the cell, outside of the nucleus and bounded by the cell membrane.

cytoskeleton   Structural matrix of a cell that is composed of tubular materials.

D

DA imbalance hypothesis of schizophrenia   Theory that altered DA function, reduced in mesocortical dopaminergic neurons and increased in mesolimbic dopaminergic neurons, leads to the symptoms observed in schizophrenics.

DA transporter (DAT)   Protein in the membrane of dopaminergic neurons that is responsible for DA uptake from the synaptic cleft.

decay   Gradual decrease in local potential as an electrical signal travels down the cell membrane.

delirium tremens   Severe effects of alcohol withdrawal characterized by irritability, headaches, agitation, hallucinations, and confusion.

Δ^9**-tetrahydrocannabinol (THC)** Psychoactive chemical found in cannabis plants; a cannabinoid.

δ**-receptor** A type of opioid receptor primarily in the forebrain that may help regulate olfaction, motor integration, reinforcement, and cognitive function.

dendrites Projections from the soma that receive signals and information from other cells.

dendritic spines Projections from dendrites that increase the receiving surface area.

denial Characteristic of alcoholics who insist that alcohol is not the source of their problems.

2-deoxyglucose (2-DG) autoradiography Technique used to determine which areas of the brain are most active by identifying the cells that are actively taking up glucose. Cells that take up the radioactively labeled 2-DG can be detected by autoradiography.

depolarization Act of neutralizing or counteracting the polarization across a cell membrane.

depolarization block Process in which the resting potential across the cell membrane is lost. The neuron cannot be excited until the membrane is repolarized.

depot binding Type of drug interaction involving binding to an inactive site, such as to proteins in the plasma, to bone, or to fat.

deprivation reversal model Theory that smoking is maintained by mood enhancement and increased concentration that occur when nicotine withdrawal symptoms are alleviated.

descending modulatory pathways Pathways, the most important of which arises from the PAG, that start at the midbrain and influence pain signals carried by the spinal cord neurons.

desensitized Altered receptor state characterized by a lack of response to an agonist.

detoxification Procedure used to treat chronic alcoholics in which drinking is stopped and withdrawal symptoms are treated (e.g., by administering a benzodiazepine) until the abstinence syndrome has ended. Similar procedures are used with other addictive drugs.

detoxified A drug user undergoing detoxification is considered to be detoxified when signs of abstinence syndrome and withdrawal end.

dexanabinol Cannabinoid, also known as HU-211, that is a noncompetitive antagonist at NMDA receptors and doesn't bind to CB_1 receptors.

dexmedetomidine (Precedex) Drug that stimulates α_2-receptors, characterized by its sedative, anxiolytic, and, analgesic effects. It is used to treat surgical patients in intensive care.

dextromethorphan Opioid-like drug that is the major antitussive agent in most over-the-counter cough medicine.

dextrorphan Bioactive metabolite of dextromethorphan that has PCP-like stimulus effects.

diazepam (Valium) A BDZ that binds to the BDZ receptor, increasing the effectiveness of GABA to open the $GABA_A$ receptor channel.

diazepam binding inhibitor (DBI) Proposed endogenous ligand for the BDZ site on $GABA_A$ receptor.

dihydrotestosterone (DHT) Metabolite of testosterone that also has androgenic effects.

5,7-dihydroxytryptamine (5,7-DHT) Neurotoxin that selectively damages serotonergic neurons.

1-(2,5-dimethoxy-4-iodophenyl)-2-aminopropane (DOI) Drug that stimulates 5-HT_{2A} receptors, producing "head-twitch" in rodents and hallucinations in humans.

dimethyltryptamine (DMT) Hallucinogenic drug found in several South American plants.

disease model Model of addiction that treats addiction as a distinct medical disorder or disease.

dissociative anesthesia An unusual type of anesthetic state characterized by environmental detachment. It is produced by certain noncompetitive NMDA receptor antagonists such as ketamine and PCP.

divergence Process by which neurons transmit their integrated signals back out to select neurons.

DNA microarray Method used to screen tissue or cell extracts for changes in the expression of many genes at the same time.

domoic acid Amino acid found in certain seafoods that causes excitotoxicity in organisms that consume it.

dopamine (DA) Neurotransmitter, related to NE and EPI, that belongs to a group called catecholamines.

dopamine β-hydroxylase (DBH) Enzyme that catalyzes the third step of NE synthesis in neurons, the conversion of DA to NE.

dopamine hypothesis of schizophrenia Theory that the DA pathway is dysregulated in schizophrenic patients, causing the symptoms observed.

dopaminergic Adjectival form of DA.

dopamine system stabilizer Antipsychotic drug that is a DA mixed agonist-antagonist.

dorsal Located toward the top of the brain and back of the body in humans.

dorsal raphe nucleus Structure located in the area of the caudal midbrain and rostral pons that contains a large number of serotonergic neurons. In conjunction with the median raphe nucleus, it is responsible for most of the serotonergic fibers in the forebrain. Together they regulate sleep, aggression, impulsiveness, and emotions.

dose–response curve Graph used to display the amount of biological change in relation to a given drug dose.

double-blind experiment Type of experiment in which neither the patient nor the observer knows the treatment received by the patient.

down-regulation Decrease in the number of receptors, which may be a consequence of chronic agonist treatment.

dronabinol   Drug that is a synthetic form of THC, sold under the trade name Marinol, used to treat nausea symptoms in chemotherapy patients.

drug action   Molecular changes associated with a drug binding to a particular target site or receptor.

drug competition   Interaction between two drugs that share a metabolic system and compete for the same metabolic enzymes.

drug depots   Inactive sites where drugs accumulate. There is no biological effect from drugs binding at these sites.

drug detoxification   Process whereby an individual eliminates a drug from the body and goes through an abstinence syndrome.

drug disposition tolerance   Type of tolerance to a drug that is characterized by a reduced amount of drug available at the target tissue, often as a result of more rapid drug metabolism. It is sometimes also called metabolic tolerance.

drug effects   Alterations in physiological or psychological functions associated with a specific drug.

drug self-administration   Technique used to measure the reinforcing properties of a drug by allowing an animal to give itself drug doses.

dry-mouth effect   State characterized by a reduction in saliva production as a result of muscarinic antagonism. Its technical name is xerostomia.

D-serine   Amino acid that is a co-agonist with glutamate for the NMDA receptor.

D-tubocurarine   Poison that targets muscle nicotinic receptors, blocking cholinergic transmission.

dual NE/5-HT modulators   Antidepressants that enhance both NE and 5-HT function, and that act on only the desired receptors.

dura mater   The outer layer of the meninges. It is the strongest of the three meninges layers.

dysphoria   An unpleasant or depressed mood.

E

effector enzymes   Enzymes of the cell membrane that may be regulated by G proteins and that cause biochemical and physiological effects in postsynaptic cells (e.g., by means of second messengers).

efficacy   Ability to produce the desired biological action (e.g., the ability of an agonist to activate its receptor).

electrical self-stimulation   A procedure whereby an animal self-administers a weak electrical shock to a specific brain area due to the reinforcing properties of the stimulation.

electroencephalography (EEG)   Technique used to measure brain activity by using electrodes taped on the scalp to obtain electrical recordings in humans. Electrodes can also be implanted surgically into the brain to monitor EEG activity in animals.

electrostatic pressure   Force drawing an ion to either side of the cell membrane in an attempt to balance or neutralize ionic charges.

elevated plus-maze   Maze type that involves a cross-shaped maze that has two open arms, two enclosed arms, and has been raised 50 cm off the floor. It is used to test a rodent's level of anxiety.

empirical validity   Term used to describe the relationship between a testing procedure done on animals and its ability to predict clinical effects on humans, regardless of the similarity between their test responses.

enablers   Friends and family members who assist an alcoholic, allowing the individual to continue to function in society without getting treatment.

endocannabinoids   Lipid-like substances that activate CB receptors. They are produced from arachidonic acid in the body.

endocrine gland   Specialized organ that secretes hormones into the bloodstream.

endocytosis   Method by which vesicles are formed within the cell by pinching off a part of the cell membrane.

endogenous ligand   Term used to describe the body's own signaling molecule for a receptor, especially in those cases in which the receptor was initially identified as the target of an exogenous substance such as a plant-derived compound or a synthetic drug.

endomorphins   Group of peptides in the CNS that have a distinct structure, selectively bind to the μ-opioid receptor, and eliminate pain.

endorphins   Group of peptides in the brain that stimulate opioid receptors, reducing pain and enhancing one's general mood.

endozepines   Small nonpeptide molecules in the brain that display BDZ-like activity on $GABA_A$ receptors.

entacapone (Comtan)   COMT inhibitor used in conjunction with L-DOPA to treat Parkinson's disease.

enzyme   A protein that functions as a biochemical catalyst.

enzyme induction   Increase in liver drug-metabolizing enzymes associated with repeated drug use.

enzyme inhibition   Reduction in liver enzyme activity associated with a specific drug.

epidural   Method that involves administration of a drug into the cerebrospinal fluid surrounding the spinal cord.

epinephrine (EPI)   Hormone related to NE that belongs to a group called catecholamines. It is secreted by the chromaffin cells of the adrenal medulla, and it produces the "fight-or-flight" response by regulating the diversion of energy and blood to muscles. Also known as adrenaline.

equilibrium potential   Point at which the electrostatic forces and the concentration gradient for an ion are balanced.

ergot   Fungus, *Claviceps purpurea*, that infects certain grains and that contains several important alkaloids from which the structure of LSD was derived.

ergotism   Disease caused by ergot-contaminated grains that can lead to death.

estradiol   Specific estrogen and a powerful female sex hormone.

estrogens   Female sex hormones secreted by the ovaries.

ethanol Proper chemical name for the type of alcohol consumed by humans. Similar to BDZs, it acts as a CNS-depressant in part by enhancing GABA$_A$ receptor activity.

euphoria Feeling of general well-being or an elevated mood.

event-related potentials Electrical changes in neuron activity in response to a sensory stimulus.

excitatory amino acid neurotransmitters Transmitters, including glutamate, aspartate, and some other amino acids, that cause an excitatory response in most neurons of the brain or spinal cord.

excitatory amino acid transporter (EAAT) Protein that transports glutamate and aspartate across the plasma membrane. There are five such transporters, designated EAAT1 to EAAT5.

excitatory postsynaptic potential (EPSP) Membrane depolarization of a postsynaptic neuron that results from neurotransmitters binding to specific receptors on the cell and that tends to increase the activity (firing) of that cell.

excitotoxicity hypothesis Theory that excessive glutamate or other excitatory amino acid exposure results in prolonged depolarization of receptive neurons, leading to their damage or death.

exocytosis Method by which vesicles release substances and neurotransmitters, characterized by fusion of the vesicle and the cell membrane, specifically the axon terminal membrane in the case of neurotransmitters. The vesicle opens toward the synaptic cleft allowing neurotransmitter molecules to diffuse out.

expectancy Term used to describe the anticipated effect of a drug and its role in drug action or perceived drug action.

exposure models Model of addiction in which changes in the brain due to chronic drug use are thought to lead to loss of control over drug-taking behavior as well as other symptoms of addiction.

expression Process that leads to manifestation of a sensitized response and that requires enhanced reactivity of DA nerve terminals in the nucleus accumbens.

expression phase The period of time after a tetanic stimulation is given, characterized by enhanced synaptic strength (i.e., LTP).

extracellular fluid Salty fluid surrounding nerve cells that provides oxygen, nutrients, and chemical signals, and that removes secreted cell waste.

extracellular recording Method of taking measurements of cell firing by inserting a fine-tipped electrode into the extracellular fluid surrounding the cell.

F

face validity Term used to describe the relationship between a testing procedure done on animals and its direct correlation to human test results or behavior. When animals and humans show the same response, a test has high face validity.

fatty acid amide hydrolase (FAAH) Enzyme that metabolizes endocannabinoids.

fatty liver Damaging effect of alcohol characterized by the accumulation of triglycerides inside liver cells.

fear-potentiated startle Enhanced response to a novel negative stimulus following a neutral stimulus as a result of previous conditioning to associate the neutral stimulus with a negative stimulus (e.g., electric shock).

fenestrations Large gaps between adjacent cells.

fenfluramine Drug similar in structure to amphetamine that stimulates 5-HT release. It is an appetite suppressor formerly used as a treatment for obesity.

first-order kinetics Term used to describe exponential elimination of drugs from the bloodstream.

first-pass effect Phenomenon in which the liver metabolizes some of a drug before it can circulate through the body, particularly when the drug has been taken orally.

fissures Deep grooves of the cerebral cortex.

flashback Reexperience of the perceptual drug effects, specifically those of a hallucinogen, following termination of drug use.

fluoxetine (Prozac) Drug that selectively blocks the 5-HT transporter. It is used as an antidepressant.

focused stereotypies Behaviors produced by high doses of psychostimulants (e.g., cocaine and amphetamine) and characterized by repetitive and aimless movement.

follicle-stimulating hormone (FSH) Hormone secreted by the anterior pituitary that helps control gonad growth and function.

forced swim test Technique used to measure depression in animals by placing them in a cylinder of water from which they cannot escape and recording the time it takes for them to abandon attempts to escape.

fornix Structure that connects the hippocampus to the mammillary bodies and the septal nuclei.

freebasing Smoking the freebase form of cocaine obtained by dissolving cocaine HCl in water, adding an alkaline solution, and then extracting with an organic solvent.

frontal Sections cut parallel to the face.

frontal lobe One of four lobes of the cerebral cortex, it is responsible for movement and executive planning.

functional MRI (fMRI) Technique used to regionally visualize brain activity by detecting the increase in blood oxygen levels through magnetic resonance measurements of oxygenated and oxygen-depleted hemoglobin.

G

GABA (γ-aminobutyric acid) Amino acid that is the principal inhibitory neurotransmitter in the CNS.

GABA aminotransferase (GABA-T) Enzyme that breaks down GABA in GABAergic neurons and astrocytes.

GABA$_A$ receptor Ionotropic receptor for GABA that allows Cl$^-$ ions to enter the cell, thereby inhibiting cell firing.

GABA$_B$ receptor Metabotropic receptor for GABA.

GABA transporter Transporters responsible for GABA uptake from the synaptic cleft into nerve cells and glia. There are three such transporters designated GAT-1, GAT-2, GAT-3.

γ-hydroxybutyrate (GHB)   Chemical similar in structure to GABA that produces sedative and anesthetic effects in users and that is used medicinally as well as recreationally.

gaseous transmitter   Substance in the gas phase that acts as a neurotransmitter in the body.

gases   Class of inhalants, such as propane and nitrous oxide, that are obtained in their gaseous form from domestic or commercial products.

gene   Portion of a chromosome that codes for a particular protein.

general anxiety disorder (GAD)   Anxiety disorder characterized by feelings of extreme apprehension that have no focus, lasting for extended and continuous periods of time.

genetic polymorphisms   Genetic variations in a population resulting in multiple forms of a particular protein.

glial cells   Supporting cells of the nervous system that insulate, protect and metabolically support neurons.

glucagon   Hormone secreted by the islets of Langerhans that, along with insulin, regulates metabolic energy sources in the body.

glucocorticoid   Hormone belonging to the steroid family that is secreted by the adrenal cortex and helps maintains blood glucose levels in the body.

glucocorticoid hypothesis   Theory that elevated glucocorticoid levels accelerate cell damage and lead to the cognitive symptoms of depression.

glutamate   The ionized form of glutamic acid. It is an excitatory amino acid neurotransmitter of the CNS.

glutamate–dopamine model of schizophrenia   Theory that a deficiency of glutamate in subcortical DA areas increases DA activity and leads to the positive symptoms of schizophrenia.

glutamatergic neurons   Neurons that use glutamate as a transmitter.

glutamic acid decarboxylase (GAD)   Enzyme that transforms glutamate into GABA.

glutaminase   Enzyme that transforms glutamine into glutamate.

glutamine   Precursor of the transmitter-related glutamate.

glutamine synthetase   Enzyme in astrocytes that converts glutamate into glutamine.

glycine   Amino acid characterized by the lack of a functional group. It is a co-agonist with glutamate for the NMDA receptor.

gonadotropin-releasing hormone (GnRH)   Hormone that stimulates FSH and LH release. It is synthesized by neurons of the hypothalamus

gonads   Glands that secrete sex-specific steroid hormones.

G proteins   Specific membrane proteins that are necessary for neurotransmitter signaling by metabotropic receptors. They operate by regulating ion channels or effector enzymes involved in the synthesis or breakdown of second messengers, ultimately causing biochemical or physiological changes in the postsynaptic cell.

G protein–coupled receptor   Slow acting receptor type composed of a single large protein in the cell membrane that activates G proteins. It may also be called a metabotropic receptor.

graded   Term used to describe the observation that the larger a stimulus, the greater the magnitude of hyperpolarization or depolarization in neurons.

growth hormone (GH)   Hormone secreted by the anterior pituitary that increases production of IGF-I in peripheral organs.

gyri   Bulges of tissue between the grooves in the cerebral cortex.

H

habituation   Learned response characterized by the loss of response to a repeatedly presented stimulus.

half-life   Time required to remove half of a drug dose from the blood. It is referred to as $t_{1/2}$.

hallucinogen   Substance that evokes hallucinations when consumed.

haloperidol   A D_2 receptor blocker that can induce catalepsy in animals when administered in high doses. It is used clinically as an antipsychotic agent.

hangover   Effect of heavy alcohol consumption that may be a sign of withdrawal, acute toxicity, or other negative effects on body regulation.

hashish   Type of cannabis derivative that is smoked or eaten.

hash oil   Potent oil that is derived from hashish and contains a high concentration of cannabinoids.

hebephrenic schizophrenia   Subtype of schizophrenia characterized by disorganized behavior and moods that are silly and immature.

hemicholinium-3 (HC-3)   Drug that blocks the choline transporter in cholinergic nerve terminals.

heteroreceptors   Axon receptors that are specific for neurotransmitters released by other cells at axoaxonic synapses. They may either decrease or increase further neurotransmitter release.

hippocampus   Subcortical structure of the limbic system that helps to establish long-term and spatial memories. The hippocampus is where LTP was first discovered and is also one of the brain areas damaged in Alzheimer's disease.

homovanillic acid (HVA)   Major metabolite formed in the breakdown of DA.

horizontal   Sections cut parallel to the horizon.

hormone   Chemical substance secreted by endocrine glands into the bloodstream, where it travels to target locations in the body.

HPLC   Abbreviation for high-performance liquid chromatography, a sensitive technique for measuring small amounts of substances (e.g., neurotransmitters or drugs) in biological samples.

5-HT transporter   Protein in the nerve terminal membrane that is responsible for 5-HT reuptake from the synaptic cleft. It is sometimes abbreviated SERT.

8-hydroxy-2-(di-*n*-propylamino)tetralin (8-OH-DPAT)
Drug that stimulates 5-HT$_{1A}$ receptors. Effects include increased appetite, reduced anxiety, reduced alcohol cravings, and a lower body temperature.

6-hydroxydopamine (6-OHDA)   Neurotoxin similar in structure to DA that damages catecholaminergic nerve terminals and is used to study catecholamine pathways.

5-hydroxyindoleacetic acid (5-HIAA)   Major metabolite of 5-HT that is produced by the action of MAO.

5-hydroxytryptamine (5-HT)   Neurotransmitter present in the central and peripheral nervous system and synthesized by the serotonergic neurons. Also known as serotonin.

5-hydroxytryptophan (5-HTP)   Intermediate formed in the synthesis of 5-HT.

hyperalgesia   Condition characterized by an increased sensitivity to pain.

hyperphagia   Condition characterized by overeating. It is one of the effects of 5-HT$_{1A}$ reception stimulation.

hyperpolarization   Act of making the inside of a cell more negative relative to the resting potential, reducing the likelihood that the cell will fire an action potential.

hypnotics   Drugs, such as benzodiazepines, that help a patient to fall asleep and stay asleep.

hypothalamic-releasing hormones   Neuropeptide hormones synthesized by neurons of the hypothalamus and carried by blood vessels to the anterior pituitary, where they control the release of many of the pituitary hormones.

hypothalamus   Structure of the diencephalon located at the base of the brain, ventral to the thalamus. It provides many functions important for survival, including the maintenance of body temperature and salt balance, regulation of hunger and thirst, and modulation of emotional responses.

hypothermia   Condition characterized by a lowering of the overall body temperature. It is one of the effects of 5-HT$_{1A}$ receptor stimulation.

I

192 IgG–saporin   Neurotoxin containing the monoclonal antibody 192 IgG, which binds to cholinergic neurons in the forebrain, and the cellular toxin saporin. It is used to selectively kill cholinergic neurons.

immunocytochemistry (ICC)   Technique that uses antibodies to determine the brain areas or neurons that contain a specific antigen such as a protein, neuropeptide, or neurotransmitter.

incentive salience   Psychological process by which drug-related stimuli gain increased prominence and attractiveness. It is an important component of the incentive-sensitization model of addiction.

incentive-sensitization model   Model of addiction based on the theory that repeated drug use leads to an increase in "wanting" the drug (i.e., craving) but no increase in drug "liking" (reward or euphoria) because only the neural system underlying drug "wanting" becomes sensitized.

indoleamines   Indole derivatives containing an amine group. They include serotonin and the hallucinogens LSD, psilocybin, psilocin, DMT, and 5-MeO-DMT.

induction   1. Increase in liver enzymes specific for drug metabolism in response to repeated drug use. 2. Process that establishes psychostimulant sensitization by activating glutamate NMDA receptors and, in some cases, D$_1$ receptors.

induction phase   Phase of LTP, during and immediately after a tetanic stimulation is given, which requires activation of NMDA receptors.

inferior   Located toward the underside of the brain in humans.

inhalants   Group of volatile substances, such as glue, that may be abused as a drug by inhaling the fumes.

inhalation   Method that involves administration of a drug through the lungs.

inhibitory postsynaptic potentials (IPSPs)   Hyperpolarizing responses of a postsynaptic cell that result from neurotransmitters binding to specific receptors on the cell and that decrease the likelihood of the cell firing an action potential.

in situ hybridization (ISH)   Technique used to locate cells that manufacture a specific protein or peptide by detecting the specific mRNA sequence coding for that substance. It can also be used to study changes in regional mRNA levels (i.e., gene expression).

insulin   Polypeptide hormone that is secreted by the islets of Langerhans and, along with glucagon, regulates glucose and metabolic energy sources in the body. It regulates glucose uptake from the bloodstream into tissues and stimulates the uptake of certain amino acids.

integration   Process whereby several small depolarizations or hyperpolarizations will add together to create one large change in membrane potential. Similarly, simultaneous depolarizations and hyperpolarizations will cancel each other out.

intercellular clefts   Small gaps between adjacent cells.

interneurons   Nerve cells in the CNS that possess short axons and mediate local information transmission.

intracellular recording   Method of taking measurements of cell firing by inserting a fine-tipped electrode into the cell.

intracerebroventricular   Method that involves administration of a drug into the cerebrospinal fluid of the ventricles.

intracranial   Method that involves administration of a drug into the brain tissue.

intramuscular   Method that involves administration of a drug into a muscle.

intravenous   Method that involves administration of a drug directly into the bloodstream by means of a vein.

inverse agonist   Substance that activates a receptor but produces the opposite effect of a typical agonist at that receptor.

in vivo voltammetry   Technique used to measure neurotransmitter release in the brain of an awake, freely moving animal by using a microelectrode to measure electrochemical responses to an applied electrical signal.

ion channels   Proteins that traverse the cell membrane and possess a water-filled pore, regulating ion movement into and out of the cell.

ionization   Condition involving the dissociation of a molecule into ions.

ionotropic receptor   Fast acting receptor type comprised of several subunits that come together in the cell membrane. The receptor has an ion channel at its center, which is regulated by neurotransmitters binding to specific sites on the receptor causing the channel to open. It may also be called a ligand-gated channel receptor.

ipsapirone   Drug that stimulates 5-HT$_{1A}$ receptors. Some of its effects include increased appetite, reduced anxiety, reduced alcohol cravings, and a lower body temperature.

ischemia   Condition characterized by an interruption of blood flow to the brain.

islets of Langerhans   Endocrine gland in the pancreas that secretes insulin and glucagons.

isoproterenol   An agonist at β-adrenergic receptors.

K

kainate receptor   An ionotropic glutamate receptor selective for the agonist kainic acid.

κ-receptor   An opioid receptor located in the striatum, amygdala, hypothalamus, and pituitary gland that may help regulate pain, perception, gut motility, dysphoria, water balance, hunger, temperature, and neuroendocrine function.

ketamine   Drug that binds to the PCP site and acts as a noncompetitive antagonist of the NMDA receptor. It is a dissociative anesthetic used in both human and veterinary medicine, and it is also used recreationally.

ketanserin   Drug that inhibits 5-HT$_{2A}$ receptors.

knockout mice   Mice that are homozygous for the targeted deletion of a specific gene. They are used to study the normal function of that gene as well as the involvement of the gene in behavioral and physiological responses to various psychoactive drugs.

L

LAAM (Orlamm)   Abbreviation for L-α-acetylmethadol. LAAM is an opioid agonist that may be substituted for methadone and has similar therapeutic results.

L-AP4 (L-2-amino-4-phosphonobutyrate)   Synthetic amino acid that is an agonist selective for glutamate autoreceptors.

lateral   Located to either side of the body.

lateral geniculate nucleus (LGN)   Portion of the thalamus that receives visual information, integrates and processes the signals, and sends them to the visual cortex.

law of thirds   Observation that schizophrenic patients' response to antipsychotic drugs falls into one of three categories in approximately a 1:1:1 ratio: The patient may show minor symptoms and lead a relatively normal life, the patient may show mild symptoms and live a slightly debilitated life, or the patient may show major symptoms and need constant help in daily life.

L-DOPA   Precursor necessary for the synthesis of DA. L-DOPA is formed by the addition of a hydroxyl group to tyrosine by the enzyme TH. It is used to treat Parkinson's disease by increasing DA formation.

learned helplessness   Condition seen in humans and animals who have had a negative experience that they could not control. Subsequent negative stimuli that could be avoided are not, since the subjects now believe they have no control over their environment.

lesioning   Process whereby brain cells are destroyed using an electrode to administer a high radio frequency current.

ligand   Molecule that selectively binds to a receptor.

ligand-gated channel   Type of ion channel that is regulated by an active ligand binding to a receptor site associated with the channel.

ligand-gated channel receptor   See *ionotropic receptor*.

light–dark crossing task   Test used to determine a rodent's level of anxiety by placing it in a two-compartment box, one side lit and the other side dark, and measuring the number of crossings between each side.

limbic cortex   Part of the limbic system located on the medial and interior surface of the cerebral hemispheres. The limbic cortex includes the cingulate.

limbic system   Neural network that integrates emotional responses and regulates behavior and learning. Some major structures include the limbic cortex, amygdala, nucleus accumbens, and hippocampus.

linkage study   Method used to locate genes responsible for a disorder, such as alcoholism or schizophrenia, by comparing similarities in the genetic loci of families with affected members.

lipids   Fatty molecules in the body. Lipids are a major component of cell membranes, and some of them also act as neurotransmitters.

lithium carbonate   Drug that stabilizes moods, preventing episodes of mania and depression, in people with bipolar disorder.

local anesthetics   Drugs that block voltage-gated Na$^+$ channels in the axonal membrane. When applied to sensory nerves, they prevent pain signals from reaching the brain.

local potentials   Small localized changes in voltage across the cell membrane.

locus   The location of a gene on a chromosome. The plural form is *loci*.

locus coeruleus (LC)   Collection of noradrenergic neurons in the reticular formation of the pons that supplies most of the NE to the cortex, limbic system, thalamus, and hypothalamus. These cells cause arousal and increased attention when active.

long-acting drugs   Drugs that have low lipid solubility, taking more than an hour to reach the brain. Slow metabolism allows for prolonged effects that persist for many hours.

long-term potentiation (LTP)   Phenomenon whereby synaptic connections are strengthened for a period of at least an hour. It requires activation of NMDA receptors for its induction and AMPA receptors for its expression.

loss of control Point at which a vulnerable person's consumption of a substance will lead to uncontrolled use and intoxication.

luteinizing hormone (LH) Hormone secreted by the anterior pituitary that helps control gonad growth and function, and increases estrogen and androgen secretion.

lysergic acid Core structural unit of all ergot alkaloids.

lysergic acid diethylamide (LSD) Hallucinogenic drug that is synthesized from lysergic acid and based on alkaloids found in ergot fungus. It is thought to produce its effects mainly by stimulating 5-HT$_{2A}$ receptors in the brain.

lysis Bursting of a cell.

M

macroelectrode Device used to electrically stimulate or record thousands of neurons in a specific brain region.

magnetic resonance imaging (MRI) Technique used to form a three-dimensional image of an organ such as the brain by taking computerized measurements of the signals emitted by atoms in the tissue as they are exposed to a strong magnetic field and activated by radio-frequency waves.

major depression Type of affective disorder characterized by extreme recurring episodes of dysphoria and negative thinking that are reflected in behavior.

mammillary body One of the termination areas of the fornix. The mammillary bodies receive fibers from the hippocampus.

MAO inhibitors (MAOIs) Class of drugs that inhibit monoamine oxidase (MAO), thereby causing an accumulation of catecholamines and serotonin in the brain. They are often used to treat clinical depression.

maternal separation Technique used to test the importance of stress as a factor in the development of depression by separating week-old animals from their mothers for brief periods daily.

mecamylamine Drug that is an antagonist for nicotinic receptors.

medial Located near the center or midline of the body.

median eminence Area in the hypothalamus that is not isolated from chemicals in the blood and where hypothalamic-releasing hormones are secreted for transport to the anterior pituitary gland.

median raphe nucleus Structure located in the area of the caudal midbrain and rostral pons that contains a large number of serotonergic neurons. In conjunction with the dorsal raphe nucleus, it is responsible for most of the serotonergic fibers in the forebrain. Together they regulate sleep, aggression, impulsiveness, and emotions.

medical model See *disease model*.

medulla Structure located in the caudal brain stem responsible for regulating heart rate, digestion, respiration, blood pressure, coughing, and vomiting.

melatonin Hormone that regulates rhythmic functions in the body. It is secreted by the pineal gland.

meninges Layers of tissue located between the bones of the skull and vertebrae and the tissue of the brain and spinal cord. They serve a protective function.

3-mercaptopropionic acid Drug that blocks GABA synthesis, inducing convulsions.

mescal button Crown of the peyote cactus, *Lophophora williamsii*, which can be dried and ingested to obtain the hallucinogenic drug mescaline.

mescaline Hallucinogenic drug produced by several cacti species, especially that of the peyote cactus, *Lophophora williamsii*.

mesocortical dopamine pathway Group of dopaminergic axons that originates in the VTA and travels to the cerebral cortex, including the prefrontal, cingulated, and entorhinal cortices. It may also be called the mesocortical tract.

mesolimbic dopamine pathway Group of dopaminergic axons that originates in the VTA and travels to structures of the limbic system, including the nucleus accumbens, septum, amygdala, and hippocampus. It may also be called the mesolimbic tract.

metabolic tolerance Type of tolerance to a drug that is characterized by a reduced amount of drug available at the target tissue, often as a result of more-rapid drug metabolism. It is sometimes also called drug disposition tolerance.

metabolites Byproducts of biochemical pathways, such as those involved in neurotransmitter or drug inactivation.

metabotropic receptors Slow-acting receptor type composed of a single large protein in the cell membrane that activates G proteins. It may also be called a G protein–coupled receptor.

methadone A long-acting opiate drug that may be substituted for other opiates in order to prevent withdrawal symptoms.

methadone maintenance program Treatment for heroin addicts that involves the substitution of heroin with methadone to prevent withdrawal symptoms and avoid a relapse.

methamphetamine Psychostimulant that acts by increasing catecholamine release from nerve terminals. It can also cause neurotoxicity at high doses.

methoxsalen Drug that inhibits metabolism of nicotine by the liver.

5-methoxy-dimethyltryptamine (5-MeO-DMT) Hallucinogenic drug found in certain South American plants. Its street name is "foxy" or "foxy methoxy."

3-methoxy-4-hydroxy-phenylglycol (MHPG) A metabolite of NE, formed primarily as a result of NE breakdown in the brain.

3,4-methylenedioxymethamphetamine (MDMA) Drug similar in structure to amphetamine that stimulates 5-HT release and is neurotoxic at high doses. It is a recreational drug that is often abused.

metoprolol Drug that selectively blocks the β_1-receptor, limiting contraction of the heart muscles. It is useful for treating hypertension.

mGluR1–mGluR8 Eight metabotropic glutamate receptors of the nervous system. They can inhibit cyclic adenosine monophosphate synthesis, activate the phosphoinositide second-messenger system, or inhibit glutamate release into the synaptic cleft.

microdialysis Technique used to measure neurotransmitter release in the brain of an awake, freely moving animal by collecting samples of extracellular fluid and then analyzing the samples biochemically using sensitive methods such as HPLC.

microelectrode Device used to electrically stimulate or record the response of a single cell.

microglia Small nonneuronal cells in the CNS that collect at points of cell damage or inflammation and demonstrate phagocytic behavior.

microsomal enzymes Enzymes in liver cells responsible for metabolizing exogenous substances such as drugs.

microtubules Tubular structures composed of proteins that form both a structural scaffold and a stationary track in the cytoplasm of cells, suitable for movement of materials along its length.

midsagittal Section taken of the brain that divides it into left and right symmetrical pieces.

mitochondrion Organelle of the cell that produces energy, in the form of ATP, from glucose. The plural form is *mitochondria*.

mixed agonist–antagonist Drug that acts as an agonist to some receptors, but an antagonist to others. Some opioid drugs have this property.

mixed nerves Collection of spinal nerves that consists of axons from both sensory and motor neurons.

MK-801 (dizocilpine) Drug that binds to the PCP site and acts as a noncompetitive antagonist of the NMDA receptor.

monoamine Refers to a compound or transmitter that contains a single amine group.

monoamine hypothesis Theory that a reduced level of monoamines in the CNS will cause depressed moods, including clinical depression.

monoamine oxidase (MAO) Enzyme responsible for metabolic breakdown of catecholamines and serotonin.

moral model Model of addiction that treats addiction as a personal and moral problem.

Morris water maze Maze type that involves repeatedly placing the animal in a pool of opaque water and testing its ability to use visual cues from outside the pool to find the escape platform. It is used to test spatial learning.

motor efferents Nerve fibers originating at the ventral horn of the spinal cord and traveling to the skeletal muscles, controlling voluntary movements.

motor neurons Nerve cells that transmit electrical signals from the CNS to muscles.

multidimensional approach Treatment that involves a combination of methods to prevent relapse, including detoxification, pharmacological support, and counseling.

multiple T-maze Maze type that contains many alleys ending in a "T" shape, which gives the animal two possible directions at each choice point.

μ-receptor A subtype of opioid receptor located in the brain and spinal cord that has a high affinity for morphine and certain other opiate drugs.

muscarine Alkaloid that stimulates muscarinic cholinergic receptors. It was first extracted from the fly agaric mushroom, *Amanita muscaria*.

muscarinic receptors Family of metabotropic cholinergic receptors that are selectively stimulated by muscarine.

muscimol Drug found in the mushroom *Amanita muscaria* that is an agonist for the $GABA_A$ receptor.

muscle relaxants Drugs, such as benzodiazepines, that reduce tension in a patient.

myasthenia gravis Neuromuscular disorder involving an attack on the muscle cholinergic receptors by one's own immune system.

myelin A fatty insulating sheath surrounding many axons that increases the speed of nerve conduction. It is produced by oligodendrocytes in the CNS and by Schwann cells in the peripheral nervous system.

N

nabilone Drug that is an analog of THC, sold under the trade name Cesamet, used to treat nausea in chemotherapy patients.

Na^+–K^+ pump Protein pump that helps to maintain the resting membrane potential by removing Na^+ from inside the cell. Three Na^+ ions are exchanged for two K^+ ions, maintaining a negative charge inside the cell.

narcolepsy Sleep disorder characterized by repeated bouts of extreme sleepiness during the daytime. Symptoms include sudden cataplexy, sleep paralysis, and dream-like hallucinations.

narcotic analgesics Class of drugs that reduce pain but do not cause unconsciousness. They create a feeling of relaxation and sleep in an individual, but in high doses can cause coma or death.

NBQX Antagonist that blocks both AMPA and kainate receptors, but has no effect on NMDA receptors.

necrosis Cell death resulting from exposure to a chemical agent (such as glutamate), disease, or other injury. It differs in several important ways from apoptosis (programmed cell death).

negative symptoms Characteristics of schizophrenia that are observed as a decline in normal function, such as reduced speech, loss of motivation, social withdrawal, and intellectual impairment.

neostigmine (Prostigmin) Synthetic analog of the drug physostigmine that cannot cross the blood–brain barrier. It is used to treat myasthenia gravis due to its ability to block AChE activity in muscle tissue.

nerve growth factor (NGF) Protein that stimulates growth and development of specific neurons in the central and peripheral nervous system. It was the first neurotrophic factor to be discovered.

NE transporter   Protein in the membrane of noradrenergic neurons that is responsible for NE reuptake from the synaptic cleft.

neural network   Interacting circuit of neurons that processes and transmits signals over a large part of the brain.

neuraxis   Imposed line through the body that starts at the base of the spinal cord and ends at the front of the brain.

neuroadaptation   Changes in brain functioning that attempt to compensate for the effects of repeated substance use.

neurodevelopmental model of schizophrenia   Theory that altered dopaminergic function and loss of nerve cells over the course of development result in the symptoms observed in schizophrenics.

neurofilaments   Tubular structures that are composed of proteins and form a scaffold in the cytoplasm of neurons.

neuroleptic malignant syndrome (NMS)   Undesired response to antipsychotic drugs characterized by fever, instability of the autonomic nervous system, rigidity, and altered consciousness.

neuromodulators   Chemicals that don't follow the typical neurotransmitter model. They may regulate neurotransmitter activity or act at distant sites from their point of release.

neuromuscular junction   Connection point between neurons and muscle cells. It has some of the characteristics of a synapse.

neurons   Nerve cells that form the brain, spinal cord, and nerves and that transmit electrical signals throughout the body.

neuropeptides   Small proteins (3 to 40 amino acids long) in the nervous system that act as neurotransmitters.

neuropharmacology   Area of pharmacology specializing in drug-induced changes to the function of cells in the nervous system.

neuropsychopharmacology   Area of pharmacology focusing on chemical substances that interact with the nervous system to restore behavior disturbed by injury, disease, or environmental factors.

neurosteroids   Family of substances that are synthesized in the brain from cholesterol and that have a steroid structure. They act as local signaling agents.

neurotoxin   Chemical that damages or kills nerve cells.

neurotransmitter   Chemical substance released by a neuron to communicate with another cell, which may be a different neuron, a muscle cell, or a hormone-producing cell in an endocrine gland.

neurotrophic factors   Proteins that encourage the growth, development, and survival of neurons. They are also involved in neuronal signaling.

neurotrophic hypothesis   Theory that low BDNF levels are responsible for a loss of dendritic branches and spines in certain neurons of depressed patients, and that antidepressants are effective because they prevent or reverse this decrease.

neurotrophin-3 (NT-3)   Protein dimer of the nervous system that stimulates early neuronal differentiation, growth, and survival.

neurotrophin-4 (NT-4)   Protein of the nervous system that stimulates early neuron differentiation, growth and survival.

nicotine   Alkaloid that is a behavioral stimulant. It is found in the tobacco plant.

nicotine replacement   Method to stop smoking that involves giving the smoker a safer nicotine source, thereby maintaining a level of nicotine in the body and reducing nicotine withdrawal symptoms.

nicotine resource model   Theory that smoking is maintained due to positive effects of nicotine such as increased concentration and greater mood control.

nicotinic cholinergic receptors (nAChRs)   Family of ionotropic receptors that are activated by ACh and selectively stimulated by nicotine. They may also be called nicotinic receptors.

nigrostriatal tract   Dopaminergic nerve tract originating at the substantia nigra and terminating in the stratum. It is important for regulation of movement and is severely damaged in Parkinson's disease.

nitric oxide (NO)   Gas that acts as a signaling molecule in the brain. Unlike typical neurotransmitters, it is not stored or released from synaptic vesicles. It may function as a retrograde messenger in LTP.

nitric oxide synthase (NOS)   Enzyme that catalyzes the formation of NO from arginine.

nitrites   Class of inhalants that are characterized by the presence of an NO_2 group and that heighten sexual arousal and pleasure.

NMDA receptor   Ionotropic glutamate receptor selective for the agonist NMDA.

nodes of Ranvier   Gaps in the myelin sheath that expose the axon to the extracellular fluid.

noncompetitive antagonist   Drug that reduces the effect of an agonist, but does not compete at the receptor site. The drug may bind to an inactive portion of the receptor, disturb the cell membrane around the receptor, or interrupt the intercellular processes initiated by the agonist–receptor association.

nondecremental   Term used to describe a potential or process that does not decay.

nonspecific actions   Characteristic actions of a drug as a result of general environmental changes in the body, which indirectly affect body functions.

nonspecific drug effects   Physical or behavioral changes not associated with the chemical activity of the drug–receptor interaction.

noradrenergic   Adjectival form of noradrenaline (norepinephrine).

norepinephrine (NE)   Neurotransmitter related to DA that belongs to a group called catecholamines. It also functions as a hormone secreted by the chromaffin cells of the adrenal medulla. Also known as noradrenaline.

nuclei Localized cluster of nerve cell bodies in the brain or spinal cord.

nucleus accumbens Structure of the limbic system that helps to modulate emotional behavior and also plays an important role in the rewarding and reinforcing effects of many abused drugs.

O

obsessions Worrying thoughts or ideas that an individual cannot easily ignore.

obsessive–compulsive disorder (OCD) Psychiatric disorder characterized by persistent thoughts of contamination, violence, sex, or religion that the individual cannot easily ignore, and that cause the individual anxiety, guilt, and shame.

occipital lobe One of four lobes of the cerebral cortex. It contains the primary visual cortex and helps integrate visual information.

oligodendroglia Glial cells that myelinate nerve axons of the CNS. Also known as oligodendrocytes.

open field test Technique used to measure locomotor activity and exploratory behavior by placing the animal on a grid and recording the number of squares traversed in a unit of time.

operant analgesia testing Technique used to test the power of an analgesic by training an animal to associate the performance of a specific behavior with the termination of a negative stimulus (e.g., an electric shock) and measuring its propensity to perform the task after given a drug dose.

operant conditioning Type of learning characterized by rewarding an organism for performing the desired response. It may also describe the apparent tolerance for a drug as a result of learning how to function while under the influence of the drug.

opponent-process model Model of addiction in which the initial positive response to a drug is followed by an opposing withdrawal response as the drug wears off.

oral Method that involves administering a drug through the mouth.

orphan receptor Receptor that is not activated by any known neurotransmitter.

orphenadrine (Norflex) Anticholinergic drug used to treat early symptoms of Parkinson's disease.

osmotic minipump Device placed just under the skin of an animal that allows a drug to be administered continuously over a set period of time.

ovaries Female-specific gonads that secrete the sex hormones estrogen and progesterone.

oxytocin Peptide hormone secreted by the posterior pituitary that induces uterine contractions during childbirth and milk letdown during lactation.

P

panic attack Feeling of extreme fear that was not preceded by a threatening stimulus.

panic disorder Disease involving repeated attacks of extreme fear, occurring either without warning or in an environment similar to previous attacks.

para-chloroamphetamine Drug similar in structure to amphetamine that stimulates 5-HT release. It is also neurotoxic at high doses.

para-chlorophenylalanine (PCPA) Drug that irreversibly inhibits tryptophan hydroxylase, blocking 5-HT synthesis.

paranoid schizophrenia Subtype of schizophrenia distinguished by delusions of greatness or persecution.

parasympathetic Division of the autonomic nervous system responsible for conserving energy, digestion, glucose and nutrient storage, slowing the heart rate, and decreasing respiration.

parasympatholytic agents Drugs that block muscarinic receptors, inhibiting the parasympathetic system. They are deadly at high doses, but at low doses they are used medicinally to dilate pupils, relax airways, counteract cholinergic agonists, and induce drowsiness.

parasympathomimetic agents Drugs that stimulate the muscarinic receptors, mimicking the effects of parasympathetic activation. Symptoms can include lacrimation, salivation, sweating, pinpoint pupils, severe abdominal pain, contraction of the smooth muscles of the viscera, and diarrhea.

parietal lobe One of four lobes of the cerebral cortex. It contains the primary somatosensory cortex and helps integrate information about body senses.

Parkinsonian symptoms Undesired response to antipsychotic drugs that resembles Parkinson's disease, including tremors, akinesia, muscle rigidity, akathesia, and lack of mood expression.

partial agonists Drugs that bind to a receptor but have low efficacy, producing weaker biological effects than a full agonist.

passive diffusion Phenomenon in which a substance, usually lipid-soluble, moves through the cell membrane without assistance by active transport.

patch clamp electrophysiology Technique used to measure the function of a single ion channel by using a micropipette to isolate the ion channel and obtain an electrical recording.

Pavlovian Reflexive and unconscious response to a stimulus.

PCP-induced psychosis Schizophrenia-like behavior observed in individuals who take high doses of PCP.

pentylenetetrazol (Metrazol) Convulsant drug that acts by blocking the function of $GABA_A$ receptors.

periaqueductal gray (PAG) Structure of the tegmentum located around the cerebral aqueduct and connecting the third and fourth ventricles. It is important for regulating pain; stimulation produces an analgesic effect.

peyote button Crown of the peyote cactus, *Lophophora williamsii*, that can be dried and ingested to obtain the hallucinogenic drug mescaline.

peyote cactus Species of cactus, *Lophophora williamsii*, that produces mescaline.

pharmacodynamics   Study of physiological and biochemical interactions of a drug with the target tissue responsible for the drug's effects.

pharmacodynamic tolerance   Type of tolerance formed by changes in nerve cell functions in response to the continued presence of a drug. Also known as cellular tolerance.

pharmacokinetic   Factors that contribute to the administration, absorption, distribution, binding, inactivation, and excretion of a drug.

pharmacology   Study of the actions of drugs and their effects on living organisms.

pharmacotherapeutic treatment   Method of disease treatment that uses drugs to modify patient behavior. It is one method used to treat alcoholism.

phencyclidine (PCP)   Drug that binds to the PCP site and acts as a noncompetitive antagonist of the NMDA receptor. It is a dissociative anesthetic that was once used medicinally but is now only taken recreationally.

phenelzine   MAO inhibitor used to treat clinical depression.

phenethylamine   Class of drugs that includes mescaline as well as NE- and amphetamine-related substances.

phenylephrine α_1-receptor agonist that causes behavioral stimulation.

phobias   Fears that are recognized as irrational.

phosphoinositide second-messenger system   Neurotransmitter signaling mechanism that activates PKC and is controlled by certain receptors for ACh, NE, and 5-HT.

phospholipid bilayer   Fatty sheet surrounding a cell that prevents most substances from passing, but allows lipid-soluble materials to pass. The sheet is composed of phospholipids aligned linearly head-to-tail, forming a tail-to-tail bilayer with the water-soluble heads facing toward the inside and outside of the cell.

phospholipids   Lipid molecules that are major constituents of the cell membrane. They are composed of a polar head and two lipid tails.

phosphorylation   Process that adds a phosphate group to a molecule.

physical dependence   Developed need for a drug, such as alcohol or opioids, by the body as a result of prolonged drug use. Termination of drug use will lead to withdrawal symptoms.

physical dependence model   Model of addiction based on physical dependence. The model emphasizes negative reinforcement, predicting that physical dependence as a result of repeated drug use will result in unpleasant withdrawal symptoms when drug use stops and will lead to relapses.

physiological antagonism   Drug interaction characterized by two drugs reducing each other's effectiveness in the body.

physostigmine (Eserine)   Drug that blocks AChE activity. Its symptoms include slurred speech, mental confusion, hallucinations, loss of reflexes, convulsions, coma, and death. It is isolated from Calabar beans.

pia mater   The innermost of the meninges. The pia mater is a thin tissue immediately surrounding the brain and spinal cord.

picrotoxin   Convulsant drug that acts by blocking the function of $GABA_A$ receptors.

pilocarpine   Extract of the shrub *Pilocarpus jaborandi* known for its ability to stimulate muscarinic receptors.

pineal gland   Specific endocrine gland that is located above the brain stem, covered by the cerebral hemispheres. It secretes melatonin.

pinocytotic vesicles   Type of vesicles that envelop and transport large molecules across the capillary wall.

pituitary gland   Endocrine gland that is located under the hypothalamus and connects to the brain by a thin stalk. It secretes TSH, ACTH, FSH, LH, GH, PRL, vasopressin, and oxytocin.

placebo   Substance that is pharmacologically inert.

polarized   Possessing an electrical charge.

pons   Band of nerve fibers within the metencephalon.

positive reinforcement model   Model of addiction that emphasizes the reinforcing power of drugs to strengthen the behaviors involved in drug seeking and consumption.

positive symptoms   Characteristics of schizophrenia that include delusions, hallucinations, disorganized speech, and bizarre behavior. They are often the more dramatic symptoms.

positron emission tomography (PET)   Imaging technique used to determine the distribution of a radioactively labeled substance in the body. It can be used to measure drug binding to neurotransmitter receptors or transporters in the brain.

posterior   Located near the back or rear of an animal.

posterior pituitary   Part of the pituitary gland that secretes vasopressin and oxytocin.

postganglionic   Relating to nerve fibers from autonomic ganglia that innervate various target organs.

postsynaptic cell   Neuron at a synapse that receives a signal from the presynaptic cell.

posttraumatic stress disorder (PTSD)   Emotional disorder that develops in response to a traumatic event, leaving the individual feeling a sense of fear, helplessness, and terror. Symptoms include sleep disturbances, avoidance of stimuli associated with the trauma, and a numbing of general emotional responses.

potency   Measure of the amount of drug necessary to produce a specific response.

potentiation   Drug interaction characterized by an increase in effectiveness greater than the collective sum of the individual drugs.

prazosin α_1-receptor antagonist that causes dilation of blood vessels and is useful for treating hypertension.

precipitated withdrawal   Method used to test dependence and withdrawal by administering an antagonist to block drug effects rapidly.

precursor   Chemical that is used to make the product formed in a biochemical pathway (e.g., tyrosine is the precursor of DOPA in the pathway for catecholamine synthesis).

prefrontal cortex   Part of the frontal lobe that receives emotional and motivational input and is necessary for logical decision making.

preganglionic   Relating to nerve fibers from the CNS that innervate autonomic ganglia.

prepulse inhibition of startle   Method to study the ability of an individual to filter out sensory stimuli by applying a weak "prepulse" stimulus shortly before the startle-inducing stimulus.

presynaptic cell   Neuron at a synapse that transmits a signal to the postsynaptic cell.

presynaptic facilitation   Signaling by the presynaptic cell to increase neurotransmitter release by the axon terminal of the postsynaptic cell.

presynaptic inhibition   Signaling by the presynaptic cell to reduce neurotransmitter release by the axon terminal of the postsynaptic cell.

primary auditory cortex   Structure that receives auditory information. It is located in the temporal lobe.

primary motor cortex   Structure located in the frontal lobe that mediates voluntary movements of the skeletal muscles.

primary somatosensory cortex   Structure located in the parietal lobe that receives information about body senses, including touch, pain, and temperature.

primary visual cortex   Structure located in the occipital lobe that receives visual information.

primers   Drug-like effects caused by drug-conditioned stimuli that remind an organism how it feels to take a drug and that promote further drug use.

prodynorphin   One of several large peptides, collectively called propeptides, that are broken down by proteases to form smaller active opioids.

proenkephalin   One of several large peptides, collectively called propeptides, that are broken down by proteases to form smaller active opioids.

progesterone   Female sex hormone secreted by the ovaries.

programmed cell death   Cell death resulting from a programmed series of biochemical events in the cell designed to eliminate unnecessary cells. Also called apoptosis.

progressive-ratio procedure   Method used to measure the relative power of drug reinforcement by steadily increasing the response to reward ratio.

prolactin (PRL)   Hormone secreted by the anterior pituitary that promotes milk production by the mammary glands.

promotor region   Section of a gene, adjacent to the coding region, that controls the rate of transcription.

pro-opiomelanocortin (POMC)   One of several large peptides, collectively called propeptides, that are broken down by proteases to form smaller active opioids.

propranolol   β-receptor antagonist. It is useful for treating hypertension due to its ability to block β-receptors in the heart, thereby limiting contraction of the heart muscles.

protein kinase A (PKA)   Enzyme that is stimulated by cAMP and that phosphorylates specific proteins as part of a neurotransmitter signaling pathway.

protein kinase C (PKC)   Enzyme that is stimulated by phosphatidylserine and Ca^{2+} and that phosphorylates specific proteins as part of a neurotransmitter signaling pathway.

protein kinase G (PKG)   Enzyme that is stimulated by cGMP and that phosphorylates specific proteins, including proteins involved in cell growth and differentiation.

protein kinases   Enzymes that catalyze the phosphorylation of other proteins.

psilocin   Metabolite of psilocybin. Psilocin is the actual psychoactive agent.

psilocybin   Hallucinogenic drug found in several mushroom species.

psychedelic   Substance that alters perceptions, state of mind or awareness.

psychedelic therapy   Therapeutic method that involved giving patients a single high dose of LSD to help them understand their problems by reaching a drug-induced spiritual state.

psycholytic therapy   Therapeutic method that employed LSD in low doses, gradually increasing the dose, in attempts to recover repressed memories or increase communication with the therapist.

psychomotor stimulants   Class of drugs characterized by sensorimotor activation. Symptoms include increased alertness, heightened arousal, and behavioral excitement.

psychopharmacology   Area of pharmacology specializing in drug-induced changes in mood, thinking, and behavior.

psychosocial treatment programs   Counseling programs that involve educating the user, promoting behavioral change and alleviating problems caused by drug use.

psychotomimetic   Substance that mimics psychosis in a subject, such as by inducing hallucinations or delusions.

pure antagonist   Drug that produces no pharmacological activity and that can prevent or reverse the effects of a drug agonist by occupying the receptor site.

pyramiding   Pattern of steroid use characterized by gradually increasing the drug dose until the middle of the cycle, then gradually decreasing the drug dose until the cycle is complete.

pyridostigmine (Mestinon)   Synthetic analog of the drug physostigmine that cannot cross the blood–brain barrier. It is used to treat myasthenia gravis due to its ability to block AChE activity in muscle tissue.

Q

quinpirole   Stimulant that increases locomotion and sniffing behavior in rodents by activating D_2 and D_3 receptors.

R

radial arm maze   Maze type composed of multiple arms leading from a central choice point. Radial arm mazes are used to test spatial learning.

radioimmunoassay (RIA)   Technique used to determine the amount of an antigen in a test sample by comparing samples with known concentrations of radioactively labeled antigen and nonlabeled antigen to the test sample.

radioligand binding   Technique used to measure the affinity and relative density of receptors for a specific drug in a particular brain area by using a radioactively labeled ligand for the receptor.

raphe nuclei   Network of cell clusters in the CNS that contain the cell bodies of serotonergic neurons. They are found almost exclusively along the midline of the brain stem.

rate-limiting enzyme   Enzyme that catalyzes the slowest step in a biochemical pathway. It determines the overall rate of product formation.

reactive depression   State of sadness that is appropriate and of a reasonable level in response to a given negative situation.

reboxetine   Antidepressant that selectively blocks the NE transporter, thereby increasing NE concentration in the synaptic cleft.

receptor binding studies   Method used to determine the density of a specific receptor in a sample.

receptor cloning   Process used to produce large amounts of identical receptor proteins in a cell line.

receptors   Proteins located on the surface of or within cells that are responsible for binding to an active ligand.

receptor subtypes   Group of receptors that respond to the same neurotransmitter but that differ from each other to varying degrees with respect to their structure, signaling mechanisms, and pharmacology.

receptor up-regulation   Increase in the number of receptors produced and maintained in a target cell.

rehabilitation   Type of program that helps an alcoholic to abstain from or decrease drinking after detoxification.

relapse   Recurrence of drug use following a period of abstinence.

relapse prevention therapy   Treatment program for drug abusers that teaches an individual how to avoid and cope with high-risk situations.

relative refractory period   Short hyperpolarizing phase after an action potential during which a more intense excitatory stimulus is necessary to obtain neuron firing.

reliability   Term used to indicate how dependable test results are and how likely the same test results are to be recorded in subsequent trials.

remission   Period in which an addict is drug free.

resensitize   Receptor state characterized by the return of receptor function and a normal response to agonist stimulation.

reserpine   Drug extracted from *Rauwolfia serpentina* (snake root) roots. It inhibits vesicular monoamine uptake by VMAT, thereby reducing monoamine levels in the central and peripheral nervous system.

reserpine-induced sedation   Animal testing method used to identify clinically useful antidepressant drugs.

respiratory center   Part of the medulla responsible for regulating respiration. Drug-induced inhibition of neuronal activity in this area can lead to death.

resting membrane potential   The difference in the electrical charge inside a neuron at rest compared to the outside. The inside of the cell is more negative, and the potential is -70 mV.

reticular formation   Collection of nuclei within the core of the pons forming a network that extends into the midbrain and medulla. These nuclei are important for arousal, attention, sleep, muscle tone, and some cardiac and respiratory reflexes.

retrograde axonal transport   Process by which waste materials are transported along microtubules from the axon terminal to the soma.

retrograde messenger   Chemical synthesized and released by a postsynaptic cell that diffuses into the nerve terminal of the presynaptic cell, often for the purpose of altering neurotransmitter release by the terminal.

reuptake   Process that involves transport of neurotransmitters out of the synaptic cleft by the same cell that released them.

reverse tolerance   Enhanced response to a particular drug after repeated drug exposure.

rimonabant   Antagonist selective for the CB_1 receptor. It is also called SR 141716.

risperidone (Risperdal)   Drug that inhibits $5\text{-}HT_{2A}$ and D_2 dopamine receptors. It is used to treat schizophrenia.

ritanserin   Drug that inhibits $5\text{-}HT_{2A}$ receptors.

rostral   Located near the front or head of an animal.

S

sagittal   Section that is taken parallel to the plane bisecting the nervous system into right and left halves.

saltatory conduction   Mode of action potential conduction characterized by jumps from one node of Ranvier to the next.

sarin   Toxin that causes irreversible inhibition of AChE. It is used as a nerve gas for chemical warfare.

saxitoxin   Poison that, once ingested, blocks voltage-gated Na^+ channels throughout the body.

SCH 23390 D_1 receptor antagonist that may induce catalepsy when administered in high doses.

Schedule of Controlled Substances   System established by the Controlled Substances Act in 1970 that classifies most substances with abuse potential into one of five schedules. Schedules I and II have the strictest guidelines.

schedule of reinforcement   Predetermined schedule used to determine when an animal will be rewarded for performing a specific behavior. A fixed ratio (FR) schedule refers to rewards given after a set number of responses; a fixed interval (FI) schedule refers to rewards given to the first response that occurs after a set amount of time has elapsed.

Schwann cells Glial cells that myelinate peripheral nerve axons.

scopolamine Drug that blocks muscarinic receptors. It is found in nightshade, *Atropa belladonna*, and in henbane, *Hyoscyamus niger*.

secondary cortex Section of the cerebral cortex containing the neuronal circuits responsible for analyzing and recognizing information from the primary cortex, and for memory storage.

secondary motor cortex Section of the frontal lobe that is located next to the primary motor cortex and is responsible for storing memories concerning motor sequences.

second messenger Substance that, when activated by signaling molecules bound to receptors in the cell membrane, will initiate biochemical processes within the cell.

section Tissue slice showing structures of the body or nervous system.

sedative–hypnotics Class of drugs that depresses nervous system activity. They are used to produce relaxation, reduce anxiety, and induce sleep.

selective D$_2$ receptor antagonists Drugs that selectively block D$_2$ receptors, including sulpiride, raclopride, and remoxipride.

selective serotonin reuptake inhibitors (SSRIs) Antidepressants used to treat major depression, panic and anxiety disorders, obsessive-compulsive disorder, obesity, and alcoholism by blocking the presynaptic membrane transporter for 5-HT.

self-administration method Test used to measure the abuse potential of a drug by allowing an animal to give itself the drug doses.

self-medication hypothesis Theory that addiction is based on an effort by the individual to treat oneself for mood or other ill feelings.

semipermeable membrane Selective membrane, such as the cell membrane, that allows some molecules to cross but prevents others from crossing.

sensitive Term used to indicate that a test uses drug doses within the normal therapeutic range.

sensitization Enhanced response to a particular drug after repeated drug exposure.

sensory afferents Signals originating at the muscles and surface tissue of the body and traveling to the spinal cord.

sensory neurons Nerve cells that are sensitive to environmental stimuli and convert the physical stimuli into electrical signals.

septal nuclei One of the terminal areas of the fornix. It receives fibers from the hippocampus.

serotonergic Adjectival form of serotonin (5-HT).

serotonin Neurotransmitter found in the central and peripheral nervous system and synthesized by serotonergic neurons. It is also known as 5-HT.

serotonin syndrome Effects associated with an overdose of SSRIs or serotonergic agonists, including severe agitation, disorientation, confusion, ataxia, muscle spasms, fever, shivering, chills, diarrhea, elevated blood pressure, and increased heart rate.

short/intermediate-acting drugs Drugs that are moderately lipid-soluble, reaching the brain within 20 to 40 minutes and lasting 5 to 8 hours. The drugs lose effectiveness over time due to liver metabolism.

side effects Undesired physical or behavioral changes associated with a particular drug.

single-photon emission computerized tomography (SPECT) Imaging technique used to view changes in regional blood flow or drug binding by using radioactively labeled compounds injected or inhaled into the body.

sinsemilla The potent marijuana produced by preventing pollination and seed production in the female cannabis plants.

SKF 38393 D$_1$ receptor agonist, it induces self-grooming behavior in rats and mice.

skull Bones that surround and protect the tissue of the brain.

social interaction test Test used to measure the level of anxiety in rodents by recording the time spent investigating other animals.

social phobia Fear of being around people due to the potential that an embarrassing event may occur.

soma Cell body of a neuron, containing all of the organelles needed to maintain the cell.

soman Toxin that causes irreversible inhibition of AChE. It is used as a nerve gas for chemical warfare.

somatodendritic autoreceptors Autoreceptors located on the dendrites or cell body that slow the rate of cell firing when activated.

specific Term used to describe the relationship between a class of drugs and the type of animal behavioral test results.

specific actions Characteristic actions of a drug on particular protein sites that are responsible for the drug's behavioral and physiological effects.

specific drug effects Physical or behavioral changes associated with biochemical interactions of a drug with the target site.

specific neurotoxin Chemical that damages a specific neural pathway leaving others intact.

spinal interneurons Nerve cells with short axons within the spinal cord.

spinal nerves Pairs of nerves originating at the spinal cord and leading to various parts of the body.

SR 141716 Antagonist selective for the CB$_1$ receptor. It is also called rimonabant.

stacking Pattern of anabolic steroid use characterized by the simultaneous use of multiple steroids, such as a short- and a long-acting steroid.

state-dependent learning Condition characterized by better performance of a particular task in a drugged state than in a nondrugged state. It can occur when the task has initially been learned in the presence of the drug.

stereotyped behaviors   Repeated, relatively invariant behaviors associated with a particular situation or drug treatment. They often occur following a high dose of a psychostimulant such as cocaine or amphetamine.

steroids   Class of hormones that are derived from cholesterol and regulate a variety of biochemical pathways.

subcutaneous   Method that involves administration of a drug just below the skin.

substance abuse   Disorder involving the overuse of a drug by an individual. It may or may not lead to substance dependence.

substance dependence   Disorder involving excessive and harmful drug use by an individual, corresponding to addiction.

substance-induced disorders   Disorders characterized by acute intoxicating effects and symptoms of withdrawal of particular substances.

substantia nigra   Collection of dopaminergic cell bodies within the tegmentum of the mesencephalon that innervate the striatum by way of the nigrostriatal tract. Damage to cells in this region leads to Parkinson's disease.

subunits   Individual protein components that must join in the cell membrane to form a complete receptor.

succinylcholine   Chemical similar to ACh that is resistant to metabolism by AChE. It is used as a muscle relaxant during some surgical procedures.

sudden sniffing death syndrome   Fatal cardiac arrhythmia associated with inhalant use.

sulci   Small grooves of the cerebral cortex. The singular form is *sulcus*.

summation   Term used to describe the observation that several small depolarizations or hyperpolarizations can add together to create one large change in membrane potential. Similarly, simultaneous depolarizations and hyperpolarizations will cancel out each other.

superior   Located near the top of the brain in humans.

supraspinal   Located above the spinal cord or spine.

susceptibility models   Models of addiction characterized by a belief that some individuals inherit a vulnerability toward uncontrolled drug use.

sympathetic   Division of the autonomic nervous system responsible for necessary energy expenditure and for triggering the "fight-or-flight" response by increasing heart rate, increasing blood pressure, stimulating adrenaline secretion, and increasing blood flow to skeletal muscles.

sympathetic chain ganglia   Clusters of cell bodies near the spinal cord that contain many of the ganglionic neurons of the sympathetic nervous system.

sympathomimetic   Substance that produces symptoms of sympathetic nervous system activation.

synapse   Structural unit of information transmission between two nerve cells. It consists of the presynaptic nerve terminal, the synaptic cleft, and a small area of the postsynaptic cell (typically associated with a dendrite or region of the cell body) that receives the incoming signal.

synaptic cleft   Small gap, about 20 nm wide, between the presynaptic and postsynaptic cells.

synaptic vesicles   Sac-like structures located in the axon terminal that are filled with molecules of neurotransmitter.

synesthesia   Mixing of sensations such that one kind of sensory stimulus creates a different kind of sensation, such as a color producing the sensation of sound.

T

tail-flick test   Technique used to measure pain sensitivity in an animal by placing a hot beam of light on the animal's tail and recording the time it takes for the animal to remove its tail from the beam.

tar   Mixture of hydrocarbons created by the vaporization of nicotine in tobacco. Tar is a major component of cigarette smoke.

tardive dyskinesia (TD)   Undesired response to antipsychotic drugs characterized by involuntary muscle movements.

tectum   Division of the midbrain. The tectum is the dorsalmost portion of the brain and contains parts of the visual and auditory systems. The nuclei are responsible for visually related reflexes.

tegmentum   Division of the midbrain. The tegmentum is composed of several important structures including the PAG, substantia nigra, and the VTA.

temporal lobe   One of four lobes of the cerebral cortex. It contains the primary auditory cortex and helps integrate auditory information.

teratogen   Substance or drug that induces abnormal fetal development, causing birth defects.

teratogenic   Adjectival form of teratogen, a substance or drug that causes birth defects.

terminal autoreceptors   Autoreceptors that are located on axon terminals and that inhibit neurotransmitter release.

terminal buttons   Small enlargements at the axon terminal, in close proximity to the dendrites of the postsynaptic cell, containing synaptic vesicles. Also known as synaptic boutons, or simply boutons.

tertiary association areas   Section of the cerebral cortex where the three sensory lobes can interact, providing a higher order of perception and memory.

testes   Male specific gonads that secrete androgens.

tetanic stimulus   Electrical stimuli delivered repeatedly, in a brief train of electrical bursts. Also referred to as tetanus.

tetanus   A train of electrical stimuli that is used experimentally to induce LTP. Also referred to as a tetanic stimulus.

tetrahydrocannabinol   See Δ^9-*tetrahydrocannabinol*.

thalamus   Structure of the diencephalon that is responsible for processing and distributing sensory and motor signals to the appropriate section of the cerebral cortex.

therapeutic effects   Desired physical or behavioral changes associated with a particular drug.

therapeutic index   The relationship between the drug dose required for the desired biological response and the drug dose that results in a toxic response. It is represented by the equation $TI = TD_{50}/ED_{50}$.

thiosemicarbazide Drug that blocks GABA synthesis, inducing convulsions.

threshold Membrane potential, typically –50 mV, at which voltage-gated Na^+ channels will open, generating an action potential.

thyroid gland Specific endocrine gland that is located in the throat and secretes T3 and T4.

thyroid-stimulating hormone (TSH) Hormone that stimulates the thyroid gland. It is secreted by the anterior pituitary.

thyrotropin-releasing hormone (TRH) Hormone that stimulates TSH release. It is synthesized by neurons of the hypothalamus.

thyroxine (T4) Hormone that is synthesized from tyrosine and helps control normal energy and metabolism in the body. It is secreted by the thyroid gland.

tiagabine (Gabitril) Drug that is a selective inhibitor of GAT-1. It is used in pharmacological studies and to treat patients with partial seizures who are resistant to standard antiepileptic drugs.

tight junctions Connection between cells characterized by a fusing of adjoining cell membranes.

T-maze Maze type that involves an alley ending in a "T" shape, giving the animal two path choices.

tolcapone (Tasmar) COMT inhibitor used in conjunction with L-DOPA to treat Parkinson's disease.

tolerance Decreased response to a drug as a direct result of repeated drug exposure.

topical Method that involves administration of a drug through a mucous membrane.

tracts Bundles of nerve axons in the CNS sharing a common origin and target.

transcription Process whereby mRNA is produced as a complementary copy of an active gene.

transcription factors Nuclear proteins that regulate gene transcription within a cell.

transdermal Method that involves administration of a drug through the skin.

transfection Process used to introduce genetic material into a cell by injecting it with a DNA sequence coding for the desired protein product.

transgenic mice Mice bred to replace one gene with another (e.g., a normal gene with a mutant version of that gene). They are used to study genetic disorders.

translation Process whereby proteins are produced using mRNA code to direct the amino acid sequence. Translation is performed by ribosomes.

transmembrane domains Parts of a protein that traverse the cell membrane.

transporter proteins Specific proteins in the cell membrane that transport molecules into and out of the cell (e.g., proteins that remove neurotransmitters from the synaptic cleft

following their release). They are sometimes just called transporters.

tranylcypromine MAO inhibitor used to treat clinical depression.

tricyclic antidepressants (TCAs) Class of antidepressants characterized by a three-ring structure. They block reuptake of NE and 5-HT, thereby increasing their concentration in the synaptic cleft.

trihexyphenidyl (Artane) Anticholinergic drug used to treat early symptoms of Parkinson's disease.

triiodothyronine (T3) Hormone that is synthesized from tyrosine and helps control normal energy and metabolism in the body. It is secreted by the thyroid gland.

trkA–trkC Types of tyrosine kinase receptors that are activated by neurotrophic factors: trkA by NGF, trkC by NT-3, and trkB by BDNF and NT4. Two activated trk receptors are needed to phosphorylate each other and trigger subsequent signaling events.

tryptophan Amino acid characterized by the presence of an indole group. It is a precursor to 5-HT.

tryptophan hydroxylase Enzyme that catalyzes the conversion of tryptophan into 5-HTP.

turnover Index of neurotransmitter activity, typically obtained by determining the level or rate of production of one or more metabolites for that transmitter.

twin studies Studies used to understand how heredity contributes to a disorder by comparing pairs of monozygotic and dizygotic twins in which at least one twin displays the disorder.

tyrosine Amino acid characterized by a phenol group. It is necessary for the synthesis of the catecholamine neurotransmitters.

tyrosine hydroxylase (TH) Enzyme that catalyzes the first step of catecholamine synthesis in neurons, the conversion of tyrosine to DOPA.

tyrosine kinase receptors Family of receptors that mediate neurotrophic factor signaling.

U

ultrashort-acting Drugs that are highly lipid-soluble, reaching the brain within seconds when administered intravenously. They lose effectiveness quickly, within about 30 minutes, as inactive drug depots form in fatty tissue.

undifferentiated schizophrenia Subtype of schizophrenia characterized by symptoms that do not match other subtypes.

up-regulation Increase in the number of receptors, which may be a consequence of denervation or of chronic antagonist treatment.

V

vanillylmandelic acid (VMA) Metabolite of NE, formed primarily by NE breakdown in the peripheral nervous system.

vasopressin Peptide hormone secreted by the posterior pituitary that increases water retention by the kidneys.

ventral Located toward the underside of the brain or front of the body in humans.

ventral tegmental area (VTA) Region containing dopaminergic cell bodies within the tegmentum of the mesencephalon (midbrain) that form the mesolimbic and mesocortical tracts.

vertebrae Bones that surround and protect the tissue of the spinal cord.

vesamicol Drug that blocks the vesicular ACh transporter.

vesicle recycling The continual release and re-formation of vesicles by exocytosis and endocytosis.

vesicular ACh transporter Vesicle membrane protein that transports ACh into synaptic vesicles.

vesicular GABA transporter (VGAT) Vesicle membrane protein that transports both GABA and glycine into synaptic vesicles.

vesicular glutamate transporter (VGLUT) Vesicle membrane protein that transports glutamate into synaptic vesicles. There are three such proteins, designated VGLUT1–VGLUT3, which differ in their location within the brain.

vesicular monoamine transporter (VMAT) Vesicle membrane protein that transports monoamines (i.e., catecholamines and 5-HT) into synaptic vesicles.

vigabatrin (Sabril) Drug that irreversibly inhibits GABA-T. It is used to treat epilepsy.

vigilance Act of being alert to important environmental stimuli.

volatile solvents Class of inhalants characterized by chemicals, such as adhesives, ink, and paint thinner, that are liquid at room temperature, but readily give off fumes that can be easily inhaled.

volume transmission Phenomenon characterized by the diffusion of a chemical signal through the extracellular fluid to reach target cells at some distance from the point of release.

voltage-gated channels Type of ion channels that are regulated by voltage differences across the cell membrane.

W

water-lick suppression test Technique used to measure anxiety in rodents by recording their propensity to lick a drinking spout that will also transmit a mild electric shock.

WAY 100635 Drug that selectively inhibits 5-HT$_{1A}$ receptors.

Wernicke–Korsakoff syndrome Symptom of thiamine deficiency characterized by confusion, disorientation, tremors, poor coordination, ataxia, and in later stages, short-term memory loss.

withdrawal See *abstinence syndrome*.

Y

yohimbine α_2-antagonist that blocks autoreceptors and increases noradrenergic cell firing. It enhances symptoms of opioid withdrawal.

Z

zero-order kinetics Term used to describe a constant rate of drug removal from the body, regardless of drug concentration in the blood.

Illustration Credits

Chapter 1   *opener* and Box 1.1: David McIntyre.

Chapter 2   *opener*: From van Praag et al., 2002; Courtesy of Fred Gage. Box 2.2: S. Mark Williams and Dale Purves, Duke University Medical Center.

Chapter 3   *opener*: Data from PDB 1OED, Miyazawa et al., 2003.

Chapter 4   *opener*: Courtesy of the Oak Ridge National Laboratory. 4.12B: © Zephyr/SPL/Photo Researchers, Inc. 4.13: © S. Mark Williams (Pyramis Studios), and Leonard E. White and James Voyvodic (Duke University). 4.15A: Courtesy of Neuroscan Labs, a division of Neurosoft, Inc.

Chapter 5   *opener*: © Simon Fraser/ Royal Victoria Infirmary, Newcastle Upon Tyne/SPL/Photo Researchers, Inc.

Chapter 6   *opener*: © Superstock/ Alamy Images. 6.12: © Karen Tweedy-Holmes/Corbis.

Chapter 7   *opener*: Courtesy of the Office of Communications, Princeton University. 7.15: © George Mccarthy/ Painet Inc.

Chapter 8   *opener*: © Viennaslide/ Painet Inc.

Chapter 9   *opener*: © Mediacolors/ Painet Inc. 9.1: Courtesy of the National Library of Medicine. 9.11: © Arthur Glauberman/Photo Researchers, Inc.

Chapter 10   *opener*: Courtesy of the National Library of Medicine. 10.1: © Heather Angel/Alamy Images.

Chapter 11   11.2: © Jean-Philippe Soule/Alamy Images. 11.5: Courtesy of the U.S. DEA. 11.16: © Stephen Psallidas/Alamy images.

Chapter 12   12.1: David McIntyre.

Chapter 13   *opener*: © David Scharf. 13.2: © Mediacolors/Painet Inc. 13.3: Courtesy of the U.S. DEA.

Chapter 14   *opener*: Courtesy of the U.S. DEA. 14.2: © Gerard Kingma/ Painet Inc. 14.3: The Tina & R. Gordon Wasson Ethnomycological Collection Archives, Harvard University, Cambridge, MA 02138. 14.4: Courtesy of the U.S. DEA. 14.9: © Ace Stock Limited/Alamy Images. 14.11: © Bent Hector (J. R.). Box 14.1: © Ken Wagner/Visuals Unlimited.

Chapter 15   *opener*: © Janine Wiedel Photolibrary/Alamy Images. 15.5: © David Hoffman Photo Library/Alamy Images. Box 15.1: David McIntyre.

Chapter 16   *opener*: © John Foxx/ Alamy Images.

Chapter 17   *opener*: © Wilmar D. Zehr/Painet Inc. 17.2: Nicolas Poussin. 17.3: Courtesy of Amy Bedell.

Chapter 18   *opener*: © L. J. Bergwerff/ Painet Inc. 18.2: Courtesy of the National Library of Medicine. Box 18.3: © The Genain quadruplets.

References

Aceto, M. D., Scates, S. M., Lowe, J. A., and Martin, B. R. (1996). Dependence on Δ^9-tetrahydrocannabinol: Studies on precipitated and abrupt withdrawal. *J. Pharmacol. Exp. Ther.,* 278, 1290–1295.

Aghajanian, G. K., and Marek, G. J. (1999). Serotonin and hallucinogens. *Neuropsychopharmacology,* 21, 16S–23S.

Agurell, S., Halldin, M., Lindgren, J.-E., Ohlsson, A., Widman, M., Gillespie, H., and Hollister, L. (1986). Pharmacokinetics and metabolism of Δ^9-tetrahydrocannabinol and other cannabinoids with emphasis on man. *Pharmacol. Rev.,* 38, 21–43.

Ahern, K., Lustig, H., and Greenberg, D. (1994). Enhancement of NMDA toxicity and calcium responses by chronic exposure of cultured cortical neurons to ethanol. *Neurosci. Lett.,* 165, 211–214.

Ahlquist, R. P. (1948). A study of adrenotropic receptors. *Am. J. Physiol.,* 153, 586–600.

Ahlquist, R. P. (1979). Adrenoreceptors. *Trends Pharmacol. Sci.,* 1, 16–17.

Ahmed, S. H., and Koob, G. F. (1997). Cocaine- but not food-seeking behavior is reinstated by stress after extinction. *Psychopharmacology,* 132, 289–295.

Aiba, A., Chen, C., Herrup, K., Rosenmund, C., Stevens, C. F., and Tonegawa, S. (1994a). Reduced hippocampal long-term potentiation and context-specific deficit in associative learning in mGluR1 mutant mice. *Cell,* 79, 365–375.

Aiba, A., Kano, M., Chen, C., Stanton, M. E., Fox, G. D., Herrup, K., Zwingman, T. A., and Tonegawa, S. (1994b). Deficient cerebellar long-term depression and impaired motor learning in mGluR1 mutant mice. *Cell,* 79, 377–388.

Alexander, G. M., Packard, M. G., and Hines, M. (1994). Testosterone has rewarding affective properties in male rats: Implications for the biological basis of sexual motivation. *Behav. Neurosci.,* 108, 424–428.

American Psychiatric Association (1994). *Diagnostic and Statistical Manual of Mental Disorders* (4th ed.). American Psychiatric Association, Washington.

American Psychiatric Association (2000). *Diagnostic and Statistical Manual of Mental Disorders* (4th ed., Text Revision). American Psychiatric Association, Washington.

Andreasen, N. C. (1990). Positive and negative symptoms: Historical and conceptual aspects. In *Modern Problems of Pharmacopsychiatry* (T. A. Ban, A. M. Freedman, C. G. Gottfries, R. Levy, P. Pinchot, and W. Poldinger, Eds.), pp. 1–42. Karger, Basel, Switzerland.

Appel, J. B., West, W. B., and Buggy, J. (2004). LSD, 5-HT (serotonin), and the evolution of a behavioral assay. *Neurosci. Biobehav. Rev.,* 27, 693–701.

Applegate, M. (1999). Cytochrome P450 isoenzymes: Nursing considerations. *Amer. Psychiatr. Nurs. Assoc.,* 5, 15–22.

Apter, A., van Praag, H. M., Plutchik, R. et al. (1990). Interrelationships among anxiety, aggression, impulsivity, and mood: A serotonergically linked cluster? *Psychiatry Res.,* 32, 191–199.

Arborelius, L., Owens, M. J., Plotsky, P. M., and Nemeroff, C. B. (1999). The role of corticotropin-releasing factor in depression and anxiety disorders. *J. Endocrinol.,* 160, 1–12.

Aston-Jones, G. (1985). Behavioral functions of locus coeruleus derived from cellular attributes. *Physiol. Psychol.,* 13, 118–126.

Aston-Jones, G., and Bloom, F. E. (1981a). Activity of norepinephrine-containing locus coeruleus neurons in behaving rats anticipates fluctuations in the sleep-waking cycle. *J. Neurosci.,* 1, 876–886.

Aston-Jones, G., and Bloom, F. E. (1981b). Norepinephrine-containing locus coeruleus neurons in behaving rats exhibit pronounced responses to non-noxious environmental stimuli. *J. Neurosci.,* 1, 887–900.

Avis, H. (1966). *Drugs and Life.* Brown and Benchmark, Guilford, CT.

Avis, H. (1996). *Drugs and Life* (3rd ed.). Brown and Benchmark, Guilford, CT.

Bahrke, M. S., Yesalis, C. E., III, and Wright, J. E. (1996). Psychological and behavioural effects of endogenous testosterone and anabolic-androgenic steroids. An update. *Sports Med.,* 22, 367–390.

Baik, J.-H., Picetti, R., Saiardi, A., Thiriet, G., Dierich, A., Depaulis, A., Le Meur, M., and Borrelli, E. (1995). Parkinsonian-like locomotor impairment in mice lacking dopamine D2 receptors. *Nature,* 377, 424–428.

Bales, R. F. (1946). Cultural differences in rates of alcoholism. *Q. J. Studies Alcohol,* 6, 480–499.

Balfour, D. J., Wright, A. E., Benwell, M. E., and Birrell, C. E. (2000). The putative role of extra-synaptic mesolimbic dopamine in the neurobiology of nicotine dependence. *Behav. Brain Res.,* 113, 73–83.

Balster, R. L., and Woolverton, W. L. (1980). Continuous-access phencyclidine self-administration by rhesus monkeys leading to physical dependence. *Psychopharmacology,* 70, 5–10.

Balster, R. L., and Woolverton, W. L. (1981). Tolerance and dependence to phencyclidine. In *PCP (Phencyclidine): Historical and Current Perspectives* (E. F. Domino, Ed.), pp. 293–306. NPP Books, Ann Arbor, Michigan.

Banerji, S., and Anderson, I. B. (2001). Abuse of Coricidin HBP cough & cold tablets: Episodes recorded by a poison center. *Am. J. Health Syst. Pharm.,* 58, 1811–1814.

Bardo, M. T., Donohew, R. L., and Harrington, N. G. (1996). Psychobiology of novelty seeking and drug seeking behavior. *Behav. Brain Res.,* 77, 23–43.

Baribeau, J., and Laurent, J. P. (1991). Longitudinal studies of clinical and ERP correlates of thought disorder and positive/negative symptoms in schizophrenia. In *Biological Basis of Schizophrenic Disorders* (T. Nakazawa, Ed.), pp. 19–30. Japan Scientific Societies Press, Karger, New York.

Barlow, D. H., and Durand, V. M. (1995). *Abnormal Psychology: An Integrative Approach.* Brooks/Cole Publishing Company, New York.

Barone, J. J., and Roberts, H. R. (1996). Caffeine consumption. *Food. Chem. Toxicol.,* 34, 119–129.

Barry, H., III, McGuire, M. S., and Krimmer, E. C. (1982). Alcohol and meprobamate resemble phenobarbital rather than chlordiazepoxide. In *Drug Discrimination: Applications in CNS Pharmacology* (F. C. Colpaert and J. F. Slangen, Eds.), pp. 219–233. Elsevier, The Netherlands.

Bartus, R. T., Dean, R. L., III, Beer, B., and Lippa, A. S. (1982). The cholinergic hypothesis of geriatric memory dysfunction. *Science,* 217, 408–414.

Basheer, R., Porkka-Heiskanen, T., Strecker, R. E., Thakkar, M. M., and McCarley, R. W. (2000). Adenosine as a biological signal mediating sleepiness following prolonged wakefulness. *Biol. Signals Receptors.,* 9, 319–327.

Basile, A. S., Fedorova, I., Zapata, A., Liu, X., Shippenberg, T., Duttaroy, A., Yamada, M., and Wess, J. (2002). Deletion of the M_5 muscarinic acetylcholine receptor attenuates morphine reinforcement and withdrawal but not morphine analgesia. *Proc. Natl. Acad. Sci. USA,* 99, 11452–11457.

Bassuk, E. L., and Gerson, S. (1978). Deinstitutionalization and mental health services. *Sci. Am.,* 444, 332–358.

Baxter, L. R., Jr., Schwartz, J. M., Bergman, K. S., Szuba, M. P., Guze, B. H., Mazziotta, J. C., Alazraki, A., Selin, C. E., Ferng, H. K., Munford, P., et al. (1992). Caudate glucose metabolic rate changes with both drug and behavior therapy for obsessive-compulsive disorder. *Arch. Gen. Psychiatry,* 49(9), 681–689.

Beal, M. F. (2003). Mitochondria, oxidative damage, and inflammation in Parkinson's disease. *Ann. N. Y. Acad. Sci.,* 991, 120–131.

Bear, M. F., Connors, B. W., and Paradiso, M. A. (2001). *Neuroscience: Exploring the Brain* (2nd ed.). Lippincott, Williams, and Wilkins, Philadelphia.

Beardsley, P., Balster, R. L., and Harris, L. S. (1996). Evaluation of the discriminative stimulus and reinforcing effects of gamma-hydroxybutyrate (GHB). *Psychopharmacology,* 127, 315–322.

Beckstead, M. J., Weiner, J. L., Eger, E. I., II, Gong, D. H., and Mihic, S. J. (2000). Glycine and γ-aminobutyric acid$_A$ receptor function is enhanced by inhaled drugs of abuse. *Mol. Pharmacol.,* 57, 1199–1205.

Beltramo, M., Stella, N., Calignano, A., Lin, S. Y., Makriyannis, A., and Piomelli, D. (1997). Functional role of high-affinity anandamide transport as revealed by selective inhibition. *Science,* 277, 1094–1097.

Benavides, J., Rumigny, J. F., Bourguignon, J. J., Cash, C., Wermuth, C. G., Mandel, P., Vincendon, G., and Maitre, M. (1982). High affinity binding site for γ-hydroxybutyric acid in rat brain. *Life Sci.,* 30, 953–961.

Berger-Sweeney, J., Heckers, S., Mesulam, M.-M., Wiley, R. G., Lappi, D. A., and Sharma, M. (1994). Differential effects on spatial navigation of immunotoxin-induced cholinergic lesions of the medial septal area and nucleus basalis magnocellularis. *J. Neurosci.,* 14, 4507–4519.

Bergman, J., Kamien, J. B., and Spealman, R. D. (1990). Antagonism of cocaine self-administration by selective dopamine D_1 and D_2 antagonists. *Behav. Pharmacol.,* 1, 355–363.

Berman, R. M., Narasimhan, M., Sanacora, G., Miano, A. P., Hoffman, R. E., Hu, X. S., Charney, D. S., and Boutros, N. N. (2000). A randomized clinical trial of repetitive transcranial magnetic stimulation in the treatment of major depression. *Biol. Psychiatry,* 47, 332–337.

Berridge, C. W., Isaac, S. O., and Espana, R. A. (2003). Additive wake-promoting actions of medial basal forebrain noradrenergic α_1- and β-receptor stimulation. *Behav. Neurosci.,* 117, 350–359.

Bertelsen, A., Harvald, B., and Hauge, M. (1977). A Danish twin study of manic-depressive disorders. *Br. J. Psychiatry,* 130, 330–351.

Bertschy, G. (1995). Methadone maintenance treatment: An update. *Eur. Arch. Psychiatr. Clin. Neurosci.,* 245, 114–124.

Bhasin, S., Storer, T. W., Berman, N., Callegari, C., Clevenger, B. A., Phillips, J., Bunnell, T., Tricker, R., Shirazi, A., and Casaburi, R. (1996). The effects of supraphysiological doses of testosterone on muscle size and strength in men. *New Engl. J. Med.,* 335, 1–7.

Bhasin, S., Woodhouse, L., Casaburi, R., Singh, A. B., Bhasin, D., Berman, N., Chen, X., Yarasheski, K. E., Magliano, L., Dzekov, C., Dzekov, J., Bross, R., Phillips, J., Sinha-Hikim, I., Shen, R., and Storer, T. W. (2001). Testosterone dose-response relationships in healthy young men. *Am. J. Physiol. Endocrinol. Metab.,* 281, E1172–E1181.

Bischof, G., Rumpf, H.-J., Hapke, U., Meyer, C., and John, U. (2001). Factors influencing remission from alcohol dependence without formal help in a representative population sample. *Addiction,* 96, 1327–1336.

Black, S. C. (2004). Cannabinoid receptor antagonists and obesity. *Curr. Opin. Invest. Drugs,* 5, 389–394.

Blier, P., and de Montigny, C. (1999). Serotonin and drug-induced therapeutic responses in major depression, obsessive-compulsive and panic disorders. *Neuropsychopharmacology,* 21, 91S–98S.

Blier, P., de Montigny, C., and Chaput, Y. (1990). A role for the serotonin system in the mechanism of action of antidepressant treatments: Preclinical evidence. *J. Clin. Psychiatry,* 51 (Suppl. 4), 4–20.

Block, R. I., Erwin, W. J., Farinpour, R., and Braverman, K. (1998). Sedative, stimulant, and other subjective effects of marijuana: Relationships to smoking techniques. *Pharmacol. Biochem. Behav.,* 59, 405–412.

Blume, S. (1991). Sexuality and stigma. *Alcohol Health Res. World,* 15, 139–145.

Boot, B. P., McGregor, I. S., and Hall, W. (2000). MDMA (Ecstasy) neurotoxicity: Assessing and communicating the risks. *Lancet,* 355, 1818–1821.

Boulay, D., Depoorte, R., Oblin, A., Sanger, D. J., Schoemaker, H., and Perrault, G. (2000). Haloperidol-induced catalepsy is absent in dopamine D_2, but maintained in dopamine D_3 receptor knock-out mice. *Eur. J. Pharmacol.,* 391, 63–73.

Bourin, M., Baker, G. B., and Bradwejn, J. (1998). Neurobiology of panic disorder. *J. Psychosom. Res.,* 44, 163–180.

Bozarth, M. A., and Wise, R. A. (1985). Toxicity associated with long-term intravenous heroin and cocaine self-administration in the rat. *JAMA,* 254, 81–83.

Bradberry, C. W. (2000). Acute and chronic dopamine dynamics in a nonhuman primate model of recreational cocaine use. *J. Neurosci.,* 20, 7109–7115.

Brady, K. T., and Sonne, S. C. (1999). The role of stress in alcohol use, alcoholism treatment, and relapse. *Alcohol Res. Health,* 23, 263–271.

Braestrup, C., and Squires, R. F. (1977). Specific benzodiazepine receptors in rat brain characterized by high-affinity [^{3}H]diazepam binding. *Proc. Natl. Acad. Sci. U.S.A.,* 74, 3805–3809.

Braff, D. L. (1993). Information processing and attention dysfunctions in schizophrenia. *Schizophr. Bull.,* 19(2), 239–242.

Brauer, L. H., and de Wit, H. (1995). Role of dopamine in *d*-amphetamine-induced euphoria in normal, healthy volunteers. *Exp. Clin. Psychopharmacol.,* 3, 371–381.

Brauer, L. H., and de Wit, H. (1997). High dose pimozide does not block amphetamine-induced euphoria in normal volunteers. *Pharmacol. Biochem. Behav.,* 56, 265–272.

Breivogel, C. S., Childers, S. R., Deadwyler, S. A., Hampson, R. E., Vogt, L. J., and Sim-Selley, L. J. (1999). Chronic Δ^9-tetrahydrocannabinol treatment produces a time-dependent loss of cannabinoid receptors and cannabinoid receptor-activated G proteins in rat brain. *J. Neurochem.,* 73, 2447–2459.

Brody, J. E. "Dietary supplements may test consumers' health." *New York Times,* September 22, 1998, section F, p. 7.

Brooks, J. S., Kessler, R. C., and Cohen, P. (1999). The onset of marijuana use from preadolescence and early adolescence to young adulthood. *Dev. Psychopathol.,* 11, 901–914.

Brower, K. J. (2002). Anabolic steroid abuse and dependence. *Curr. Psychiatr. Rep.,* 4, 377–387.

Brower, K. J., Blow, F. C., Young, J. P., and Hill, E. M. (1991). Symptoms and correlates of anabolic-androgenic steroid dependence. *Br. J. Addict.,* 86, 759–768.

Brower, K. J., Eliopulos, G. A., Blow, F. C., Catlin, D. H., and Beresford, T. P. (1990). Evidence for physical and psychological dependence on anabolic androgenic steroids in eight weight lifters. *Am. J. Psychiatry,* 147, 510–512.

Brown, S.-L., Steinberg, R. L., and van Praag, H. M. (1994). The pathogenesis of depression: Reconsideration of neurotransmitter data. In *Handbook of Depression and Anxiety* (J. A. den Boer and J. M. Ad Sitsen, Eds.), pp. 317–347. Marcel Dekker, New York.

Brown, W. A. (1998). The placebo effect. *Sci. Am.* 278, 90–95.

Browndyke, J. N., Tucker, K. A., Woods, S. P., Beauvals, J., Cohen, R. A., Gottschalk, P. C., and Kosten, T. R. (2004). Examining the effect of cerebral perfusion abnormality magnitude on cognitive performance in recently abstinent chronic cocaine abusers. *J. Neuroimaging,* 14, 162–169.

Bruhn, J. G., De Smet, P. A. G. M., El-Seedi, H. R., and Beck, O. (2002). Mescaline use for 5700 years. *Lancet,* 359, 1866.

Buchsbaum, M. S. (1990). The frontal lobes, basal ganglia, and temporal lobes as sites for schizophrenia. *Schizophr. Bull.,* 16, 379–390.

Buckholtz, N. S., Zhou, D., Freedman, D. X., and Potter, W. Z. (1990). Lysergic acid diethylamide (LSD) administration selectively downregulates serotonin$_2$ receptors in rat brain. *Neuropsychopharmacology,* 3, 137–148.

Budney, A. J., Higgins, S. T., Radonovich, K. J., and Novy, P. L. (2000). Adding voucher-based incentives to coping skills and motivational enhancement improves outcomes during treatment for marijuana dependence. *J. Consult. Clin. Psychol.,* 68, 1051–1061.

Budney, A. J., Moore, B. A., Vandrey, R. G., and Hughes, J. R. (2003). The time course and significance of cannabis withdrawal. *J. Abnorm. Psychol.,* 112, 393–402.

Bunney, B. G., Bunney, W. E., and Carlsson, A. (1995). Schizophrenia and glutamate. In *Psychopharmacology: The Fourth Generation of Progress* (F. E. Bloom and D. J. Kupfer, Eds.), pp. 1205–1214. Raven Press, New York.

Burglass, M. E., and Shaffer, H. (1984). Diagnosis in the addictions I: Conceptual problems. *Adv. Alcohol Subst. Abuse,* 3, 19–34.

Burns, R. S., Chiueh, C. C., Markey, S. P., Ebert, M. H., Jacobowitz, D. M., and Kopin, I. J. (1983). A primate model of parkinsonism: Selective destruction of dopaminergic neurons in the pars compacta of the substantia nigra by *N*-methyl-4-phenyl-1,2,3,6-tetrahydropyridine. *Proc. Natl. Acad. Sci. USA,* 80, 4546–4550.

Byck, R. (Ed.) (1974). *The Cocaine Papers by Sigmund Freud.* Stonehill, New York.

Bzdega, T., Chin, H., Kim, H., HoJung, H., Kozak, C. A., and Klee, W. A. (1993). Regional expression and chromosomal localization of the "delta" opiate receptor gene. *Proc. Natl. Acad. Sci. USA,* 90, 9305–9399.

Cabral, G. A., and Pettit, D. A. D. (1998). Drugs and immunity: Cannabinoids and their role in decreased resistance to infectious disease. *J. Neuroimmunol.,* 83, 116–123.

Caine, S. B., Negus, S. S., Mello, N. K., Patel, S., Bristow, L., Kulagowski, J., Vallone, D., Saiardi, A., and Borrelli, E. (2002). Role of dopamine D2-like receptors in cocaine self-administration: Studies with D2 receptor mutant mice and novel D2 receptor antagonists. *J. Neurosci.,* 22, 2977–2988.

Calabrese, J. R., Bowden, C., and Woyshville, M. J. (1995). Lithium and the anticonvulsants in the treatment of bipolar disorder. In *Psychopharmacology: The Fourth Generation of Progress* (F. E. Bloom and D. J. Kupfer, Eds.), pp. 1099–1111. Raven Press, New York.

Caldecott-Hazard, S., Morgan, D. G., DeLeon-Jones, F., Overstreet, D. H., and Hanowsky, D. (1991). Clinical and biochemical aspects of depressive disorders: II. Transmitter/receptor theories. *Synapse,* 9, 251–301.

Calhoun, S. R., Galloway, G. P., and Smith, D. E. (1998). Abuse potential of dronabinol (Marinol®). *J. Psychoactive Drugs,* 30, 187–196.

Calignano, A., La Rana, G., Giuffrida, A., and Piomelli, D. (1998). Control of pain initiation by endogenous cannabinoids. *Nature,* 394, 277–281.

Campbell, W. G., and Hodgins, D. C. (1993). Alcohol-related blackouts in a medical practice. *Am. J. Drug Alcohol Abuse,* 19, 369–376.

Carai, M. A., Colombo, G., Brunetti, G., Melis, S., Serra, S., Vacca, G., Mastinu, S., Pistuddi, A. M., Solinas, C., Cignarella, G., Minardi, G., and Gessa, G. L. (2001). Role of GABA$_B$ receptors in the sedative/hypnotic effects of γ-hydroxybutyric acid. *Eur. J. Pharmacol.,* 428, 315–321.

Carleton, P. L. (1983). *A Primer of Behavioral Pharmacology.* W. H. Freeman, New York.

Carlezon, W. A., Jr., and Wise, R. A. (1996). Rewarding actions of phencyclidine and related drugs in nucleus accumbens shell and frontal cortex. *J. Neurosci.,* 16, 3112–3122.

Carlsson, A. (2001). A paradigm shift in brain research. *Science,* 294, 1021–1024.

Carlsson, A., Lindqvist, M., and Magnusson, T. (1957). 3,4-Dihydrozypheylalanine and 5-hydroxytryptophan as reserpine antagonists. *Nature,* 180, 1200.

Carrera, M. R. A., Ashley, J. A., Wirsching, P., Koob, G. F., and Janda, K. D. (2001). A second-generation vaccine protects against the psychoactive effects of cocaine. *Proc. Natl. Acad. Sci. U.S.A.,* 98, 1988–1992.

Carroll, C. R. (1996). *Drugs in Modern Society* (4th ed.). Brown and Benchmark, Guilford, CT.

Carroll, M. E., Krattiger, K. L., Gieske, D., and Sadoff, D. A. (1990). Cocaine-base smoking in rhesus monkeys: Reinforcing and physiological effects. *Psychopharmacology, 102,* 443–450.

Carson, R. C., and Sanislow, C. A. (1993). The schizophrenias. In *Comprehensive Handbook of Psychopathology* (P. B. Sutker and H. E. Adams, Eds.), pp. 295–333. Plenum Press, New York.

Carter, L. P., Flores, L. R., Wu, H., Chen, W., Unzeitig, A. W., Coop, A., and France, C. P. (2003). The role of GABA$_B$ receptors in the discriminative stimulus effects of γ-hydroxybutyrate in rats: Time course and antagonism studies. *J. Pharmacol. Exp. Ther., 305,* 668–674.

Carter, R. J., Lione, L. A., Humby, T., Mangiarini, L., Mahal, A., Bates, G. P., Dunnett, S. B., and Morton, A. J. (1999). Characterization of progressive motor deficits in mice transgenic for the human Huntington's disease mutation. *J. Neurosci., 19,* 3248–3257.

Carvey, P. M. (1998). *Drug Action in the Central Nervous System.* Oxford University Press, New York.

Casey, D. E. (1995). Tardive dyskinesia: Pathophysiology. In *Psychopharmacology: The Fourth Generation of Progress* (F. E. Bloom and D. J. Kupfer, Eds.), pp. 1497–1502. Raven Press, New York.

Castagnoli, K., Steyn, S. J., Magnin, G., Van Der Schyf, C. J., Fourie, I., Khalil, A., and Castognoli, N., Jr. (2002). Studies on the interactions of tobacco leaf and tobacco smoke constituents and monoamine oxidase. *Neurotoxicol. Res., 4,* 151–160.

Castañé, A., Valjent, E., Ledent, C., Parmentier, M., Maldonado, R., and Valverde, O. (2002). Lack of CB1 cannabinoid receptors modified nicotine behavioural responses, but not nicotine abstinence. *Neuropharmacology, 43,* 857–867.

Castelli, M. P., Mocci, I., Langlois, X., Gommeren, W., Luyten, W. H. M. L., Leysen, J. E., and Gessa, G. L. (2000). Quantitative autoradiographic distribution of γ-hydroxybutyric acid binding sites in human and monkey brain. *Mol. Brain Res., 78,* 91–99.

Centers for Disease Control and Prevention (2004). Targeting tobacco use: The nation's leading cause of death. http://www.cdc.gov/nccdphp/aag/pdf/aag_osh2004.pdf, accessed 3/25/2004.

Chait, L. D., and Burke, K. A. (1994). Preference for high- versus low-potency marijuana. *Pharmacol. Biochem. Behav., 49,* 643–647.

Chait, L. D., and Zacny, J. P. (1992). Reinforcing and subjective effects of oral Δ⁹-THC and smoked marijuana in humans. *Psychopharmacology, 107,* 255–262.

Charney, D. S., Grillon, C. C. G., and Bremner, J. D. (1998). The neurobiological basis of anxiety and fear: Circuits, mechanisms, and neurochemical interactions (part II). *Neuroscientist, 4,* 122–132.

Charney, D. S., Krystal, J. H., Delgado, P. L., and Heninger, G. R. (1990). Serotonin-specific drugs for anxiety and depressive disorders. *Ann. Rev. Med., 41,* 437–446.

Chausmer, A. L., Elmer, G. I., Rubinstein, M., Low, M. J., Grandy, D. K., and Katz, J. I. (2002). Cocaine-induced locomotor activity and cocaine discrimination in dopamine D2 receptor mutant mice. *Psychopharmacology, 163,* 54–61.

Chen, A. C., Shirayama, Y., Shin, K. H., Neve, R. L., and Duman, R. S. (2001). Expression of the cAMP response element binding protein (CREB) in hippocampus produces an antidepressant effect. *Biol. Psychiatry, 49,* 753–762.

Chen, K., and Kandel, D. B. (1995). The natural history of drug use from adolescence to the mid-thirties in a general population sample. *Am. J. Public Health, 85,* 41–47.

Chermack, S. T., and Giancola, P. R. (1997). The relation between alcohol and aggression: An integrated biopsychosocial conceptualization. *Clin. Psychol. Rev., 17,* 621–649.

Childers, S. R., and Breivogel, C. S. (1998). Cannabis and endogenous cannabinoid systems. *Drug Alcohol Depend., 51,* 173–187.

Childress, A. R., McLellan, T., and O'Brien, C. P. (1986). Abstinent opiate abusers exhibit conditioned craving, conditioned withdrawal and reductions in both through extinction. *Br. J. Addict., 81,* 655–660.

Childress, A. R., Mozley, P. D., McElgin, W., Fitzgerald, J., Reivich, M., and O'Brien, C. P. (1999). Limbic activation during cue-induced cocaine craving. *Am. J. Psychiatry, 156,* 11–18.

Chin, R. L., Sporer, K. A., Cullison, B., Dyer, J. E., and Wu, T. D. (1998). Clinical course of γ-hydroxybutyrate overdose. *Ann. Emerg. Med., 31,* 716–722.

Cloninger, C. R. (1987). Neurogenetic adaptive mechanisms in alcoholism. *Science, 236,* 410–416.

Compton, D. R., Dewey, W. L., and Martin, B. R. (1990). Cannabis dependence and tolerance production. *Adv. Alcohol Subst. Abuse, 9,* 129–147.

Compton, P. A., Ling, W., Charuvastra, V. C., and Wesson, D. R. (1995). Buprenorphine as a pharmacotherapy for cocaine abuse: A review of the evidence. *J. Addictive Dis., 14,* 97–114.

Conquet, F., Bashir, Z. I., Davies, C. H., Daniel, H., Ferraguti, F., Bordi, F., Franz-Bacon, K., Reggiani, A., Matarese, V., Condé, F., Collingridge, G. L., and Crépel, F. (1994). Motor deficit and impairment of synaptic plasticity in mice lacking mGluR1. *Nature, 372,* 237–243.

Cook, C. D., Aceto, M. D., Coop, A., and Beardsley, P. M. (2002). Effects of the putative antagonist NCS382 on the behavioral pharmacological actions of gamma-hydroxybutyrate in mice. *Psychopharmacology, 160,* 99–106.

Cordero-Erausquin, M., Marubio, L. M., Klink, R., and Changeux, J.-P. (2000). Nicotinic receptor function: New perspectives from knockout mice. *Trends Pharmacol. Sci., 21,* 211–217.

Corrigall, W. A., Franklin, K. B., Coen, K. M., and Clarke, P. B. (1992). The mesolimbic dopaminergic system is implicated in the reinforcing effects of nicotine. *Psychopharmacology, 107,* 285–289.

Costa, E., and Guidotti, A. (1991). Diazepam binding inhibitor (DBI): A peptide with multiple biological actions. *Life Sci., 49,* 325–344.

Costa, E., and Guidotti, A. (1996). Benzodiazepines on trial: A research strategy for their rehabilitation. *Trends Pharmacol. Sci., 17,* 192–2000.

Costall, B., and Naylor, R. J. (1991). Anxiolytic effects of 5-H$_3$ antagonists in animals. In *5-HT$_{1A}$ Agonists, 5-HT$_3$ Antagonists and Benzodiazepines: Their Comparative Behavioral Pharmacology* (R. J. Rodgers and S. J. Cooper, Eds.), pp. 133–157. Wiley, New York.

Cotman, C. W., and McGaugh, J. L. (1980). *Behavioral Neuroscience.* Academic Press, New York.

Cottraux, J., Note, I. D., Cungi, C., Legeron, P., Heim, F., et al. (1995). A controlled study of cognitive behaviour therapy with buspirone or placebo in panic disorder with agoraphobia. *Br. J. Psychiatry, 167,* 635–641.

Craig, K., Gomez, H. F., McManus, J. L., and Bania, T. C. (2000). Severe gamma-hydroxybutyrate withdrawal: A case report and literature review. *J. Emerg. Med., 18,* 65–70.

Cravatt, B. F., Demarest, K., Patricelli, M. P., Bracey, M. H., Giang, D. K., Martin, B. R., and Lichtman, A. H. (2001). Supersensitivity to anandamide and enhanced endogenous cannabinoid signaling in mice lacking fatty acid amide hydrolase. *Proc. Natl. Acad. Sci. USA, 98,* 9371–9376.

Crawley, J. N. (1996). Unusual behavioral phenotypes of inbred mouse strains. *Trends Neurosci.,* 19, 181–182.

Creese, I., Burt, D. R., and Snyder, S. H. (1976). Dopamine receptor binding predicts clinical and pharmacological potencies of antischizophrenic drugs. *Science,* 192, 481–483.

Crow, T. J. (1980). Molecular pathology of schizophrenia: More than one disease process? *Br. Med. J.,* 280, 66–68.

Csernansky, J. G., King, R. J., Faustman, W. O., Moses, J. A., Poscher, M. E., and Faull, K. F. (1990). 5-HIAA in cerebrospinal fluid and deficit schizophrenic characteristics. *Br. J. Psychiatry,* 156, 501–507.

Curran, H. V., and Morgan, C. (2000). Cognitive, dissociative and psychotogenic effects of ketamine in recreational users on the night of drug use and 3 days later. *Addiction,* 95, 575–590.

Curran, H. V., Brignell, C., Fletcher, S., Middleton, P., and Henry, J. (2002). Cognitive and subjective dose-response effects of acute oral Δ^9-tetrahydrocannabinol (THC) in infrequent cannabis users. *Psychopharmacology,* 164, 61–70.

Dackis, C. A., and Gold, M. S. (1985). New concepts in cocaine addiction: The dopamine depletion hypothesis. *Neurosci. Biobehav. Rev.,* 9, 469–477.

Dahchour, A., and DeWitte, P. (2000). Ethanol and amino acids in the central nervous system: Assessment of the pharmacological actions of acamprosate. *Prog. Neurobiol.,* 60, 343–362.

Dahlström, A., and Fuxe, K. (1964). Evidence for the existence of monoamine-containing neurons in the central nervous system. I. Demonstration of monoamines in the cell bodies of brainstem neurons. *Acta Physiol. Scand.,* 62 (Suppl. 232), 1–55.

Dalgarno, P. J., and Shewan, D. (1996). Illicit use of ketamine in Scotland. *J. Psychoactive Drugs,* 28, 191–199.

Daly, J. W., and Fredholm, B. B. (1998). Caffeine—an atypical drug of dependence. *Drug Alcohol Depend.,* 51, 199–206.

Damasio, H., Grabowski, T., Frank, R., Galaburga, A. M., et al. (1994). The return of Phineas Gage: Clues about the brain from the skull of a famous patient. *Science,* 264, 1102–1105.

Dambisya, Y. M., and Lee, T. L. (1996). Role of nitric oxide in the induction and expression of morphine tolerance and dependence in mice. *Br. J. Pharmacol.,* 117, 914–918.

Davis, K. L., Kahn, R. S., Ko, G., and Davidson, M. (1991). Dopamine in schizophrenia: A review and reconceptualization. *Am. J. Psychiatry,* 148, 1474–1486.

Davis, M. (1997). Neurobiology of fear responses: The role of the amygdala. *J. Neuropsychiatry Clin. Neurosci.,* 9, 382–402.

Davis, W. (1985). *The Serpent and the Rainbow.* Warner Books, New York.

Davison, G. C. and Neale, J. M. (2001). *Abnormal Psychology.* (8th ed.). John Wiley and Sons, New York.

de Fonseca, F. R., Carrera, M. R. A., Navarro, M., Koob, G. F., and Weiss, F. (1997). Activation of corticotropin-releasing factor in the limbic system during cannabinoid withdrawal. *Science,* 276, 2054.

de Lint, J., and Schmidt, W. (1968). The distribution of alcohol consumption in Ontario. *Q. J. Studies Alcohol,* 29, 968–973.

de Montigny, C. (1981). Enhancement of the 5-HT neurotransmission by antidepressant treatments. *J. Physiol.,* 77, 455–461.

De Vries, T., Homberg, J. R., Binnekade, R., Raasø, H., and Schoffelmeer, A. N. M. (2003). Cannabinoid modulation of the reinforcing and motivational properties of heroin and heroin-associated cues in rats. *Psychopharmacology,* 168, 164–169.

De Vries, T., Shaham, Y., Homberg, J. R., Crombag, H., Schuurman, K., Dieben, J., Vandershuren, L. J. M. J., and Schoffelmeer, A. N. M. (2001). A cannabinoid mechanism in relapse to cocaine seeking. *Nat. Med.,* 7, 1151–1154.

Deitcher, D. L., Ueda, A., Stewart, B. A., Burgess, R. W., Kidokoro, Y., and Schwarz, T. L. (1998). Distinct requirements for evoked and spontaneous release of neurotransmitter are revealed by mutations in the *Drosophila* gene *neuronal-synaptobrevin. J. Neurosci.,* 18, 2028–2039.

Delgado, P. L., Charney, D. S., Price, L. H., Aghajanian, G. K., Landis, H., and Heninger, G. R. (1990). Serotonin function and the mechanism of antidepressant action. *Arch. Gen. Psychiatry,* 47, 411–418.

DeLisi, L. E., Hoff, A. L., Schwartz, J. E., Shields, G. W., Halthore, S. N., Gupta, S. M., Henn, F. A., and Anand, A. K. (1991). Brain morphology in first-episode schizophrenic-like psychotic patients: A quantitative magnetic resonance imaging study. *Biol. Psychiatry,* 29, 159–175.

Deng, S. X., de Prada, P., and Landry, D. W. (2002). Anticocaine catalytic antibodies. *J. Immunol. Methods,* 269, 299–310.

Deroche, V., Piazza, P. V., Casolini, P., Maccari, S., Le Moal, M., and Simon, H. (1992). Stress-induced sensitization to amphetamine and morphine psychomotor effects depend on stress-induced corticosterone secretion. *Brain Res.,* 598, 343–348.

Devane, W. A., Dysarz, F. A., III, Johnson, M. R., Melvin, L. S., and Howlett, A. C. (1988). Determination and characterization of a cannabinoid receptor in rat brain. *Mol. Pharmacol.,* 34, 605–613.

Devane, W. A., Hanus, L., Breuer, A., Pertwee, R. G., Stevenson, L. A., Griffin, G., Gibson, D., Mandelbaum, A., Etinger, A., and Mechoulam, R. (1992). Isolation and structure of a brain constituent that binds to the cannabinoid receptor. *Science,* 258, 1946–1949.

DeWied, D. (1980). Hormonal influences on motivation, learning, memory, and psychosis. In *Neuroendocrinology* (D. T. Krieger and J. C. Hughes, Eds.), pp. 198. Sinauer Associates, Sunderland, MA.

Diamond, I., and Gordon, A. (1997). Cellular and molecular neuroscience of alcoholism. *Physiol. Rev.,* 77, 1–20.

Diana, M., Melis, M., Muntoni, A. L., and Gessa, G. L. (1998). Mesolimbic dopaminergic decline after cannabinoid withdrawal. *Proc. Natl. Acad. Sci. USA,* 95, 10269–10273.

Diana, M., Pistis, M., Carboni, S., Gessa, G. L., and Rossetti, Z. L. (1993). Profound decrement of mesolimbic dopaminergic neuronal activity during ethanol withdrawal syndrome in rats: Electrophysiological and biochemical evidence. *Proc. Natl. Acad. Sci. U.S.A.,* 90, 7966–7969.

Diaz, J. (1997). *How Drugs Influence Behavior.* Prentice-Hall, Upper Saddle River, New Jersey.

DiChiara, G. (1997). Alcohol and dopamine. *Alcohol Health Res. World,* 21, 108–114.

DiChiara, G., and North, R. A. (1992). Neurobiology of opiate abuse. *Trends Pharmacol. Sci.,* 13, 185–193.

Dinwiddie, S. H. (1994). Abuse of inhalants: A review. *Addiction,* 89, 925–939.

Dole, V. P., and Nyswander, M. E. (1965). A medical treatment for diacetylmorphine (heroin) addiction. *JAMA,* 193, 646–650.

Domino, E. F. (2001). Nicotine induced behavioral locomotor sensitization. *Prog. Neuro-Psychopharmacol. Biol. Psychiatry,* 25, 59–71.

Domino, E. F., Chodoff, P., and Corssen, G. (1965). Pharmacologic effects of CI-581, a new dissociative anesthetic, in man. *Clin. Pharmacol. Ther.,* 6, 279–291.

Donovan, J. E., and Jessor, R. (1985). Structure of problem behavior in adolescence and young adulthood. *J. Consult. Clin. Psychol.,* 53, 890–904.

Dougherty, D. D., Bonab, A. A., Spencer, T. J., Rauch, S. L., Madras, B. K., and Fischman, A. J. (1999). Dopamine transporter density in patients with attention deficit hyperactivity disorder. *Lancet,* 354, 2132.

Drago, J., Gerfen, C. R., Lachowicz, J. E., Steiner, H., Hollon, T. R., Love, P. E., Ooi, G. T., Grinberg, A., Lee, E. J., Huang, S. P., Bartlett, P. F., Jose, P. A., Sibley, D. R., and Westphal, H. (1994). Altered striatal function in a mouse mutant lacking D_{1A} dopamine receptors. *Proc. Natl. Acad. Sci. USA,* 91, 12564–12568.

Dresel, S., Krause, J., Krause, K. H., LaFougere, C., Brinkbaumer, K., Kung, H. F., Hahn, K., and Tatsch, K. (2000). Attention deficit hyperactivity disorder: Binding of [99mTc]TRODAT-1 to the dopamine transporter before and after methylphenidate treatment. *Eur. J. Nucl. Med.,* 27, 1518–1524.

Drevets, W. C., Gautier, C., Price, J. C., Kupfer, D. J., Kinahan, P. E., Grace, A. A., Price, J. L., and Mathis, C. A. (2001). Amphetamine-induced dopamine release in human ventral striatum correlates with euphoria. *Biol. Psychiatry,* 49, 81–96.

Drugan, R. C., Basile, A. S., Ha, J. H., and Ferland, R. J. (1994). The protective effects of stress control may be mediated by increased brain levels of benzodiazepine receptor agonists. *Brain Res.,* 661, 127–136.

Duggan, A. W., and Fleetwood-Walker, S. M. (1993). Opioids and sensory processing in the central nervous system. In *Opioids I,* Handbook of Experimental Pharmacology, Vol. 104 (A. Herz, Ed.), pp. 731–771. Springer-Verlag, New York.

Duggan, A. W., Hall, J. G., and Headly, P. M. (1976). Morphine, enkephalin and the substantia gelatinosa. *Nature,* 264, 456–458.

Dulawa, S. C., Grandy, D. K., Low, M. J., Paulus, M. P., and Geyer, M. A. (1999). Dopamine D4 receptor–knock-out mice exhibit reduced exploration of novel stimuli. *J. Neurosci.,* 19, 9550–9556.

Duman, R. S., Malberg, J., and Thome. J. (1999). Neural plasticity to stress and anitdepressant treatment. *Biol. Psychiatry,* 46, 1181–1191.

Dyer, J. E. (1991). γ-Hydroxybutyrate: A health-food product producing coma and seizure-like activity. *Am. J. Emerg. Med.,* 9, 321–324.

Dyer, J. E., Roth, B., and Hyma, B. A. (2001). Gamma-hydroxybutyrate withdrawal syndrome. *Ann. Emerg. Med.,* 37, 147–153.

Enoch, M.-A., and Goldman, D. (1999). Genetics of alcoholism and substance abuse. *Psychiatr. Clin. North Am.,* 22, 289–299.

Epping-Jordan, M. P., Watkins, S. S., Koob, G. F., and Markou, A. (1998). Dramatic decreases in brain reward function during nicotine withdrawal. *Nature,* 393, 76–79.

Erb, S., Shaham, Y., and Stewart, J. (1996). Stress reinstates cocaine-seeking behavior after prolonged extinction and a drug-free period. *Psychopharmacology,* 128, 408–412.

Erb, S., Shaham, Y., and Stewart, J. (1998). The role of corticotropin-releasing factor and corticosterone in stress- and cocaine-induced relapse to cocaine seeking in rats. *J. Neurosci.,* 18, 5529–5536.

Esposito, R. U., Porrino, L. J., and Seeger, T. F. (1989). Brain stimulation reward measurement and mapping by psychophysical techniques and quantitative 2-(^{14}C)deoxyglucose autoradiography. In *Methods of Assessing the Reinforcing Properties of Abused Drugs* (M. A. Bozartth, Ed.), pp. 421–447. Springer-Verlag, New York.

Evans, A. C., and Raistrick, D. (1987). Phenomenology of intoxication with toluene-based adhesives and butane gas. *Br. J. Psychiatry,* 150, 769–773.

Evans, C. J., Keith, D. E., Jr., Morrison, H., Magendzo, K., and Edwards, R. H. (1992). Cloning of a delta opioid receptor by functional expression. *Science,* 258, 1952–1955.

Evans, D. A. P., Manley, K. A., and McKusick, V. C. (1996). Genetic control of isoniazid metabolism. *Br. Med. J.,* 2, 485–491.

Fà, M., Carcangiu, G., Passino, N., Ghiglieri, V., Gessa, G. L., and Mereu, G. (2000). Cigarette smoke inhalation stimulates dopaminergic neurons in rats. *NeuroReport,* 11, 3637–3639.

Fadda, F., and Rossetti, Z. (1998). Chronic ethanol consumption: From neuroadaptation to neurodegeneration. *Prog. Neurobiol.,* 56, 385–431.

Farde, L. (1996). The advantage of using positron emission tomography in drug research. *Trends Neurosci.,* 19, 211–214.

Farde, L., Nordstrom, A.-L., Wiesel, F.-A., Pauli, S., Halldin, C., and Sedvall, G. (1992). Positron emission tomographic analysis of central D_1 and D_2 dopamine receptor occupancy in patients treated with classical neuroleptics and clozapine. *Arch. Gen. Psychiatry,* 49, 538–544.

Farkas, G., and Rosen, R. C. (1976). The effects of ethanol on male sexual arousal. *J. Stud. Alcohol,* 37, 265–272.

Fattore, L., Cossu, G., Martellotta, C. M., and Fratta, W. (2001). Intravenous self-administration of the cannabinoid CB1 receptor agonist WIN 55,212-2 in rats. *Psychopharmacology,* 156, 410–416.

Faulkner, J. M. (1933). Nicotine poisoning by absorption through the skin. *JAMA,* 100, 1664–1665.

Felder, C. C., and Glass, M. (1998). Cannabinoid receptors and their endogenous agonists. *Annu. Rev. Pharmacol.,* 38, 179–200.

Fergusson, D. M., Horwood, L. J., and Beautrais, A. L. (2003a). Cannabis and educational achievement. *Addiction,* 98, 1681–1692.

Fergusson, D. M., Horwood, L. J., Lynskey, M. T., and Madden, P. A. F. (2003b). Early reactions to cannabis predict later dependence. *Arch. Gen. Psychiatry,* 60, 1033–1039.

Fernstrom, J. D., and Wurtman, R. J. (1972). Brain serotonin content: Physiological regulation by plasma neutral amino acids. *Science,* 178, 149–152.

Ferrara, S. D., Giorgetti, R., Zamcaner, S., Orlando, R., Tagliabracci, A., Cavarzeran, F., and Palatini, P. (1999). Effects of single dose of gamma-hydroxybutyric acid and lorazepam on psychomotor performance and subjective feelings in healthy volunteers. *Eur. J. Clin. Pharmacol.,* 54, 821–827.

Ferrarese, C., Alho, H., Guidotti, A., and Costa, E. (1987). Co-localization and co-release of GABA and putative allosteric modulators of GABA receptor. *Neuropharmacology,* 26, 1011–1018.

Ferrero, P., Conti-Tronconi, B., and Guidotti, A. (1986a). DBI, an anxiogenic neuropeptide found in human brain. In *GABAergic Transmission and Anxiety* (G. Biggio and E. Costa, Eds.), pp. 177–185. Raven Press, New York.

Ferrero, P., Santi, M. R., Conti-Tronconi, B., Costa, E., and Guidotti, A. (1986b). Study of an octadecaneuropeptide derived from diazepam binding inhibitor (DBI): Biological activity and presence in rat brain. *Proc. Natl. Acad. Sci. U.S.A.,* 83, 827–831.

Fibiger, H. C., Phillips, A. G., and Brown, E. E. (1992). The neurobiology of cocaine-induced reinforcement. *Ciba Found. Symp.,* 166, 96–111.

Fingerhood, M. I., Sullivan, J. T., Testa, M., and Jasinski, D. R. (1997). Abuse liability of testosterone. *J. Psychopharmacol.,* 11, 59–63.

Fink, M. (1987). Convulsive therapy in affective disorders: A decade of understanding and acceptance. In *Psychopharmacology: The Third Generation of Progress* (H. Y. Meltzer, Ed.), pp. 1077–1083. Raven Press, New York.

Finney, J. W., Hahn, A. C., and Moos, R. H. (1996). The effectiveness of inpatient and outpatient treatment for alcohol abuse:

The need to focus on mediators and moderators of setting effects. *Addiction,* 91, 1773–1796.

Fischer, C. A., Hatzidimitriou, G., Katz, J. L., and Ricaurte, G. A. (1995). Reorganization of ascending serotonin axon projections in animals previously exposed to the recreational drug 3,4-methylenedioxymethamphetamine. *J. Neurosci.,* 15, 5476–5485.

Fischer, M., Kaech, S., Knutti, D., and Matus, A. (1998). Rapid actin-based plasticity in dendritic spines. *Neuron,* 20, 847–854.

Fischman, A. J., Bonab, A. A., Babich, J. W., Palmer, E. P., Alpert, N. M., Elmaleh, D. R., Callahan, R. J., Barrow, S. A., Graham, W., Meltzer, P. C., Hanson, R. N., and Madras, B. K. (1998). Rapid detection of Parkinson's disease by SPECT with altropane: A selective ligand for dopamine transporters. *Synapse,* 29, 128–141.

Foltin, R. W., Fischman, M. W., and Byrne, M. F. (1988). Effects of smoked marijuana on food intake and body weight of humans living in a residential laboratory. *Appetite,* 11, 1–14.

Fonnum, F. (1987). Biochemistry, anatomy, and pharmacology of GABA neurons. In *Psychopharmacology: The Third Generation of Progress* (H. Y. Meltzer, Ed.), pp. 173–182. Raven Press, New York.

Foulds, J., Stapleton, J. A., Bell, N., Swettenham, J., Jarvis, M. J., and Russell, M. A. H. (1997). Mood and physiological effects of subcutaneous nicotine in smokers and never-smokers. *Drug Alcohol Depend.,* 44, 105–115.

Foulds, J., Stapleton, J., Swettenham, J., Bell, N., McSorley, K., and Russell, M. A. H. (1996). Cognitive performance effects of subcutaneous nicotine in smokers and never-smokers. *Psychopharmacology,* 127, 31–38.

Fowler, J. S., Logan, J., Wang, G. J., and Volkow, N. D. (2003a). Monoamine oxidase and cigarette smoking. *Neurotoxicology,* 24, 75–82.

Fowler, J. S., Logan, J., Wang, G. J., Volkow, N. D., Telang, F., Zhu, W., Franceschi, D., Pappas, N., Ferrieri, R., Shea, C., Garza, V., Xu, Y., Schlyer, D., Gatley, S. J., Ding, Y. S., Alexoff, D., Warner, D., Netusil, N., Carter, P., Jayne, M., King, P., and Vaska, P. (2003b). Low monoamine oxidase B in peripheral organs in smokers. *Proc. Natl. Acad. Sci. USA,* 100, 11600–11605.

Fowler, J. S., Wang, G.-J., Volkow, N. D., Franceschi, D., Logan, J., Pappas, N., Shea, C., MacGregor, R. R., and Garza, V. (1999). Smoking a single cigarette does not produce a measurable reduction in brain MAO B in non-smokers. *Nicotine Tobacco Res.,* 1, 325–329.

Francis, D. D., Caldji, C., Champagne, F., Plotsky, P. M., and Meaney, M. J. (1999). The role of corticotropin-releasing factor–norepinephrine systems in mediating the effects of early experience on the development of behavioral and endocrine responses to stress. *Biol. Psychiatry,* 46, 1153–1166.

Franke, W. W., and Berendonk, B. (1997). Hormonal doping and androgenization of athletes: A secret program of the German Democratic Republic government. *Clin. Chem.,* 43, 1262–1279.

Franklin, T. R., Acton, P. D., Maldjian, J. A., Gray, J. D., Croft, J. R., Dackis, C. A., O'Brien, C. P., and Childress, A. R. (2002). Decreased gray matter concentration in the insular, orbitofrontal, cingulate, and temporal cortices of cocaine patients. *Biol. Psychiatry,* 51, 134–142.

Freeza, M., Padova, C., Terpin, M., Baranona, E., and Lieber, C. (1990). High blood alcohol levels in women. The role of decreased gastric alcohol dehydrogenase activity and first-pass metabolism. *New Engl. J. Med.,* 322, 95–99.

Fremeau, R. T., Jr., Toyer, M. D., Pahner, I., Nygaard, G. O., Tran, C. H., Reimer, R. J., Bellocchio, E. E., Fortin, D., Storm-Mathisen, J., and Edwards, R. H. (2001). The expression of vesicular glutamate transporters defines two classes of excitatory synapse. *Neuron,* 31, 247–260.

Friedhoff, A. J., and Silva, R. R. (1995). The effects of neuroleptics on plasma homovanillic acid. In *Psychopharmacology: The Fourth Generation of Progress* (F. E. Bloom and D. J. Kupfer, Eds.), pp. 1229–1234. Raven Press, New York.

Friedman, A., Kaufer, D., Shemer, J., Hendler, I., Soreq, H., Tur-Kaspa, I. (1996). Pyridostigmine brain penetration under stress enhances neuronal excitability and induces early immediate transcriptional response. *Nat. Med.,* 2, 1382–1385.

Friedman, J., Westlake, R., and Furman, M. (1996). "Grievous bodily harm": Gamma-hydroxybutyrate abuse leading to Wernicke-Korsakoff syndrome. *Neurology,* 46, 469–471.

Froelich, J. C. (1997). Opioid peptides. *Alcohol Health Res. World,* 21, 132–143.

Frye, C. A., Park, D., Tanaka, M., Rosellini, R., and Svare, B. (2001). The testosterone metabolite and neurosteroid 3α-androstanediol may mediate the effects of testosterone on conditioned place preference. *Psychoneuroendocrinology,* 26, 731–750.

Frye, C. A., Rhodes, M. E., Rosellini, R., and Svare, B. (2002). The nucleus accumbens as a site of action for rewarding properties of testosterone and its 5α-reduced metabolites. *Pharmacol. Biochem. Behav.,* 74, 119–127.

Fuller, R. K., and Hiller-Sturmhofel, S. (1999). Alcoholism treatment in the United States. *Alcohol Health Res. World,* 23, 69–77.

Funada, M., Sato, M., Makino, Y., and Wada, K. (2002). Evaluation of rewarding effect of toluene by the conditioned place preference procedure in mice. *Brain Res. Protocols,* 10, 47–54.

Fuxe, K., Agnati, L. F., Kalia, M., Goldstein, M., Andersson, K., and Häfstrand, A. (1985). Dopaminergic systems in the brain and pituitary. In *Basic and Clinical Aspects of Neuroscience: The Dopaminergic System* (E. Flückiger, E. E. Müller, and M. O. Thorner, Eds.), pp. 11–25. Springer-Verlag, Berlin.

Galloway, G. P., Frederick, S. L., Staggers, F. E., Jr., Gonzales, M., Stalcup, S. A., and Smith, D. E. (1997). Gamma-hydroxybutyrate: An emerging drug of abuse that causes physical dependence. *Addiction,* 92, 89–96.

Garbutt, J. C., West, S. L., Carey, T. S., Lohr, K. N., and Crews, F. T. (1999). Pharmacological treatment of alcohol dependence: A review of the evidence. *JAMA,* 281, 1318–1325.

Garrett, B. E., and Griffiths, R. R. (1998). Physical dependence increases the relative reinforcing effects of caffeine versus placebo. *Psychopharmacology,* 139, 195–202.

Garris, P. A., Kilpatrick, M., Bunin, M. A., Michael, D., Walker, Q. D., and Wightman, R. M. (1999). Dissociation of dopamine release in the nucleus accumbens from intracranial self-stimulation. *Nature,* 398, 67–69.

Gavaghan, H. (1994). NIH panel rejects Persian Gulf Syndrome. *Nature,* 369, 8.

Gawin, F. H., and Kleber, H. D. (1986). Abstinence symptomatology and psychiatric diagnosis in cocaine abusers. Clinical observations. *Arch. Gen. Psychiatry,* 43, 107–113.

Gawin, F. H., and Kleber, H. D. (1988). Evolving conceptualizations of cocaine dependence. *Yale J. Biol. Med.,* 61, 123–136.

Gaziano, J. M., and Hennekens, C. (1995). Moderate alcohol intake, increased levels of high density lipoprotein and its subfractions, and decreased risk of myocardial infarction. *New Engl. J. Med.,* 329, 1829–1834.

Gehlbach, S. H., Williams, W. A., Perry, L. D., and Woodall, J. S. (1974). Green-tobacco sickness. An illness of tobacco harvesters. *JAMA,* 229, 1880–1883.

George, M. S., Nahas, Z., Molloy, M., Speer, A. M., Oliver, N. C., Li, X.-B., Arana, G. W., Risch, S. C., and Ballenger, J. C. (2000). A controlled trial of daily left prefrontal cortex TMS for treating depression. *Biol. Psychiatry,* 48, 962–970.

George, T. P., and O'Malley, S. S. (2004). Current pharmacological treatments for nicotine dependence. *Trends Pharmacol. Sci.,* 25, 42–48.

George, W. H., and Norris, J. (1991). Alcohol, disinhibition, sexual arousal, and deviant sexual behavior. *Alcohol Health Res. World,* 15, 133–138.

Gerasimov, M. R., Ferrieri, R. A., Schiffer, W. K., Logan, J., Gatley, S. J., Gifford, A. N., Alexoff, D. A., Marsteller, D. A., Shea, C., Garza, W., Carter, P., King, P., Ashby, C. R., Jr., Vitkun, S., and Dewey, S. L. (2002). Study of brain uptake and biodistribution of [^{11}C]toluene in non-human primates and mice. *Life Sci.,* 70, 2811–2828.

Gerlach, J. (1991). New antipsychotics: Classification, efficacy, and adverse effects. *Schizophr. Bull.,* 17, 289–309.

Gerlai, R. (1996). Gene-targeting studies of mammalian behavior: Is it the mutation or the background genotype? *Trends Neurosci.,* 19, 177–181.

Gerra, G., Zaimovic, A., Ferri, M., Zambelli, U., Timpano, M., Neri, E., Marzocchi, G. F., Delsignore, R., and Brambilla, F. (2000). Long-lasting effects of (±)3,4-methylene-dioxymethamphetamine (Ecstasy) on serotonin system function in humans. *Biol. Psychiatry,* 47, 127–136.

Gerrits, M., and Vanree, J. (1996). Effects of nucleus accumbens dopamine depletion on motivational aspects involved in initiation of cocaine and heroin self-administration in rats. *Brain Res.,* 713, 114–124.

Ghozland, S., Matthes, H. W. D., Simonin, F., Filliol, D., Kieffer, B. L., and Maldonado, R. (2002). Motivational effects of cannabinoids are mediated by μ-opioid and κ-opioid receptors. *J. Neurosci.,* 22, 1146–1154.

Gibbons, B. (1992). Alcohol: The legal drug. *National Geographic,* 181 (2), 3–35.

Giros, B., Jaber, M., Jones, S. R., Wightman, R. M., and Caron, M. G. (1996). Hyperlocomotion and indifference to cocaine and amphetamine in mice lacking the dopamine transporter. *Nature,* 379, 606–612.

Glazer, W. M., Morgenstern, H., and Doucette, J. T. (1993). Predicting the long-term risk of tardive dyskinesia in outpatients maintained on neuroleptic medications. *J. Clin. Psychiatry,* 54, 133–139.

Goeders, N. E., and Smith, J. E. (1983). Cortical dopaminergic involvement in cocaine reinforcement. *Science,* 221, 773–775.

Gold, L. H., Geyer, M. A., and Koob, G. F. (1989). Neurochemical mechanisms involved in behavioral effects of amphetamines and related designer drugs. *NIDA Res. Monogr.,* 104, 101–126.

Gold, M. S. (1989). Opiates. In *Drugs of Abuse* (A. J. Giannini and A. E. Slaby, Eds.), pp. 127–145. Medical Economics Books, Oradell, New Jersey.

Goldman-Rakic, P. S. (1987). Circuitry of the prefrontal cortex and the regulation of behavior by representational memory. In *Handbook of Physiology,* Section 1, The Nervous System, Vol. 5, Higher Functions of the Brain, Part I (F. Plum, Ed.), pp. 373–417. American Physiological Society, Bethesda, MD.

Goldstein, A. (1989). *Molecular and Cellular Aspects of the Drug Addictions.* Springer-Verlag, New York.

Goldstein, D. B. (1972). Relationship of alcohol dose to intensity of withdrawal signs in mice. *J. Pharmacol. Exp. Ther.,* 180, 203–210.

Goldstein, M. (1987). Psychosocial issues. *Schizophr. Bull.,* 13, 171–186.

Goldstein, M. J. (1995). Psychoeducation and relapse prevention. An update. In *Critical Issues in the Treatment of Schizophrenia*

(N. Brunello, G. Racagni, S. Z. Langer, and J. Mendlewicz, Eds.), pp. 134–141. Karger, New York.

Golub, A., and Johnson, B. D. (1994). The shifting importance of alcohol and marijuana as gateway substances among serious drug abusers. *J. Stud. Alcohol,* 55, 607–614.

Goode, E. (1993). *Drugs in American Society.* McGraw-Hill, New York.

Gordis, E. (1991). *Alcohol Research: Promise for the Decade.* NIAAA, Rockville, MD.

Gottesman, I. I. (1991). *Schizophrenia Genesis.* W. H. Freeman, New York.

Goudie, A. J., and Leathley, M. J. (1993). Drug discrimination assays. In *Behavioural Neuroscience: A Practical Approach,* Vol. 2 (A. Sahgal, Ed.), pp. 145–168. Oxford University Press, New York.

Gourlay, S. G., and Benowitz, N. L. (1997). Arteriovenous differences in plasma concentration of nicotine and catecholamines and related cardiovascular effects after smoking, nicotine nasal spray, and intravenous nicotine. *Clin. Pharmacol. Ther.,* 62, 453–463.

Grace, A. A. (1992). The depolarization block hypothesis of neuroleptic action: Implications for the etiology and treatment of schizophrenia. *J. Neural Transm.,* 36 (Suppl.), 91–131.

Gray, H. (1966). *Anatomy of the Human Body* (28th ed.). Lea and Febiger, Philadelphia.

Green, B., Kavanagh, D., and Young, R. (2003). Being stoned: A review of self-reported cannabis effects. *Drug Alcohol Rev.,* 22, 453–460.

Greer, G., and Tolbert, R. (1986). Subjective reports of the effects of MDMA in a clinical setting. *J. Psychoactive Drugs,* 18, 319–327.

Griesar, W. S., Zajdel, D. P., and Oken, B. S. (2002). Nicotine effects on alertness and spatial attention in non-smokers. *Nicotine Tobacco Res.,* 4, 185–194.

Griffiths, R. R., and Mumford, G. K. (1995). Caffeine: A drug of abuse? In *Psychopharmacology: The Fourth Generation of Progress* (F. E. Bloom and D. J. Kupfer, Eds.), pp. 1699–1713. Raven Press, New York.

Griffiths, R. R., Evans, S. M., Heishman, S. J., Preston, K. L., Sannerud, C. A., Wolf, B., and Woodson, P. P. (1990). Low-dose caffeine physical dependence in humans. *J. Pharmacol. Exp. Ther.,* 255, 1123–1132.

Griffiths, R. R., Lamb, R. J., Sannerud, C. A., Ator, N., and Brady, J. V. (1991). Self-injection of barbiturates and benzodiazepines. *Psychopharmacology,* 103, 154–161.

Grilly, D. M. (1998). *Drugs and Human Behavior.* (3rd ed.) Allyn and Bacon, Boston.

Grilly, D. M. (2002). *Drugs and Human Behavior.* (4th ed.) Allyn and Bacon, Boston.

Grobin, A. C., Matthews, D. B., Devaud, L. L., and Morrow, A. L. (1998). The role of GABA$_A$ receptors in the acute and chronic effects of ethanol. *Psychopharmacology,* 139, 2–19.

Gruber, A. J., and Pope, H. G., Jr. (2002). Marijuana use among adolescents. *Pediatr. Clin. North Am.,* 49, 389–413.

Grunhaus, L., Dannon, P. N., Schreiber, S., Dolberg, O. H., Amiaz, R., Ziv, R., and Lefkifker, E. (2000). Repetitive transcranial magnetic stimulation is as effective as electroconvulsive therapy in the treatment of nondelusional major depressive disorder: An open study. *Biol. Psychiatry,* 47, 314–324.

Guay, D. R. (1995). The emerging role of valproate in bipolar disorder and other psychiatric disorders. *Pharmacotherapy,* 15, 631–647.

Guidotti, A., Forchetti, C. M., Corda, M. G., Konkel, D., Bennett, C. D., and Costa, E. (1983). Isolation, characterization, and purification to homogeneity of an endogenous polypeptide with agonistic action on benzodiazepine receptors. *Proc. Natl. Acad. Sci. U.S.A.,* 80, 3531–3535.

Gur, R. E. (1995). Functional brain-imaging studies in schizophrenia. In *Psychopharmacology: The Fourth Generation of Progress* (F. E. Bloom and D. J. Kupfer, Eds.), pp. 1185–1192. Raven Press, New York.

Haley, R. W., Hom, J., Roland, P. S., Bryan, W. W., Van Ness, P. C., Bonte, F. J., Devous, M. D., Sr., Mathews, D., Fleckenstein, J. L., Wians, F. H., Jr., Wolfe, G. I., and Kurt, T. L. (1997). Evaluation of neurological function in Gulf War veterans. A blinded case-control study. *JAMA,* 277, 223–230.

Halpern, J. H., and Pope, H. G., Jr. (2003). Hallucinogen persisting perception disorder: What do we know after 50 years? *Drug Alcohol Depend.,* 69, 109–119.

Hamilton, L. W., and Timmons, C. R. (1990). *Principles of Behavioral Pharmacology: A Biopsychological Perspective.* Prentice-Hall, Englewood, New Jersey.

Haney, M., Bisaga, A., and Foltin, R. W. (2003). Interaction between naltrexone and oral THC in heavy marijuana smokers. *Psychopharmacology,* 166, 77–85.

Haney, M., Hart, C. L., Vosburg, S. K., Nasser, J., Bennett, A., Zubaran, C., and Foltin, R. W. (2004). Marijuana withdrawal in humans: Effects of oral THC or divalproex. *Neuropsychopharmacology,* 29, 158–170.

Haney, M., Ward, A. S., Foltin, R. W., and Fischman, M. W. (2001). Effects of ecopipam, a selective D1 antagonist, on smoked cocaine self-administration by humans. *Psychopharmacology,* 155, 330–337.

Hardy, J., and Selkoe, D. J. (2002). The amyloid hypothesis of Alzheimer's disease: Progress and problems on the road to therapeutics. *Science,* 297, 353–356.

Harney, J., Scarbrough, K., Rosewell, K. L., and Wise, P. M. (1996). In vivo antisense antagonism of vasoactive intestinal peptide in the suprachiasmatic nuclei causes aging-like changes in the estradiol-induced luteinizing hormone and prolactin surges. *Endocrinology,* 137, 3696–3701.

Hart, C. L., van Gorp, W., Haney, M., Foltin, R. W., and Fischman, M. W. (2001). Effects of acute smoked marijuana on complex cognitive performance. *Neuropsychopharmacology,* 25, 757–765.

Harvey, D. M., Yasar, S., Heishman, S. J., Panlilio, L. V., Henningfield, J. E., and Goldberg, S. R. (2004). Nicotine serves as an effective reinforcer of intravenous drug-taking behavior in human cigarette smokers. *Psychopharmacology,* 175, 134–142.

Harvey, K. V., and Balon, R. (1995). Augmentation with buspirone: A review. *Ann. Clin. Psychiatry,* 7, 143–147.

Hatzidimitriou, G., McCann, U. D., and Ricaurte, G. A. (1999). Altered serotonin innervation patterns in the forebrain of monkeys treated with (±)3,4-methylenedioxymethamphetamine seven years previously: Factors influencing abnormal recovery. *J. Neurosci.,* 19, 5096–5107.

Hechler, V., Ratomponirina, C., and Maitre, M. (1997). γ-Hydroxybutyrate conversion into GABA induces displacement of $GABA_B$ binding that is blocked by valproate and ethosuximide. *J. Pharmacol. Exp. Ther.,* 281, 753–760.

Hechler, V., Weissmann, D., Mach, E., Pujol, J.-F., and Maitre, M. (1987). Regional distribution of high-affinity γ-[^{3}H]hydroxybutyrate binding sites as determined by quantitative autoradiography. *J. Neurochem.,* 49, 1025–1032.

Heisler, L. K., Chu, H.-M., Brennan, T. J., Danao, J. A., Bajwa, P., Parsons, L. H., and Tecott, L. H. (1998). Elevated anxiety and antidepressant-like responses in serotonin $5-HT_{1A}$ receptor mutant mice. *Proc. Natl. Acad. Sci. USA,* 95, 15049–15054.

Helton, D. R., Modlin, D. L., Tizzano, J. P., and Rasmussen, K. (1993). Nicotine withdrawal: A behavioral assessment using schedule controlled responding, locomotor activity, and sensorimotor reactivity. *Psychopharmacology,* 113, 205–210.

Hendershott, J. (1969). Steroids: Breakfast of champions. *Track and Field News,* I April, 3.

Heninger, G. R., Delgado, P. L., and Charney, D. S. (1996). The revised monoamine theory of depression: A modulatory role for monoamines, based on new findings from monoamine depletion experiments in humans. *Pharmacopsychiatry,* 29, 2–11.

Hering-Hanit, R., and Gadoth, N. (2003). Caffeine-induced headache in children and adolescents. *Cephalagia,* 23, 332–335.

Herz, A. (1997). Endogenous opioid systems and alcohol addiction. *Psychopharmacology,* 129, 99–111.

Hidalgo, R. B., and Davidson, J. R. T. (2000). Selective serotonin reuptake inhibitors in post-traumatic stress disorder. *J. Psychopharmacol.,* 14, 70–76.

Higgins, S. T., Budney, A. J., and Bickel, W. K. (1994). Applying behavioral concepts and principles to the treatment of cocaine dependence. *Drug Alcohol Depend.,* 34, 87–97.

Hildebrand, B. E., Nomikos, G. G., Bondjers, C., Nisell, M., and Svensson, T. H. (1997). Behavioral manifestations of the nicotine abstinence syndrome in the rat: Peripheral versus central mechanisms. *Psychopharmacology,* 129, 348–356.

Hildebrand, B. E., Nomikos, G. G., Hertel, P., Schilström, B., and Svensson, T. H. (1998). Reduced dopamine output in the nucleus accumbens but not in the medial prefrontal cortex in rats displaying a mecamylamine-precipitated nicotine withdrawal syndrome. *Brain Res.,* 779, 214–225.

Hildebrand, B. E., Panagis, G., Svensson, T. H., and Nomikos, G. G. (1999). Behavioral and biochemical manifestations of mecamylamine-precipitated nicotine withdrawal in the rat: Role of nicotinic receptors in the ventral tegmental area. *Neuropsychopharmacology,* 21, 560–574.

Hilts, P. J. "Is nicotine addictive? It depends on whose criteria you use." *New York Times,* August 2, 1994, section C, p. 3.

Himmelsbach, C. K. (1943). Can the euphoric, analgesic and physical dependence effects of drugs be separated? With reference to physical dependence. *Fed. Proc.,* 2, 201–203.

Hobbs, W. R., Rall, T. W., and Verdoorn, T. A. (1996). Hypnotics and sedatives: Ethanol. In *The Pharmacological Basis of Therapeutics* (A. G. Gilman, L. S. Goodman, J. G. Hardman, L. E. Limbird, P. B. Molinoff, and R. W. Rudon, Eds.), pp. 361–396. McGraw-Hill, New York.

Hoebel, B. G., Monaco, A. P., Hernandez, L., Aulisi, E. F., Stanley, B. G., and Lenard, L. (1983). Self-injection of amphetamine directly into the brain. *Psychopharmacology,* 81, 158–163.

Hoffman, A. (1979). How LSD originated. *J. Psychoactive Drugs,* 11, 53–60.

Hollinger, M. A. (1995). The criminalization of drug use in the United States. A brief historical perspective. *Res. Commun. Alcohol Subst. Abuse,* 16, 1–23.

Hollinger, M. A. (1997). *Introduction to Pharmacology.* Taylor and Francis, Washington.

Hollon, T. R., Bek, M. J., Lachowicz, J. E., Ariano, M. A., Mezey, E., Ramachandran, R., Wersinger, S. R., Soares-da-Silva, P., Liu, Z. F., Grinberg, A., Drago, J., Young, W. S., III, Westphal, H., Jose, P. A., and Sibley, D. R. (2002). Mice lacking D_5 dopamine receptors have increased sympathetic tone and are hypertensive. *J. Neurosci.,* 22, 10801–10810.

Howard, R., Castle, D., Wessely, S., and Murray, R. (1993). A comparative study of 470 cases of early-onset and late-onset schizophrenia. *Br. J. Psychiatry,* 163, 352–357.

Huestis, M. A., Gorelick, D. A., Heishman, S. J., Preston, K. L., Nelson, R. A., Moolchan, E. T., and Frank, R. A. (2001). Blockade of effects of smoked marijuana by the CB1-selective cannabinoid receptor antagonist SR141716. *Arch. Gen. Psychiatry, 58,* 322–328.

Hughes, J. (1975). Search for the endogenous ligand of the opiate receptor. *Neurosci. Res. Prog. Bull., 13,* 55–58.

Hughes, J. R., Gust, S. W., Skoog, K., Keenan, R. M., and Fenwick, J. W. (1991). Symptoms of tobacco withdrawal. A replication and extension. *Arch. Gen. Psychiatry, 48,* 52–59.

Hunt, G. M., and Azrin, N. H. (1973). A community-reinforcement approach to alcoholism. *Behav. Res. Ther., 11,* 91–104.

Ichise, T., Kano, M., Hashimoto, K., Yanagihara, D., Nakao, K., Shigemoto, R., Katsuki, M., and Aiba, A. (2000). mGluR1 in cerebellar Purkinje cells essential for long-term depression, synapse elimination, and motor coordination. *Science, 288,* 1832–1835.

Ikonomidou, C., Bittigau, P., Ishimaru, M., Wozniak, D., Koch, C., Genz, K., Price, M., Stefovska, V., Tenkova, T., Dikranian, K., and Olney, J. (2000). Ethanol-induced apoptotic neurodegeneration and fetal alcohol syndrome. *Science, 287,* 1056–1060.

Inada, T., Polk, K., Purser, C., Hume, A., Hoskins, B., Ho, I. K., and Rockhold, R. W. (1992). Behavioral and neurochemical effects of continuous infusion of cocaine in rats. *Neuropharmacology, 31,* 701–708.

International Assembly of NCSS (2004). *IA Update Newsletter, 3,* 2.

Inturrisi, C. E. (1997). Preclinical evidence for a role of glutamatergic systems in opioid tolerance and dependence. *Semin. Neurosci., 9,* 110–119.

Itzhak, Y. (1997). Modulation of cocaine- and methamphetamine-induced behavioral sensitization by inhibition of brain nitric oxide synthase. *J. Pharmacol. Exp. Ther., 282,* 521–527.

Itzhak, Y., Ali, S. F., Martin, J. L., Black, M. D., and Huang, P. L. (1998). Resistance of neuronal nitric oxide synthase-deficient mice to cocaine-induced locomotor sensitization. *Psychopharmacology, 140,* 378–386.

Itzhak, Y., and Ali, S. F. (2002). Repeated administration of gamma-hydroxybutyric acid (GHB) to mice. Assessment of the sedative and rewarding effects of GHB. *Ann. N. Y. Acad. Sci., 965,* 451–460.

Iversen, L. (2003). Cannabis and the brain. *Brain, 126,* 1252–1270.

Iversen, L. L. (2000). *The Science of Marijuana.* Oxford University Press, New York.

Jacobs, B. L., and Fornal, C. A. (1993). 5-HT and motor control. *Trends Neurosci., 16,* 346–352.

Jacobs, E. H., Smith, A. B., de Vries, T. J., and Schoffelmeer, A. N. M. (2003). Neuroadaptive effects of active versus passive drug administration in addiction research. *Trends Pharmacol. Sci., 24,* 566–573.

Jacobs, I. G., Roszler, M. H., Kelly, J. K., Klein, M. A., and Kling, G. A. (1989). Cocaine abuse: Neurovascular complications. *Radiology, 170,* 223–227.

Jacobs, M. J., Zigmond, M. J., Finlay, J. M., and Sved, A. F. (1995). Neurochemical studies of central noradrenergic responses to acute and chronic stress. In *Neurobiological and Clinical Consequences of Stress: From Normal Adaptation to PTSD* (M. J. Friedman, D. S. Charney, and A. Y. Deutch, Eds.), pp. 45–60. Lippincott-Raven, Philadelphia.

Jacobson, S. (1972). Neurocytology. In *An Introduction to the Neurosciences* (B. A. Curtis, S. Jacobson, and E. M. Marcus, Eds.), pp. 36–71. Saunders, Philadelphia.

James, J. E. (2004). Critical review of dietary caffeine and blood pressure: A relationship that should be taken more seriously. *Psychosom. Med., 66,* 63–71.

Jansen, K. L. R. (2000). A review of the nonmedical use of ketamine: Use, users and consequences. *J. Psychoactive Drugs, 32,* 419–433.

Jansen, K. L. R. (2001). *Ketamine: Dreams and Realities.* Multidisciplinary Association for Psychedelic Studies, Sarasota, Florida.

Jansen, K. L. R., and Darracot-Cankovic, R. (2001). The nonmedical use of ketamine, part two: A review of problem use and dependence. *J. Psychoactive Drugs, 33,* 151–158.

Javitt, D. C., and Zukin, S. R. (1991). Recent advances in the phencyclidine model of schizophrenia. *Am. J. Psychiatry, 148,* 1301–1308.

Jellinek, E. M. (1960). *The Disease Concept of Alcoholism.* Hillhouse Press, New Haven, Connecticut.

Jentsch, J. D., Redmond, D. E., Jr., Elsworth, J. D., Taylor, J. R., Youngren, K. D., and Roth, R. H. (1997). Enduring cognitive deficits and cortical dopamine dysfunction in monkeys after long-term administration of phencyclidine. *Science, 277,* 953–955.

Jentsch, J. D., Taylor, J. R., and Roth, R. H. (2000). Phencyclidine model of frontal cortical dysfunction in nonhuman primates. *Neuroscientist, 6,* 263–270.

Jibson, M. D., and Tandon, R. (1998). New atypical antipsychotic medications. *J. Psychiatr. Res., 32,* 215–228.

Jones, B. J., Paterson, I. A., and Roberts, M. H. T. (1986). Microinjections of methyl-β-carboline-carboxylate into the dorsal raphe nucleus: Behavioral consequences. *Pharmacol. Biochem. Behav., 24,* 1487–1489.

Jones, K. L., Smith, D. W., Ulleland, C. N., and Streissguth, P. (1973). Pattern of malformation in offspring of chronic alcoholic mothers. *Lancet, 7815,* 1267–71.

Jones, R. T. (1990). The pharmacology of cocaine smoking in humans. *NIDA Res. Monogr., 99,* 30–41.

Jorenby, D. E., Leischow, S. J., Nides, M. A., Rennard, S. I., Johnston, J. A., Hughes, A. R., Smith, S. S., Muramoto, M. L., Daughton, D. M., Doan, K., Fiore, M. C., and Baker, T. B. (1999). A controlled trial of sustained-release bupropion, a nicotine patch, or both for smoking cessation. *New Engl. J. Med., 340,* 685–691.

Julien, R. M. (1998). *A Primer of Drug Action: A Concise, Nontechnical Guide to the Actions, Uses, and Side Effects of Psychoactive Drugs* (8th ed.). W. H. Freeman, New York.

Julien, R. M. (2002). *A Primer of Drug Action.* (10th ed.). Worth Publishers, New York.

Jung, J. (2001). *Psychology of Alcohol and Other Drugs: A Research Perspective.* Sage Publications, London.

Justinova, Z., Tanda, G., Munzar, P., and Goldberg, S. R. (2004). The opioid antagonist naltrexone reduces the reinforcing effects of Δ⁹-tetrahydrocannabinol (THC) in squirrel monkeys. *Psychopharmacology, 173,* 186–194.

Justinova, Z., Tanda, G., Redhi, G. H., and Goldberg, S. R. (2003). Self-administration of Δ⁹-tetrahydrocannabinol (THC) by drug naive squirrel monkeys. *Psychopharmacology, 169,* 135–140.

Kahn, R. S., and Davis, K. L. (1995). New developments in dopamine and schizophrenia. In *Psychopharmacology: The Fourth Generation of Progress* (F. E. Bloom and D. J. Kupfer, Eds.), pp. 1193–1204. Raven Press, New York.

Kales, A., Scharf, M. B., and Kales, J. D. (1978). Rebound insomnia: A new clinical syndrome. *Science, 201* 1039–1041.

Kalman, D. (2002). The subjective effects of nicotine: Methodological issues, a review of experimental studies, and recommendations for future research. *Nicotine Tobacco Res.,* 4, 25–70.

Kandel, D., and Yamaguchi, K. (1993). From beer to crack: Developmental patterns of drug involvement. *Am. J. Public Health,* 83, 851–855.

Kandel, D., Yamaguchi, K., and Chen, K. (1992). Stages of progression in drug involvement from adolescence to adulthood: Further evidence for the gateway theory. *J. Stud. Alcohol,* 53, 447–457.

Kandel, E. R. (2000). Disorders of mood: Depression, mania, and anxiety disorders. In *Principles of Neural Science* (4th ed.) (E. R. Kandel , J. H. Schwartz, and T. M. Jessell, Eds.), pp. 1209–1226. McGraw-Hill, New York.

Kaneyuki, H., Yokoo, H., Tsuda, A., et al. (1991). Psychological stress increases dopamine turnover selectively in mesoprefrontal dopamine neurons of rats: Reversal by diazepine. *Brain Res.,* 557, 154–161.

Kantak, K. M. (2003). Vaccines against drugs of abuse: A viable treatment option? *Drugs,* 63, 341–352.

Karch, S. B. (1998). *A Brief History of Cocaine.* CRC Press, Boca Raton, Florida.

Katz, D. L., and Pope, H. G., Jr. (1990). Anabolic-androgenic steroid-induced mental status changes. *NIDA Res. Monogr.,* 102, 215–223.

Kebabian, J. W., and Calne, D. B. (1979). Multiple receptors for dopamine. *Nature,* 277, 93–96.

Kelly, D. D. (1991) Sleep, and dreaming. In *Principles of Neural Science* (3rd ed.) (E.R. Kandel, J. H. Schwartz, and T. M. Jessell, Eds.), pp. 792–804. Elsevier, New York.

Kelly, M. A., Rubinstein, M., Phillips, T. J., Lessov, C. N., Burkhart-Kasch, S., Zhang, G., Bunzow, J., Fang, Y., Gerhardt, G. A., Grandy, D. K., and Low, M. J. (1998). Locomotor activity in D2 dopamine receptor-deficient mice is determined by gene dosage, genetic background, and developmental adaptations. *J. Neurosci.,* 18, 3470–3479.

Keshavan, M. S., Anderson, S., and Pettegrew, J. W. (1994). Is schizophrenia due to excessive synaptic pruning in the prefrontal cortex? The Feinberg hypothesis revisited. *J. Psychiatr. Res.,* 28, 239–265.

Kessler, R. C., Nelson, C. B., McGonagle, K. A., et al. (1996). Comorbidity of DSM-III-R major depressive disorder in the general population: Results from the US National Comorbidity Survey. *Br. J. Psychiatry,* 168 (Suppl. 30), 17–30.

Kieffer, B. L., Befort, K., Gaveriaux-Ruff, C., and Hirth, C. G. (1992). The "mu"-opioid receptor: Isolation of a cDNA by expression cloning and pharmacological characterization. *Proc. Natl. Acad. Sci. U.S.A.,* 89, 12048–12052.

Kirk, J. M., and de Wit, H. (1999). Responses to oral Δ^9-tetrahydrocannabinol in frequent and infrequent marijuana users. *Pharmacol. Biochem. Behav.,* 63, 137–142.

Kirk, J. M., Doty, P., and de Wit, H. (1998). Effects of expectancies on subjective responses to oral Δ^9-tetrahydrocannabinol. *Pharmacol. Biochem. Behav.,* 59, 287–293.

Klein, D. C., and Seligman, M. E. P. (1976). Reversal of performance deficits and perceptual deficits in learned helplessness and depression. *J. Abnorm. Psychol.,* 85, 11–26.

Klein, S. B. (2000). *Biological Psychology.* Prentice-Hall, Upper Saddle River, New Jersey.

Klingemann, H. K.-H. (1992). Coping and maintenance strategies of spontaneous remitters from problem use of alcohol and heroin in Switzerland. *Int. J. Addict.,* 27, 1359–1388.

Knott, V., Bosman, M., Mahoney, C., Ilivitsky, V., and Quirt, K. (1999). Transdermal nicotine: Single dose effects on mood, EEG, performance, and event-related potentials. *Pharmacol. Biochem. Behav.,* 63, 253–261.

Kolb, B., and Wishaw, I. Q. (1989). Plasticity in the neocortex: Mechanisms underlying recovery from early brain damage. *Prog. Neurobiol.,* 32, 242.

Koob, G. F., and Le Moal, M. (1997). Drug abuse: Hedonic homeostatic dysregulation. *Science,* 278, 52–58.

Koob, G. F., Maldonado, R., and Stinus, L. (1992). Neural substrates of opiate withdrawal. *Trends Neurosci.,* 15, 186–191.

Koob, G. F., Sanna, P. P., and Bloom, F. E. (1998). Neuroscience of addiction. *Neuron,* 21, 467–476.

Kosten, T. R., Rosen, M., Bond, J., Settles, M., Roberts, J. S. C., Shields, J., Jack, L., and Fox, B. (2002). Human therapeutic cocaine vaccine: Safety and immunogenicity. *Vaccine,* 20, 1196–1204.

Kosterlitz, H. W., and Waterfield, A. A. (1975). In vitro models in the study of structure-activity relationships of narcotic analgestis. *Annu. Rev. Pharmacol.,* 15, 29–47.

Kosterlitz, H. W., Lydon, R. J., and Watt, A. J. (1970). The effects of adrenaline, noradrenaline, and isoprenaline on inhibitory α- and β-adrenoreceptors in the longitudinal muscle of the guinea pig ileum. *Br. J. Pharmacol.,* 39, 398–413.

Koukkou, M., and Lehmann, D. (1976). Human EEG spectra before and during cannabis hallucinations. *Biol. Psychiatry,* 11, 663–677.

Kouri, E. M., and Pope, H. G., Jr. (2000). Abstinence symptoms during withdrawal from chronic marijuana use. *Exp. Clin. Psychopharmacol.,* 8, 483–492.

Kouri, E. M., Pope, H. G., Jr., and Lukas, S. E. (1999). Changes in aggressive behavior during withdrawal from long-term marijuana use. *Psychopharmacology,* 143, 302–308.

Kovelman, J. A., and Scheibel, A. B. (1984). A neurohistologic correlate of schizophrenia. *Biol. Psychiatry,* 19, 1601–1621.

Krakowski, M. (1997). Neurologic and neuropsychologic correlates of violence. *Psychiatr. Ann.,* 27, 674–677.

Krause, K. H., Dresel, S. H., Krause, J., Kung, H. F., and Tatsch, K. (2000). Increased striatal dopamine transporter in adult patients with attention deficit hyperactivity disorder: Effects of methylphenidate as measured by single photon emission computed tomography. *Neurosci. Lett.,* 285, 107–110.

Kuczenski, R., and Segal, D. S. (2002). Exposure of adolescent rats to oral methylphenidate: Preferential effects on extracellular norepinephrine and absence of sensitization and cross-sensitization to methamphetamine. *J. Neurosci.,* 22, 7264–7271.

Kuhar, M. J., Ritz, M. C., and Boja, J. W. (1991). The dopamine hypothesis of the reinforcing effects of cocaine. *Trends Neurosci.,* 14, 299–302.

Lahti, A. C., Koffel, B., LaPorte, D., and Tamminga, C. A. (1995). Subanesthetic doses of ketamine stimulate psychosis in schizophrenia. *Neuropsychopharmacology,* 13, 9–19.

Lane, R., and Baldwin, D. (1997). Selective serotonin reuptake inhibitor-induced serotonin syndrome: Review. *J. Clin. Psychopharmacol.,* 17, 208–221.

Lang, A. R., Goeckner, D. J., Adesso, V. J., and Marlatt, G. A. (1975). Effects of alcohol on aggression in male social drinkers. *J. Abnorm. Psychol.,* 84, 508–518.

Langlais, P. J., and Savage, L. M. (1995). Thiamine deficiency in rats produces cognitive and memory deficits on spatial tasks correlated with tissue loss in diencephalon, cortex and white matter. *Behav. Brain Res.,* 68, 75–89.

Langston, J. W., and Palfreman, J. (1995). *The Case of the Frozen Addicts.* Pantheon Books, New York.

Laruelle, M. Abi-Darghani, A., Gile R., Kegeles, L., and Innis, R. (1999). Increased dopamine transmission in schizophrenia: Relationship to illness phases. *Biol. Psychiatry,* 46, 56–72.

Lathe, R. (1996). Mice, gene targeting and behaviour: More than just genetic background. *Trends Neurosci.,* 19, 183–186.

Le, A. D., Poulos, C. X., and Cappell, H. (1979). Conditioned tolerance to the hypothermic effect of ethyl alcohol. *Science,* 206, 1109–1110.

Leary, T. (1984). Personal computers/personal freedom. In *Digital Deli* (S. Ditlea, Ed.), pp. 359–361. Workman Publishing Co., New York.

Le Blanc, A. E., Lalant, H., and Gibbins, R. J. (1976). Acquisition and loss of behaviorally augmented tolerance to ethanol in the rat. *Psychopharmacology,* 48, 153–158.

Le Blanc, A. E., Lalant, H., and Gibbins, R. J. (1975). Acute tolerance to ethanol in the rat. *Psychopharmacologia,* 41, 43–46.

Ledent, C., Valverde, O., Cossu, G., Petitet, F., Aubert, J.-F., Beslot, F., Böhme, G. A., Imperato, A., Pedrazzini, T., Roques, B. P., Vassart, G., Fratta, W., and Parmentier, M. (1999). Unresponsiveness to cannabinoids and reduced addictive effects of opiates in CB$_1$ receptor knockout mice. *Science,* 283, 401–404.

LeDoux, J. E. (1995). Emotion: Clues from the brain. *Ann. Rev. Psychol.,* 46, 209–235.

LeDoux, J. E. (1996). *The Emotional Brain.* Simon and Schuster, New York.

Lee, M. A., and Shlain, B. (1992). *Acid Dreams. The Complete Social History of LSD: The CIA, the Sixties, and Beyond.* Grove Press, New York.

Leibowitz, S. F., and Alexander, J. T. (1998). Hypothalamic serotonin in control of eating behavior, meal size, and body weight. *Biol. Psychiatry,* 44, 851–864.

Leonard, H. L., Swedo, S. E., Rapoport, J. L., Koby, E. V., Lenane, M. C., Cheslow, D. L., and Hamburger, S. D. (1989). Treatment of obsessive-compulsive disorder with clomipramine and desipramine in children and adolescents: A double blind crossover comparison. *Arch. Gen. Psychiatry,* 46, 1088–1092.

Leshner, A. I. (1997). Addiction is a brain disease, and it matters. *Science,* 278, 45–47.

Levin, E. D. (1996). Nicotinic agonist and antagonist effects on memory. *Drug Dev. Res.,* 38, 188–195.

Levin, E. D., Rezvani, A. H., Montoya, D., Rose, J. E., and Swartzwelder, H. S. (2003). Adolescent-onset nicotine self-administration modeled in female rats. *Psychopharmacology,* 169, 141–149.

Levin, J. D. (1989). *Alcoholism: A Bio-psycho-social Approach.* Hemisphere, New York.

Levine, R. R. (1973). *Pharmacology: Drug Actions and Reactions.* Little, Brown, and Co., Boston.

Lewis, D. A., and Levitt, P. (2002). Schizophrenia as a disorder of neurodevelopment. *Annu. Rev. Neurosci.,* 25, 409–432.

Leza, J. C., Lizasoain, I., Cuellar, B., Moro, M. A., and Lorenzo, P. (1996). Correlation between brain nitric oxide synthase activity and opiate withdrawal. *Naunyn-Schmiedeberg's Arch. Pharmacol.,* 353, 349–354.

Lichtman, A. H., Dimen, K. R., and Martin, B. R. (1995). Systemic or intrahippocampal cannabinoid administration impairs spatial memory in rats. *Psychopharmacology,* 119, 282–290.

Lickey, M. E., and Gordon, B. (1991). *Medicine and Mental Illness.* W. H. Freeman, New York.

Lieberman, J. A., Jody, D., Alvir, J. M. J., Ashtari, M., Levy, D. L., Bogerts, B., Degreef, G., Mayeroff, D. I., and Cooper, T. (1993). Brain morphology, dopamine, and eye-tracking abnormalities in first-episode schizophrenia. *Arch. Gen. Psychiatry,* 50, 357–368.

Liebowitz, M. R., Schneier, F., Campeas, R., Hollander, E., Hatterer, J., Fyer, A., Gorman, J., Papp, L., Davies, S., Gully, R., and Klein, D. F. (1992). Phenelzine vs. atenolol in social phobia: A placebo controlled comparison. *Arch. Gen. Psychiatry,* 49, 290–300.

Lin, C. L., Bristol, L. A., Jin, L., Dykes-Hoberg, M., Crawford, T., Clawson, L., and Rothstein, J. D. (1998). Aberrant RNA processing in a neurodegenerative disease: The cause for absent EAAT2, a glutamate transporter, in amyotrophic lateral sclerosis. *Neuron,* 20, 589–602.

Lindenmayer, J.-P. (1994). Risperidone: Efficacy and side effects. *J. Clin. Psychiatry,* 12, 53–58.

Lindgren, J. E., Ohlsson, A., Agurell, S., Hollister, L., and Gillespie, H. (1981). Clinical effects and plasma levels of Δ^9-tetrahydrocannabinol (Δ^9-THC) in heavy and light users of cannabis. *Psychopharmacology,* 74, 208–212.

Loewi, O. (1960). An autobiographic sketch. *Persp. Biol. Med.,* 4, 3–25.

Lucas, D. R., and Newhouse, J. P. (1957). The toxic effect of sodium L-glutamate on the inner layers of the retina. *Arch. Ophthalmol.,* 58, 193–201.

Luo, Z., and Geschwind, D. (2001). Microarray applications in neuroscience. *Neurobiol. Disease,* 8, 183–193.

Lynskey, M., and Hall, W. (2000). The effects of adolescent cannabis use on educational attainment: A review. *Addiction,* 95, 1621–1630.

Lynskey, M. T., Coffey, C., Degenhardt, L., Carlin, J. B., and Patton, G. (2003). A longitudinal study of the effects of adolescent cannabis use on high school completion. *Addiction,* 98, 685–692.

Lyons, D., Porrino, L. F., and Hiller-Sturmhofel, S. (1995). Visualizing neural pathways affected by alcohol in animals. *Alcohol Health Res. World,* 19, 300–306.

MacAndrew, C., and Edgerton, R. B. (1969). *Drunken Comportment: A Social Explanation.* Aldine, Chicago.

Mackesy-Amiti, M. E., Fendrich, M., and Goldstein, P. J. (1997). Sequence of drug use among serious drug users: Typical vs. atypical progression. *Drug Alcohol Depend.,* 45, 185–196.

Madden, T. E., and Johnson, S. W. (1998). Gamma-hydroxybutyrate is a GABA$_B$ receptor agonist that increases a potassium conductance in rat ventral tegmental dopamine neurons. *J. Pharmacol. Exp. Ther.,* 287, 261–265.

Maddux, J. F., and Desmond, D. P. (1981). *Careers of Opioid Users.* Praeger Publishers, New York.

Maitre, M., Hechler, V., Vayer, P., Gobaille, S., Cash, C. D., Schmitt, M., and Bourguignon, J. J. (1990). A specific γ-hydroxybutyrate receptor ligand possesses both antagonistic and anticonvulsant properties. *J. Pharmacol. Exp. Ther.,* 255, 657–663.

Malizia, A. L., Cunningham, V. J., Bell, C. J., Liddle, P. F., Jones, T., et al. (1998). Decreased brain GABA(A)-benzodiazepine receptor binding in panic disorder: Preliminary results from a quantitative PET study. *Arch. Gen. Psychiatry,* 55, 715–720.

Mangini, M. (1998). Treatment of alcoholism using psychedelic drugs: A review of the program of research. *J. Psychoactive Drugs,* 30, 381–418.

Mansour, A., and Watson, S. J. (1993). Anatomical distribution of opioid receptors in mammalians: An overview. In *Opioids I,* Handbook of Experimental Pharmacology, Vol. 104 (A. Herz, Ed.), pp. 79–106. Springer-Verlag, New York.

Mansour, A., Khachaturian, H., Lewis, M. E., Akil, H., and Watson, S. J. (1988). Anatomy of CNS opioid receptors. *Trends Neurosci., 7,* 308–314.

Mao, J., Price, D. D., Phillips, L. L., Lu, J., and Mayer, D. J. (1995). Increases in protein kinase C immunoreactivity in the spinal cord of rats associated with tolerance to the analgesic effects of morphine. *Brain Res., 677,* 257–267.

Marcotte, E., Srivastava, L., and Quirion, R. (2001). DNA microarrays in neuropsychopharmacology. *Trends Pharmacol. Sci., 22,* 426–436.

Marlatt, G. A., and Rohsenow, D. J. (1980). Cognitive processes in alcohol use: Expectancy and the balanced placebo design. In *Advances in Substance Abuse: Behavioral and Biological Research* (N. K. Mello, Ed.), pp. 159–199. JAI, Greenwich, Connecticut.

Marsicano, G., Wotjak, C. T., Azad, S. C., Bisogno, T., Rammes, G., Cascio, M. G., Hermann, H., Tang, J., Hofmann, C., Zieglgänsberger, W., Di Marzo, V., and Lutz, B. (2002). The endogenous cannabinoid system controls extinction of aversive memories. *Nature, 418,* 530–534.

Martellotta, M. C., Cossu, G., Fattore, L., Gessa, G. L., and Fratta, W. (1998a). Self-administration of the cannabinoid receptor agonist WIN 55,212-2 in drug-naive mice. *Neuroscience, 85,* 327–330.

Martellotta, M. C., Cossu, G., Fattore, L., Gessa, G. L., and Fratta, W. V. (1998b). Intravenous self-administration of gamma-hydroxybutyric acid in drug-naive mice. *Eur. Neuropsychopharmacology, 8,* 293–296.

Martellotta, M. C., Fattore, L., Cossu, G., and Fratta, W. (1997). Rewarding properties of gamma-hydroxybutyric acid: An evaluation through place preference paradigm. *Psychopharmacology, 132,* 1–5.

Martin, W. R., Eades, C. G., Thompson, J. A., Huppler, R. E., and Gilbert, P.E. (1976). The effects of morphine and naloxone-like drugs in the non-dependent and morphine dependent chronic spinal dog. *J. Pharmacol. Exp. Ther., 197,* 517–532.

Martuza, R. L., Chiocca, E. A., Jenike, M. A., Giriunas, I. E., et al. (1990). Stereotactic radiofrequency thermal cingulotomy for obsessive compulsive disorder. *J. Neuropsychiatry Clin. Neurosci., 2,* 331–336.

Mateo, Y., Budygin, E. A., John, C. E., and Jones, S. R. (2004). Role of serotonin in cocaine effects in mice with reduced dopamine transporter function. *Proc. Natl. Acad. Sci. U.S.A., 101,* 372–377.

Mathivet, P., Bernasconi, R., De Barry, J., Marescaux, C., and Bittiger, H. (1997). Binding characteristics of γ-hydroxybutyric acid as a weak but selective GABA$_B$ receptor agonist. *Eur. J. Pharmacol., 321,* 67–75.

Matsuda, L. A., Lolait, S. J., Brownstein, M. J., Young, A. C., and Bonner, T. I. (1990). Structure of a cannabinoid receptor and functional expression of the cloned cDNA. *Nature, 346,* 561–564.

Mayberg, H. S., and Frost, J. J. (1990). Opiate receptors. In *Quantitative Imaging: Neuroreceptors, Neurotransmitters, and Enzymes* (J. J. Frost and H. N. Wagner, Jr., Eds.), pp. 81–95. Raven Press, New York.

Mayhew, K. P., Flay, B. R., and Mott, J. A. (2000). Stages in the development of adolescent smoking. *Drug Alcohol Depend., 59* (Suppl. 1), S61–S81.

McBride, W. J., and Li, T.-K. (1998). Animal models of alcoholism: Neurobiology of high alcohol-drinking behavior in rodents. *Crit. Rev. Neurobiol., 12,* 339–369.

McCann, U. D., and Ricaurte, G. A. (2004). Amphetamine neurotoxicity: Accomplishments and remaining challenges. *Neurosci. Biobehav. Rev., 27,* 821–826.

McCann, U. D., Wong, D. F., Yokoi, F., Villemagne, V., Dannals, R. F., and Ricaurte, G. A. (1998). Reduced striatal dopamine transporter density in abstinent methamphetamine and methcathinone users: Evidence from positron emission tomography studies with [^{11}C]WIN-35,428. *J. Neurosci., 18,* 8417–8422.

McDaniel, C. H., and Miotto, K. A. (2001). Gamma-hydroxybutyrate (GHB) and gamma butyrolactone (GBL) withdrawal: Five case studies. *J. Psychoactive Drugs, 33,* 143–149.

McEwen, B. S., Frankfurt, M., Kuroda, Y., Magarinos, A. M., McKittrick, C., and Watanabe, Y. (1994). Dysregulation of the hypothalamo-pituitary-adrenal axis in depressive illness: Interactions between antidepressants, glucocorticoids, serotonin and excitatory amino acids. In *Critical Issues in the Treatment of Affective Disorders* (S. Z. Langer, N. Bunello, G. Racagni, and J. Mendlewicz, Eds.), pp. 75–81. Karger, Basel, Switzerland.

McGuire, P. K., Shah, G. M. S., and Murray, R. M. (1993). Increased blood flow in Broca's area during auditory hallucinations in schizophrenia. *Lancet, 342,* 703–706.

McKim, W. A. (2000). *Drugs and Behavior: An Introduction to Behavioral Pharmacology* (4th ed.). Prentice-Hall, Upper Saddle River, New Jersey.

McNeece, C. A., and DiNitto, D. M. (1998). *Chemical Dependency.* Allyn and Bacon, Boston.

McRae, A. L., Budney, A. J., and Brady, K. T. (2003). Treatment of marijuana dependence: A review of the literature. *J. Subst. Abuse Treatment, 24,* 369–376.

Mechoulam, R., Panikashvili, D., and Shohami, E. (2002). Cannabinoids and brain injury: Therapeutic implications. *Trends Mol. Med., 8,* 58–61.

Mehta, A. K., Muschaweck, N. M., Maeda, D. Y., Coop, A., and Ticku, M. J. (2001). Binding characteristics of the γ-hydroxybutyric acid receptor antagonist [^{3}H](2*E*)-(5-hydroxy-5,7,8,9-tetrahydro-6*H*-benzo[*a*][7]annulen-6-ylidene) ethanoic acid in the rat brain. *J. Pharmacol. Exp. Ther., 299,* 1148–1153.

Meisch, R. A., and Stewart, R. B. (1994). Ethanol as a reinforcer: A review of laboratory studies of non-human primates. *Behav. Pharmacol., 5,* 425–440.

Meltzer, H. Y. (1995). Atypical antipsychotic drugs. In *Psychopharmacology: The Fourth Generation of Progress* (F. E. Bloom and D. J. Kupfer, Eds.), pp. 1277–1286. Raven Press, New York.

Meltzer, H. Y. (1999). The role of serotonin in antipsychotic drug action. *Neuropsychopharmacology, 21*(2S), 106S–115S.

Miczek, K. A., and Mutschler, N. H. (1996). Activational effects of social stress on IV cocaine self-administration in rats. *Psychopharmacology, 128,* 256–264.

Midgley, S. J., Heather, N., and Davies, J. B. (1999). Dependence-producing potential of anabolic-androgenic steroids. *Addict. Res., 7,* 539–550.

Mihic, S. J., and Harris, R. A. (1997). GABA and the GABA$_A$ receptor. *Alcohol Health Res. World, 21,* 127–131.

Mindus, P., Rasmussen, S. A., and Lindquist, C. (1994). Neurosurgical treatment for refractory obsessive-compulsive disorder: Implications for understanding frontal lobe function. *J. Neuropsychiatry, 6,* 467–477.

Mirnics, K., Middleton, F. A., Marquez, A., Lewis, D. A., and Levitt, P. (2000). Molecular characterization of schizophrenia viewed by microarray analysis of gene expression in prefrontal cortex. *Neuron, 28,* 53–67.

Mirsky, I. E., Piker, P., Rosenbaum, M., and Lederer, H. (1941). "Adaptation" of the central nervous system to various concentrations of alcohol in the blood. *Q. J. Studies Alcohol,* 2, 35–45.

Miyazawa, A., Fujiyoshi, Y., and Unwin, N. (2003). Structure and gating mechanism of the acetylcholine receptor pore. *Nature,* 423, 949–955.

Moore, B. A., and Budney, A. J. (2003). Relapse in outpatient treatment for marijuana dependence. *J. Subst. Abuse Treatment,* 25, 85–89.

Moratalla, R., Xu, M., Tonegawa, S., and Graybiel, A. M. (1996). Cellular responses to psychomotor stimulant and neuroleptic drugs are abnormal in mice lacking the D1 dopamine receptor. *Proc. Natl. Acad. Sci. USA,* 93, 14928–14933.

Morgan, H. W. (1981). *Drugs in America. A Social History, 1800–1980.* Syracuse University Press, Syracuse, New York.

Morral, A. R., McCaffrey, D. F., and Paddock, S. M. (2002). Reassessing the marijuana gateway effect. *Addiction,* 97, 1493–1504.

Morrow, A. L. (1995). Regulation of GABA$_A$ receptor function and gene expression in the central nervous system. In *International Review of Neurobiology,* Vol. 38 (R. J. Bradley and R. A. Harris, Eds.), pp. 1–41. Academic Press, New York.

Mottram, D. R., and George, A. J. (2000). Anabolic steroids. *Baillieres Best Pract. Res. Clin. Endocrinol. Metab.,* 14, 55–69.

Muir, J. L., Dunnett, S. B., Robbins, T. W., and Everitt, B. J. (1992). Attentional functions of the forebrain cholinergic systems: Effects of intraventricular hemicholinium, physostigmine, basal forebrain lesions and intracortical grafts on a multiple-choice serial reaction time task. *Exp. Brain Res.,* 89, 611–622.

Musto, D. F. (1991). Opium, cocaine and marijuana in American history. *Sci. Am.,* 265, 40–47.

Naassila, M., Pierrefiche, O., Ledent, C., and Daoust, M. (2004). Decreased alcohol self-administration and increased alcohol sensitivity and withdrawal in CB1 receptor knockout mice. *Neuropharmacology,* 46, 243–253.

Nahas, G. G. (1975). *Marijuana—Deceptive Weed.* Raven Press, New York.

Nahas, G. G., Sutin, K. M., Harvey, D., and Agurell, S. (Eds.) (1999). *Marihuana and Medicine.* Humana Press, Totowa, New Jersey.

National Institute on Alcoholism and Alcohol Abuse. (1983). *Fifth special report to the U.S. Congress on alcohol and health.* Government Printing Office, Washington, D.C.

Navarro, M., Carrera, M. R. A., Fratta, W., Valverde, O., Cossu, G., Fattore, L., Chowen, J. A., Gómez, R., del Arco, I., Villanúa, M. A., Maldonado, R., Koob, G. F., and de Fonseca, F. R. (2001). Functional interaction between opioid and cannabinoid receptors in drug self-administration. *J. Neurosci.,* 21, 5344–5350.

Nelson, D. L., Lucaites, V. L., Wainscott, D. B., and Glennon, R. A. (1999). Comparisons of hallucinogenic phenylisopropylamine binding affinities at cloned human 5-HT$_{2A}$, 5-HT$_{2B}$, and 5-HT$_{2C}$ receptors. *Naunyn-Schmiedeberg's Arch. Pharmacol.,* 359, 1–6.

Nemeroff, C. B. (1998). The neurobiology of depression. *Sci. Am.,* 278, 42–49.

Nestler, E. J., Alreja, M., and Aghajanian, G. K. (1994). Molecular and cellular mechanisms of opiate action: Studies in the rat locus coeruleus. *Brain Res. Bull.,* 35, 521–528.

Nestler, E. J., Barrot, M., KiLeone, R. J., Eisch, A. J., Gold, S. J., and Monteggia, L. M. (2002). Neurobiology of depression. *Neuron,* 34, 13–25.

Newcomer, J. W., Farber, N. B., Jevtovic-Todorovic, V., Selke, G., Melson, A. K., Hershey, T., Craft, S., and Olney, J. W. (1998). Ketamine-induced NMDA receptor hypofunction as a model of memory impairment and psychosis. *Neuropsychopharmacology,* 20, 106–118.

Nichols, D. E. (1986). Differences between the mechanism of action of MDMA, MBDB, and the classic hallucinogens. Identification of a new therapeutic class: Entactogens. *J. Psychoactive Drugs,* 18, 305–313.

Nichols, D. E. (1997). Role of serotoninergic neurons and 5-HT receptors in the action of hallucinogens. In *Serotoninergic Neurons and 5-HT Receptors in the CNS.* Handbook of Experimental Pharmacology, Vol. 129 (H. G. Baumgarten and M. Göthert, Eds.), pp. 563–585. Springer-Verlag, Berlin.

Nichols, D. E. (2004). Hallucinogens. *Pharmacol. Ther.,* 101, 131–181.

Nicholson, K. L., and Balster, R. L. (2001). GHB: A new and novel drug of abuse. *Drug Alcohol Depend.,* 63, 1–22.

Nicholson, K. L., Hayes, B. A., and Balster, R. L. (1999). Evaluation of the reinforcing properties and phencyclidine-like discriminative stimulus effects of dextromethorphan and dextrorphan in rats and rhesus monkeys. *Psychopharmacology,* 146, 49–59.

Ninan, P. T. (1999). The functional anatomy, neurochemistry, and pharmacology of anxiety. *J. Clin. Psychiatry,* 60 (Suppl. 22), 12–17.

Noonan, W. C., Miller, W. R., and Feeney, D. M. (2000). Dextromethorphan abuse among youth. *Arch. Fam. Med.,* 9, 791–792.

Nowinski, J. (1996). Facilitating 12-step recovery from substance abuse and addiction. In *Treating Substance Abuse: Theory and Technique* (F. Rotgers, D. S. Keller, and J. Morgenstern, Eds.), pp. 37–67. Guilford Press, New York.

Nutt, D. J., Bell, C. J., and Malizia, A. L. (1998). Brain mechanisms of social anxiety disorder. *J. Clin. Psychiatry,* 59 (Suppl. 17), 4–9.

O'Brien, C. P. (1993). Opioid addiction. In *Opioids II,* Handbook of Experimental Pharmacology (A. Herz, Ed.), pp. 803–824. Springer-Verlag, New York.

O'Brien, C. P. (1994). Treatment of alcoholism as a chronic disorder. In *Toward a Molecular Basis of Alcohol Use and Abuse* (B. Jansson, H. Jönvall, U. Rydberg, L. Terenius, and B. L. Vallee, Eds.), pp. 349–359, Birkhäuser, Verlag, Basel, Switzerland.

OECD. (1978). *Road research: New research on the role of alcohol and drugs in road accidents.* A report prepared by an Organization for Economic Co-operation and Development (OECD) road research group.

Oldendorf, W. H. (1975). Permeability of the blood–brain barrier. In *The Nervous System,* Vol. 1. (D. B. Tower, Ed.), pp. 279–289. Raven Press, New York.

Olney, J. W. (1969). Brain lesions, obesity, and other disturbances in mice treated with monosodium glutamate. *Science,* 164, 719–721.

Olney, J. W., Ho, O. L., and Rhee, V. (1971). Cytotoxic effects of acidic and sulphur containing amino acids on the infant mouse central nervous system. *Exp. Brain Res.,* 14, 61–76.

Osborn, E., Grey, C., and Reznikoff, M. (1986). Psychosocial adjustment, modality choice, and outcome in naltrexone versus methadone treatment. *Am. J. Drug Alcohol Abuse,* 12, 383–388.

Overton, D. A. (1984). State dependent learning and drug discriminations. In *Handbook of Psychopharmacology,* Vol. 18 (L. L. Iversen, S. D. Iversen, and S. H. Snyder, Eds.), pp. 59–112. Plenum Press, New York.

Packard, M. G., Cornell, A. H., and Alexander, G. M. (1997). Rewarding affective properties of intra-nucleus accumbens injections of testosterone. *Behav. Neurosci.,* 111, 219–224.

Packard, M. G., Schroeder, J. P., and Alexander, G. M. (1998). Expression of testosterone conditioned place preference is blocked by peripheral or intra-accumbens injection of α-flupenthixol. *Horm. Behav., 34,* 39–47.

Parker, D. A., Harford, T. C., and Rosenstock, I. M. (1994). Alcohol, other drugs, and sexual risk-taking among young adults. *J. Subst. Abuse, 6,* 87–93.

Parrott, A. C. (1999). Does cigarette smoking *cause* stress? *Am. Psychologist,* 54, 817–820.

Parrott, A. C. (2001). Human psychopharmacology of Ecstasy (MDMA): A review of 15 years of empirical research. *Hum. Psychopharmacol. Clin. Exp., 16,* 557–577.

Parrott, A. C., and Kaye, F. J. (1999). Daily uplifts, hassles, stresses and cognitive failures: In cigarette smokers, abstaining smokers, and non-smokers. *Behav. Pharmacol., 10,* 639–646.

Pauls, D. L., Alsobrook, J. P., Goodman, W., Rasmussen, S., and Leckman, J. F. (1995). A family study of obsessive-compulsive disorder. *Am. J. Psychiatry, 152,* 76–84.

Perkins, K. A., Donny, E., and Cagguila, A. R. (1999). Sex differences in nicotine effects and self-administration: Review of human and animal evidence. *Nicotine Tobacco Res., 1,* 301–305.

Perkins, K. A., Gerlach, D., Broge, M., Grobe, J. E., Sanders, M., Fonte, C., Vender, J., Cherry, C., and Wilson, A. (2001). Dissociation of nicotine tolerance from tobacco dependence in humans. *J. Pharmacol. Exp. Ther., 296,* 849–856.

Pert, C. B., and Snyder, S. H. (1973). Properties of opiate receptor binding in rat brain. *Proc. Natl. Acad. Sci. U.S.A., 70,* 2243–2247.

Peters, A., Palay, S. L., and Webster, H. deF. (1991). *The Fine Structure of the Nervous System: Neurons and their Supporting Cells* (3rd ed.). Oxford University Press, New York.

Petersen, R. C. (1977). Cocaine: An overview. *NIDA Res. Monogr., 13,* 17–34.

Petraitis, J., Flay, B. R., and Miller, T. Q. (1995). Reviewing theories of adolescent substance use: Organizing pieces in the puzzle. *Psychol. Bull., 117,* 67–86.

Petty, M. A., Neumann-Haefelin, C., Kalisch, J., Sarhan, S., Wettstein, J. G., and Juretschke, H.-P. (2003). In vivo neuroprotective effects of ACEA 1021 confirmed by magnetic resonance imaging in ischemic stroke. *Eur. J. Pharmacol., 474,* 53–62.

Pfefferbaum, A., and Sullivan, E. V. (2004). Diffusion MR imaging in psychiatry and ageing. In *Physiological Magnetic Resonance in Clinical Neuroscience* (J. Gillard, A. Waldman, and P. Barker, Eds), Chapter 33. Cambridge University Press, Cambridge, U.K.

Pflug, B. (1988). Sleep deprivation in treatment of depression. In *Affective Disorders—Directions in Psychiatry* (Monogr. series, No. 3), pp. 175–185. W. W. Norton, New York.

Philippu, A. (1984). Use of push–pull cannulae to determine the release of endogenous neurotransmitters in distinct brain areas of anaesthetized and freely moving animals. In *Measurement of Neurotransmitter Release In Vivo* (C. A. Marsden, Ed.), pp. 3–38. Wiley, New York.

Phillips, T. J., Brown, K. J., Burkhart-Kasch, S., Wenger, C. D., Kelly, M. A., Rubinstein, M., Grandy, D. K., and Low, M. J. (1998). Alcohol preference and sensitivity are markedly reduced in mice lacking dopamine D_2 receptors. *Nat. Neurosci., 1,* 610–615.

Piazza, P. V., and Le Moal, M. (1996). Pathophysiological basis of vulnerability to drug abuse: Role of an interaction between stress, glucocorticoids, and dopaminergic neurons. *Annu. Rev. Pharmacol. Toxicol., 36,* 359–378.

Piazza, P. V., Maccari, S., Deminière, J. -M., Le Moal, M., Mormède, P., and Simon, H. (1991.) Corticosterone levels determine individual vulnerability to amphetamine self-administration. *Proc. Natl. Acad. Sci. USA, 88,* 2088–2092.

Piazza, P., and Le Moal, M. (1998). The role of stress in drug self-administration. *Trends Pharmacol. Sci., 19,* 67–74.

Picciotto, M. R., Zoli, M., Rimondini, R., Léna, C., Marubio, L. M., Pich, E. M., Fuxe, K., and Changeux, J.-P. (1998). Acetylcholine receptors containing the β2 subunit are involved in the reinforcing properties of nicotine. *Nature, 391,* 173–177.

Picciotto, M. R., Zoli, M., Zachariou, V., and Changeux, J.-P. (1997). Contribution of nicotinic acetylcholine receptors containing the β2-subunit to the behavioural effects of nicotine. *Biochem. Soc. Trans., 25,* 824–829.

Pidoplichko, V. I., DeBiasi, M., Williams, J. T., and Dani, J. A. (1997). Nicotine activates and desensitizes midbrain dopamine neurons. *Nature, 390,* 401–404.

Pilla, M., Perachon, S., Sautel, F., Garrido, F., Mann, A., Wermuth, C. G., Schwartz, J.-C., Everitt, B. J., and Sokoloff, P. (1999). Selective inhibition of cocaine-seeking behaviour by a partial dopamine D_3 receptor agonist. *Nature, 400,* 371–375.

Pinder, R. M. (1997). Designing a new generation of antidepressant drugs. *Acta Psychiatr. Scand., 96* (Suppl. 391), 7–13.

Pinel, J. P. J. (2000). *Biopsychology* (4th ed.). Allyn and Bacon, Boston.

Piomelli, D. (2003). The molecular logic of endocannabinoid signaling. *Nat. Rev. Neurosci., 4,* 873–884.

Platt, D. M., Rowlett, J. K., and Spealman, R. D. (2002). Behavioral effects of cocaine and dopaminergic strategies for preclinical medication development. *Psychopharmacology, 163,* 265–282.

Ploner, M., Gross, J., Timmermann, L., and Schnitzler, A. (2002). Cortical representation of first and second pain sensation in humans. *Proc. Natl. Acad. Sci. U.S.A., 99,* 12444–12448.

Pope, H. G., Jr., Gruber, A. J., Hudson, J. I., Huestis, M. A., and Yurgelun-Todd, D. (2001a). Neuropsychological performance in long-term cannabis users. *Arch. Gen. Psychiatry, 58,* 909–915.

Pope, H. G., Jr., Gruber, A. J., and Yurgelun-Todd, D. (2001b). Residual neuropsychologic effects of cannabis. *Curr. Psychiatr. Rep., 3,* 507–512.

Pope, H. G., Jr., Kouri, E. M., and Hudson, J. I. (2000). Effects of supraphysiological doses of testosterone on mood and aggression in normal men. A randomized controlled trial. *Arch. Gen. Psychiatry, 57,* 133–140.

Porsolt, R. D., Anton, G., Blavet, N., and Jalfre, M. (1978). Behavioral despair in rats: A new model sensitive to antidepressant treatments. *Eur. J. Pharmacol., 47,* 379–391.

Posner, M. I., and Raichle, M. E. (1994). *Images of Mind.* W. H. Freeman, New York.

Post, R. M., Ballenger, J. C., Uhde, T., and Bunney, W. (1984). Efficacy of carbamazapine in manic-depressive illness: Implications for underlying mechanisms. In *Neurobiology of Mood Disorders* (R. M. Post and J. C. Ballenger, Eds.), pp. 777–816. Williams and Wilkins, Baltimore.

Post, R. M., and Contel, N. R. (1983). Human and animal studies of cocaine: Implications for the development of behavioral pathology. In *Stimulants: Neurochemical, Behavioral, and Clinical Perspectives* (I. Creese, Ed.), pp. 169–203. Raven Press, New York.

Post, R. M., and Weiss, S. R. B. (1988). Psychomotor stimulant vs. local anesthetic effects of cocaine: Role of behavioral sensitization and kindling. *NIDA Res. Monogr., 88,* 217–238.

Purves, D., Augustine, G. J., Fitzpatrick, D. , Hall, W. C., LaMantia, A. S., McNamara, J. O., and Williams, S. M. (2004). *Neuroscience* (3rd ed.). Sinauer Associates, Sunderland, MA.

Quirion, R., and Pilapil, C. (1991). Distribution of multiple opioid receptors in the human brain. In *Receptors in the Human*

Nervous System (F. A. O. Mendelsohn, Ed.), pp. 103–121. Academic Press, New York.

Racz, I., Bilkei-Gorzo, A., Toth, Z. E., Michel, K., Palkovits, M., and Zimmer, A. (2003). A critical role for the cannabinoid CB_1 receptors in alcohol dependence and stress-stimulated ethanol drinking. *J. Neurosci.,* 23, 2453–2458.

Rago, L., Kiivet, R. A., Harro, J., and Pold, M. (1988). Behavioral differences in an elevated plus maze: Correlation between anxiety and decreased number of GABA and benzodiazepine receptors in mouse cerebral cortex. *Naunyn-Schmiedeberg's Arch. Pharmacol.,* 337, 3675–3678.

Rainville, P. (2002). Brain mechanisms of pain affect and pain modulation. *Curr. Opinion Neurobiol.,* 12, 195–204.

Rainville, P. Duncan, G. H., Price, D. D., Carrier, B., and Bushnell, M. C. (1997). Pain affect encoded in human anterior cingulate but not somatosensory cortex. *Science,* 277, 968–971.

Ramaekers, J. G., Berghaus, G., van Laar, M., and Drummer, O. H. (2004). Dose related risk of motor vehicle crashes after cannabis use. *Drug Alcohol Depend.,* 73, 109–119.

Randall, C. L., Ekblad, U., and Anton, R. F. (1990). Perspectives on the pathophysiology of fetal alcohol syndrome. *Alcohol. Clin. Exp. Res.,* 14, 807–812.

Rapoport, J. L. (1989). The biology of obsessions and compulsions. *Sci. Am.* 260, 83–89.

Rapoport, J. L., Buchsbaum, M. S., Zahn, T. P., Weingartner, H., Ludlow, C., and Mikkelsen, E. J. (1978). Dextroamphetamine: Cognitive and behavioral effects in normal prepubertal boys. *Science,* 199, 560–563.

Rauch, S. L., and Jenike, M. A. (1993). Neurobiological models of obsessive-compulsive disorder. *Psychosomatics,* 34, 20–32.

Rauch, S. L., and Jenike, M. A. (1998). Pharmacological treatment of obsessive-compulsive disorder. In *A Guide to Treatments That Work* (P. E. Nathan and J. M. Gorman, Eds.), pp. 358–376. Oxford University Press, New York.

Ray, O., and Ksir, C. (1999). *Drugs, Society, and Human Behavior* (8th ed.). WCB/McGraw-Hill, Boston.

Redgrave, P., Prescott, T. J., and Gurney, K. (1999). Is the short-latency dopamine response too short to signal reward error? *Trends Neurosci.,* 22, 146–151.

Reisine, T., and Pasternak, G. (1996). Opioid analgesics and antagonists. In *The Pharmacological Basis of Therapeutics* (A. G. Gilman, L. S. Goodman, J. G. Hardman, L. E. Limbard, P. B. Molinoff, and R. W. Ruddon, Eds.), pp. 521–555. McGraw-Hill, New York.

Richards, J. G., Schoch, P., and Jenck, F. (1991). Benzodiazepine receptors and their ligands. In *5-HT_{1A} Agonists, 5-HT_3 Antagonists and Benzodiazepines: Their Comparative Behavioural Pharmacology* (R. J. Rogers and S. J. Cooper, Eds.), pp. 1–30. Wiley, New York.

Richardson, J. D., Aanonsen, L., and Hargreaves, K. M. (1998). Hypoactivity of the spinal cannabinoid system results in NMDA-dependent hyperalgesia. *J. Neurosci.,* 18, 451–457.

Richelson, E. (1995). Cholinergic transduction. In *Psychopharmacology: The Fourth Generation of Progress* (F. E. Bloom and D. J. Kupfer, Eds.), pp. 125–134. Raven Press, New York.

Riegel, A. C., and French, E. D. (2002). Abused inhalants and central reward pathways. *Ann. N. Y. Acad. Sci.,* 965, 281–291.

Ritchie, J. M., (1975). Central nervous system stimulants. In *The Pharmacological Basis of Therapeutics* (5th ed.) (L. Goodman and A. Gilman, Eds.), pp. 367–378. Macmillan, New York.

Ritz, M. C., Cone, E. J., and Kuhar, M. J. (1990). Cocaine inhibition of ligand binding at dopamine, norepinephrine and serotonin transporters: A structure-activity study. *Life Sci.,* 46, 635–645.

Roberts, A. J., McDonald, J. S., Heyser, C. J., Kieffer, B. L., Matthes, H. W. D., Koob, G. F., and Gold, L. H. (2000). μ-Opioid receptor knockout mice do not self-administer alcohol. *J. Pharmacol. Exp. Ther.,* 293, 1002–1008.

Robins, L. N., Helzer, J. E., and Davis, D. H. (1975). Narcotic use in southeast Asia and afterward. An interview study of 898 Vietnam returnees. *Arch. Gen. Psychiatry,* 32, 955–961.

Robins, L. N., Helzer, J. E., Weissman, M. M., Orvaschel, H., Gruenber, E., Burke, J. D., Jr., and Regier, D. A. (1984). Lifetime prevalence of specific psychiatric disorders in three sites. *Arch. Gen. Psychiatry,* 41, 949–958.

Robinson, M. L., Houtsmuller, E. J., Moolchan, E. T., and Pickworth, W. B. (2000). Placebo cigarettes in smoking research. *Exp. Clin. Psychopharmacol.,* 8, 326–332.

Robinson, T. E., and Berridge, K. C. (1993). The neural basis of drug craving: An incentive-sensitization theory of addiction. *Brain Res. Rev.,* 18, 247–291.

Robinson, T. E., and Berridge, K. C. (2000). The psychology and neurobiology of addiction: An incentive-sensitization view. *Addiction,* 95 (Suppl. 2), S91–S117.

Robinson, T. E., and Berridge, K. C. (2001). Incentive-sensitization and addiction. *Addiction,* 96, 103–114.

Rocha, B. A. (2003). Stimulant and reinforcing effects of cocaine in monoamine transporter knockout mice. *Eur. J. Pharmacol.,* 479, 107–115.

Rocha, B. A., Fumagalli, F., Gainetdinov, R. R., Jones, S. R., Ator, R., Giros, B., Miller, G. W., and Caron, M. G. (1998). Cocaine self-administration in dopamine-transporter knockout mice. *Nat. Neurosci.,* 1, 132–137.

Roffman, M., Reddy, C., and Lal, H. (1972). Alleviation of morphine withdrawal symptoms by conditional stimuli: Possible explanation for "drug hunger" and "relapse." In *Drug Addiction: Experimental Pharmacology* (J. M. Singh, L. Miller, and H. Lal, Eds.), pp. 223–226. Futura, Mt. Kisco, New York.

Rogers, P. J., and Dernoncourt, C. (1998). Regular caffeine consumption: A balance of adverse and beneficial effects for mood and psychomotor performance. *Pharmacol. Biochem. Behav.,* 59, 1039–1045.

Roine, R., Gentry, T., Hernandez-Munoz, R., Baraona, E., and Lieber, C. (1990). Aspirin increases blood alcohol concentrations in humans after ingestion of ethanol. *JAMA,* 264, 2406–2408.

Romach, M. K., Glue, P., Kampman, K., Kaplan, H. L., Somer, G. R., Poole, S., Clarke, L., Coffin, V., Cornish, J., O'Brien, C. P., and Sellers, E. M. (1999). Attenuation of the euphoric effects of cocaine by the dopamine D1/D5 antagonist ecopipam (SCH 39166). *Arch. Gen. Psychiatry,* 56, 1101–1106.

Romanul, F. C. A. (1970). Examination of the brain and spinal cord. In *Neuropathology. Methods and Diagnosis* (C. G. Tedeschi, Ed.), pp. 131–214. Little, Brown, and Co., Boston.

Rosenberg, H. (1993). Prediction of controlled drinking by alcoholics and problem drinkers. *Psychol. Bull.,* 113, 129–139.

Rosenberg, N. L., Grigsby, J., Dreisbach, J., Busenbark, D., and Grigsby, P. (2002). Neuropsychologic impairment and MRI abnormalities associated with chronic solvent abuse. *Clin. Toxicol.,* 40, 21–34.

Rosenbloom, M. J., Pfefferbaum, A., and Sullivan, E. V. (1995). Structural brain alterations associated with alcoholism. *Alcohol Health Res. World,* 19, 266–272.

Rosenthal, D. (Ed.) (1963). *The Genain Quadruplets: A Case Study and Theoretical Analysis of Heredity and Environment in Schizophrenia.* Basic Books, New York.

Rotgers, F. (1996). Behavioral theory of substance abuse treatment: Bringing science to bear on practice. In *Treating Substance*

Abuse: Theory and Technique (F. Rotgers, D. S. Keller, and J. Morgenstern, Eds.), pp. 174–201. Guilford Press, New York.

Rothman, K. J., and Michels, K. B. (1994). The continuing unethical use of placebo controls. *New Engl. J. Med.,* 331 , 394–398.

Rothstein, J. D., Dykes-Hoberg, M., Pardo, C. A., Bristol, L. A., Jin, L., Kuncl, R. W., Kanai, Y., Hediger, M. A., Wang, D. F., Schielke, J. P., and Welty, D. F. (1996). Knockout of glutamate transporters reveals a major role for astroglial transport in excitotoxicity and clearance of glutamate. *Neuron,* 16, 675–686.

Rothstein, J. D., Garland, W., Puia, G., Guidotti, A., Weber, R. J., and Costa, E. (1992). Purification and characterization of naturally occurring benzodiazepine receptor ligands in rat and human brain. *J. Neurochem.,* 58, 2102–2115.

Rougé-Pont, F., Marinelli, M., Le Moal, M., Simon, H., and Piazza, P. V. (1995). Stress-induced sensitization and glucocorticoids. II. Sensitization of the increase in extracellular dopamine induced by cocaine depends on stress-induced corticosterone secretion. *J. Neurosci.,* 15, 7189–7195.

Roy-Byrne, P. P., and Cowley, D. S. (1998). Pharmacological treatment of panic, generalized anxiety, and phobic disorders. In *A Guide to Treatments That Work* (P. E. Nathan and J. M. Gorman, Eds.), pp. 319–338. Oxford University Press, New York.

Rubinstein, M., Phillips, T. J., Bunzow, J. R., Falzone, T. L., Dziewczapolski, G., Zhang, G., Fang, Y., Larson, J. L., McDougall, J. A., Chester, J. A., Saez, C., Pugsley, T. A., Gershanik, O., Low, M. J., and Grandy, D. K. (1997). Mice lacking dopamine D4 receptors are supersensitive to ethanol, cocaine, and methamphetamine. *Cell,* 90, 991–1001.

Rudgley, R. (1999). *The Encyclopaedia of Psychoactive Substances.* St. Martin's Press, New York.

Rugh, J. T. (1896). Profound toxic effects from the drinking of large amounts of strong coffee. *Med. Surg. Reporter,* 75, 549–550.

Sánchez, M. P., Dietl, M. M., De Blas, A. L., and Palacios, J. M. (1991). Mapping of benzodiazepine-like immunoreactivity in the rat brain as revealed by a monoclonal antibody to benzodiazepines. *J. Chem. Neuroanat.,* 4, 111–121.

Sanders, S. K., and Shekhar, A. (1995). Anxiolytic effects of chlordiazepoxide blocked by injection of GABA$_A$ and benzodiazepine receptor antagonists in the region of the anterior basolateral amygdala of rats. *Biol. Psychiatry,* 37, 473–476.

Sanger, D. J., Benavides, J., Perrault, G., Morel, E., Cohen, C., Joly, D., et al. (1994). Recent developments in the behavioral pharmacology of benzodiazepine (omega) receptors: Evidence for the functional significance of receptor subtypes. *Neurosci. Biobehav. Rev.,* 18, 355–372.

Sapolsky, R. M. (1996). Why stress is bad for your brain. *Science,* 273, 749–750.

Satel, S. L., Price, L. H., Palumbo, J. M., McDougle, C. J., Krystal, J. H., Gawin, F., Charney, D. S., Heninger, G. R., and Kleber, H. D. (1991). Clinical phenomenology and neurobiology of cocaine abstinence: A prospective inpatient study. *Am. J. Psychiatry,* 448, 1712–1716.

Saxena, S., and Rauch, S. L. (2000). Functional neuroimaging and the neuroanatomy of obsessive-compulsive disorder. *Psychiatr. Clin. North Am.,* 23, 563–586.

Saxena, S., Brody, A. L., Ho, M. L., Alborzian, S., Maidment, K. M., Zohrabi, N., Ho, M. K., Huang, S. C., Wu, H. M., and Baxter, L. R. (2002). Differential cerebral metabolic changes with paroxetine treatment of obsessive-compulsive disorder vs. major depression. *Arch. Gen. Psychiatry,* 59, 250–261.

Schaffer Library of Drug Policy. http://www.druglibrary.org/schaffer/index.htm, accessed 5/4/04.

Schaler, J. A. (2000). *Addiction Is a Choice.* Open Court, Peru, Illinois.

Schildkraut, J. J. (1965). The catecholamine hypothesis of affective disorders: A review of supporting evidence. *Am. J. Psychiatry,* 122, 509–522.

Schmauss, C., Doherty, C., and Yaksh, T. L. (1983). The analgesic effects of intrathecally administered partial agonist nalbuphine hydrochloride. *Eur. J. Pharmacol.,* 86, 1–7.

Schuckit, M. A. (1994). Low level of response to alcohol as predictor of alcoholism. *Am. J. Psychol.,* 151, 184–189.

Schuckit, M. A. (2000). Genetics of the risk for alcoholism. *Am. J. Addict.,* 9, 103–112.

Schulteis, G., Markou, A., Cole, M., and Koob, G. F. (1995). Decreased brain reward produced by ethanol withdrawal. *Proc. Natl. Acad. Sci. U.S.A.,* 92, 5880–5884.

Schultz, W. (1998). Predictive reward signal of dopamine neurons. *J. Neurophysiol.,* 80, 1–27.

Sedvall, G. (1992). The current status of PET scanning with respect to schizophrenia. *Neuropsychopharmacology,* 7, 41–54.

Seeman, P. (1990). Atypical neuroleptics: Role of multiple receptors, endogenous dopamine, and receptor linkage. *Acta Psychiatr. Scand.,* 82 (Suppl. 358), 14–20.

Segal, M., Korkotian, E., and Murphy, D. (2000). Dendritic spine formation and pruning: Common cellular mechanisms? *Trends Neurosci.,* 23, 53–57.

Self, D. W., and Nestler, E. J. (1995). Molecular mechanisms of drug reinforcement and addiction. *Annu. Rev. Neurosci.,* 18, 463–495.

Seligman, M. E. P. (1975). *Helplessness: On Depression, Development and Death.* W. H. Freeman, San Francisco.

Sepinwall, J., and Cook, L. (1980). Mechanism of action of the benzodiazepines: Behavioral aspect. *Fed. Proc.,* 39, 3024–3031.

Shannon, J. R., Flattem, N. L., Jordan, J., Jacob, G., Black, B. K., Biaggioni, I., Blakely, R. D., and Robertson, D. (2000). Orthostatic intolerance and tachycardia associated with norepinephrine transporter deficiency. *New Engl. J. Med.,* 342, 541–549.

Sharma, S. K., Klee, W. A., and Nirenberg, M. (1975). Dual regulation of adenylate cyclase accounts for narcotic dependence and tolerance. *Proc. Natl. Acad. Sci. U.S.A.,* 72, 3092–3096.

Shaw, G. K., Waller, S., Majumdar, S. K., Alberts, J. L., Latham, C. J., and Dunn, G. (1994). Tiapride in the prevention of relapse in recently detoxified alcoholics. *Br. J. Psychiatry,* 165, 515–523.

Sheehan, D. V. (1999). Venlafaxine extended release (XR) in the treatment of generalized anxiety disorder. *J. Clin. Psychiatry,* 60 (Suppl. 22), 23–28.

Sheffield-Moore, M., Urban, R. J., Wolf, S. E., Jiang, J., Catlin, D. H., Herndon, D. N., Wolfe, R. R., and Ferando, A. A. (1999). Short-term oxandrolone administration stimulates net muscle protein synthesis in young men. *J. Clin. Endocrinol. Metab.,* 84, 2705–2711.

Sher, K. J., Trull, T. J., Bartholow, B. D., and Vieth, A. (1999). Personality and alcoholism: Issues, methods, and etiological processes. In *Psychological Theories of Drinking and Alcoholism* (2nd ed.) (K. E. Leonard and H. T. Blane, Eds.), pp. 54–105. Guilford Press, New York.

Sherwood, N. (1993). Effects of nicotine on human psychomotor performance. *Hum. Psychopharmacol.,* 8, 155–184.

Shippenberg, T. S. (1993). Motivational effects of opioids. In *Opioids II,* Handbook of Behavioral Neurology, Vol. 104 (A. Herz, Ed.), pp. 633–650. Springer-Verlag, New York.

Shippenberg, T. S., Herz, A., Spanagel, R., and Bals-Kubik, R. (1991). Neural substrates mediating the motivational effects of opioids. *Biol. Psychiatry,* 2, 33–35.

Shirayama, Y., Chen, A. C.-H., Nakagawa, S., Russell, D. S., and Duman, R. S. (2002). Brain derived neurotrophic factor produces antidepressant effects in behavioral models of depression. *J. Neurosci.* 22, 3251–3261.

Siegel, R. K. (1989). *Intoxication: Life in Pursuit of Artificial Paradise.* Pocket Books, New York.

Siegel, S. (1975). Evidence from rats that morphine tolerance is a learned response. *J. Comp. Physiol. Psychol.,* 89, 498–506.

Siegel, S. 1978. A pavlovian conditioning analysis of morphine tolerance. In *Behavioral Tolerance: Research and Treatment Implications.* (N. A. Krasnegor, Ed.) NIDA Research Monograph 18, U. S. Department of Health, Education and Welfare, Public Health Service, National Institute of Drug Abuse, Washington, D.C.

Siegel, S. (1985). Drug-anticipatory responses in animals. In *Placebo: Theory, Research and Mechanisms* (L. White, B. Tursky, and B. Schwartz, Eds.), pp. 288–305. Guilford Press, New York.

Siegel, S. (1989). Pharmacological conditioning and drug effects. In *Psychoactive Drugs: Tolerance and Sensitization* (A. J. Goudie, and M. W. Emmett-Oglesby, Eds.), pp. 115–180. Humana Press, Clifton, New Jersey.

Siegelbaum, S. A., and Koester, J. (1991). Ion Channels. In *Principles of Neural Science* (3rd ed.) (E. R. Kandel, J. H. Schwartz, and T. M. Jessell, Eds.), pp. 66–79. Elsevier, New York.

Siever, L. J., Kalus, O. F., and Keefe, R. S. E. (1993). The boundaries of schizophrenia. *Psychiatr. Clin. North Am.,* 16, 217–244.

Silbersweig, D. A., Stern, E., Frith, C., Cahill, C., Holmes, A., Grootoouk, S., Seaward, J., McKenna, P., Chua, S. E., Schnoor, L., Jones, T., and Frackowiak, R. S. J. (1995). A functional neuroanatomy of hallucinations in schizophrenia. *Nature,* 378, 176–179.

Simon, E. J. (1991). Opioid receptors and endogenous opioid peptides. *Med. Res. Rev.,* 11, 357–374.

Simpson, D. D., Joe, G. W., and Bracy, S. A. (1982). Six-year follow-up of opioid addicts after administration to treatment. *Arch. Gen. Psychiatry,* 39, 1318–1326.

Sinha-Hikim, I., Artaza, J., Woodhouse, L., Gonzalez-Cadavid, N., Singh, A. B., Lee, M. I., Storer, T. W., Casaburi, R., Shen, R., and Bhasin, S. (2002). Testosterone-induced increase in muscle size in healthy young men is associated with muscle fiber hypertrophy. *Am. J. Physiol. Endocrinol. Metab.,* 283, E154–E164.

Smith, A., Sturgess, W., and Gallagher, J. (1999). Effects of a low dose of caffeine given in different drinks on mood and performance. *Hum. Psychopharmacol. Clin. Exp.,* 14, 473–482.

Smith, C. G., and Asch, R. H. (1987). Drug abuse and reproduction. *Fertil. Steril.,* 48, 355–373.

Smith, K. A., Fairburn, C. G., and Cowen, P. J. (1997). Relapse of depression after rapid depletion of tryptophan. *Lancet,* 349, 915–919.

Smith, S. S., and Fiore, M. C., (1999). The epidemiology of tobacco use, dependence, and cessation in the United States. *Primary Care,* 26, 433–461.

Snead, O. C., III (2000). Evidence for a G protein-coupled gamma-hydroxybutyric acid receptor. *J. Neurochem.,* 75, 1986–1996.

Snyder, S. H. (1977). Opiate receptors and internal opiates. *Sci. Am.,* 236, 44–56.

Sobell, L. C., Ellingstad, T. P., and Sobell, M. B. (2000). Natural recovery from alcohol and drug problems: Methodological review of the research with suggestions for future directions. *Addiction,* 95, 749–764.

Solomon, R. L. (1977). An opponent-process theory of acquired motivation: The affective dynamics of addiction. In *Psychopathology: Experimental Models* (J. D. Maser and M. E. P. Seligman, Eds.), pp. 66–103. W. H. Freeman, San Francisco.

Solomon, R. L., and Corbit, J. D. (1974). An opponent-process theory of motivation. I. Temporal dynamics of affect. *Psych. Rev.,* 81, 119–145.

Solowij, N. (1998). *Cannabis and Cognitive Functioning.* Cambridge University Press, Cambridge, U.K.

Solowij, N., Stephens, R. S., Roffman, R. A., Babor, T., Kadden, R., Miller, M., Christiansen, K., McRee, B., Vendetti, J., and the Marijuana Treatment Project Research Group (2002). Cognitive functioning of long-term heavy cannabis users seeking treatment. *JAMA,* 287, 1123–1131.

Somani, S. M., and Gupta, P. (1988). Caffeine: A new look at an age-old drug. *Int. J. Clin. Pharmacol. Ther. Toxicol.,* 26, 521–533.

Sora, I., Hall, F. S., Andrews, A. M., Itokawa, M., Li, X.-F., Wei, H.-B., Wichems, C., Lesch, K.-P., Murphy, D. L., and Uhl, G. R. (2001). Molecular mechanisms of cocaine reward: Combined dopamine and serotonin transporter knockouts eliminate cocaine place preference. *Proc. Natl. Acad. Sci. U.S.A.,* 98, 5300–5305.

Sora, I., Wichems, C., Takahashi, N., Li, X.-F., Zeng, Z., Revay, R., Lesch, K.-P., Murphy, D. L., and Uhl, G. R. (1998). Cocaine reward models: Conditioned place preference can be established in dopamine- and in serotonin-transporter knockout mice. *Proc. Natl. Acad. Sci. U.S.A.,* 95, 7699–7704.

Southwick, S. M., Bremner, J. D., Rasmusson, A., Morgan, C. A., III, Arnsten, A., and Charney, D. S. (1999). Role of norepinephrine in the pathophysiology and treatment of posttraumatic stress disorder. *Biol. Psychiatry,* 46, 1192–1204.

Spencer, D. G., Jr., and Lal, H. (1983). Effects of anticholinergic drugs on learning and memory. *Drug Dev. Res.,* 3, 489–502.

Stein, D. J. (2000). Advances in the neurobiology of obsessive-compulsive disorder. *Psychiatr. Clin. North Am.,* 23, 545–561.

Steiner, H., Fuchs, S., and Accili, D. (1998). D_3 dopamine receptor-deficient mouse: Evidence for reduced anxiety. *Physiol. Behav.,* 63, 137–141.

Stewart, J. (2000). Pathways to relapse: The neurobiology of drug- and stress-induced relapse to drug-taking. *J. Psychiatry Neurosci.,* 25, 125–136.

Stewart, R. B., and Li, T.-K. (1997). The neurobiology of alcoholism in genetically selected rat models. *Alcohol Health Res. World,* 21, 169–176.

Stine, S. M., Southwick, S. M., Petrakis, I. L., Kosten, T. R., Charney, D. S., and Krystal, J. H. (2002). Yohimbine-induced withdrawal and anxiety symptoms in opioid-dependent patients. *Biol. Psychiatry,* 51, 642–651.

Stolerman, I. (1992). Drugs of abuse: Behavioural principles, methods and terms. *Trends Pharmacol. Sci.,* 13, 170–176.

Stolerman, I. P., Mirza, N. R., and Shoaib, M. (1995). Nicotine psychopharmacology: Addiction, cognition and neuroadaptation. *Med. Res. Rev.,* 15, 47–72.

Substance Abuse and Mental Health Services Administration. (2003). *2002 National Household Survey on Drug Use and Health.* http://www.samhsa.gov/centers/clearinghouse/clearinghouses.html, accessed 3/24/2004.

Substance Abuse and Mental Health Services Administration. (2003). *Results from the 2002 National Household Survey on Drug Use and Health: National Findings.* http://www.oas.samhsa.gov/nhsda.htm#NHSDAinfo, accessed 05/17/04.

Substance Abuse and Mental Health Services Administration, Office of Applied Statistics. (2002). *Emergency Department Trends from the Drug Abuse Warning Network, Final Estimates*

1994–2001. DAWN Series D-21, DHHS Publication No. (SMA) 02-3635. Rockville, MD.

Sulik, K. K., Johnston, M. C., and Webb, M. A. (1981). Fetal alcohol syndrome: Embryogenesis in a mouse model. *Science,* 214, 936–938.

Sullivan, E. V. (2000). Human brain vulnerability to alcoholism: Evidence from neuroimaging studies. *NIAAA Res. Monogr.,* 34, 477–508.

Sullivan, G. M., Coplan, J. D., Kent, J. M., and Gorman, J. M. (1999). The noradrenergic system in pathological anxiety: A focus on panic with relevance to generalized anxiety and phobias. *Biol. Psychiatry,* 46, 1205–1218.

Sulser, F. (1989). New perspectives on the molecular pharmacology of affective disorders. *Eur. Arch. Psychiatr. Neurol. Sci.,* 238, 231–239.

Swerdlow, J. L. (2000). Nature's Rx. *National Geographic,* 197 (4), 98–117.

Swerdlow, N. R., and Geyer, M. A. (1998). Using an animal model of deficient sensorimotor gating to study the pathophysiology and new treatments of schizophrenia. *Schizophr. Bull.,* 24, 285–301.

Swift, R. M. (1999). Drug therapy for alcohol dependence. *New Engl. J. Med.,* 340, 1482–1490.

Tanda, G., Munzar, P., and Goldberg, S. R. (2000). Self-administration behavior is maintained by the psychoactive ingredient of marijuana in squirrel monkeys. *Nat. Neurosci.,* 3, 1073–1074.

Tanda, G., Pontieri, F. E., and Di Chiara, G. (1997). Cannabinoid and heroin activation of mesolimbic dopamine transmission by a common μ1 opioid receptor mechanism. *Science,* 276, 2048–2050.

Tang, Y.-P., Shimizu, E., Dube, G. R., Rampon, C., Kerchner, G. A., Zhuo, M., Liu, G., and Tsien, J. Z. (1999). Genetic enhancement of learning and memory in mice. *Nature,* 401, 63–69.

Tashkin, D. P., Baldwin, G. C., Sarafian, T., Dubinett, S., and Roth, M. D. (2002). Respiratory and immunologic consequences of marijuana smoking. *J. Clin. Pharmacol.,* 42 (Suppl. 11), 71S–81S.

Terenius, L., and Wahlstrom, A. (1974). Inhibitor(s) of narcotic receptor binding in brain extracts and cerebrospinal fluid. *Acta Pharmacol. Toxicol.,* 35 (Suppl. 1), 87 (Abst.).

Thakkar, M. M., Delgiacco, R. A., Strecker, R. E., and McCarley, R. W. (2003). Adenosinergic inhibition of basal forebrain wakefulness-active neurons: A simultaneous unit recording and microdialysis study in freely behaving cats. *Neuroscience,* 122, 1107–1113.

Thannickal, T. C., Moore, R. Y., Nienhuis, R., Ramanathan, L., et al. (2000). Reduced number of hypocretin neurons in human narcolepsy. *Neuron,* 27, 469–474.

Thomas, C. L. (Ed.) (1993). *Taber's Cyclopedic Medical Dictionary.* F. A. Davis, Philadelphia.

Thombs, D. L. (1999). *Introduction to Addictive Behaviors* (2nd ed.). Guilford Press, New York.

Tiffany, S. T., Drobes, D. J., and Cepeda-Benito, A. (1992). Contribution of associative and nonassociative processes to the development of morphine tolerance. *Psychopharmacology,* 109, 185–190.

Time Out (2000). April 12–19, 20.

Timpone, J. G., Wright, D. J., Li, N., Egorin, M. J., Enama, M. E., Mayers, J., and Galetto, G. (1997). The safety and pharmacokinetics of single-agent and combination therapy with megestrol acetate and dronabinol for the treatment of HIV wasting syndrome. The DATRI 004 Study Group. Division of AIDS Treatment Research Initiative. *AIDS Res. Hum. Retroviruses,* 13, 305–315.

Toomey, R., Lyons, M. J., Eisen, S. A., Xian, H., Chantarujikapong, S., Seidman, L. J., Faraone, S. V., and Tsuang, M. T. (2003). A twin study of the neuropsychological consequences of stimulant abuse. *Arch. Gen. Psychiatry,* 60, 303–310.

Treit, D. (1985). Animal models for the study of anti-anxiety agents: A review. *Neurosci. Biochem. Rev.,* 9, 203–222.

Trujillo, K. A. (2000). Are NMDA receptors involved in opiate-induced neural and behavioral plasticity? *Psychopharmacology,* 151, 121–141.

Trujillo, K. A., and Akil, H. (1991). Opiate tolerance and dependence: Recent findings and synthesis. *New Biologist,* 3, 915–923.

Tsou, K., Patrick, S. L., and Walker, J. M. (1995). Physical withdrawal in rats tolerant to Δ^9-tetrahydrocannabinol precipitated by a cannabinoid receptor antagonist. *Eur. J. Pharmacol.,* 280, R13–R15.

Tsuang, M. (2000). Schizophrenia: Genes and environment. *Biol. Psychiatry,* 47, 210–220.

Tyndale, R. F., and Sellers, E. M. (2001). Variable CYP2A6-mediated nicotine metabolism alters smoking behavior and risk. *Drug Metab. Dispos.,* 29, 548–552.

United States Department of Health and Human Services. (1990). *Seventh annual report to the U.S. Congress on alcohol and health from the Secretary of Health and Human Services.* NIAAA, Rockville, MD.

United States Department of Health, Education, and Welfare. Public Health Service. National Institute of Mental Health. (1968). *1943–1966 Bibliography on Psychotomimetics.* U.S. Government Printing Office, Washington. D.C..

Uhl, G. R., Hall, F. S., and Sora, I. (2002). Cocaine, reward, movement and monoamine transporters. *Mol. Psychiatry,* 7, 21–26.

Ulas, J., and Cotman, C. W. (1993). Excitatory amino acid receptors in schizophrenia. *Schizophr. Bull.,* 19, 105–117.

Ungerstedt, U. (1984). Measurement of neurotransmitter release by intracranial dialysis. In *Measurement of Neurotransmitter Release In Vivo* (C. A. Marsden, Ed.), pp. 81–106. Wiley, New York.

Vaillant, G. E. (1995). *The Natural History of Alcoholism Revisited.* Harvard University Press, Cambridge, Massachusetts.

Vale, W., Banker, G., and Hall, Z. W. (1992). The neuronal cytoskeleton. In *An Introduction to Molecular Neurobiology* (Z. W. Hall, Ed.), pp. 247–280. Sinauer Associates, Sunderland, MA.

Valjent, E., and Maldonado, R. (2000). A behavioural model to reveal place preference to Δ^9-tetrahydrocannabinol in mice. *Psychopharmacology,* 147, 436–438.

Vanderschuren, L. J. M. J., and Kalivas, P. W. (2000). Alterations in dopaminergic and glutamatergic transmission in the induction and expression of behavioral sensitization: A critical review of preclinical studies. *Psychopharmacology,* 151, 99–120.

van Praag, H., Schinder, A. F., Christie, B. R., Toni, N., Palmer, T. D., and Gage, F. H. (2002). Functional neurogenesis in the adult hippocampus. *Nature,* 415, 1030–1034.

Varty, G. B., and Higgins, G. A. (1995). Examination of drug-induced and isolation-induced disruptions of prepulse inhibition as models to screen antipsychotic drugs. *Psychopharmacology,* 122, 15–26.

Varvel, S. A., and Lichtman, A. H. (2002). Evaluation of CB1 receptor knockout mice in the Morris water maze. *J. Pharmacol. Exp. Ther.,* 301, 915–924.

Verheul, R., and van den Brink, W. (2000). The role of personality pathology in the aetiology and treatment of substance disorders. *Curr. Opinion Psychiatry,* 13, 163–169.

Vogel, J .B., Beer, B., and Clody, D. E. (1971). A simple and reliable conflict procedure for the testing of antianxiety agents. *Psychopharmacology,* 2, 1–7.

Volkow, N. D., Chang, L., Wang, G.-J., Fowler, J. S., Leonido-Yee, M., Franceschi, D., Sedler, M. J., Gatley, S. J., Hitzemann, R., and Ding, Y.-S. (2001a). Association of dopamine transporter reduction with psychomotor impairment in methamphetamine abusers. *Am. J. Psychiatry,* 158, 377–382.

Volkow, N. D., Fowler, J. S., Wang, G.-J., Hitzemann, R., Logan, J., Schlyer, D. J., Dewey, S. L., and Wolf, A. P. (1993). Decreased dopamine D$_2$ receptor availability is associated with reduced frontal metabolism in cocaine abusers. *Synapse,* 14, 169–177.

Volkow, N. D., Wang, G.-J., Fischman, M. W., Foltin, R., Fowler, J. S., Franceschi, D., Franceschi, M., Logan, J., Gatley, S. J., Wong, C., Ding, Y.-S., Hitzemann, R., and Pappas, N. (2000). Effects of route of administration on cocaine induced dopamine transporter blockade in the human brain. *Life Sci.,* 67, 1507–1515.

Volkow, N. D., Fowler, J. S., and Wang, G.-J. (1999a). Imaging studies on the role of dopamine in cocaine reinforcement and addiction in humans. *J. Psychopharmacol.,* 13, 337–345.

Volkow, N. D., Wang, G.-J., Fowler, J. S., Gatley, S. J., Logan, J., Ding, Y.-S., Dewey, S. L., Hitzemann, R., Gifford, A. N., and Pappas, N. R. (1999b). Blockade of striatal dopamine transporters by intravenous methylphenidate is not sufficient to induce self-reports of "high." *J. Pharmacol. Exp. Ther.,* 288, 14–20.

Volkow, N. D., Wang, G.-J., Fowler, J. S., Logan, J., Gatley, S. J., Wong, C., Hitzemann, R., and Pappas, N. R. (1999). Reinforcing effects of psychostimulants in humans are associated with increases in brain dopamine and occupancy of D$_2$ receptors. *J. Pharmacol. Exp. Ther.,* 291, 409–415.

Volkow, N. D., Wang, G.-J., Fowler, J. S., Gatley, S. J., Logan, J., Ding, Y.-S., Hitzeman, R., and Pappas, N. (1998). Dopamine transporter occupancies in the human brain induced by therapeutic doses of oral methylphenidate. *Am. J. Psychiatry,* 155, 1325–1331.

Volkow, N. D., Wang, G.-J., Fowler, J. S., Logan, J., Gatley, S. J., Hitzemann, R., Chen, A. D., Dewey, S. L., and Pappas, N. (1997). Decreased striatal dopaminergic responsiveness in detoxified cocaine-dependent subjects. *Nature,* 386, 830–833.

Volkow, N. D., Wang, G.-J., Fowler, J. S., Logan, J., Gerasimov, M., Maynard, L., Ding, Y.-S., Gatley, S. J., Gifford, A., and Franceschi, D. (2001). Therapeutic doses of oral methylphenidate significantly increase extracellular dopamine in the human brain. *J. Neurosci.,* 21, RC121, 1–5.

Vollenweider, F. X., and Geyer, M. A. (2001). A systems model of altered consciousness: Integrating natural and drug-induced psychoses. *Brain Res. Bull.,* 56, 495–507.

Vollenweider, F. X., Vollenweider-Scherpenhuyzen, M. F. I., Bäbler, A., Vogel, H., and Hell, D. (1998). Psilocybin induces schizophrenia-like psychosis in humans via a serotonin-2 agonist action. *NeuroReport,* 9, 3897–3902.

Vorel, S. R., Ashby, C. R., Jr., Paul, M., Liu, X., Hayes, R., Hagan, J. J., Middlemiss, D. N., Stemp, G., and Gardner, E. L. (2002). Dopamine D$_3$ receptor antagonism inhibits cocaine-seeking and cocaine-enhanced brain reward in rats. *J. Neurosci.,* 22, 9595–9603.

Waldorf, D. (1983). Natural recovery from opiate addiction: Some social-psychological processes of untreated recovery. *J. Drug Issues,* 13, 237–280.

Wall, T. L., and Ehlers, C. L. (1995). Genetic influences affecting alcohol use among Asians. *Alcohol Health Res. World,* 19, 184–189.

Walters, G. D. (2000). Spontaneous remission from alcohol, tobacco, and other drug abuse: Seeking quantitative answers to qualitative questions. *Am. J. Drug Alcohol Abuse,* 26, 443–460.

Walters, G. D., and Gilbert, A. (2000). Defining addiction: Contrasting views of clients and experts. *Addiction Res.* 8, 211–220.

Wang, G.-J., Volkow, N. D., Hitzemann, R. J., Wong, C., Angrist, B., Burr, G., Pascani, K., Pappas, N., Lu, A., and Cooper, T. (1997). Behavioral and cardiovascular effects of intravenous methylphenidate in normal subjects and cocaine abusers. *Eur. Addict. Res.,* 3, 49–54.

Wasson, R. G. (1957). Seeking the magic mushroom. *Life,* 42 (19), 100–115.

Watson, S. J., Benson, J. A., and Joy, J. E. (2000). Marijuana and medicine: Assessing the science base. A summary of the 1999 Institute of Medicine report. *Arch. Gen. Psychiatry,* 57, 547–552.

Wechsler, H., Dowdall, G. W., Davenport, A., and Castillo, S. (1995). Correlates of college student binge drinking. *Am. J. Public Health,* 85, 921–926.

Wechsler, H., Moeykens, B., Davenport, A., Castillo, S., and Hanson, J. (1995). The adverse impact of heavy episodic drinkers on other college students. *J. Stud. Alcohol,* 56, 628–634.

Weddington, W. W., Brown, B. S., Haertzen, C. A., Cone, E. J., Dax, E. M., Herning, R. I., and Michaelson, B. S. (1990). Changes in mood, craving, and sleep during short-term abstinence reported by male cocaine addicts. *Arch. Gen. Psychiatry,* 47, 861–868.

Weeks, J. R., and Collins, R. J. (1987). Screening for drug reinforcement using intravenous self-administration in the rat. In *Methods of Assessing the Reinforcing Properties of Abused Drugs* (M. A. Bozarth, Ed.) pp. 35–43. Springer-Verlag, New York.

Wei, F., Wang, G. D., Kerchner, G. A., Kim, S. J., Xu, H. M., Chen, Z. F., and Zhuo, M. (2001). Genetic enhancement of inflammatory pain by forebrain NR2B overexpression. *Nat. Neurosci.,* 4, 164–169.

Weinberger, D. R. (1987). Implications of normal brain development for the pathogenesis of schizophrenia. *Arch. Gen. Psychiatry,* 44, 660–669.

Weinberger, D. R. (1995). Neurodevelopmental perspectives on schizophrenia. In *Psychopharmacology: The Fourth Generation of Progress* (F. E. Bloom and D. J. Kupfer, Eds.), pp. 1171–1183. Raven Press, New York.

Weintraub, M., Sundaresan, P. R., Madan, M., Schuster, B., Balder, A., Lasagna, L., and Cox, C. (1992). Long-term weight control study I (weeks 0 to 34). *Clin. Pharmacol. Ther.,* 51, 586–594.

Wellman, P. J., Davies, B. T., Morien, A., and McMahon, L. (1993). Modulation of feeding by hypothalamic paraventricular nucleus α$_1$- and α$_2$-adrenergic receptors. *Life Sci.,* 53, 669–679.

Wenger, J. R., Tiffany, T. M., Bombardier, C., Nicoins, K., and Woods, S. C. (1981). Ethanol tolerance in the rat is learned. *Science,* 213, 575–576.

Wikler, A. (1973). Dynamics of drug dependence: Implications of a conditioning theory for research and treatment. *Arch. Gen. Psychiatry,* 28, 611–616.

Wikler, A. (1980). *Opioid Dependence.* Plenum Press, New York.

Williams, B. F., Howard, V. F., and McLaughlin, T. F. (1994). Fetal alcohol syndrome: Developmental characteristics and directions for further research. *Educ. Treatment Child.,* 17, 86–97.

Williams, C. M., Rogers, P. J., and Kirkham, T. C. (1998). Hyperphagia in pre-fed rats following oral Δ^9-THC. *Physiol. Behav.,* 65, 343–346.

Willner, P. (1995). Dopaminergic mechanisms in depression and mania. In *Psychopharmacology: The Fourth Generation of Progress* (F. E. Bloom and D. J. Kupfer, Eds.), pp. 921–932. Raven Press, New York.

Wilson, G. T., and Lawson, P. W. (1976a). Expectancies, alcohol, and sexual arousal in male social drinkers. *J. Abnorm. Psychol.*, 85, 587–594.

Wilson, G. T., and Lawson, D. W. (1976b). The effects of alcohol on sexual arousal in women. *J. Abnorm. Psychol.*, 85, 489–497.

Wilson, R. I., and Nicoll, R. A. (2002). Endocannabinoid signaling in the brain. *Science,* 296, 678–682.

Windle, M., and Davies, P. T. (1999). Developmental theory and research. In *Psychological Theories of Drinking and Alcoholism* (2nd ed.) (K. E. Leonard and H. T. Blane, Eds.), pp. 164–202. Guilford Press, New York.

Winter, J. C., Fiorella, D. J., Timineri, D. M., Filipink, R. A., Helsley, S. E., and Rabin, R. A. (1999). Serotonergic receptor subtypes and hallucinogen-induced stimulus control. *Pharmacol. Biochem. Behav.,* 64, 283–293.

Wittchen, H.-U., Zhao, S., Kessler, R. C., and Eaton, W. W. (1994). DSM-III-R generalized anxiety disorder in the National Comorbidity Survey. *Arch. Gen. Psychiatry,* 51, 355–364.

Wolfe, B. L., and Meyers, R. J. (1999). Cost-effective alcohol treatment: The community reinforcement approach. *Cognitive Behav. Pract.,* 6, 105–109.

Woods, J. H., France, C. P., Winger, G., Bertalmio, A. J., and Schwarz-Stevens, K. (1993). Opioid abuse liability assessment in rhesus monkeys. In *Opioids II,* Handbook of Experimental Pharmacology, Vol. 104 (A. Herz, Ed.), pp. 609–632. Springer-Verlag, New York.

Woods, J. H., Katz, J. L., and Winger, G. (1995). Abuse and therapeutic use of benzodiazepines and benzodiazepine-like drugs. In *Psychopharmacology: The Fourth Generation of Progress* (F. E. Bloom and D. J. Kupfer, Eds.), pp. 1777–1789. Raven Press, New York.

Woolverton, W. L., Rowlett, J. K., Winger, G., Woods, J. H., Gerak, L. R., and France, C. P. (1999). Evaluation of the reinforcing and discriminative stimulus effects of γ-hydroxybutyrate in rhesus monkeys. *Drug Alcohol Depend.,* 54, 137–143.

Wrenn, C. C., and Wiley, R. G. (1998). The behavioral functions of the cholinergic basal forebrain: Lessons from 192 IgG-saporin. *Int. J. Dev. Neurosci.,* 16, 595–602.

Wu, J. C., and Bunney, W. E. (1990). The biological basis of an antidepressant response to sleep deprivation and relapse: Review and hypothesis. *Am. J. Psychiatry,* 147, 14–21.

Wu, T.-C., Tashkin, D. P., Djahed, B., and Rose, J. E. (1988). Pulmonary hazards of smoking marijuana as compared with tobacco. *New Engl. J. Med.,* 318, 347–351.

Wurtman, R. J., Wurtman, J. J., Regan, M. M., McDermott, J. M., Tsay, R. H., and Breu, J. J. (2003). Effects of normal meals rich in carbohydrate or proteins on plasma tryptophan and tyrosine ratios. *Am. J. Clin. Nutr.,* 77, 128–132.

Xu, F., Gainetdinov, R. R., Wetsel, W. C., Jones, S. R., Bohn, L. M., Miller, G. W., Wang, Y.-M., and Caron, M. G. (2000). Mice lacking the norepinephrine transporter are supersensitive to psychostimulants. *Nat. Neurosci.,* 3, 465–471.

Xu, M., Guo, Y., Vorhees, C. V., and Zhang, J. (2000). Behavioral responses to cocaine and amphetamine administration in mice lacking the dopamine D1 receptor. *Brain Res.,* 852, 198–207.

Xu, M., Hu, X.-T., Cooper, D. C., Moratalla, R., Graybiel, A. M., White, F. J., and Tonegawa, S. (1994). Elimination of cocaine-induced hyperactivity and dopamine-mediated neurophysiolog-ical effects in dopamine D1 receptor mutant mice. *Cell,* 79, 945–955.

Yehuda, R., Bierer, L. M., Schmeidler, J., Aferiat, D. H., Breslau, I., and Dolan, S. (2000). Low cortisol and risk for PTSD in adult offspring of holocaust survivors. *Am. J. Psychiatry,* 157, 1252–1259.

Yehuda, R., Marshall, R., and Giller, E. L. (1998). Psychopharmacological treatment of post-traumatic stress disorder. In *A Guide to Treatments That Work* (P. E. Nathan and J. M. Gorman, Eds.), pp. 377–407. Oxford University Press, New York.

Young, A. M., and Goudie, A. J. (1995). Adaptive processes regulating tolerance to behavioral effects of drugs. In *Psychopharmacology: The Fourth Generation of Progress* (F. E. Bloom and D. J. Kupfer, Eds.) pp. 733–742. Raven Press, New York.

Young, E. A. (1993). Induction of the intermediate lobe POMC system with chronic swim stress and β-adrenergic modulation of this induction. *Neuroendocrinology,* 52, 405–411.

Young, L. J., Lim, M. M., Gingrich, B., and Insel, T. R. (2001). Cellular mechanisms of social attachment. *Horm. Behav.,* 40, 133–138.

Zadina, J. E., Martin-Schild, S., Gerall, A. A., Kastin, A. J., Hackler, L., Ge, L. J., and Zhang, X. (1999). Endomorphins: Novel endogenous mu-opiate receptor agonists in regions of high mu-opiate receptor density. *Ann. N. Y. Acad. Sci.,* 897, 136–144.

Zahn, T. P., Rapoport, J. L., and Thompson, C. L. (1980). Autonomic and behavioral effects of dextroamphetamine and placebo in normal and hyperactive prepubertal boys. *J. Abnorm. Child Psychol.,* 8, 145–160.

Zajecka, J. (1993). Pharmacology, pharmacokinetics, and safety issues of mood-stabilizing agents. *Psychiatr. Ann.,* 23, 79–85.

Zajecka, J., Tracy, K. A., and Mitchell, S. (1997). Discontinuation symptoms after treatment with serotonin reuptake inhibitors: A literature review, *J. Clin. Psychiatry,* 58, 291–297.

Zald, D. H., and Kim, S. W. (1996). Anatomy and function of the orbital frontal cortex: Anatomy, neurocircuitry, and obsessive-compulsive disorder. *J. Neuropsychiatry,* 8, 125–138.

Zhou, Q.-Y., and Palmiter, R. D. (1995). Dopamine-deficient mice are severely hypoactive, adipsic, and aphagic. *Cell,* 83, 1197–1209.

Zilberman, M. L., Tavares, H., Blume, S. B., and el-Guebaly, N. (2003). Substance use disorders: Sex differences and psychiatric comorbidities. *Can. J. Psychiatry,* 48, 5–13.

Zimmer, A., Zimmer, A. M., Hohmann, A. G., Herkenham, M., and Bonner, T. I. (1999). Increased mortality, hypoactivity, and hypoalgesia in cannabinoid CB1 receptor knockout mice. *Proc. Natl. Acad. Sci. USA,* 96, 5780–5785.

Zinberg, N. E., and Jacobson, R. C. (1976). The natural history of "chipping." *Am. J. Psychiatry,* 33, 37–40.

Zivin, J. A. (2000) Understanding clinical trials. *Sci. Am.* 282(4), 69–75.

Zobel, A. W., Nickel, T., Kunzel, H. E., Ackl, N., Sonntag, A., Ising, M., and Holsboer, F. (2000). Effects of the high-affinity corticotropin-releasing hormone receptor 1 antagonist R121919 in major depression: The first 20 patients treated. *J. Psychiatr. Res.,* 34, 171–181.

Zubieta, J. K., Smith, Y. R., Bueller, J. A., Xu, Y., Kilbourn, M. R., Jewett, D. M., Meyer, C. R., Koeppe, R. A., and Stohler, C. S. (2001). Regional μ opioid receptor regulation of sensory and affective dimensions of pain. *Science,* 293, 311–315.

Author Index

Moeykens, B., 238
Moghaddam, B., 182
Molloy, M., 399
Monaco, A. P., 282
Monteggia, L. M., 408
Montoya, D., 309
Moolchan, E. T., 335, 336
Moore, B. A., 341, 342, 343
Moos, R. H., 242
Moratalla, R., 131, 285
Morel, E., 427
Morgan, C., 362
Morgan, D. G., 405
Morgan, H. W., 187, 189
Morien, A., 135
Mormède, P., 86
Morral, A. R., 194
Morrison, H., 252
Morrow, A. L., 234
Morton, A. J., 104
Moses, J. A., 456
Mott, J. A., 314
Mozley, P. D., 197, 266
Muir, J. L., 141
Mumford, G. K., 321
Muntoni, A. L., 342
Munzar, P., 339
Muramoto, M. L., 318
Murphy, D. L., 282, 283
Murray, R., 442
Murray, R. M., 444
Muschaweck, N. M., 373
Musto, D. F., 272
Mutschler, N. H., 85

N
Naassila, M., 340
Nahas, G. G., 333, 334
Nahas, Z., 399
Nakao, K., 169
Narasimhan, M., 399
Nasser, J., 343
Navarro, M., 340, 342
Naylor, R. J. 428
Negus, S. S., 285
Nelson, D. L., 354
Nelson, R. A., 335, 336
Nemeroff, C. B., 394, 408
Neri, E., 86
Nestler, E. J., 265, 266, 408
Netusil, N., 316
Neumann-Haefelin, C., 175
Neve, K. A., 137
Neve, R. L., 137, 407
Newcomer, J. W., 362

Newhouse, J. P., 173
Nichols, D. E., 354, 356
Nicholson, K. L., 361, 373, 383
Nickel, T., 407
Nicoins, K., 222
Nicoll, R. A., 332
Nides, M. A., 318
Ninan, P. T., 412, 434, 438
Nirenberg, M., 265
Nisell, M., 312
Nomikos, G. G., 312
Noonan, W. C., 361
Nordstrom, A.-L., 454
North, R. A., 255
Novy, P. L., 342
Nowinksi, J., 186
Nutt, D., 160
Nutt, D. J., 414
Nyswander, M. E., 269

O
Oblin, A., 131
O'Brien, C. P., 197, 242, 266, 269, 270, 285, 290
Ohlsson, A., 330, 336, 341
Oken, B. S., 308
Oldendorf, W. H., 15
Oliver, N. C., 399
Olney, J. W., 173
Olney, J., 221
Olney, J. W., 173, 362
O'Malley, S. S., 317
Ooi, G. T., 130
Orlando, R., 370
Osborn, E., 270
Overstreet, D. H., 405
Overton, D. A., 30

P
Packard, M. G., 381, 382
Paddock, S. M., 194
Padova, C., 219
Palacios, J. M., 181
Palatini, P., 370
Palay, S. L., 64
Palfreman, J., 119
Palkovits, M., 340
Palmer, E. P., 127
Palmiter, R. D., 130
Palumbo, J. M., 288
Panagis, G., 312
Panikashvili, D., 334
Panlilio, L. V., 309
Pappas, N., 284, 289, 298, 316
Pappas, N. R., 284
Paradiso, M. A., 98

Pardo, C. A., 165
Park, D., 381
Parker, D. A., 224
Parmentier, M., 337, 340
Parrott, A. C., 298, 299, 315
Parsons, L. H., 158, 159
Pascani, K., 298
Passino, N., 309
Patel, S., 285
Paterson, I. A., 221
Patrick, S. L., 341
Patten, B. M., 363
Patton, G., 343
Paul, M., 285
Pauli, S., 454
Paulus, M. P., 131
Pedrazzini, T., 337, 340
Perachon, S., 285
Perkins, K. A., 314, 316
Perrault, G., 131, 427
Perry, L. D., 311
Pert, C. B., 249
Pertwee, R. G., 332
Peters, A., 64
Petersen, R. C., 276
Petitet, F., 337, 340
Petraitis, J., 207, 208
Petrakis, I. L., 123
Petrovic, P., 272
Pettegrew, J. W., 462
Pettersson, K. M., 272
Pettit, D. A. D., 345
Petty, M. A., 175
Pfefferbaum, A., 228
Pflug, B., 393
Philippu, A., 93
Phillips, A. G., 285
Phillips, J., 377
Phillips, L. L., 268
Phillips, T. J., 130, 131
Piazza, P., 85, 86, 210
Piazza, P. V., 86
Picciotto, M. R., 106, 308, 309
Picetti, R., 130
Pich, E. M., 106, 309
Pidoplichko, V. I., 310
Pierrefiche, O., 340
Piker, P., 223
Pilapil, C., 250
Pilla, M., 285
Pinder, R. M., 399
Piomelli, D., 332, 338
Pistis, M., 234, 235
Pistuddi, A. M., 372, 373

Subject Index

About the Book

Editor: Graig Donini

Project Editors: Kathaleen Emerson and Sydney Carroll

Production Manager: Christopher Small

Electronic Book Production: Joan Gemme

Illustration Program: Pyramis Studios

Copy Editor: Mark Via

Indexer: Robie Grant

Photo Researcher: David McIntyre

Book and Cover Design: Jefferson Johnson

Book Manufacturer: Courier Companies, Inc.